Reoperative Hand Surgery

Scott F.M. Duncan
Editor

Reoperative Hand Surgery

Springer

Editor
Scott F.M. Duncan, MD, MPH
Department of Orthopedic Surgery
Ochsner Health System
New Orleans, LA, USA

ISBN 978-1-4614-2372-0 ISBN 978-1-4614-2373-7 (eBook)
DOI 10.1007/978-1-4614-2373-7
Springer New York Dordrecht Heidelberg London

Library of Congress Control Number: 2012933438

Printed on acid-free paper

Springer is part of Springer Science+Business Media (www.springer.com)

Preface

The purpose of this book is to present some reoperative options for challenging problems that face the reconstructive hand surgeon after failed primary surgery. We have tried to do this as a one-volume book that is very concise and discusses some of the more common issues that hand surgeons may face in performing revision surgery. Even though there are several books dealing with hand surgery and other problems of the upper extremity, this book is unique in that it looks specifically at the problem of what to do when the original index procedure did not go as planned. We have included topics that involve the hand, wrist, forearm, and elbow. We have also included some sections in the book to look at some of the psycological and social factors that also go into the decision process whether to reoperate or not. My hope with this book is that it will give the busy hand and upper extremity surgeon easily accessible information relating to the evaluation, diagnosis, and possible surgical interventions for the diagnoses discussed.

Hand and upper extremity surgery has a diversity of different procedures to accomplish common goals. There are usually pros and cons to each type of procedure. Complications are a known risk of surgery and do occur despite the best efforts of the surgeon. The purpose of this book is to help hand surgeons manage some of these issues when they do arise in the patients that we all care for.

The chapters are tightly focused so that the important aspects to consider for reoperation can be quickly reviewed. There is also a component of the chapters that discusses how to avoid other pitfalls and to minimize as well as manage any complications that may occur with the reoperative procedures.

The authors that have graciously contributed their expertise to this book are all well known in the hand surgery world. The book has a straightforward table of contents and index which should allow the reader to easily locate the topic which they wish to review. We have purposely minimized the historical aspects and reviews of the literature in this book as these can be found in other hand surgery text books, but again have focused our core competency for this text to be reoperative considerations in those patients who have had previous surgery.

The book is filled with original art work to help describe and demonstrate how to perform some of these reoperative procedures. Our goal is that the artwork should be simple and straightforward but yet detailed enough to convey the important steps and aspects for the surgical intervention that it is outlining. It is my personal hope that in future editions of this book the number of topics will continue to expand and that the current topics will continue to be refined. This first edition represents the hard work of authors, editors, and publishers alike and will hopefully come to serve for the betterment of the patients under our care.

New Orleans, LA, USA Scott F.M. Duncan

Contents

Contributors

Kane L. Anderson, MS, MD Section of Hand and Micro Surgery, Department of Orthopaedics and Sports Medicine, University of Washington, Seattle, WA, USA

James H. Calandruccio, MS, MD Department of Orthopedic Surgery, University of Tennessee—Campbell Clinic, Germantown, TN, USA

Kevin C. Chung, MD Department of Surgery, University of Michigan Health System, Ann Arbor, MI, USA

Scott F.M. Duncan, MD, MPH Department of Orthopedic Surgery, Ochsner Health System, New Orleans, LA, USA

George S.M. Dyer, MD Department of Orthopedic Surgery, Harvard Medical School and Brigham and Women's Hospital, Boston, MA, USA

Scott G. Edwards, MD Center for Hand and Elbow Specialists, Georgetown University Hospital, Washington, DC, USA

Kristen Fleager, MD Department of Orthopaedic Surgery, Stanford Hospitals and Clinics, Redwood City, CA, USA

Jeffrey B. Friedrich, MD Department of Surgery, Division of Plastic Surgery, University of Washington, Seattle, WA, USA

A. Ylenia Giuffrida, MD Hackensack University Medical Center, Hackensack, NJ, USA

Ranjan Gupta, MD Department of Orthopedic Surgery, University of California, Irvine, Orange, CA, USA

Steven C. Haase, MD, FACS Section of Plastic Surgery, University of Michigan Health System, Ann Arbor, MI, USA

Douglas P. Hanel, MD Department of Orthopedics and Sports Medicine, Harborview Medical Center, University of Washington, Seattle, WA, USA

Scott E. Hecox, MD Department of Orthopedic Surgery, University of Tennessee—Campbell Clinic, Germantown, TN, USA

Nathan A. Hoekzema, MD Orthopedic Center, Mayo Clinic Health System, Eau Claire, WI, USA

Shushan Jacob, MD Department of Orthopedic Surgery, Division of Hand and Microsurgery, UT Southwestern Medical Center, Dallas, TX, USA

Jesse B. Jupiter, MD Department of Orthopedic Surgery, Harvard Medical School and Massachusetts General Hospital, Boston, MA, USA

Ryosuke Kakinoki, MD, PhD Department of Orthopedic Surgery, Kyoto University Hospital, Kyoto, Japan

Jason R. Kang, BS Department of Orthopedic Surgery, University of California, Irvine, Orange, CA, USA

Jeffrey C. King, MD Division of Hand and Elbow Surgery, Michigan State University College of Human Medicine and Kalamazoo Center for Medical Studies, Kalamazoo, MI, USA

Amy L. Ladd, MD Department of Orthopaedic Surgery, Stanford Hospitals and Clinics, Redwood City, CA, USA

Susan E. Mackinnon, MD Department of Surgery, Washington University School of Medicine, St. Louis, MO, USA

Paul Maloof, MD Department of Orthopedics, University of Medicine and Dentistry of New Jersey and University Hospital, Newark, NJ, USA

Roy A. Meals, MD Department of Orthopedic Surgery, University of California, Los Angeles, Los Angeles, CA, USA

Scott A. Mitchell, MD, MPH Department of Orthopedic Surgery, University of California, Los Angeles, Los Angeles, CA, USA

Jose A. Ortiz, Jr., MD Orthopedics Center, Mayo Clinic Health System, Eau Claire, WI, USA

A. Lee Osterman, MD Department of Orthopedic Surgery, Philadelphia Hand Center, Thomas Jefferson University, King of Prussia, PA, USA

Rick F. Papandrea, MD Partner, Orthopaedic Associates of WI, Waukesha, WI, USA

Vipul P. Patel, MD Department of Orthopedic Surgery, Crystal Run Healthcare, Middletown, NY, USA

William C. Pederson, MD, FACS The Hand Center of San Antonio, The University of Texas Health Science Center at San Antonio, San Antonio, TX, USA

Kevin J. Renfree, MD Department of Orthopedic Surgery, Mayo Clinic Hospital, Phoenix, AZ, USA

David Ring, MD, PhD Massachusetts General Hospital, Boston, MA, USA

Marco Rizzo, MD Department of Orthopedic Surgery, Mayo Clinic College of Medicine, Rochester, MN, USA

Nicholas E. Rose, MD California Orthopedic Specialists, Newport Beach, CA, USA

Douglas M. Sammer, MD Department of Plastic and Reconstructive Surgery, University of Texas Southwestern Medical School, Dallas, TX, USA

Robert E. Schlenker, MD Department of Surgery, Division of Plastic Surgery, University of Washington, Seattle, WA, USA

Alexander Y. Shin, MD Department of Orthopedic Surgery, Mayo Clinic College of Medicine, Rochester, MN, USA

Virak Tan, MD Department of Orthopedics, University of Medicine and Dentistry of New Jersey and University Hospital, Newark, NJ, USA

S.C. Tay, MD, MS Department of Hand Surgery, Singapore General Hospital, Singapore

Department of Orthopedic Surgery, Mayo Clinic College of Medicine, Rochester, MN, USA

Tsu-Min Tsai, MD Department of Hand and Microsurgery, Christine M. Kleinert Institute of Hand and Microsurgery, University of Louisville School of Medicine, Louisville, KY, USA

Jennifer Moriatis Wolf, MD Department of Orthopaedic Surgery, University of Connecticut Health Center, New England Musculoskelatal Institute, Farmington, CT, USA

Scott Wolfe, MD Weill Medical College of Cornell University, Hospital for Special Surgery, New York, NY, USA

Considerations in Reoperative Hand Surgery

1

Scott F.M. Duncan

Abstract

The reoperative hand surgeon is a unique individual. The surgeon who is willing to take on these types of cases, whether they be their own complications or patients who have been referred in from colleagues, faces some unique challenges when compared to dealing with the patient who has not previously been operated on for that particular disease or diagnosis. These patients have unique psychological and social considerations that are compounded by the need for further surgical intervention. Some of these patients may be overtly hostile, and others may have very unrealistic expectations. However, many patients will be very grateful for the surgeon who is willing to rise to the occasion and who has the caring temperament to help guide these patients through their diagnostic and decision-making process. Some patients who think they need surgery in actuality do not; moreover, some patients that would not benefit from further surgery will still want to have surgery performed in the hopes of having some improvement or change in their outcome. This chapter is for those surgeons who understand the unique role of the reoperative surgeon and wish to explore some of the insights needed to try and be more effective.

Keywords

Reoperative • Surgeon • Psychological • Challenges

Introduction

There are many different reasons for reoperating on a patient. The usual reasons for reoperation come from complications. Other times, things such as recurrent disease come about necessitating further surgery. In other situations, there may be continuation or worsening of a biologic process such as Dupuytren's disease. Finally, there are those cases where the outcome by various measures has been less than optimal, and the surgeon and patient wish to see if these results can be optimized with further surgery. In some circumstances, the procedures do not really represent a reoperation, but rather are the planned sequences in a series of staged procedures needed to reconstruct or correct hand and upper extremity dysfunction. Any hand and upper extremity surgeon who has had to perform reoperative surgery in anatomic areas that have undergone previous surgery can vouch for the difficulty in dealing with tissues that have already undergone scarring.

Most hand surgeons learn how to perform reoperative surgery (to a degree) through their fellowship training, but much of reoperative surgery is learned while engaging in the practice of hand surgery. Some of this learning curve comes about from trial and error in finding out what has worked for them or colleagues, as well as what has not yielded positive results. As the surgeon ages, he or she may find themselves not only mentoring a younger group of hand surgeons, but also being referred patients who potentially could benefit from reoperative surgery. However, no surgeon is free from the possibility of unanticipated surgical outcomes and the

S.F.M. Duncan, MD, MPH (✉)
Department of Orthopedic Surgery, Ochsner Health System, Ochsner Medical Center, 1514 Jefferson Highway, New Orleans, LA 70121, USA
e-mail: duncan.academic@gmail.com

S.F.M. Duncan (ed.), *Reoperative Hand Surgery*,
DOI 10.1007/978-1-4614-2373-7_1, © Springer Science+Business Media, LLC 2012

need for reoperative surgery in their own patients. Much of what is known about treating hand surgery complications is passed down through verbal communication, but not necessarily written down in the same way that primary surgical procedures are written down and described in textbooks. Most hand and upper extremity surgery procedures are meant to be single procedures that the patient recovers from with time, therapy, and normal biological healing. However, some upper extremity surgery procedures are meant to be staged and these staged procedures are frequently done in order to facilitate the healing of one aspect of the anatomy so that another aspect of the anatomy is not detrimentally affected by the other procedure.

In some cases, the outcome is not as satisfactory as the patient and surgeon would like. An example of this would be a flexor tendon repair that has developed tendon adhesions. While the flexor tendon or tendons may have healed, unfortunately the patient's functional use of the hand and finger is restricted because of these adhesions. In these cases, because of less than satisfactory outcome, it is reasonable to consider performing a flexor tenolysis in order to try and better optimize the patient's usage of the extremity. It is a commonly known fact among surgeons that operative rates go up after national meetings. The thought behind this is that surgeons may elect to try newly seen surgical techniques before they have expertise in judgment that only comes with practice and experience with the technique. These potential complications from the new procedures create a "bump" in the incidence of reoperative upper extremity surgery. Other times, the issue may be subtler. Sometimes they keloid or scar that is deemed cosmetically unacceptable by the patient may require a "touch-up" surgery.

As mentioned previously, a common reason for reoperation is recurrence of disease. Hand surgery examples of this are Dupuytren's disease as well as giant cell tumor of the tendon sheath. Other examples can be recurrent scarring in flexor and extensor tendons after injury and/or surgery. Unfortunately, the worse case scenario is recurrence of malignancy in the extremity after the attempt at limb-sparing or limb-salvaging techniques. In the hand, if there is a recurrent malignancy, usually a more aggressive surgical approach is required, and this may necessitate loss of limb.

All surgery carries the possibility for potential risk of complications, and many of these complications may require further operative treatment. In hand surgery cases, a failed microsurgical anastomosis and a replant may necessitate an emergent trip back to the operating room. In other cases, a hematoma, seroma, or infection may require an urgent, but not necessarily an emergent trip to the operative suite for decompression. Complications can occur both in the immediate phase or the late phase following surgery. At no point during the postoperative period is the patient completely immune from potential complications. Technical difficulties or errors can result in complications; however, in many cases it is actually host factors. The host compromising issues are diabetes, tobacco use, immunodeficiency, and osteoporosis, among others. Any repeat procedure needs to be weighed against the potential risk of making the problem worse with further intervention.

In planning the reoperative surgery, the surgeon needs to perform a thorough analysis of the pros and cons of proceeding, as well as be able to technically perform the reoperative procedure. Considerations such as circulation to the devitalized previously operated tissue, potential further or worsening of scar tissue, possible internal fixation, and postoperative therapy all need to be made in the planning stages. And then if things were not difficult enough, the surgeon needs to consider potential complications in treating the complications. The obvious goals of the secondary procedure are to fix the underlying problem(s) and to try to avoid any recurrence of those same issues, as well as to try and mitigate the formation of any new complications. All three of these variables need to be incorporated into the treatment plan, as they may all potentially have an effect on the ultimate outcome. In forming the reoperative plan: (1) The surgeon must think creatively and try to avoid the temptation of merely repeating the original plan that proved to not work in the first place; (2) It is especially tempting for the surgeon who is treating a patient who had surgery done elsewhere to fall into the trap that their surgical skills are superior to the other surgeons; (3) The reoperative surgeon always needs to take a step back and think about different ways to attack the problem.

Patient Expectations

One of the challenges for the reoperative surgeon is trying to explain to the patient why further surgery or surgeries are needed. One of the key aspects is setting a realistic level of expectation from the patient. This is especially true for a patient who is disappointed and frustrated by the previous surgical management and the patient's perceived failure of that surgery. The specific goals of reoperative hand surgery are usually more specific and focused and commonly deal with a very narrow problem. However, multiple problems may require multiple staged procedures and some quality time should be spent trying to counsel the patient in this regard.

Scar Tissue

Scarring while part of the normal healing of soft tissues can also be part of the problem for the reoperative hand surgeon. Scars and scarring can also be important to consider in that they can make it difficult to place new skin incisions in many cases. When a scar is operated on, it has a tendency to further retract, which can make wound closure problematic.

These potential problems with tissue management need to be anticipated. Scar tissue may form thick dense areas, but scar tissue can also heal in a process that leaves tissues thin and atrophic. Both extremes can be challenging for soft tissue management. A poorly planned incision, as part of a secondary procedure, can create ischemic zones with subsequent soft tissue necrosis. In some cases, this may not be visible by the naked eye. However, the necrotic soft tissues under the skin will result in worsening of any scar problems and may ultimately sabotage the reoperative procedure. Anatomical structures are forever changed when the scalpel incises them. An example of this is incision of muscle fascia. Once muscle fascia is incised, it is impossible, if not dangerous, to try and close it. However, the cosmetic appearance of the overlying tissues will be very different to the patient. Tissue characteristics change with surgical intervention, and this includes skin, fat, muscle, and bone. All of these structures change and are usually more difficult to work with after previous surgical intervention. Furthermore, this scar tissue can make finding neurovascular structures more difficult. This can translate into a potential increased risk for neurovascular injury or compromise to the upper extremity.

Implications for the surgeon mean that any reopening of a wound in the first 4 days is usually quite easy and only needs blunt dissection. Reoperating during this early phase where there is a copious amount of angiogenesis can be difficult, as frequently there can be oozing and bleeding and it is sometimes difficult to obtain adequate hemostasis. Also, in reoperating on wounds that are in various stages of healing, the surgeon can find it difficult to obtain good suture purchase. Frequently, the sutures will cut out or will just slice through the weak and fibrotic soft tissues. Usually, the time between about 20 and 60 days after previous surgery is the time where the most bleeding and densest adhesions may be found. Usually after 90 days, the soft tissues have matured enough such that the tissues are less hemorrhagic and are more supple and compliant. Therefore, in our practice we frequently try to delay any reoperative procedures (when possible) until after 3 months of healing. The intricate upper extremity surgical techniques are even more important in the reoperative cases. Gentle dissection with careful soft tissue and bone handling can potentially be the difference in whether the surgery is of benefit or not.

The Patient

Patients who are undergoing reoperative procedures have a different perspective on their disease as well as on the surgeon. Sometimes the patient is nervous, but at the same time grateful for someone who can potentially help him or her with what they potentially perceive as something that went wrong. Other times, the patient may be quite angry and hostile, even though you as the evaluating surgeon have never previously met them and have never done anything to them. These patient/surgeon interactions take more time to thoroughly review the patient's history, the accompanying data, as well as to perform a thorough exam. However, frequently the most important part is actually the counseling that ensues after the evaluation. These patients are usually hungry for information, and in general, want as much knowledge as possible in regard to options. In trying to place oneself in the patient's position, they are in a vulnerable position and feel like they are at the mercy of the surgeon's potential skills without really knowing whether the surgeon truly has the skill or not. There may be even some feelings of victimization, and these may be expressed as outright anger and hostility. Others may be very sad and tearful in the face of more surgery. Most have genuine fears of undergoing another anesthesia, the postoperative pain, more scarring, and potential further complications that may necessitate even more surgical intervention. It is important to spend some time with these patients counseling them as well as educating them. It is probably most important to actually demonstrate a caring attitude and to address whatever concerns they raise during the visit. Sometimes patients, especially those who have faced a complication, may feel abandoned by the primary surgeon, and this anger can sometimes quickly come to the surface. Sometimes just spending the time with the patient and reassuring them that their previous hand surgeon is an excellent-treating surgeon and is capable of taking care of the problem, is enough to reassure the patient and is helpful in salvaging the patient/surgeon relationship (from the index procedure).

It is important to try and set realistic expectations. As mentioned earlier in this chapter, some patients may have unrealistic expectations that their hand or arm can be made completely whole or completely normal. It is not uncommon to have a patient semijokingly state "Doc, just cut it all off and give me a new one." Some of these people are clearly joking, but others may have some hope that this can actually be done. Those patients, who have a thorough explanation of possible complications, as well as potential pitfalls and problems, may be less frustrated or angry if the need for reoperation arises. This time spent counseling the patient in regard to realistic expectations is truly "time well spent." The other issue, though, is despite setting realistic expectations, one must continue to try and inspire hope for the patient as well. Hope frequently will get them engaged in wellness behavior, and this is key in the patient potentially arising from the reoperative surgery in a better physical and mental state.

The Surgeon

It is easy in retrospect to look at unanticipated outcomes and complications with derision. However, the reoperative surgeon should avoid casting judgment. The reoperative surgeon should be there to help facilitate healing, not to act as "judge, jury, and hangman." It is important to try and be honest and realistic with the patient. Do not deny there is an issue if one clearly exists. However, sometimes when the risks and benefits are thoroughly explained to the patient, they may see that the potential risks outweigh the potential benefits. This is where it is important to have unrealistic expectations adjusted to more realistic ones. Try to avoid blaming the patient. However, it is reasonable to educate the patient that things like smoking, diabetes, and other health issues do influence how bones, tendons, and other soft tissues about the hand and upper extremity heal. Sometimes these factors are controllable, such as smoking; other times they are manageable, such as diabetes; and other times it may be due to genetic factors such as collagen disorders which are beyond anyone's control.

It is difficult in a busy practice to always have the time needed to spend with the patient. However, the reoperative patient does deserve extra time, and office staff should be educated as to potentially schedule these patients for longer visits. These patients need more attention, need to be shown the utmost respect, and certainly need to have our emotional engagement for the difficulties that they are facing. These patients need a chance to verbalize their concerns and frustrations, and in some case their anger. Frequently once this is out on the table, a productive relationship can then move forward. Sometimes patients will complain of pain that may seem out of proportion to the problem at hand. However, sometimes this is how a patient may verbalize their unhappiness with their surgical outcome. Unfortunately, there may be some problems that are not amenable to repeat surgical intervention. Most patients can frequently understand this, although occasionally the surgeon may run into a patient who is convinced that just one more surgery will make them better. If you do not see something that you think you can help the patient with, there is nothing wrong with stating such and potentially offering them even another opinion. The reoperative surgeon also needs to be aware of the "SHAFT Syndrome" patient [1]. These patients want to be operated on and they can pose a real challenge, as they will frequently doctor shop until they find a surgeon who is willing to use a scalpel on them.

It is important in these reoperative cases to understand the social and economic implications of further surgery. This can have impacts not only upon the family, but also on employment as well as hobbies and recreation. Patients may be having stressors at home or from family members because of the decreased work and income. Patients may have feelings of guilt because of the need or their decision to proceed with further surgery. It can be very helpful to have a spouse, significant other, or other family member present during these consultations. There is a lot of information that is frequently discussed and provided by the surgeon, and patients may only remember a small portion of this [2]. By having a second person present, frequently a better discussion can occur at home and potentially even further questions can come from these discussions allowing the surgeon to further clarify and educate.

The surgical plan should be thoroughly outlined to the patient. The patient needs to understand that there could be further surgeries needed with additional time away from work, as well as the additional personal financial cost of surgery. Sometimes these are covered by the patient's own health insurance or short-term disability policy, but other times they are not. The patient may be frustrated when multiple previous surgeries have failed and now an entirely new course of action must be taken. Again, this goes into the education and counseling of these patients.

Fortunately in most cases, the patients prefer to have any further needed surgery performed by the original surgeon. However, patients may decide to switch surgeons for various reasons. These can be as simple as the patient has moved or, in the worse case, the patient has lost confidence in the treating surgeon. Sometimes the patient is seeing a different surgeon on the advice of an attorney or insurance company, which is frequently seen with the worker's compensation patient. Other times, the patient may be specifically referred by another orthopedic, plastic, or hand surgeon in order to provide another opinion or to assume care. If you are seeing a patient because another surgeon has asked for the consult, it is wise to try and clarify whether you are assuming care of the patient or whether they just want you to provide advice to the original surgeon, as well as counseling to the patient.

Patient Categories

It is not unreasonable for the reoperative surgeon to consider the patient's motivation. In most cases, patients are coming to you because they desire a caring, as well as skilled surgeon to take over their care. However, occasionally there will be patients who have secondary gain issues. These patients who have either a financial or psychological benefit to remaining impaired or disabled will not be made better by further surgery. Remember that your role is to provide your opinion and what you think can or cannot be reasonably done by you. You do not have to be a hero despite the fact that is what the patient may be looking for.

There are specific types of patients that can be categorized. We have talked somewhat about the angry patient, and this is not an uncommon problem for the reoperative surgeon. Usually by allowing the patient to present and verbalize their feelings, a new relationship can then begin. However, if the surgeon detects that the patient really is not moving past their anger, it may be reasonable to consider having them work with a psychologist. Fortunately most people, if appropriate time is spent with them, begin to develop some trust for their new doctor, and especially when they see that a potential treatment timetable is available, they may be more positive in moving forward rather than staying in the depths of their anger. The other type of patient is the dissatisfied patient. Sometimes the dissatisfaction is appropriate in that the outcome was not as anticipated or the outcome and surgery were made problematic with complications. However, the other type of dissatisfied patient is one with purely unrealistic expectations. In these cases, it can be beneficial to remind the patient that they are better than they were prior to the index procedure (only state that if that is truly the case). However, other patients have justifiable reasons for the dissatisfaction and usually listening to their concerns and explaining possible solutions will help the patient move past this.

The other category of patient is the one with a psychiatric disorder. Sometimes these patients, such as the "SHAFT syndrome" patient, have a need to continue to have further surgeries [1]. This can usually be seen in their medical record that they have had numerous procedures that are by far greater than what the average person would normally have performed. If the patient's history is significant for having had multiple other hand and upper extremity surgeons decline operating on the patient, this should cause the reoperative surgeon to only proceed with extreme caution. Many of these patients would benefit from psychiatric intervention, but most will refuse to go or potentially become angry at the suggestion. The patient who suffers from depression or is having postoperative depression may be predisposed to symptom magnification. This does not negate the fact that they may require or benefit from further surgery. However, it is important to have this depression managed so that it does not potentially interfere with their recovery and their ability to engage and comply with a therapy program. In patients who are having pain, it is important to try and rule out any mechanical cause, but once the evaluation has ruled out anything that necessitates surgical intervention, it is appropriate to refer these patients for other intervention. If they have evidence of complex regional pain syndrome, this may require a team approach involving anesthesia and stellate ganglion blocks, as well as therapy and desensitization techniques. Frequently, medications such as Neurontin or Lyrica may be of benefit. Occasionally, antidepressants are helpful in these scenarios as well. The key with all relationships is to try and maintain open communication. This lets the patient know that the surgeon cares and that the surgeon will "walk the walk" with them. It also allows the patient to feel more comfortable about verbalizing any concerns that they may have about the surgery or with the surgeon themselves.

Informed Consent

One of the most critical aspects from a medical/legal standpoint for the reoperative hand and upper extremity surgeon is the informed consent. There are considered to be five types of information needed to convey informed consent. These are: diagnosis, nature and purpose of the proposed surgery, alternative treatment options, including operative and nonoperative, as well as those that the surgeon does not perform, risks, complications, potential outcomes, and potential results with no treatment. The discussion of the informed consent should be dictated or otherwise documented in the patient's clinical medical record. This documentation should go into the exact detail that was discussed in clinic, just in case that it is reviewed at a later time for legal reasons.

Final Thoughts

One of the key components of reoperative hand and upper extremity surgery is realizing that not every patient who has difficulties or complications postoperatively necessarily needs another operation. As outlined in one of our later chapters in this book, sometimes not proceeding with any further surgical intervention actually is in the best interest of the patient. As previously discussed, it is important to take one's time in reassuring the patient and discussing these nonoperative options with the patient. If the patient is unwilling to accept the advice of the surgeon at that time, or does not believe in the sincerity of the surgeon, it is reasonable to offer that patient other opinions. Second or third opinions can give the benefit of time in that the patient has time to think about things and both parties avoid hurrying into a surgical intervention that is counterintuitive to the instincts of the reoperative surgeon.

The surgeon needs to make sure that the patient understands that you are there for them. They should understand that the offer of another opinion does not mean that you are abandoning them, brushing them off, or pushing them off to another surgeon. Moreover, I think many surgeons would vouch for this: that those patients who needed additional surgery because of a complication or less-than-desired outcome frequently can become some of your most devoted patients and can provide you much in the way of good public relations. One of the other common temptations in the face of a complication is to try and see the patient fewer times or to have an assistant deal with the patient. In contrast, you should actually see that patient more than you would potentially even need to, and the operative or reoperative surgeon should be the one dealing with that patient when and if at all possible. This shows to the patient that you truly care and have a vested interest in their recovery. One of the key components is to have a sincere and demonstrated empathy for the patient's condition. It is best to let them know what you will be on this "train ride" together for as long as they wish.

The reoperative surgeon needs to demonstrate that they share in the patient's frustration, but at the same time that they are capable and confident to take care of the problem. The professional ethics regarding reoperative surgery need to remain collegial. The reoperative surgeon should not issue any disparaging remarks or exhibit any types of body language that would be perceived by the patient as signs of malpractice. The patient should not be utilized as a tool in any type of personal vendetta against another surgeon and colleague. While some patients may not see through this, many will and may report your comments or body language back to the originating surgeon, potentially causing you more grief in the long term. The patient is already in a vulnerable position, and unprofessional comments do not elevate the espousing surgeon to any higher level, but instead lowers their stature, as they have not helped the patient emotionally or psychologically with those comments. It is reasonable to ask the patient permission to speak with the original surgeon. This can usually be to the patient's benefit in that the reoperative surgeon would like to have as much information as possible. However, the reoperative surgeon needs to remember to obtain permission for that depending on the context. One technique to allay a patient's concern about what might be said with any communication is to have a telephone call with the other physician in the patient's presence.

Summary

In summary, the key is good communication. The patient and surgeon need to be able to have frank and forthright discussions. The hand and upper extremity surgeon needs to demonstrate a caring bedside manner and provide the needed information to the patient to help facilitate their decision. The patient should be actively engaged in participating in the decision-making process. All questions, no matter how small or peripheral, need to be answered to the best of the surgeon's ability. Education about the surgery, as well as potential further complications and setting realistic expectations, will go a long way in maximizing the patient's satisfaction and outcome.

References

1. Kasdan ML, Soergel TM, Johnson AL, Lewis K, White WL. Expanded profile of the SHAFT syndrome. J Hand Surg Am. 1998;23(1):26–31.
2. Madan AK, Tichansky DS. Patients postoperatively forget aspects of preoperative patient education. Obes Surg. 2005;15(7):1066–9.

Reoperative Dupuytren Contracture

2

James H. Calandruccio and Scott E. Hecox

Abstract

Dupuytren disease (DD) is a challenging clinical problem even with primary surgical cases. However, in the face of recurrence, the surgeon is frequently left with a more challenging and complex problem. Soft tissues may be more adherent because of scar formation, and the anatomy may be distorted making identification of structures such as the nerves and vessels more problematic. Furthermore, the flexor pulley system can be damaged while trying to remove some of these recurrent cords and adherent scar risking potential bow-stringing of the flexor tendons. This chapter outlines some of the options for reoperation on recurrent DD. This type of surgery takes not only skill, but extreme patience on the part of the surgeon as the dissection can be quite tedious. Fortunately, patients are usually grateful for the improvement in function that is obtained.

Keywords

Dupuytren disease • Recurrence • Reoperation • Cord

Key Points

- Allocate ample surgical time for each finger
- Mark out diseased tissue intended for procedure
- Draw out intended incision(s)
- Dissect disease from proximal to distal
- Identify proper digital and dorsal sensory branches and arteries
- Assume that digital nerves may be drawn superficially and toward midline of involved finger(s)
- Control bleeding prior to closure
- Rearrange skin to reduce lines of tension
- Do not close wounds tightly
- Splint operated fingers in as much extension as reasonable

Introduction

Painless finger and thumb flexion and web space contractures in Dupuytren disease (DD) are common in the northern European population especially those of Celtic descent [1–3]. The disease is inherited via an autosomal dominant gene with variable penetrance yielding tremendous diversity in onset, expression rate, and clinical manifestations. These manifestations have been linked to expression of the ZF9 polymorphism of TGF-b1. The variation in expression of TGF-b1 causes differential transformation from fibroblast to myofibroblast. Moreover, nonmuscle myosin contractile proteins appear to suggest that both myofibroblasts and fibroblasts play a role in DD. Therefore, recurrence of Dupuytren contractures following surgery does not necessarily indicate an inadequate initial operative procedure, but more appropriately cord resurgence from persistent cellular deposits triggered by as yet poorly defined mechanisms and disease extension in previously normal-appearing tissue [4, 5].

Reoperation for Dupuytren contractures should follow a careful assessment of the functional limitation imposed by the contracture and the recent activity of the disease process.

J.H. Calandruccio, MS, MD (✉) • S.E. Hecox, MD
Department of Orthopedic Surgery,
University of Tennessee—Campbell Clinic,
Germantown, TN 38138, USA
e-mail: Norwal@aol.com

S.F.M. Duncan (ed.), *Reoperative Hand Surgery*,
DOI 10.1007/978-1-4614-2373-7_2, © Springer Science+Business Media, LLC 2012

Successful contracture correction accompanied by permanently supple fingers and palms occurs in a minority of patients, and nodularity and cord recurrence are common. Correction of the metacarpophalangeal contractures is almost uniformly achieved. However, loss of proximal interphalangeal joint (PIPJ) contracture correction is very frequent, and repeat surgical intervention may be indicated in one third of males and one fourth of females [6–8].

Indications and Contraindications

The time elapsed since the initial surgery and the rate and degree of contracture recurrence are important determinants in considering repeat surgical intervention. Recurrent metacarpophalangeal joint (MPJ) and PIPJ contractures of 30° may be enough to warrant additional surgery [1, 3]. The surgical indications are commonly problematic finger and thumb MPJ and PIPJ and web space contractures that compromise vocational and avocational activities. The ideal reoperative patient with well-defined cords, moderate degrees of contractures, good quality skin, and normal sensory function is rare. More commonly, the reoperative patient has multiple zones of scar tissue, poorly defined cords, severe contractures, and previously grafted skin. Palmar flexion contracture forces must also be addressed in patients with MPJ contractures. Concomitant release of the fixed deforming palmar contractures, especially of the MP joints, is a prerequisite for satisfactory soft tissue balancing.

On the contrary, diffusely thickened skin, web space contractures, sensory neuropathies, vascular insufficiency, and poor quality skin represent some factors that may contraindicate additional surgery. Poor return of motion follows PIPJ contracture release in patients with either joint arthrofibrosis, to arthritic deformity, and those with a prior surgical release. Fusion for significant PIPJ contractures in such individuals can be considered, especially on the ulnar side of the hand.

Preoperative History and Considerations

Reoperation for DD will render a more functional hand only if preservation of sensation and ability to make a composite fist accompany flexion contracture and web space contracture release. The prior surgical notes ideally should be reviewed, and the disease onset and rapidity of progression since the initial procedure noted. A detailed sensory examination should be performed on the entire hand and regions of altered or absent sensation recorded. A critical component of reoperation is to carefully isolate and protect all digital nerves, especially the small finger ulnar and index radial digital nerves during the dissection on the borders of the hand. Sensory nerve protection is assisted by correlation of the skin crease surface anatomy to the underlying neurovascular structures (Fig. 2.1).

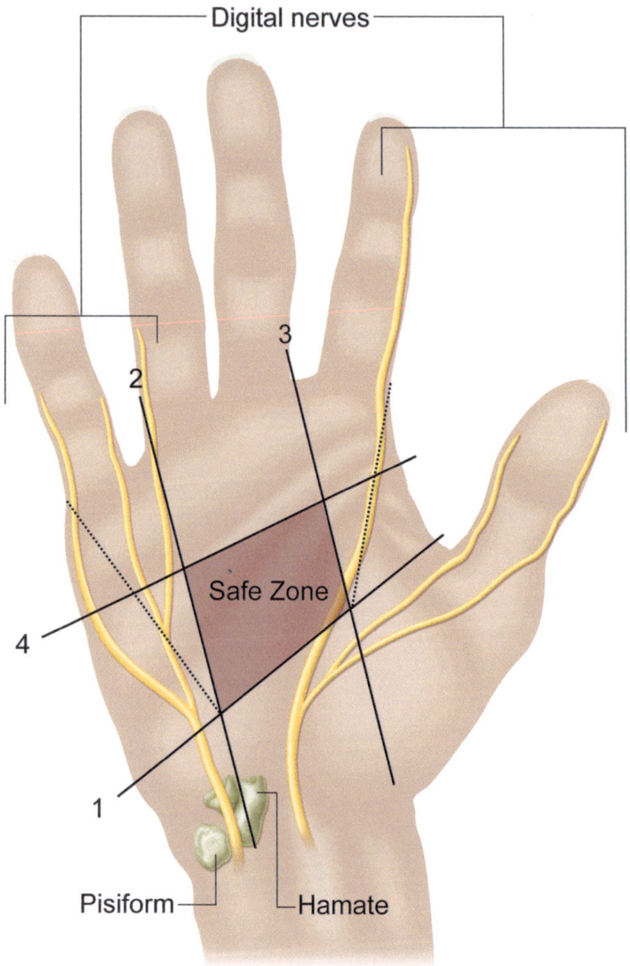

Fig. 2.1 Correlation of digital nerves to skin surface creases. The small finger ulnar digital nerve courses obliquely across the hand under the *line* drawn from the small finger ulnar palmar digital crease to the intersection point of Kaplan's cardinal line and one parallel to the ulnar border of the ring finger. Similarly, the index radial digital nerve courses obliquely across the hand under the *line* drawn from the index finger radial palmar digital crease to the intersection point of Kaplan's cardinal line and one parallel to the radial border of the middle finger

Tips and Pearls

Digital nerve and artery: The most problematic complications following repeat DD surgery, digital nerve and/or artery injury can be reduced when the operative procedure is considered a task of isolation. External neurolysis of each digital nerve can be performed along with careful dissection of arterial structures. Dissection should be from proximal to distal and the nerves located in disease-free palmar areas and gently manipulated as they are excavated from dense scar tissue. As the digital nerves may be drawn midline and

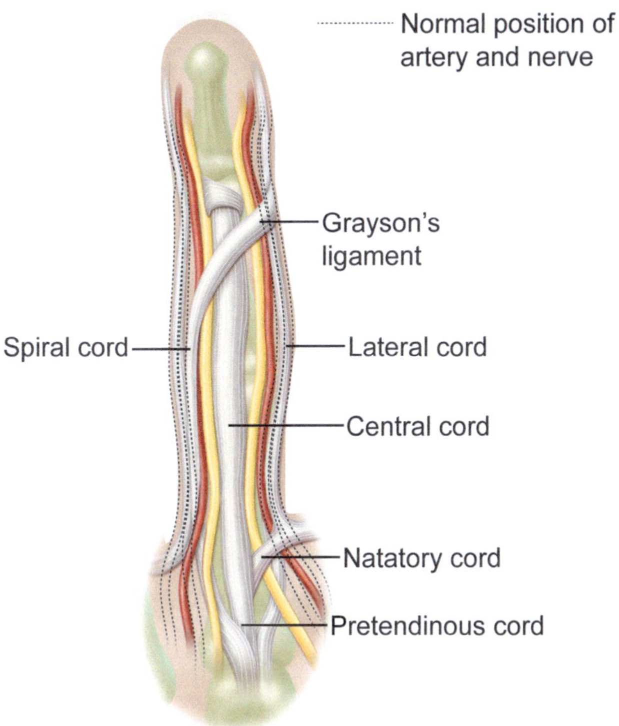

Fig. 2.2 Digital nerve displacement in Dupuytren disease. Abnormal structures composing the spiral cord causing medial and volar nerve displacement

superficially from their normal anatomic locations, the nerves are best followed when possible from their deep origins and on the side of the nerve away from the midline of the finger (Fig. 2.2). When the disease process extends dorsally, the digits' dorsal sensory branches should also be followed in a proximal to distal direction. However, in some cases, a distal to proximal dissection will be needed. The surgeon should be versed in microsurgery, in case the need for arterial or nerve repair arises.

PIP contracture: PIP joint contractures may be considered secondary to extrinsic (skin or DD fibrous elements) or intrinsic (flexor sheath, tendon adhesions, volar plate, collateral ligament, and joint surface pathology) causes. Only after the pathologic fibrous elements of DD are excised and the skin contractures released by whatever means can an underlying intrinsic PIP joint contracture be evaluated. Sometimes gentle manipulation into extension is sufficient to have the remaining volar constraints give way to achieve the desired extension. Persistent firm endpoints and resistance to passive correction of remaining PIP joint contractures presents a possible need for addressing the intrinsic joint contracture. Efforts should be made to try passive extension of the PIPJ joint because suboptimal outcomes accompany formal contracture release [9]. Intrinsic joint release often results in decreased PIP joint flexion and modest improvement in extension. Therefore, PIP joint intrinsic release is performed by a superficial to deep sequential release of the soft tissue PIP joint pathoanatomy: limited flexor sheath release over the PIP joint (A3 pulley), evaluation of FDS and FDP mobility within the tendon sheath, volar plate release, and finally collateral ligament release and/or partial excision. Passive manipulation should follow each step in the release sequence and the process terminated when the desired PIP joint extension is achieved. Temporary pinning of the PIP joint in extension for 1–2 weeks may be beneficial prior to a structured therapy program. Significant PIP joint surface irregularities are evaluated by bi-planar preoperative X-rays, and degenerative joint disease with significant contractures may be better treated by fusion in a functional position, especially on the ulnar border of the hand [1, 10].

Web space contracture: Inability to separate the fingers is most commonly secondary to natatory cord involvement, but may also be from adjacent finger central cords' continuity with a single common pretendinous cord. Excision of the pretendinous and/or central cords allows evaluation for the presence of a natatory cord. This cord should be excised by careful delineation and dissection of this interdigital cord from the overlying web space skin. Lacerations into the web space skin may result in further contracture and form prominent scars and should be avoided whenever possible.

Patient medical condition: Contracture release surgery should not overshadow concerns for a patient's general medical condition. The adage "there is no condition so bad that it cannot be made worse by another operation" should certainly be recalled in certain circumstances of recurrent DD. Many conditions are common denominators for a poor outcome including but not limited to patients who smoke excessively as well those with medical conditions resulting in peripheral vascular disease and poor healing capacity. Moreover, disease affecting the hand such as MP osteoarthritis or rheumatoid joint pathology will render suboptimal outcome when the procedure addresses only the DD pathology.

Operative Approach

Surgical approaches to recurrent DD require outlining all the problem areas to be addressed by the surgical procedure. Previous surgical scars may be disregarded in most cases; however, incorporation of portions of the previous incisions when possible may be advantageous and improve the final appearance of the wounds. Extensile palmar and digital incisions should be fashioned to allow excision of as much of the diseased tissue as possible. Usually, the palmar incision allows for multiple pretendinous cords to be excised. When multiple digits are involved, similar incisions in the adjacent digits should be used when possible. PIPJ contractures

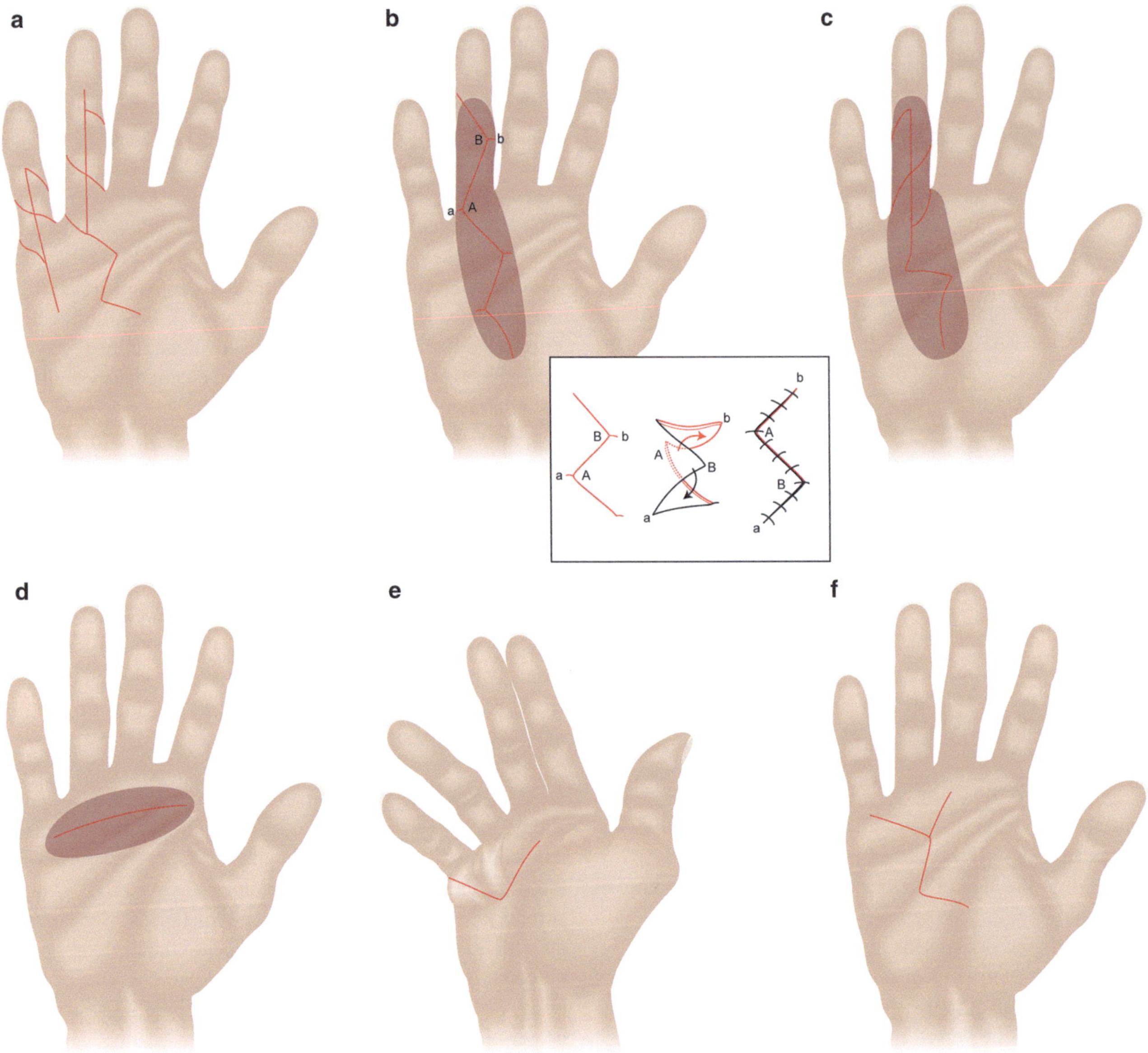

Fig. 2.3 Common skin incisions for Dupuytren cord excision. (**a**) Longitudinal incisions here shown in the ring and small fingers are converted to multiple z-plasty flaps. (**b**) Bruner incision. (**c**) Combination of z-plasty flaps and an extensile palmar incision alternating directions obliquely across palmar flexion creases. (**d**) Transverse palmar incision. (**e**) Distally based V-shaped incision. (**f**) Distally based V-shaped incision with proximal palmar extension

of more than 45° are more easily approached through straight midline volar incisions converted to z-plasties (Fig. 2.3). Sometimes the skin is inseparable and/or indistinguishable from the underlying disease, especially in reoperative regions, and the skin flaps should be designed to reduce devascularization and skin loss.

The scope of procedures for recurrent DD is essentially the same as for the initial intervention, including subcutaneous fasciotomy (scalpel, needle, or enzymatic release), fasciectomy (limited, selective, or complete), nodule fasciectomy and skin grafting, arthrodesis, and amputation [5]. The procedure chosen for reoperation may not be similar to that chosen for the first procedure. Disease extension in regions remote from that previously excised may need to be addressed and require a much more extensive approach, multiple incisions, and possibly a combination of procedures.

Regional or general anesthesia is preferred for partial selective fasciectomy, complete or total fasciectomy, and nodule fasciectomy and skin grafting procedures as surgical times may be lengthy. Allocating an hour per finger is not unreasonable, and patient motion from tourniquet pain may interfere and compromise the operation when the whole arm is not anesthetized.

Subcutaneous Fasciotomy

Clostridial collagenase injection aponeurotomy has now become available for widespread use. It may become a popular procedure as less than 5% recurrence and minimal untoward effects at 4-year follow-up have been reported [11]. A prospective, randomized, double-blind, placebo-controlled, multicenter trial involving 308 patients reported improvement over placebo injection in regard to contracture reduction and motion improvement. The treatment included manipulation the day following the injections and up to three injections over 30-day intervals. Serious side effects were rare, but did include two tendon ruptures. Most side effects were local or regional and transient. The utility of this office-based procedure may be soon approaching more widespread clinical application.

Needle aponeurotomy has been reported to give satisfactory short-term results in a group of 74 releases at 32-month follow-up [7, 8]. However, in this group the recurrence rate was 65% where recurrence was defined as loss of 30° or more from the immediate postsurgical correction. Although sensory disturbance was noted in only two fingers, digital nerve stretch injury in addition to needle trauma remains a concern. The multiple site release along taut cords may gain more initial contracture correction beyond the distal palmar area (pretendinous cord insertion site) and shorten the recovery period. This may be performed as an office procedure and repeated as necessary to gain extension.

Percutaneous fasciotomy is ideally suited for patients with well-defined cords in the palm [7, 8]. This procedure may be performed in the office under local anesthesia with an 11 or 15 blade. The involved finger is extended with the physician's nondominant hand, while the scalpel blade (held parallel with the skin) is then slid between the skin and cord. The blade is then turned ninety degrees to be perpendicular to the taut cord, and the finger is more forcefully extended (Fig. 2.4). A sudden release of the MP joint contracture follows cord division. Multiple cords in multiple fingers are released in similar fashion, and multiple sites proximal to the distal palmar flexion crease may be released as well. Neurovascular injury can be minimized by avoiding scalpel blade penetration deep into the palm and cord release more distally where the digital nerve course and location are less certain.

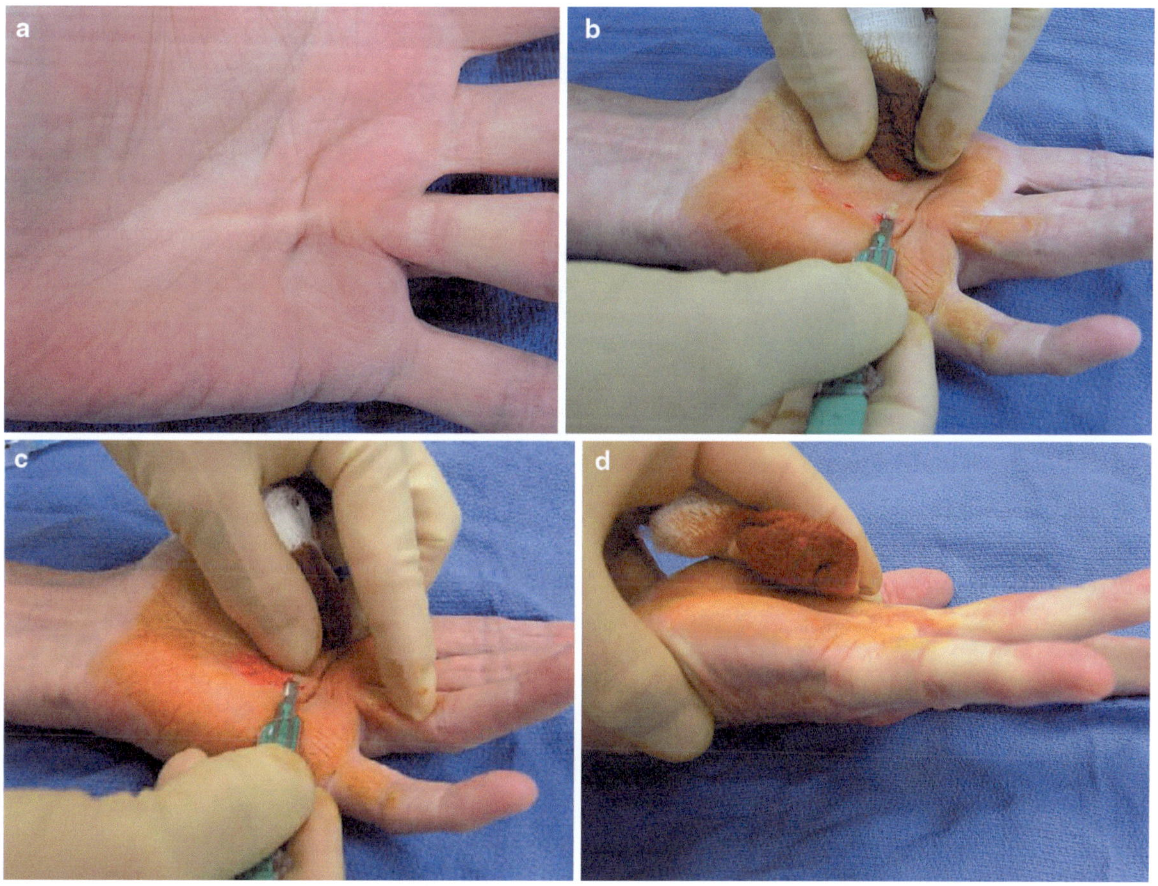

Fig. 2.4 Percutaneous release of Dupuytren cord. (**a**) Well-defined ring finger pretendinous cord with a 60° MP joint contracture. (**b**) Scalpel blade is inserted between the skin and the pretendinous cord. (**c**) The finger is forcefully extended effectively delivering more superficially the abnormal cord onto the blade held at 90° to the cord. (**d**) The resultant MP joint extension achieved

Partial Selective Fasciectomy

Repeat partial selective fasciectomy is probably the most frequently performed procedure for recurrent DD contractures [5]. The diseased tissue is removed as completely as possible and also parts of the uninvolved aponeurosis. The range of reported recurrence varies widely: In an exhaustive review of the literature, McGrouther [12] found percentages of recurrence between 2 and 63%. On average, the recurrence rate might be 40–50%. Another variant of this technique is nodule fasciectomy, which removes only the nodule (sometimes also the cord) and leaves in place the aponeurosis that is not considered as critical to disease development. Depending on the disease's stage, cords will be cut but not fully excised (subcutaneous fasciotomy). Discontinuity in the retracted aponeurotic cords similarly can be created without wide resection of the fascia and segmental aponeurectomy probably has recurrence rates similar to partial fasciectomy [7, 13, 14].

Partial selective fasciectomy procedures are designed to remove pathologic tissue-affecting regions considered problematic to the patient. Prior to incision, the problem areas are mapped out with a marking pen, such as placing dots along the cords and nodules to be excised (Fig. 2.5). The incision choice is at the surgeon's discretion as a multitude of skin incisions allow safe access to the DD. An incision made directly overlying the pretendinous and central cords in the finger(s) midline is an extensile approach facilitating longitudinal digital nerve and cord dissection. Often this longitudinal incision in the palm will permit adjacent pretendinous cord excision.

Tips and Pearls

Design and conversion of the longitudinal incision(s) to z-plasties should be done only after the surgeon has accomplished the cord and nodule excision. Direct disease adherence to the skin in recurrent cases is common distal to the web spaces and parts of the skin may be unsatisfactory for the base of a rotational flap. Thus, the flaps should be drawn to keep the healthiest skin flaps for the bases. The flaps should be sutured relatively tension-free and the z-plasty flaps need not recreate the normal flexion creases in the fingers; they merely need to course obliquely across them. The skin need not be completely closed and transverse areas left open intentionally are techniques to reduce tension and allow drainage.

Partial selective fasciectomy may be performed by a series of transverse incisions in certain disease configurations. A liberal length transverse incision in the palm proximal to the proximal palmar flexion crease or between it and the distal palmar flexion crease will expose pretendinous

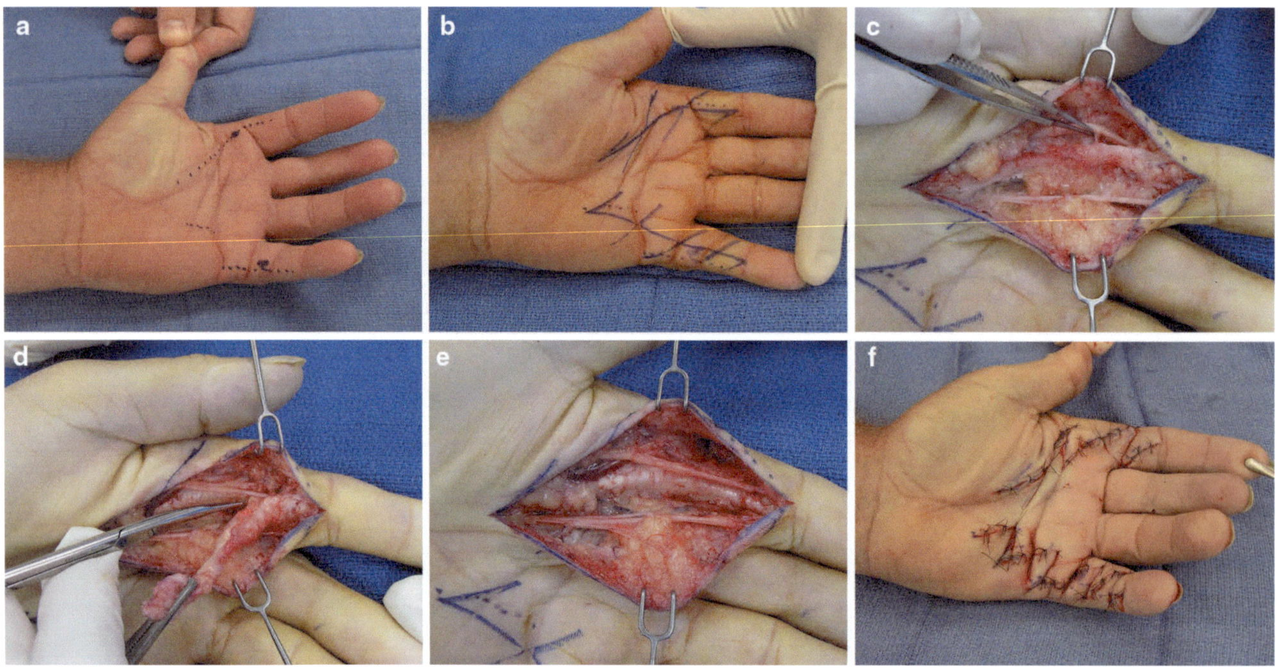

Fig. 2.5 Selective fasciectomy. (**a**) The taut cords to be excised are *dotted* and the nodules marked with a *skin pen*. (**b**) Markings of the preliminarily planned z-plasty flaps. (**c**) The palmar and digital cords are exposed through the longitudinal incision. (**d**) Proximal to distal dissection of the cord revealing well-protected digital nerves. (**e**) Index finger after visible disease and prior to skin rearrangement. (**f**) Following meticulous hemostasis, the z-plasty wounds are closed

cords adequately. Transverse incisions in the palmar digital and PIPJ flexion creases may also be used to trace the neurovascular bundles prior to excision of the offending tensile disease tissues. Persistent PIP joint contractures may be released as previously described and the wounds left to heal secondarily.

Total Fasciectomy

Total fasciectomy removes all of the diseased tissue and often also the aponeurosis, which is sometimes believed to be the source of the disease. Due to higher risk of functional loss of the hand, this technique has become less popular in the last few decades. Even with this extensive excision, recurrence rate estimated 20–40% after 5 years [4].

Dermofasciectomy

Nodule fasciectomy with skin grafting (dermofasciectomy) is intended to use the purported myofibroblast inhibitory property of a full thickness skin graft to reduce recurrent DD contractures [6]. In this procedure, the diseased fascia plus the overlying skin is replaced by upper arm or groin skin grafts. Although the reasons for recurrence are not always known, in a comparative series Rousch and Stern [5] found the recurrence rate for this procedure higher than in those with local flaps.

Gonzalez [10] analyzed 100 such procedures where skin grafts were used as gap bridges and found that full function was achieved by 21 days in 85% of patients. Skin graft loss was rare when motion began 10 days postoperatively and indicated immediate cross-finger flaps when the skin grafts were lost.

Dynamic External Stretching

There are some devices available such as the Agee Digit Widget™ (Hand Biomechanics Lab; Sacramento, CA), which provide an extension torque that can be controlled by the surgeon (Fig. 2.6). Such devices are usually installed dorsally or laterally. This can be used to slowly stretch the soft tissues over a 4–6 week period. Fasciectomy can then more easily be performed with the finger in straighter alignment. The risk of neuropraxia from sudden stretching of the digital nerves is also theoretically reduced. Moreover, vascular compromise that can be seen from stretching of the digital arteries after fasciectomy or contracture release is also theoretically reduced. There are numerous case reports describing finger compromise from vascular injury after suddenly stretching a finger after Dupuytren excision [15, 16].

Optimizing Outcomes

Optimizing outcomes when performing a repeat operative procedure for recurrent DD contractures requires strict adherence to those same factors as when performing the initial procedure. Most importantly, the disease process should be in a later stage when the likelihood of recurrence will be less. Broad collagen fibers in the fibrotic or residual phase are usually more distinct from the surrounding tissue than those in either the proliferative or fibrocellular phase. Regardless of the procedure or surgical technique chosen, the fundamental elements for successful outcomes remain excision, separation, and/or unlinking the contractile soft tissue chain. Healing by secondary intention, z-plasty and skin grafting accompanying open procedures are excellent methods to accomplish this goal, while less invasive methods may not fully address the dermal components.

Therapeutic involvement should ideally be initiated within the first week for wound management and tailoring a therapy program to maintain the extension achieved from the intervention as well as begin the process of regaining digital flexion. Interval extension splinting between instructed exercises and active patient participation is requisite for satisfactory results. A postoperative schedule is individualized, as some patients require more intense and frequent visits to work through the recovery process.

Complications and Side Effects

Reduction in PIPJ motion following joint release is common especially with repeat surgical intervention for a PIPJ flexion contracture, especially in osteoarthritic joints and joints with prolonged immobilization. Temporary pinning of the PIPJ in extension is sometimes beneficial during the first 7–14 days following surgery. Loss of PIP joint flexion is common in those joints immobilized in extension longer than 2 weeks.

Flexor tendon adhesions in conjunction with PIPJ arthrofibrosis present rare but very difficult postoperative sequelae, for which an adequate solution may not be possible. Digital nerve lacerations are more likely with reoperation for DD, especially when postsurgical scarring is combined with cord redevelopment. More often, sensory neuropraxias occur even with gentle digital nerve dissection and stretch from the extension achieved intraoperatively. Neuropraxias often resolve in 6–12 weeks.

Digital artery injury probably occurs with some regularity and its effect is uncertain. The digital arteries should be protected, especially the larger vessel which is on the side of the finger towards the midline of the hand. Vessels more at risk for injury are those associated with spiral or digital cords distal to the MPJ where emphasis on digital nerve protection

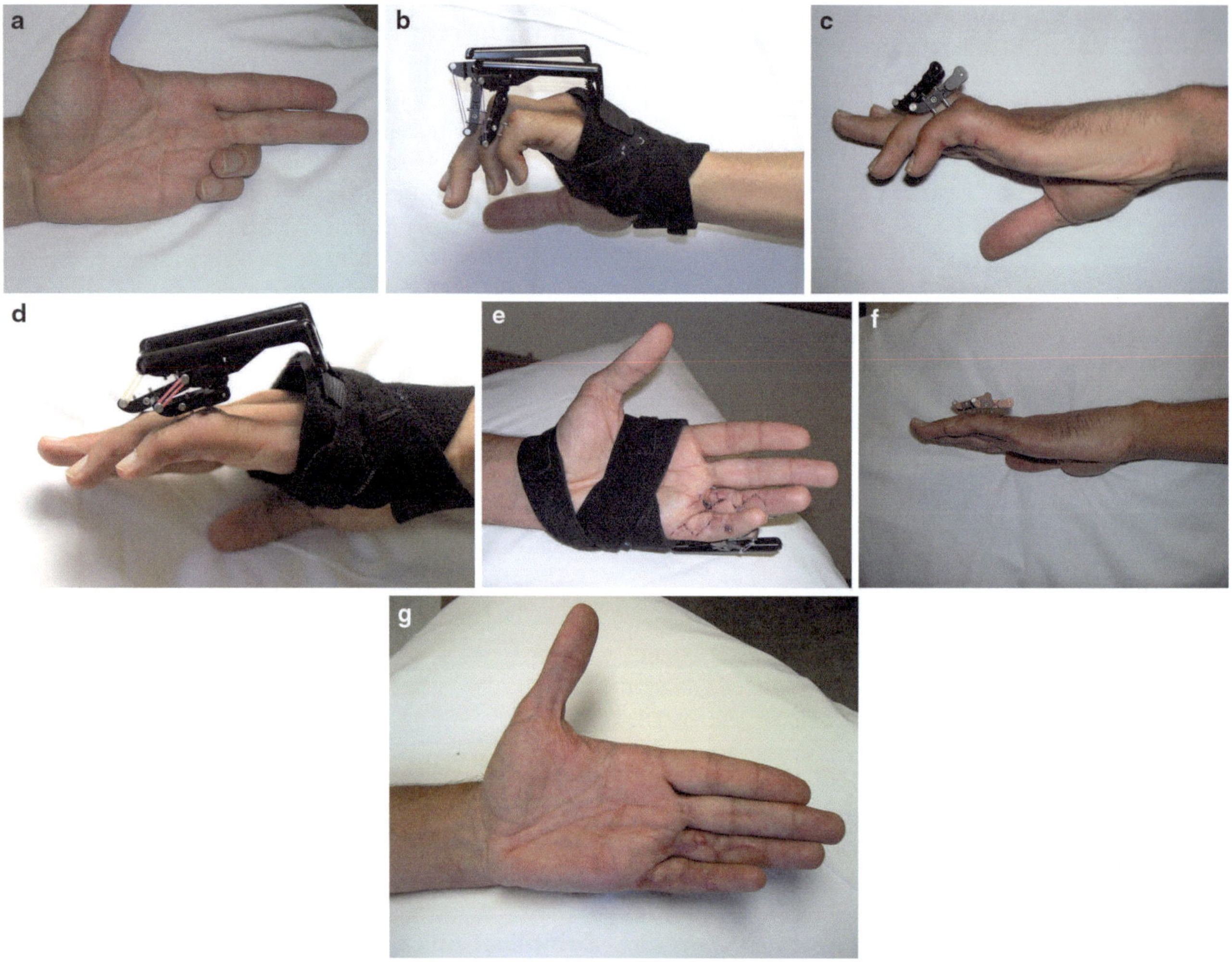

Fig. 2.6 Agee Digit Widget showing the dorsal placement with dynamic stretch of soft tissues over an extended period of time. (**a**) The pre-op view is from the palm side. This was his full extension and the scar shows that he had prior surgery on that hand. (**b**) The next view is with the two DW on after 1 week of extension torque. At the time of DW application, Dr. Agee made two small incisions on the little finger and one on the ring to cut the bands. (**c**) The patient has worn the DW for 3 weeks. (**d**) The patient has worn the DW for 6 weeks and is now scheduled for a fasciectomy. (**e**) The patient is now 10 days postfasciectomy and the DW extension torque is resumed. There was a 10-day "rest" period after fasciectomy to let the skin incisions heal. (**f**) This view is at 7 weeks postfasciectomy. (**g**) Final extension view. This example case is courtesy of Dr. John Agee

may take focus off the nearby digital artery. Vascular compromise is a possible complication and a "white finger" distal to the PIPJ can exist for a period of time especially when significant flexion contractures are released. Usually the pulp turgor and capillary refill return within 20–30 min and dressing removal and splint and/or pin removal to allow the finger to flex seldom are necessary. However, if it does not improve, then further action must be taken. This may include flexing the digit as well as microsurgical repair or reconstruction.

Skin tip necrosis is a frequent finding in patients with marginal circulation. Older patients, smokers, and those with other comorbid factors may have loss of the end portions of their skin flaps and wound healing by secondary intention usually ensues.

Postoperative Care

Soft noncompressive dressings over nonadherent gauzes are applied to the surgical areas and a volar-formed digital splint is used to keep the digit(s) in as much extension as safely possible. Hand-based splints adequately immobilize the MPJs and PIPJs sufficiently. The uninvolved portions of the hand may be left free for use in the recovery period. Hand elevation for several days is advised, and the first postoperative visit is within 7 days from surgery, frequently with a therapist.

The first postoperative visit can be made with a knowledgeable therapist who follows the surgeon's specific postoperative protocol. All dressings are removed and sterile technique is followed for range of motion exercises. Efforts to achieve greater extension are concomitant with a program to regain digital flexion. Patients benefit from a structured therapy plan and are usually seen on regular visits for the first 6 weeks after surgery. Night-time extension splints are worn for several months, and normal use of the hand is encouraged as soon as the wounds permit; however, the resultant edema, scar thickening, and stiffness often prevent palmar impaction activities for 3–6 months following reoperation for DD.

Conclusion

Fundamental research on the initiation and progression of DD has not significantly altered its clinical management [3]. The disease is clearly genetically transmitted with variable expression and its course altered by the health status of each patient. Reoperation for Dupuytren contractures does not necessarily represent a technical failure of the initial or previous procedures, but merely the manifestations and transformation of tissue which had previously appeared normal. Minimally invasive procedures such as clostridial collagenase injections and percutaneous releases appear to simplify contracture management yet they have their own set of complications [7, 8, 11, 13, 14].

The surgical approach for excision of pathological elements is less important than the skin rearrangement to uncouple regions of skin tension. This is most feasibly accomplished with either secondary intention skin healing or gap skin grafting. Selective fasciectomy continues to be the most common procedure designed for both initial and recurrent DD management. However, management of DD is undergoing rapid change and the minimally invasive techniques are becoming more accepted and widely utilized.

References

1. Calandruccio JH. Dupuytren contracture. Chap. 72 in Part XVIII: "The hand". In: Canale ST, Beaty JH, editors. Campbell's operative orthopaedics. 11th ed. Philadelphia: Mosby Elsevier; 2008. p. 4273–84.
2. Russ R. The surgical aspects of Dupuytren's contraction. Am J Med Sci. 1908;135:856.
3. Rayan GM. Dupuytren disease: anatomy, pathology, presentation, and treatment. J Bone Joint Surg Am. 2007;89:189–98.
4. Rodrigo JJ, et al. Treatment of Dupuytren's contracture. Long-term results after fasciotomy and fascial excision. J Bone Joint Surg. 1976;58(3):380–7.
5. Rousch TF, Stern PJ. Results following surgery for recurrent Dupuytren's disease. J Hand Surg [Am]. 2000;25:291–6.
6. Ketchum LD, Hixson FD. Dermofasciectomy and full-thickness grafts in the treatment of Dupuytren's contracture. J Hand Surg [Am]. 1987;12:659–64.
7. van Rijssen AL, et al. A comparison of the direct outcomes of percutaneous needle fasciotomy and limited fasciectomy for Dupuytren's disease: a 6-week follow-up study. J Hand Surg. 2006;31A(5):717–25.
8. Van Russen AL, Werker PMN. Percutaneous needle fasciotomy in Dupuytren's disease. J Hand Surg. 2006;31(5):498–501.
9. Cools H, Verstreken J. The open palm technique in the treatment of Dupuytren's disease. Acta Orthop Belg. 1994;60(4):413–20.
10. Gonzalez RI. Dupuytren's contracture of the fingers: a simplified approach to surgical treatment. California Medicine. West J Med. 1971;115(2):25–31.
11. Hurst LC, et al. Injectable collagenase *Clostridium histolyticum* for Dupuytren's contracture. New Engl J Med. 2009;361(10):968–79.
12. McFarlane RM, McGrouther DA, Flint MH, editors. Dupuytren's disease: biology and treatment. Edinburgh: Churchill Livingstone; 1990.
13. Badalamente M, et al. Collagen as a clinical target: nonoperative treatment of Dupuytren's disease. J Hand Surg. 2002;27A(5):788–98.
14. Badalamente M, Hurst L. Efficacy and safety of injectable mixed collagenase subtypes in the treatment of Dupuytren's contracture. J Hand Surg. 2007;32A(6):767–74.
15. Boyer MI, Gelberman RH. Complications of the operative treatment of Dupuytren's disease. Hand Clin. 1999;15(1):161–6, viii.
16. Chung KC, Segalman KA. Microvascular solution for vascular complication in surgery for Dupuytren's contracture: a case report. J Hand Surg Am. 1996;21(4):711–3.

Options for Failed Flexor Tendon Surgery

3

A. Ylenia Giuffrida and Scott Wolfe

Abstract

Reconstructive flexor tendon surgery can be extremely difficult. The zone of failure will determine the potential reconstructive options that are available. For the thumb, tendon grafts as well as potential flexor digitorum superficialis tendon transfer are options for reconstruction. In the digits fusion as well as 2-stage tendon reconstructions are options. If the flexor tendon sheath is still intact, a single-stage tendon graft can sometimes be successful. These surgeries can be fraught with complications including failure of the graft to heal, rupture of the graft, scarring of the graft, and hand stiffness. These types of surgeries really should be performed by someone who performs hand surgery on a regular basis or who has specialized training in hand surgery. Both skill and creative thinking are required to succeed in these reconstructions. However, even in the best of hands, these cases may not turn out as the patient and surgeon had hoped. This chapter discusses the options available for reconstructing the finger or thumb that has failed initial repair.

Keywords

Flexor • Tendon • Reconstruction • Failed • Repair

Key Points

- Proper patient selection is essential
- Adhere to the basic tenets of flexor tendon surgery to avoid unnecessary dissection, scarring, and adhesions
- A course of preoperative therapy can provide valuable information about patient motivation in addition to maximizing motion
- When possible, delay surgery until soft tissue scarring has matured
- Digital vascular status should be determined preoperatively with a digital Allen's test or advanced imaging, and digits with tenuous blood supply should not be reoperated
- Tensioning of tendon grafts is critical to overall hand function and should not be over- or undertensioned
- A team effort with surgeon, patient, and hand therapist is essential
- Always be prepared for an intraoperative change in plans to a more complicated reconstructive procedure if indicated, having the appropriate equipment available

A.Y. Giuffrida, MD
Hackensack University Medical Center, Hackensack, NJ, USA
e-mail: aygiuffrida@gmail.com

S. Wolfe, MD (✉)
Weill Medical College of Cornell University, Hospital for Special Surgery, 523 E. 72nd Street, 4th Floor Hand Center, New York, NY 06830, USA
e-mail: wolfes@hss.edu; wolfesw@gmail.com

S.F.M. Duncan (ed.), *Reoperative Hand Surgery*,
DOI 10.1007/978-1-4614-2373-7_3, © Springer Science+Business Media, LLC 2012

Introduction

Failed flexor tendon repair can be among the most challenging complications in hand surgery to address. The technical difficulty of the surgery, the proximity to important neurovascular structures, the presence of scar tissue and attenuated anatomical structures, coupled with a paucity of experience by many hand surgeons in this area make this one of hand surgery's most challenging problems. By the same token, if successful, restoration of the flexor tendon system can be one of the most elegant and gratifying of all hand surgical procedures.

The evolution of flexor tendon surgery has been dramatic over the last 40 years. Development of strong repair techniques and early motion protocols are among the major advances. Several principles have become standard, such as the use of braided nonabsorbable core sutures and monofilament epitendinous sutures. Repairs should have at minimum four strands crossing the repair site, all with equal tension. Unfortunately, there exist many factors which are variable and beyond the control of the surgeon, and result in less than predictable results for all patients. One of such problems is adhesion formation—adhesions between tendons, between sheath and tendon, and occasionally between bone and tendon. Adhesions prevent the essential gliding function of tendons from developing. In addition, the changes which occur in the surrounding soft tissues as a result of surgical intervention compound the challenge of tendon healing in this sometimes hostile environment.

Recent basic science research has emerged which may suggest that tendon healing can be modulated by various biologic and mechanical factors. Until these concepts can be put into practice, we are left to utilize the techniques developed over the last several decades, with careful attention to selection of surgical candidates, to optimize outcomes of flexor tendon surgery. Perhaps the next decade will bring us the tissue engineering applications we need to overcome the limitations we currently have in achieving more predictable successful results.

This chapter is organized into rerepair techniques by zone of injury, beginning at the fingertip and moving proximally. Rehabilitation protocols specific to zones of injury and repair technique are presented. Appropriate rehabilitation protocols are designed to increase the tensile strength of repairs and prevent adhesions while protecting the repair integrity.

A team approach involving the physician, hand therapist, and patient is essential and cannot be overemphasized. This system should be put in place prior to embarking on any flexor tendon reoperation.

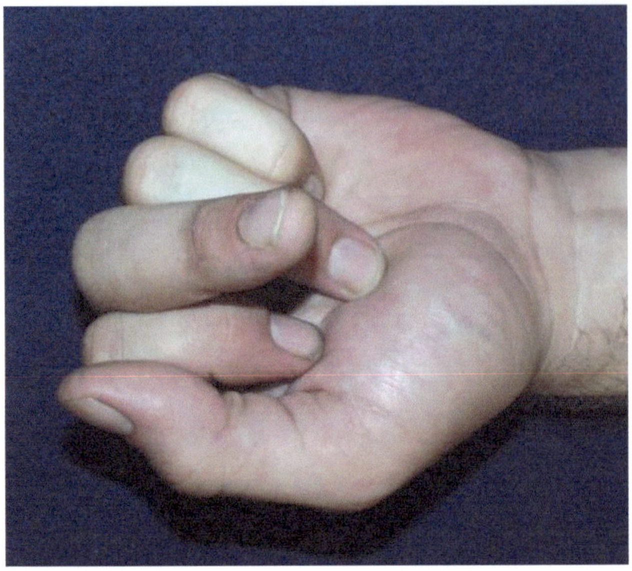

Fig. 3.1 Loss of flexion posture of the DIPJ may signify rerupture or repair site elongation

Zone I Failed Primary Repair

Preoperative History and Considerations

Rerupture of repaired FDP tendons in Zone I can be readily diagnosed once the loss of distal interphalangeal flexion posture or loss of active DIPJ flexion occurs (Fig. 3.1), but rarely is this the case. Repair site elongation can present similarly with a more gradual loss of flexion posture. A careful physical examination is essential because, unfortunately, imaging modalities such as ultrasound [1, 2] and MRI [3–5] can yield inconsistent results. If loss of flexion posture and active flexion occurs, or if the dorsal button becomes loose within 3 weeks of repair, it may be assumed that elongation or rerupture has occurred. The repair site continues to gain strength between 3 and 6 weeks, so it is not unusual for repair failure to occur at this stage with an overaggressive rehabilitation program. Serial physical examinations over the rehabilitation period can provide the best information in making this diagnosis.

Passive DIPJ motion should be evaluated and compared to active motion. If passive motion is limited, there is little utility in restoring the FDP insertion.

Indications and Contraindications for Rerepair

The best candidates for rerepair of the FDP tendon are young patients with supple DIP joints that demonstrate a need for DIP flexion in the ulnar digits of the hand (i.e., ring and small fingers) to restore power grip, or to prevent hyperextension of the DIP joint. If FDS function has been compromised or if PIP flexion is limited, the FDP becomes even more important to restore. Manual laborers, unmotivated patients, and relatively older, low functioning patients make poor candidates for restoration of FDP function.

Despite the simplicity in its name, rerepair can be a challenging procedure. The surgeon and patient should always be prepared for a more involved operation, i.e., reconstruction, should the tissues be found at reoperation to not support or be too short for a rerepair.

Indications
- Young, motivated patients
- Intact passive DIPJ motion
- Ring or small finger involvement
- Symptomatic DIPJ hyperextension

Contraindications
- Elderly, low functioning, or unmotivated patients
- DIPJ arthritis or injury
- Advancement more than 1 cm

Operative Approach for Rerepair

A general or regional anesthetic is preferred over local anesthesia, to allow maximal comfort and prevent any tourniquet discomfort by the patient. A hand table attachment should be positioned so that the arm lies at 90° from the patient's body. A brachial tourniquet is used to allow full and natural excursion of the forearm musculature, and exsanguination is performed with an elastic bandage.

The original incision is generally used to expose the insertion site of the FDP, the neurovascular bundles, and the A4 pulley. Proximal extension may be carried out in order to find a proximally retracted tendon stump. Knowledge of the location of the tendon stump at the time of repair of the original injury may be helpful in that an intact vincula may prevent retraction proximal to the PIP joint, limiting the necessary exposure. An effort should be made to avoid unnecessary dissection and exposure of the tendon sheath. If the tendon does not easily advance to the repair site with a gentle milking maneuver, the authors recommend using the retrieval method described by Sourmelis and McGrouther [6]. The surgeon should have a low threshold for opening the sheath more proximally for tendon retrieval, in order to prevent unnecessary scarring within the sheath by passing instruments blindly into it in attempts to retrieve a retracted tendon. If the sheath is opened proximally, the tendon stump should be brought out of the sheath in its resting location, between the nearest pulleys, with a transverse incision in the sheath. A pediatric feeding tube should be advanced retrograde from the repair site (Fig. 3.2), through the sheath beneath the pulley system, to the area of the tendon stump. The stump should be sutured to the tube, and the tube pulled from the repair site to deliver the tendon stump in an atraumatic fashion. Once the tendon stump is delivered, it should be secured with a 25 gauge needle transfixed in the soft tissues (Fig. 3.3). Old sutures should be removed and any devitalized tissue should be debrided, taking care not to overshorten the tendon. Repair site elongation is not an uncommon finding (Fig. 3.4), and attenuated tissue should be removed, as it does not have the mechanical properties to assure a strong rerepair.

The tendon can then be passed underneath the A4 pulley if not already done so. A pulley-plasty or partial release of the A4 pulley may have already been performed at the primary operation, allowing more facile passage of the stump. A cervical dilator can be used if necessary to create more space beneath the pulley.

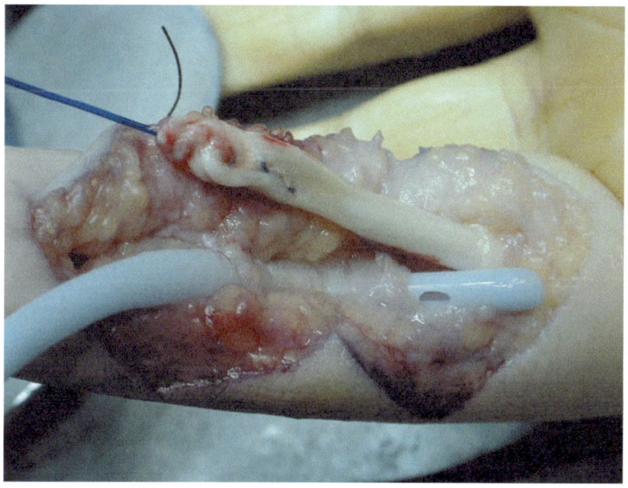

Fig. 3.2 Retrograde passage of a pediatric feeding tube can assist in retrieval and threading a tendon through the pulley system

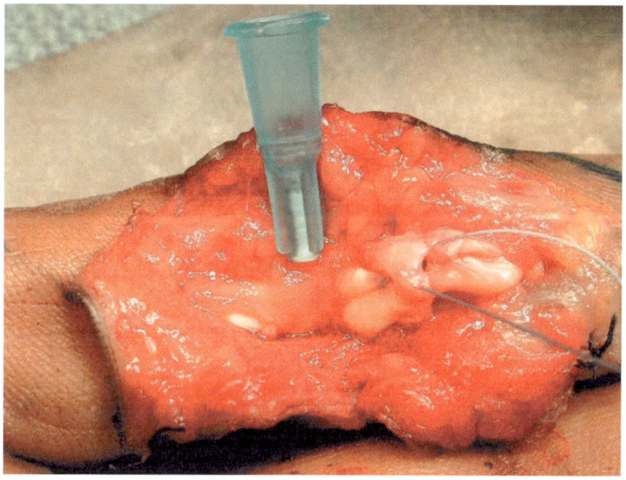

Fig. 3.3 Transfixion of the tendon stump with a 25-guage needle will facilitate placement of core sutures with minimal additional manipulation of tissues

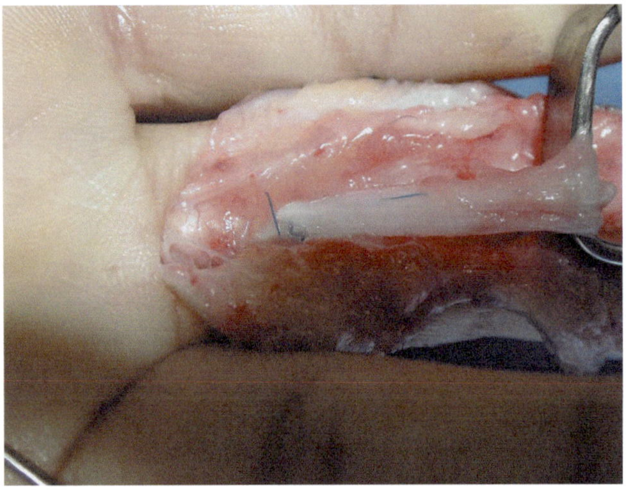

Fig. 3.4 Repair site elongation is a common reason for clinical failure of tendon repair. All attenuated tissues must be debrided down to normal tendon to ensure a strong rerepair

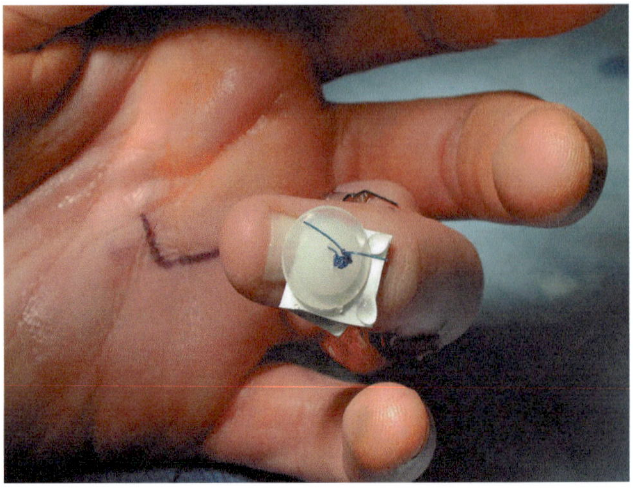

Fig. 3.5 The bolster should consist of a nonadherent layer (Xeroform or Adaptik) followed by a layer of felt, then the button. It should be positioned distal to the lunula to avoid later fingernail deformity. Note the exaggerated flexed posture of the digit after the suture is tied

Methods of reattachment are similar to that of primary repair. The type of repair depends on the length and condition of the remaining distal stump. If there is less than 1 cm remaining, an advancement should be performed [7]. The insertion site at the base of the proximal phalanx should be debrided of any scar tissue in preparation for reattachment. The authors suggest a 4-strand Kessler or Becker repair if possible for revision situations, using a 3-0 or 4-0 braided suture to prevent elastic stretch and gapping at the repair site. Two strands each should be passed through two drill holes in the distal phalanx, exiting through the nail plate several millimeters distal to the lunula. Alternatively, the sutures can be passed around the ulnar and radial aspects of the distal phalanx with a Keith needle instead of through drill holes. The sutures should be tied over a button resting on a small sheet of xeroform and Mexican felt for padding (Fig. 3.5). The tendon stump should be directly observed docking into the distal phalanx as the suture is tied, to ensure good repair tension (Fig. 3.6). Additional fixation with a micro suture anchor into the base of the distal phalanx is optional; however, careful attention must be paid to the size of the anchor, as the distal phalanges, especially the small and ring, are often too small to accept the device.

If there is more than 1 cm of distal tendon stump remaining, a primary repair can be reattempted with a 3-0 braided polyester suture such as Ethibond, and a 6-0 volar locked epitendinous repair with prolene suture. When the cascade of the digits is examined, the repaired digit should be in slightly more flexion than the others (Fig. 3.5), with the knowledge that over time the repair and/or the musculotendinous unit will usually lengthen slightly. The A4 pulley should be examined for successful gliding of the repair site sutures. The repair should be protected by placing the wrist and MP joints in flexion for the remainder of the procedure. Skin closure should be carried out with a combination of 5-0 nylon and 6-0 chromic sutures after the tourniquet is let down and hemostasis is achieved. The forearm can be pronated and supinated to provide adequate exposure for closure of the incisions with the wrist and MP joints continually held in flexion. A dorsal block splint is applied with the wrist in 30° of flexion, the MP joints in 60–70° of flexion, and the remainder of the digits in some degree of flexion. The hand must be protected in the event that the patient emerges violently from general anesthesia.

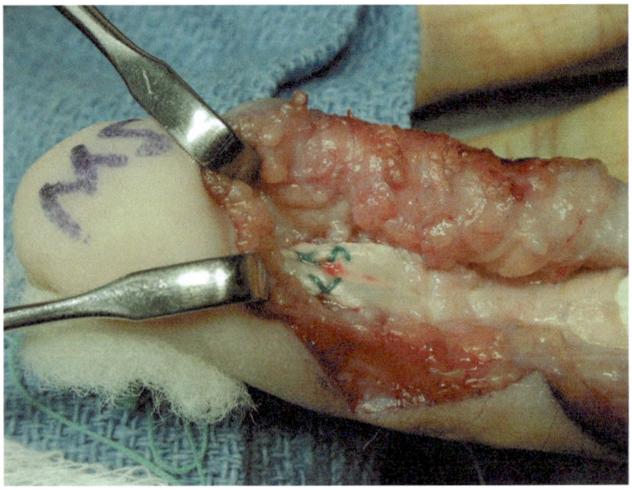

Fig. 3.6 Direct observation of the tendon stump docking should be performed while tying the bolster in order to ensure appropriate contact and tensioning

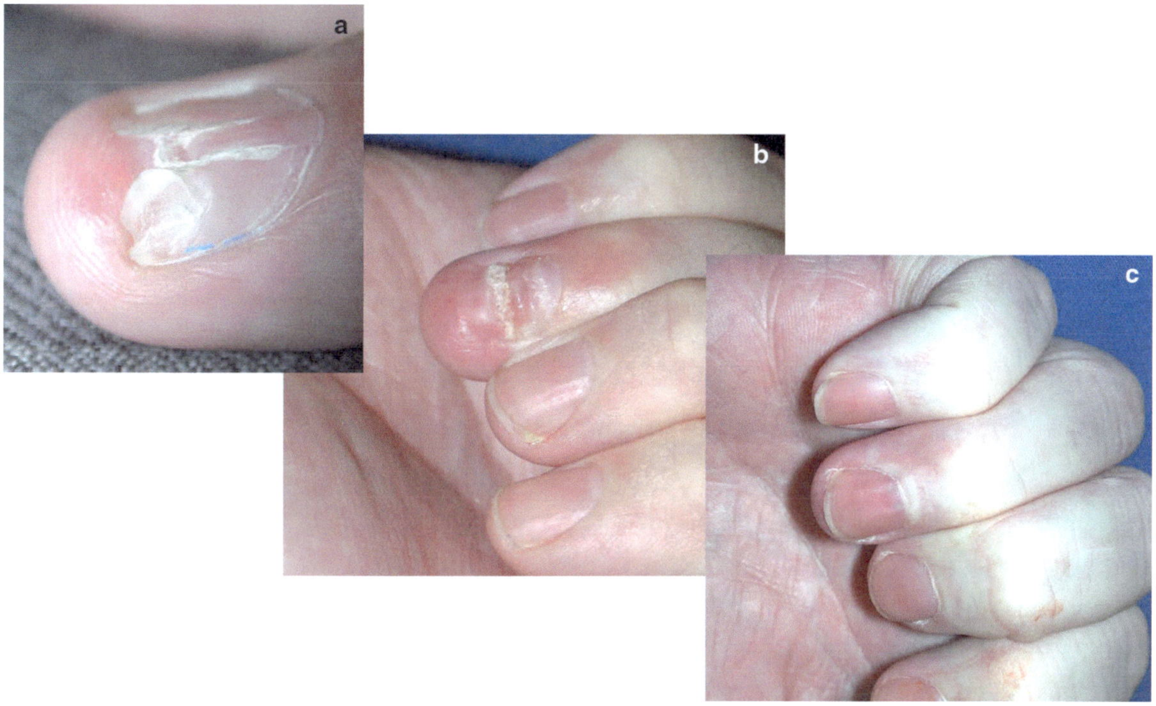

Fig. 3.7 (**a**) Nail plate deformities can occur with prolonged button retention, or with passage of suture material or wires through the germinal matrix. These deformities can be expected to improve with time. (**b**) Appearance of the nail plate at 3 months. (**c**) Appearance of the nail plate at 12 months

Optimizing Outcomes

- A successful result is more likely if rerepair is performed within 3 weeks of original repair.
- Do not advance more than 1 cm, due to the risk of overtightening.
- Directly observe the repair site through full ROM to ensure the repair or sutures do not catch on the A4 pulley.

Complications and Side Effects

Special attention should be paid to the problem of overtightening the FDP in the long, ring, and small fingers, as advancement of a short tendon can lead to the problem of quadriga [7, 8], or loss of flexion power of the adjacent digits. Quadriga can be avoided by using a tendon graft to restore proper tension to the FDP tendon. Nail plate deformities (Fig. 3.7a–c) are not unusual if the button is retained for a long period of time, or if the germinal matrix is injured during passage of sutures. PIPJ flexion contractures may develop, and their treatment with stretching and ROM must not compromise the integrity of the repair.

Postoperative Care

Postoperative rehabilitation should begin several days after repair. The patient should be placed in a dorsal block splint with the wrist flexed to 20–30° and the MP joints flexed to 40–60°. Passive and early active ROM of the wrist and digits should be instructed with strict guidelines. Combined wrist flexion–MPJ extension, and wrist extension–MPJ flexion should avoid excessive tension and subsequent gap formation at the repair site while allowing maximal tendon excursion [9–11]. Adhesion formation is less common when the repair occurs outside of Zone II; thus, the surgeon should err on the conservative side of motion protocols in order to prevent undue tension on the repair site. The button is removed after 6–8 weeks and active motion with gradual resistance is begun. Full return to sports activities is not recommended for at least 4–6 months.

Indications and Contraindications for Single-Stage Tendon Graft

In a previously operated patient, single-stage tendon graft reconstruction is a good surgical option for the same patient who is an ideal candidate for rerepair as described previously, but has a residual tendon stump which is too short for primary rerepair and requires an advancement greater than 1 cm. This can happen under several circumstances. First, if an excessive time period, i.e., more than 4 weeks, has passed between rerupture and attempted rerepair, the musculotendinous unit can contract and be unable to be advanced to the DIPJ. Second, if the original repair was a tendon–tendon repair, the residual tissues may not support another primary repair, and a graft may be necessary to bridge this gap.

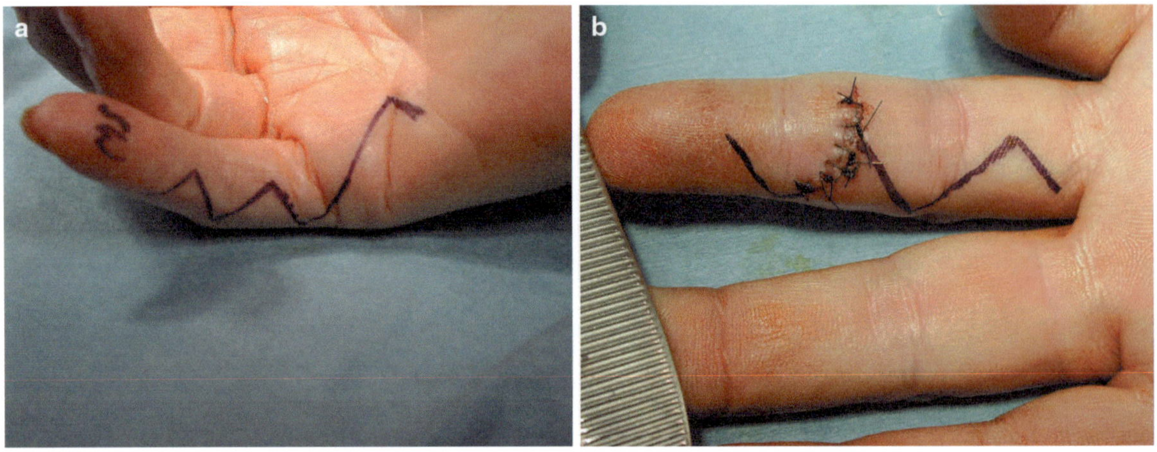

Fig. 3.8 (**a**, **b**) A volar oblique Bruner-type incision can provide the advantages a Bruner incision, without placing the suture line directly volar to the flexor sheath, theoretically minimizing scar above the sheath area. In addition, it can provide better visualization and access to an injured digital artery or nerve

This technique is especially useful for patients who have limited PIPJ flexion due to FDS dysfunction or deficiency.

Grafting introduces a new set of possible complications which must be discussed with the patient preoperatively. Because the proximal junction of the graft is usually placed at or near the FDS insertion, there is potential for dysfunction of the FDS to result. Older patients and manual laborers with a well functioning FDS and a DIP joint that does not hyperextend should be treated conservatively due to the risk of additional impairment of the FDS to that digit [12–14].

Single-stage grafting is contraindicated in children who are too young to cooperate in a rehabilitation protocol, elderly patients, and digits with neurovascular compromise [15]. It is also not recommended in digits that require additional procedures such as joint contracture release and/or pulley reconstruction.

Indications

- Injury requiring FDP advancement more than 1 cm
- Limited active PIPJ flexion due to FDS injury or insufficiency, with supple joint
- Ring or small finger involvement
- Symptomatic DIPJ hyperextension
- Delayed treatment of a Zone 2 injury

Contraindications

- Elderly, children, low functioning, or unmotivated patients
- DIPJ arthritis or injury
- Limited PROM, pulley compromise, immature scar tissue
- Neurovascular compromise
- Digits requiring secondary procedures such as joint contracture release

Preoperatively, the patient should have a well-healed zone of injury or previous surgery with mature and supple scar, no joint contractures, intact pulleys, and full passive range of motion. The digit should be well vascularized with at least one digital nerve intact.

Operative Approach for Single-Stage Tendon Grafting

The patient should be placed in the supine position with the arm on a hand table and a brachial tourniquet applied to allow harvest of the Palmaris tendon. The ipsilateral lower extremity should be prepped and draped if harvest of the Plantaris tendon is to be performed. The original incision, preferably a Bruner-type or volar oblique Bruner-type incision (Fig. 3.8a, b), is utilized to expose the area from the FDS insertion to the FDP insertion. If an FDP tendon stump exists and is in good condition, it should be preserved. The A4 and other annular and cruciate pulleys should be preserved as well as any undamaged areas of sheath. An incision in the palm should be made at the level of the lumbrical origin on the FDP. The FDP should be transected just distal to the lumbrical origin and prepared for grafting. The scarred FDP avulsion segment should be removed from the field.

Next, the tendon harvest should be performed. For a single digit palm-to-fingertip graft, the authors prefer Palmaris tendon [16], due to its thin shape and ease of harvest in the same surgical field [18]. The patient should always be examined preoperatively for presence of the Palmaris tendon, which can be absent in 16% of patients unilaterally and 8% bilaterally [19]. The palmaris tendon can be insufficient in some patients, and preoperative MRI or ultrasound can be helpful in questionable cases. Harvest of the Palmaris is performed by making a 1–2 cm transverse incision at the wrist and identifying the tendon subcutaneously and verifying its insertion into the palmar fascia. Extreme caution should be exercised to protect the median nerve, as there are rare cases of erroneous harvest of this nerve when attempting to harvest the palmaris tendon [20, 21]. Several small transverse incisions may be made more proximally to aid in identification and differentiation of the tendon from the median nerve and surrounding tendons. The tendon is transected and tagged with a suture. Tension is applied and the tendon is dissected from the surrounding connective tissues for several centimeters. A tendon stripper is then used to truncate the tendon from its musculotendinous junction. If a tendon stripper is not available, the tendon can be truncated with a scalpel through a stab incision at the musculotendinous junction. The graft is kept hydrated with a saline gauze until the time of implantation (Fig. 3.9).

In multiple-digit or forearm-to-fingertip grafts, or if the tendon sheath is expected to be narrow, the Plantaris tendon should be used due to its longer length and thinner diameter [17]. The tendon is located with blunt dissection at its position anteromedial to the Achilles tendon via a longitudinal incision medially (Fig. 3.10a–d). The tendon is truncated at its insertion and tagged with a suture for harvest. Blunt dissection is again used to loosen the tendon from surrounding tissues. A tendon stripper is placed, while holding gentle traction on the graft, and advanced proximally until it severs the graft at

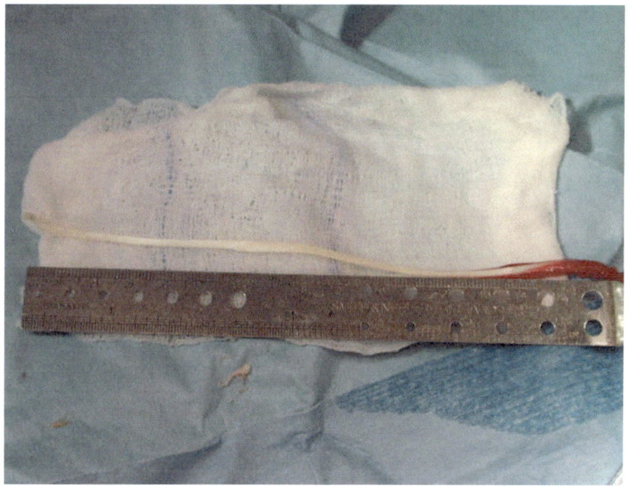

Fig. 3.9 A 10–15 cm Palmaris graft can usually be obtained with a tendon stripper

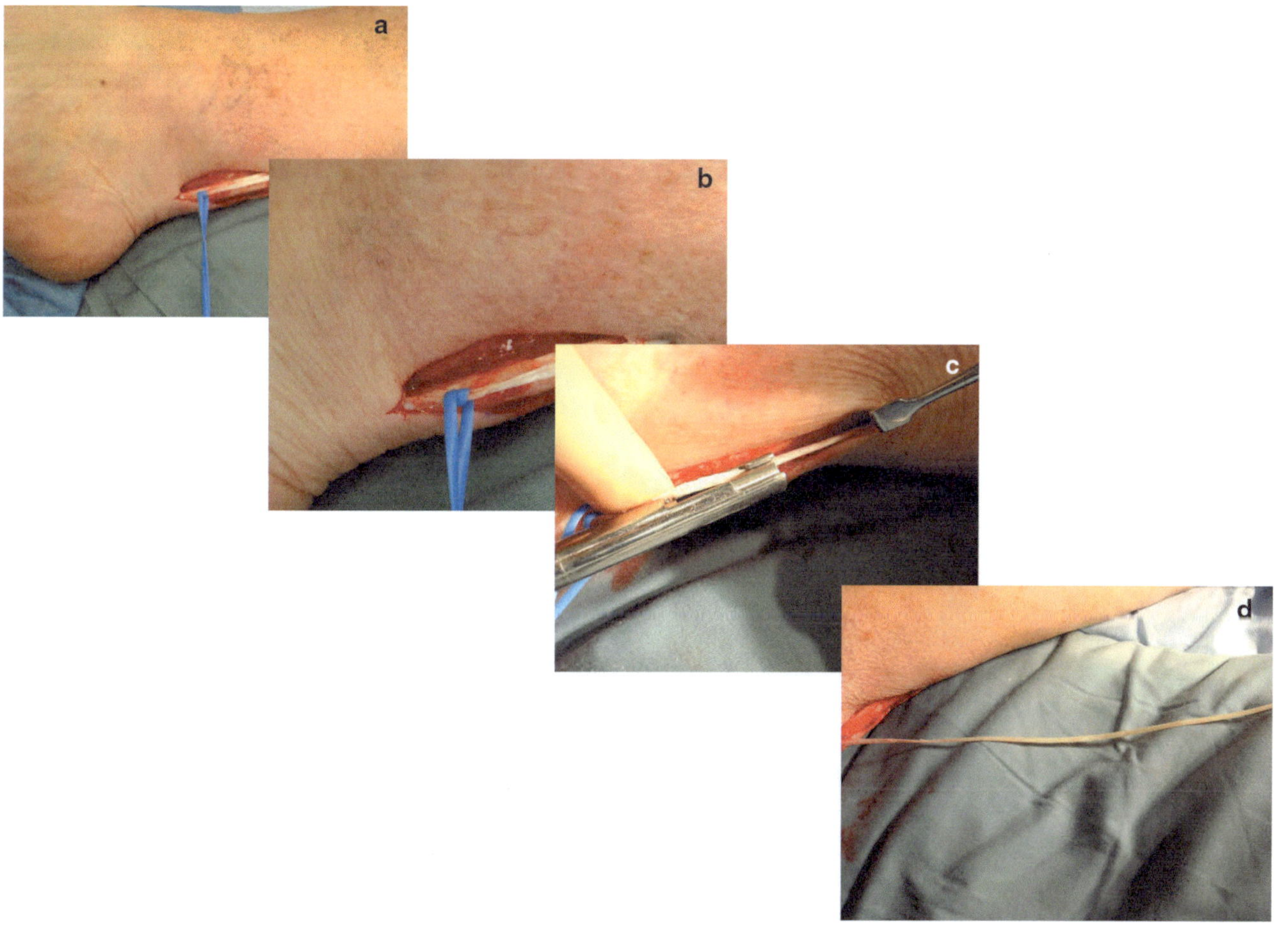

Fig. 3.10 (**a–d**) Plantaris harvest is performed by locating the tendon anteromedial to the Achilles, bluntly dissecting it proximally, truncating it at the insertion, and using a tendon stripper to amputate it at the musculotendinous junction. This tendon is usually longer and thinner than the palmaris tendon

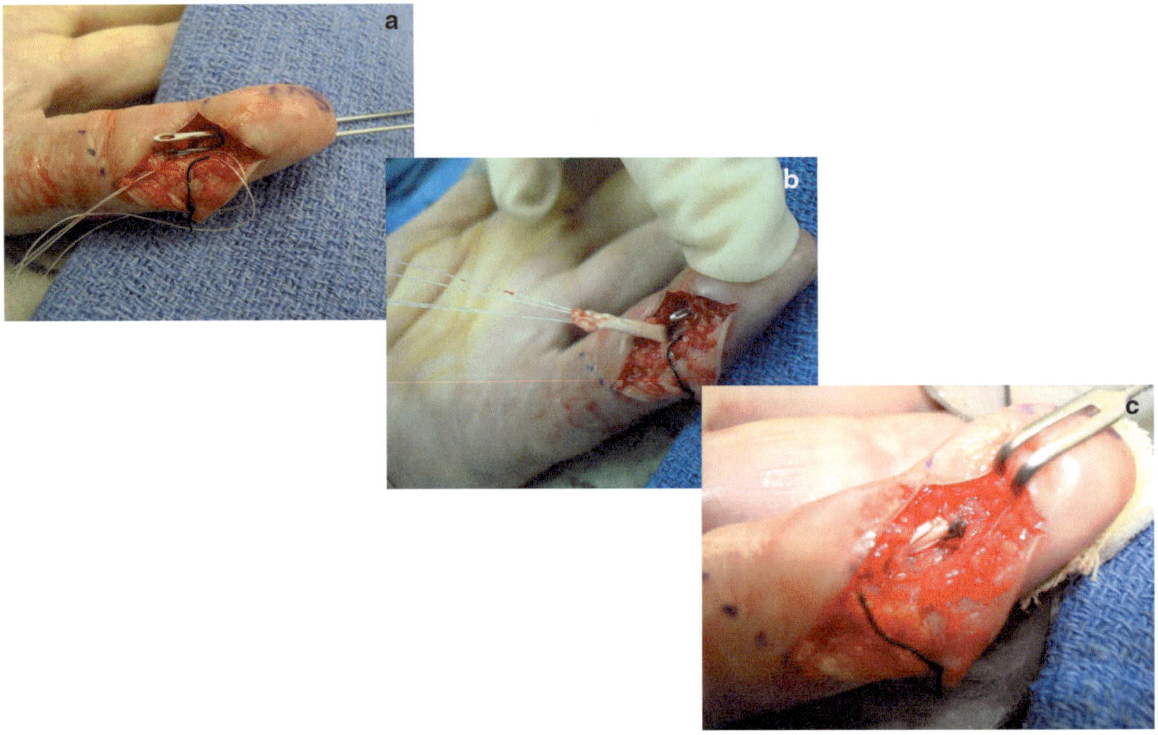

Fig. 3.11 Fixation of the distal junction and incision closure is performed before the proximal junction is tensioned. (**a**, **b**)When a native tendon stump is insufficient for fixation, the graft can be secured by passing the sutures around the distal phalanx and out through the nail plate with two Keith needles. (**c**) The graft can be secured to the remainder of the native tendon stump with braided polyester suture

the musculotendinous junction. The graft is kept hydrated with a saline gauze until the time of implantation.

When the proximal and distal junctions are ready for the graft, the graft is weaved underneath the pulley system by passing its grasping suture retrograde using a tendon grabber, wire loop, or pediatric feeding tube, and pulling the graft though the sheath. It should pass easily, but may need to be guided using a freer elevator. Care must be taken to avoid any unnecessary trauma to the sheath or pulley system. The graft can be passed either through the decussation of the intact FDS insertions, or to the side of the decussation. On occasion, release of one slip of the FDS to accommodate the graft can be performed without loss of PIP flexion or strength. The proximal end is clamped or pinned with a 25 gauge needle to prevent inadvertent withdrawal. The authors prefer to fix the distal junction first, as tensioning of the graft is much easier from the proximal junction. In addition, this will allow distal skin closure before the digit assumes a flexed posture after tensioning. If there exists an FDP tendon stump, the graft can be directly weaved and sutured to the stump with 3-0 braided polyester suture, with additional sutures passed around or through the distal phalanx and tied over a button on the nail plate distal to the lunula. If there is no tendon stump, the graft can be advanced according to the technique described in the previous rerepair section, and tied over a button (Fig. 3.11a–c). Micro suture anchors can provide additional fixation, but are not required.

Tensioning is performed after firm fixation is obtained at the distal junction, and the distal skin incisions are closed. The proximal end of the graft is pulled proximally to tension the graft with the wrist in a neutral position (Fig. 3.12a). Ideally, the tension should be enough to create slightly more digital flexion than expected for the cascade, in order to accommodate for postoperative lengthening of the graft and musculotendinous unit. Placing a slightly long graft may have the unintended consequence of lumbrical plus finger [22], while a slightly short graft will result in quadriga [8]. The proximal junction is secured with an interweaving technique [23, 24] using 3-0 braided polyester suture. A minimum of 4–5 weaves is recommended, and the remainder of the graft is truncated. Tension can be readjusted from this junction (Fig. 3.12b, c). The tenodesis effect should be utilized to determine appropriate tensioning when the wrist is flexed (Fig. 3.13a) and extended (Fig. 3.13b).

Proximal skin incisions are closed with 5-0 nylon and 6-0 chromic sutures after the tourniquet is deflated and hemostasis is achieved. A plaster splint is applied with the wrist at 20–30° of flexion, the MP joints at 40–60° of flexion, and the digits in some degree of flexion.

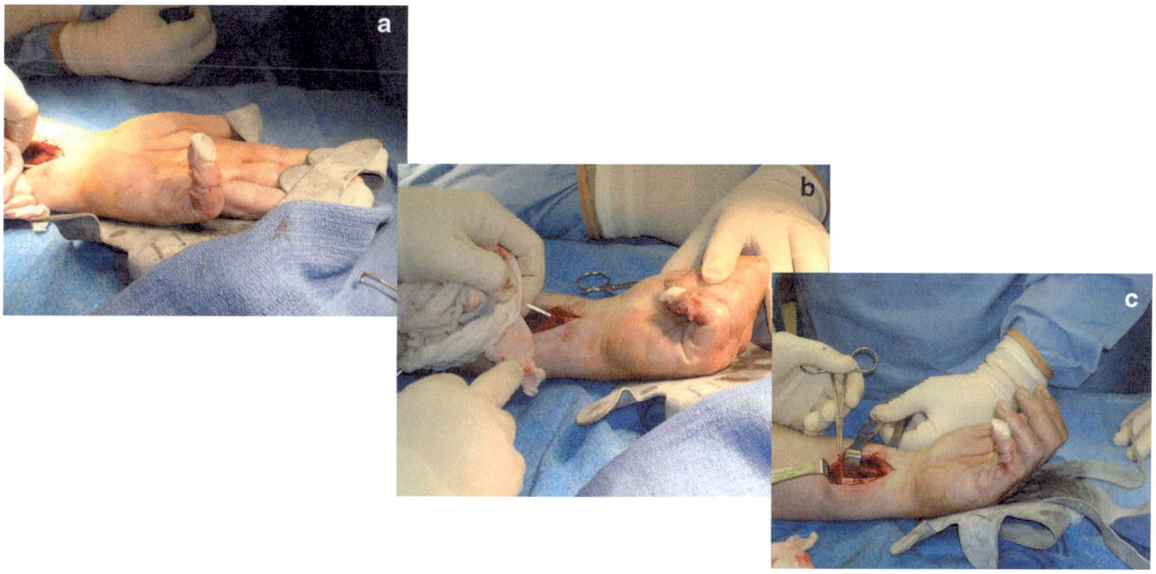

Fig. 3.12 (**a–c**) With the button secured and the wound closed, the graft can be tensioned from the distal forearm or palmar incision. Flexion should be determined and a Pulvertaft weave with 4–5 weaves should be secured with a braided polyester suture. Tension can then be readjusted from this junction after assessing finger position with wrist flexion and extension

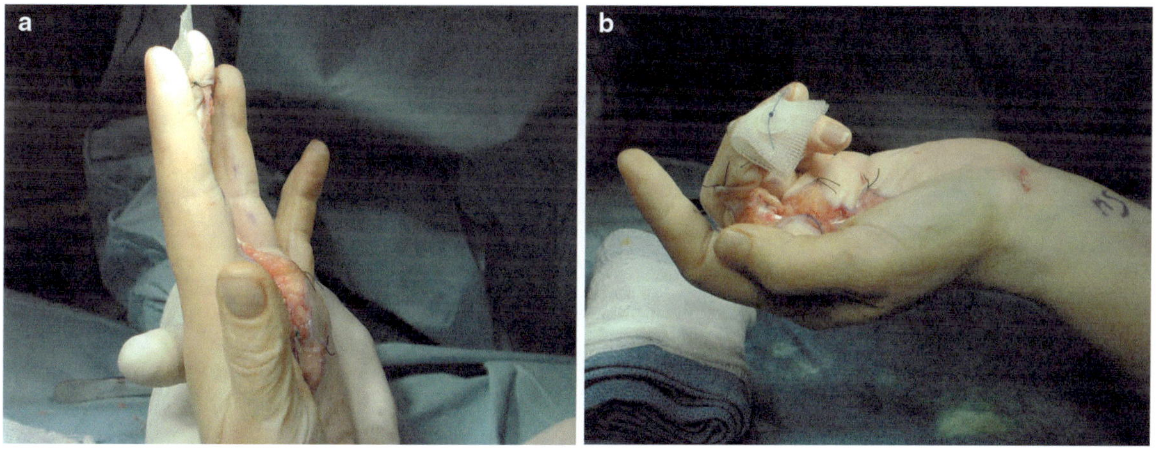

Fig. 3.13 The tenodesis effect in wrist flexion (**a**) and extension (**b**) is a necessary maneuver to determine the appropriate graft tension

Optimizing Outcomes

- Tensioning from the proximal junction after skin closure distally
- Use four or more interweaves to secure the proximal junction
- Avoidance of unnecessary trauma to the tendon sheath
- Avoid sacrificing an intact FDS insertion to accommodate the graft
- Intraoperative ROM to ensure no catching or interference of the repair sites on adjacent structures

Complications and Side Effects

Special attention should be paid to the problem of overtightening the FDP, which can lead to the problem of quadriga [7, 8]. Some degree of lengthening can be expected from the musculotendinous unit, but this should not be overestimated. Nail plate deformities are not unusual if the button is retained for a long period of time, or if the sterile matrix is injured during passage of sutures (Fig. 3.7a–c). Joint contractures can be treated with passive stretching and splinting after 6–8 weeks, and their treatment must not compromise the integrity of the graft. If excessive scarring or pulley incompetence is found intraoperatively, a 2-stage technique should be utilized.

Postoperative Care

Rehabilitation should begin within the first few days after surgery, with passive and active motion as described in the previous section, as long as the junctions are secure. A static dorsal blocking splint should be worn at all times except during

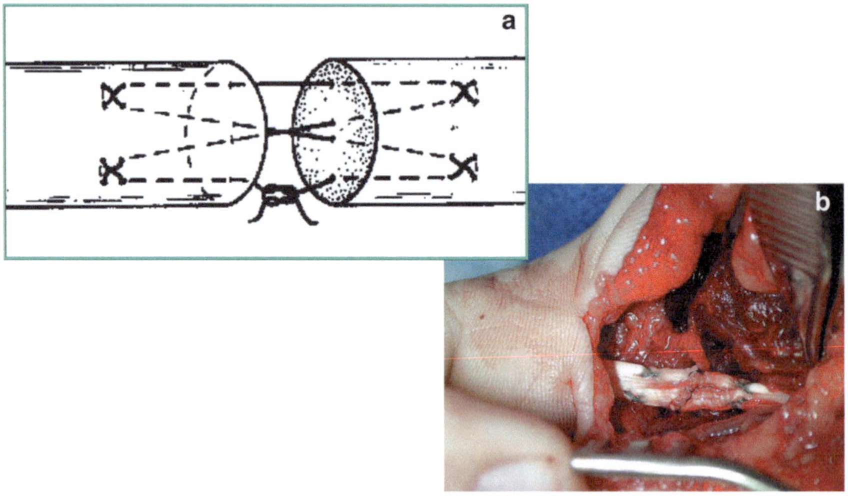

Fig. 3.14 (**a**, **b**) Locking Cruciate stitch

therapy for the first 6 weeks. Synchronous wrist flexion/MPJ extension and wrist extension/MPJ flexion will protect the graft from undue tension and encourage gliding. Short arc active motion as well as place-and-hold and straight-fist exercises can begin to encourage differential glide between the graft and FDS [25]. The button can be removed after 6 weeks, and active motion begun with gradual initiation of resistance.

Indications and Contraindications for FDS Finger

For the patient who is not an ideal candidate for rerepair or single-stage grafting because of age or motivation, who has a stiff, unstable, or arthritic DIP joint, and who has difficulty with active PIP joint flexion with a presumably intact FDS tendon, the FDS finger may be a good surgical option. This procedure is also a good salvage operation for the low-demand patient with digital pulley disruption and bowstringing, or the patient who underwent FDP grafting and had a distal insertion site rupture which cannot be repaired. Often a DIP joint arthrodesis is added in the properly indicated patient.

Indications

- Active patient with FDP laceration and stiff, unstable, or arthritic DIPJ (need to perform a DIPJ arthrodesis in addition)
- Well functioning FDS tendon with full PIP motion
- Low demand patient with FDP laceration and pulley failure or inadequacy causing bowstringing
- Salvage for distal repair site rupture of FDP graft

Contraindications

- Nonfunctional FDS or FDP motor
- Stiff PIPJ and MPJ

Operative Approach for FDS Finger

Surgical repair is carried out with the patient in the supine position with the arm at 90° to the body on a hand table, with a brachial tourniquet. General or regional anesthesia is preferred, although this operation can be performed under local anesthesia with short-acting sedation. The limb is exsanguinated with an elastic bandage and the tourniquet is raised. The original incision is utilized, whether a midlateral, volar, or volar oblique Bruner-type, and extended to include the area around the PIP joint. The proximal FDP tendon stump is identified and debrided of any devitalized or scarred tissue, leaving enough to properly tension it to the middle phalanx. If there is a remnant of the FDS insertion sites, but the FDS is not functioning to flex the PIP joint, they are used to suture directly to the FDP tendon with 3-0 braided polyester suture. The FDP is tensioned with the wrist in a neutral position and the digit falling into line with the natural cascade of the hand. This repair can be reinforced with suture of the pulley remnants and/or periosteum. If there is no FDS remnant, the FDP can be grasped with a 3-0 monofilament suture or fine-gauge wire and advanced to the middle phalanx through drill holes, tying sutures over a button and some Mexican felt padding over the dorsal skin (Fig. 3.13b). Alternatively, a micro suture anchor can be used to secure the FDP tendon to the middle phalanx, to avoid any dorsal skin complications. If DIPJ arthrodesis is indicated, it should be performed prior to securing the FDP tendon to avoid any compromise or manipulation of the repair site.

Optimizing Outcomes

- Proper tension must be restored for this digit to be functional.

Complications and Side Effects

Complications are related to improper tensioning and development of stiff joints. Dorsal skin compromise beneath the button can also occur and must be monitored.

Postoperative Care

Rehabilitation is similar to that of a free tendon graft. Early protected motion can be started with the wrist flexed to 20–30°, the MCP joints flexed to 40–60°, and the PIP joints allowed to extend to neutral. The DIPJ should be protected if it is fused. Button removal and active motion should begin at 6 weeks.

Indications and Contraindications for DIPJ Arthrodesis

Arthrodesis is a great surgical option for patients who are troubled by hyperextension of the DIPJ, manual laborers, older patients who are not candidates for grafting, and patients who may not be compliant with any rehabilitation protocol.

Indications

- Hyperextensible, unstable, or arthritic DIPJ with intact FDS

Contraindications

- Poor circulation to the digit

Operative Approach for DIPJ Arthrodesis

Typically, the approach to DIPJ arthrodesis is through a dorsal incision; however, in a patient who has a previous volar or midlateral incision, it may be prudent to use the existing surgical incision to avoid any potential vascular compromise to the fingertip. The neurovascular bundles should be identified and protected if using a volar or midlateral approach, and the cartilaginous surfaces should be removed in an atraumatic fashion. The joint should be positioned in 20–30° of flexion, depending on the digit and which position would best suit the patient's needs. Fixation is dependent on surgeon preference, with options including two 0.035 Kirschner wires placed across the fusion site or a single headless compression screw if the size of the phalanges allows. A single digital splint bandage is applied and the fusion site is protected until healing.

Optimizing Outcomes

- Ensure maximal bony opposition of surfaces in a functional degree of flexion
- Ensure stable fixation

Complications and Side Effects

Nonunion or pin site infections are common complications. Patients with a malpositioned arthrodesis will often note this deformity and express dissatisfaction. Fingertip hyperesthesia may persist and nonunion must be ruled out with radiographs or advanced imaging.

Postoperative Care

Healing may take in excess of 8 weeks in digits that have less than optimal circulation. Hand therapy may be required if loss of PIP or MCP motion occurs, or if the fingertip remains overly sensitive.

Zone II Failed Primary Repair

Preoperative History and Considerations

Zone II reoperation can be the most challenging of hand surgical procedures. Careful evaluation of patient with previous Zone II flexor tendon repair is mandatory, and early recognition of problems is necessary for prompt diagnosis and treatment.

Zone II repairs of the FDS and FDP can adhere both to surrounding structures as well as to each other. Active and passive ROM should be tested, as well as differential glide between the two tendons. Serial examinations can give the examiner the best information about the progress of therapy. Patients who fail to improve ROM at least 5–10% each week should be considered for tenolysis.

Of paramount importance is the diagnosis of concomitant injuries to the digit, including digital artery and nerve lacerations. The surgeon must be prepared for repair, or protection of previous repair, of these structures in addition to tendons.

Imaging studies have little role evaluating the integrity of tendon repairs due to the abundance of scar tissue and its potential to obscure the native anatomy in this region.

Indications and Contraindications for Rerepair

Rerepair can be considered in the patient who is within 3 weeks of initial repair, and experiences a sudden or gradual loss of flexion strength or posture. At time periods later than 3 weeks, rerepair can be considered if a sudden loss of flexion occurs.

Indications

- Sudden failure of primary repair more than 3 weeks post-op
- Gradual failure of primary repair sooner than 3 weeks post-op

Contraindications

- Significant neurovascular injury or pulley incompetence
- Patients unwilling to cooperate with required postoperative hand therapy

Operative Approach for Rerepair

Original surgical incisions should be utilized and extended if needed, in order to provide adequate exposure. A volar oblique Bruner incision can be helpful in the event one neurovascular bundle needs to be explored. Minimal sheath dissection should be performed, and the tendon ends should be debrided of suture material and scar tissue prior to rerepair. In the case of repair site elongation, the attenuated tissue must be excised (Fig. 3.4). A 3-0 or 4-0 core suture should be utilized and a 4-strand repair should be performed. The authors prefer the locking cruciate stitch [1] because of its strength (Fig. 3.14a, b). A locking epitendinous repair with 6-0 prolene should be carried out, and gliding should be observed. There is a tendency for rerepairs to result in slightly more tension than the neighboring digits, due to loss of tissue at the repair site. A dorsal blocking splint should be applied with the wrist in 20–30° flexion, the MCP joints in 40–60° flexion, and the IP joints in neutral.

Optimizing Outcomes

- If tendon tissue quality is poor at the repair site and debridement leads to overtightening, a single-stage graft must be considered.
- Handle tissues gently to minimize additional trauma to the multiply operated digit.

Complications and Side Effects

Although rerepairs can be successful, poor tendon tissue quality may again result in rerupture. Consideration must then be made to single-stage grafting. Stiffness should be improved with therapy, taking care not to compromise the repairs.

Postoperative Care

A flexor tendon splint should be placed, with the wrist in 20–30° of flexion, the MP joints at 60–70° of flexion, and the distal digits in neutral. Early rehabilitation should be initiated as the strength of the repair dictates. Typical Zone II rehab protocols should be instituted, with active wrist flexion and extension "tenodesis" motion, coupled with passive digital flexion and extension, and vice versa. Place and hold exercises should be initiated at the first week. Differential glide between the FDP and FDS should be encouraged with flat fist and hook fist exercises. All therapy should be supervised until the patient can demonstrate competence in executing the protocol and understanding of activity limitations. Splinting can be discontinued at 6 weeks with a gradual return to active motion. Return to sports should not be allowed for 6 months.

Indications and Contraindications for Single-Stage Tendon Graft

Single-stage grafting is a good technique for the patient with a Zone II flexor tendon laceration who is referred late, or who was unable to receive appropriate surgical treatment in the first 3–4 weeks after injury. The single-stage tendon graft is also a good back-up procedure for the patient who is considered for rerepair but has insufficient residual tendon length to carry this out. Knowledge of the mechanism of injury (crush vs. sharp laceration), or of the condition of the tendons at original surgery is helpful. If the palm exhibits excessive scar tissue and thus a hostile environment for tendon gliding and healing, it may be wise to bypass the palm by placing a tendon graft in which the anastomosis sites are distal and proximal to this unfavorable region. A tendon graft requires an intact pulley system, mature scar, supple joints, adequate vascularity, and at least one intact digital nerve. Any patient who does not meet these criteria should be considered for 2-stage grafting, and all potential candidates for this procedure should be advised preoperatively of the possibility of conversion to a 2-stage graft depending on findings at surgery.

Patients should be made aware of the required postoperative therapy, and unmotivated patients, or the very young or old patients, should be carefully scrutinized for their level of compliance prior to embarking on this type of reconstructive procedure. Very often, a prescribed course of preoperative hand therapy, aimed at maximizing range of motion and softening scar, can be helpful at gauging a patient's level of commitment to improvement.

Indications

- Subacute, chronic, or failed repair of Zone II flexor tendon laceration
- Back-up procedure for rerepair candidates with poor residual tendon quality

Contraindications

- Poor patient compliance
- Pulley system compromise requiring reconstruction
- Insensate, poorly vascular, or stiff digits

Operative Approach for Single-Stage Tendon Graft

The surgical procedure is similar to that described for Zone I single-stage tendon grafting (see page 22), with some important differences for Zone II injuries. Although both the FDP and FDS tendons may be lacerated, only one tendon, the FDP, is reconstructed per digit. A palm-to-finger or a forearm-to-finger graft can be chosen depending on intraoperative condition of the palmar scar tissue. As previously mentioned, attempted repair of an FDP tendon which has lost some length, and/or is overtightened, can lead to the problem of quadriga [8], especially in the ulnar three digits.

The patient should be placed in the supine position with the arm on a hand table and a brachial tourniquet applied to allow harvest of the Palmaris tendon (see page 22). The ipsilateral lower extremity should be prepped and draped if harvest of the Plantaris tendon is to be performed (see page 23). The original incision is utilized to expose the area from the mid-palm to the FDP insertion. The FDP insertion is commonly in good condition, and the last centimeter should be preserved to facilitate a good distal graft junction site repair. The A4 and other annular and cruciate pulleys should be preserved as well as any undamaged areas of sheath. The proximal incision should be extended to expose the entire zone of injury. If the condition of the FDP at the level of the lumbrical origin is satisfactory to become the proximal graft junction, and can accommodate a Pulvertaft weave, the FDP should be transected just distal to the lumbrical origin. A weave technique is not mandatory, but can allow greater strength than an end-to-end technique and can allow more facile tensioning of the segment. The FDS, if in good condition, can also be a satisfactory motor for the tendon graft at this level. If the palm is not an adequate environment for the junction, plans should be made to make the proximal graft junction in the distal forearm, requiring a Plantaris graft. The scarred residual FDP segment should be removed from the field.

Likewise, a segment of the FDS should also be removed to accommodate the graft and to reduce potential adhesion formation. One centimeter of FDS at the insertion site (both slips) should be left intact to confer some stability to the PIP region and provide a bed for gliding of the grafted tendon within the sheath. The proximal FDS tendon stump should be evaluated for a potential motor for the graft if the FDP is found to be inadequate. If the FDS is not needed, it can be pulled taut, truncated, and allowed to retract into the forearm.

Preparation of the distal forearm, if necessary, for the proximal graft junction site is straightforward. A longitudinal or curvilinear incision can be made over the ulnar aspect of the flexor tendon mass, and the FDP to the involved finger should be identified and pulled out through the incision. It should be truncated in an area where the weave will not cause interference or impingement on surrounding structures such as the flexor retinaculum, antebrachial fascia, or transverse carpal ligament. It should be tagged to prevent withdrawal.

Next, the tendon harvest should be performed. This technique is described in the single-stage tendon grafting for Zone I section (see page 22 for Palmaris, page 23 for Plantaris).

When the proximal and distal junctions are ready for the graft, the graft is weaved underneath the pulley system by passing its grasping suture retrograde using a tendon grabber or a wire loop, and pulling the graft though the sheath. A pediatric feeding tube can also be used to pull the graft through the sheath. It should pass easily, but may need to be guided using a Freer elevator. Care must be taken to avoid any unnecessary trauma to the sheath or pulley system. The graft can be passed either through the decussation of the intact FDS insertions, or to the side of the decussation. Release of one slip of the FDS to accommodate the graft is not recommended. The proximal end is clamped to prevent inadvertent withdrawal. The authors prefer to secure the distal junction first, as tensioning of the graft and skin closure is much easier from the proximal junction (Fig. 3.12a–c). The graft can be directly weaved and sutured to the stump with 3-0 braided polyester suture, with additional sutures passed around or through the distal phalanx and tied over a button on the nail plate distal to the lunula. Micro suture anchors can provide additional fixation, but are not required.

Tensioning is performed after firm fixation is obtained at the distal junction. The proximal end of the graft is pulled proximally to tension the graft with the wrist in a neutral position. Ideally, the tension should be enough to create slightly more digital flexion than expected for the cascade, in order to accommodate for postoperative lengthening of the graft and musculotendinous unit. Tensioning is critical because a graft which is too long may have the unintended consequence of lumbrical plus finger [22], and that which is too short might cause quadriga [8]. The proximal junction is secured either in the palm or in the distal forearm with an interweaving technique [23, 24] using 3-0 braided polyester suture. A minimum of 4–5 weaves is recommended, and the remainder of the graft is truncated. An end-to-end repair technique can be used if the junction is in the palm; however, these repairs tend to be less strong than a traditional weave technique.

Skin incisions are closed with 5-0 nylon and 6-0 chromic sutures after the tourniquet is deflated and hemostasis is achieved. A plaster splint is applied with the wrist at 30° of flexion, the MP joints at 60–70° of flexion, and the digits in some degree of flexion.

Optimizing Outcomes

- Choosing the appropriate donor graft (palmaris vs. plantaris vs. long toe flexor) for length and width
- Tensioning from the proximal junction after skin closure distally
- Use four or more interweaves to secure the proximal junction
- Avoidance of unnecessary trauma to the tendon sheath

- Maintain 1 cm of intact FDS insertion to preserve some stability to the PIPJ
- Intraoperative ROM to ensure no catching or interference of the repair sites on adjacent structures

Complications and Side Effects

Complications related to poor tensioning of the graft are avoidable with careful intraoperative examination. Some degree of lengthening can be expected from the musculotendinous unit, but this should not be overestimated. Rupture of a junction must be taken back to the operating room for rerepair. Nail plate deformities are not unusual if the button is retained for a long period of time, or if the sterile matrix is injured during passage of sutures (Fig. 3.7a–c). Joint contractures can be treated with passive stretching and splinting after 6–8 weeks, and their treatment must not compromise the integrity of the graft. Adhesion formation refractory to hand therapy may be treated with tenolysis after the proximal and distal junctions have healed. If excessive scarring or pulley incompetence is found intraoperatively, a 2-stage technique should be utilized.

Postoperative Care

Rehabilitation should begin within the first few days after surgery, with passive motion as described in the previous section. Short arc active motion as well as place-and-hold, flat fist and hook fist exercises can begin in a supervised setting to encourage differential glide between the graft and FDS. Joint contractures can be treated with passive stretching and splinting after 6–8 weeks. The button can be removed after 6–8 weeks and active motion gradually begun. Sports activities should be restricted until after 6 months time.

Indications and Contraindications for 2-Stage Tendon Reconstruction

Two-stage reconstruction is preferred when patients considered for single-stage grafting demonstrate excessive scar tissue, an inadequate pulley system, and/or joint contractures requiring surgical release. These concomitant procedures can compromise the integrity of a single-stage tendon graft and should be performed during the first of two stages, the second being placement of the tendon graft. Some patients will require a third procedure for tenolysis, and this must be conveyed before any reconstructive endeavor is attempted.

Two-stage reconstruction is contraindicated in any patient unwilling or unable to comply with a rigorous postoperative therapy program, or any patient with neurovascular compromise. Very often, a prescribed course of preoperative therapy to maximize range of motion and soften scars can give the surgeon an idea of the patient's level of compliance.

Indications

- Patients considered for single-stage grafting, but with excessive scar tissue, an inadequate pulley system, and/or joint contractures requiring surgical release

Contraindications

- Active infection
- Neurovascular compromise or insensate digit
- Patients unable to comply with therapy protocols or prolonged duration of treatment

Operative Approach for 2-Stage Tendon Grafting

Stage I

The patient is placed in the supine position with the arm at 90° from the body, positioned on a hand table, with a brachial tourniquet. The arm is exsanguinated with an elastic bandage. Ideally a volar or oblique volar Bruner-type incision is utilized to expose the digital sheath from the insertion of the FDP to the level of the lumbrical origin in the palm. Care is taken not to disturb the flexor sheath or pulley system. The FDP is identified distally and transected 1 cm from its insertion, if possible, leaving a stump behind for graft reattachment. Proximally the FDP is transected just distal to the lumbrical origin. The FDS is truncated just proximal to its insertion site if possible. A second curvilinear incision is made at the distal forearm, and the FDS tendon is identified, withdrawn, and transected. Care must be taken to preserve the flexor retinaculum. After transection of the FDS, any undamaged tendon material may be put aside and preserved for pulley reconstruction procedures.

If any joint contractures remain, they should be addressed by surgically releasing the volar plate and accessory collateral ligaments. The silicone tendon implant trials are then utilized to determine the appropriate size to be opened. The size should be large enough to allow smooth gliding of the implant, but small enough to form a snug fit to prevent bowstringing of the eventual graft. The appropriate graft is chosen and opened onto the sterile field. Care must be taken in handling of the implant, so as not to scrape or damage its smooth surface. It is threaded through the sheath and pulley system, allowing evaluation of the integrity and mechanical efficiency of the structures which remain. The A2 and A4 pulleys are the minimum requirement for a successful outcome, although a complete system is ideal. Pulley reconstruction should be carried out with the nondiseased portion of the tendon excised.

The distal insertion site of the silicone graft should be repaired first, with a grasping figure-of-eight suture, ensuring penetration of the Dacron tape within the silicone graft.

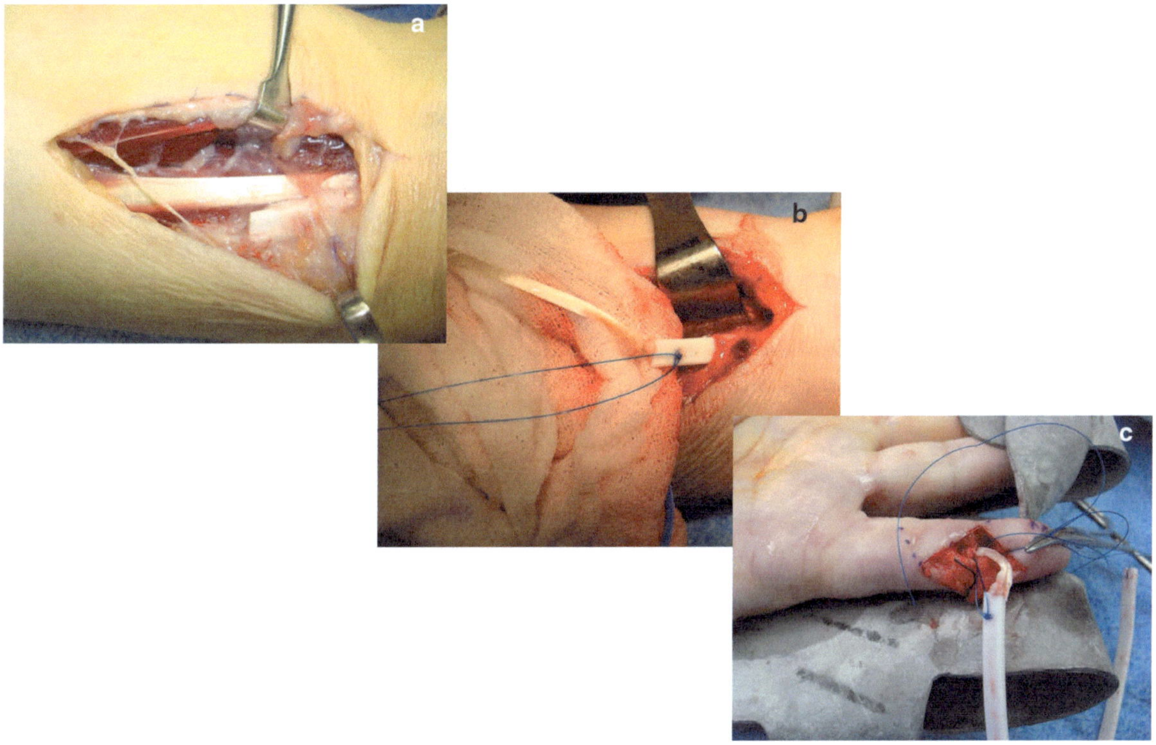

Fig. 3.15 (**a**) The silicone rod is located in the forearm through the previous incision, and (**b**) the graft is sutured to the silicone rod in the forearm. (**c**) the silicone rod is advanced in an antegrade direction to pull the graft into position. This approach is atraumatic and eliminates the need for reexposure of the entire sheath

The graft should be secured to the remaining 1 cm stump of the FDP, with an additional two sutures placed into the periosteum and local tissues. The proximal end of the silicone graft should pass through the palm and into the distal forearm, in the space between the FDP and FDS to the involved finger. It should not be sutured to any surrounding tissue. The hand and digits should be taken through maximal flexion and extension to ensure that the silicone graft does not buckle or dislodge from its space. It can be trimmed to accomplish these goals without passing too far proximally into the forearm. The graft can be pulled in tension to evaluate the pulley reconstructions and joint ROM, and any final adjustments can be made. The wounds are closed with 5-0 nylon and 6-0 chromic sutures, and the hand is splinted with the wrist in 30° of flexion and the MCP joints in 60° of flexion.

Postoperative rehabilitation between Stage 1 and 2 begins on the first few postoperative days. Patients should be instructed in passive ROM of the digits with the wrist in flexion, to allow maximal proximal migration of the silicone rod and prevent dislodgement. Special attention should be paid to patients requiring joint contracture releases, and therapy should maximize and maintain functional ROM.

Stage 2

Typically the second stage is performed after soft tissue healing has reached an equilibrium, after 3 months. At this time, passive digital ROM has plateaued and the silicone rod should have created itself a smooth gliding sheath. Inflammation and synovitis ideally should no longer be present. There is no maximum time at which the silicone rod must be exchanged for a tendon graft, but a theoretical risk of detachment exists at the distal insertion which would render the rod free-floating. Prior to Stage 2, the patient should be examined for the presence of potential donor tendons. The appropriate length should be estimated, and the Plantaris or long toe extensor or flexor should be used if a long graft is needed.

The patient should be placed supine on the operating table with the arm positioned 90° from the body, with a brachial tourniquet placed. If a Plantaris graft is used, the ipsilateral lower extremity should be prepped as well. The authors prefer the Palmaris, if it is present and sufficiently long, due to its ease of harvest and presence in the operating field. The limb is exsanguinated, and the distal incision is reopened to expose the area between the FDP stump/silicone rod complex and the A4 pulley, taking care to preserve both of these structures. The distal forearm incision is also reopened to expose the proximal end of the rod in its sheath. Care is taken to preserve the sheath and the flexor retinaculum. The motor is identified, usually either the FDP to the long, ring, and small fingers or the FDS to the involved finger. For the index finger, the FDP or FDS can be prepared.

After harvest of the donor tendon, it is then sutured to the proximal end of the silicone rod (Fig. 3.15a), and the rod is advanced antegrade after detachment of the distal insertional sutures to deliver the tendon graft in an atraumatic fashion into the sheath (Fig. 3.15b). The silicone rod can be discarded. The distal insertion fixation can be performed with either direct suture or a transosseous technique, depending on the presence or absence of the FDP stump as described previously for single-stage grafting. The finger incision is then closed. Active ROM can be tested by pulling tension on the graft through the forearm incision (Fig. 3.12a–c).

The proximal junction is then sutured with a weave technique, with a minimum of 4–5 weaves. If the profundus mass to the long, ring, and small fingers is used as a motor, the interweave may be bulky. The digits should be passively extended to ensure the proximal junction does not inhibit excursion by impinging on any crossing structures such as the flexor retinaculum. If this is the case, the impinging structure should be carefully trimmed to allow full excursion.

In the rare event that the FDP tendon to the involved finger is uninjured and was previously truncated in the palm distal to the lumbrical origin, the proximal junction can be placed in the palm. This can be technically more challenging, and care must be taken to perform minimal dissection of the sheath in order to minimize scar and adhesion potential postoperatively.

All remaining incisions are closed after hemostasis is achieved. A bulky dorsal block splint should be placed with the wrist in neutral, the MCP joints flexed to 45°, and the IP joints in neutral.

Postoperative rehabilitation should begin within a few days, and should be fully supervised for the first several weeks. Passive ROM is begun early, adding short-arc active motion and place-and-hold flexion exercises at 2 weeks, and resistance at 6 weeks. This protocol can be altered depending on the quality of the repair and the formation of adhesions postoperatively.

Indications and Contraindications for Paneva-Holevich Tenoplasty

Paneva-Holevich described this 2-stage technique in 1969, whereby the patient's own FDS tendon was employed as a pedicled graft to be utilized at the second stage, eliminating the need to harvest a graft. This procedure has other advantages, including allowing the junctions to heal in stages, providing an intrasynovial graft if one otherwise would not be available, and potentially being a better size match for the injured tendon.

Indications for this novel procedure include acute, chronic, or failed repair of Zone II lacerations of both the FDS and FDP in a motivated patient with full passive digital flexion and full active digital extension, soft and mature scar, intact pulleys, good vascularity, and at least one functional digital nerve. Acute injuries amenable to primary repair should be treated with primary repair, so as not to delay recovery with a 2-staged procedure and the wide surgical exposure required of the second stage, although good results have been obtained with this group [26]. The use of this procedure in the acute setting may be limited to grossly contaminated injuries in Zone II with tendon loss or extensive damage distal to the lumbrical origin, although implantation of a foreign body (silicone rod) is not recommended in the setting of gross contamination.

Indications

- Chronic, or failed repair of Zone II FDP and FDS injuries
- Acute Zone II FDP and FDS injuries with tendon loss or extensive tendon damage distal to the lumbrical origin

Contraindications

- Insensate or poorly vascular digits
- Extensive tendon loss or damage proximal to the lumbrical origin
- Active infection

Operative Approach for Paneva-Holevich Tenoplasty

Stage 1

The surgical incision is made in the palm at the level of the lumbrical origin from the FDP to the involved digit (Fig. 3.16a), which must have full passive motion preoperatively (Fig. 3.16b). The scarred mass in Zone II is carefully dissected and removed (Fig. 3.17a, b). Both tendons are removed from the flexor sheath, preserving pulleys if possible. Any PIP contracture must be released at this time. A silicone rod, sized to match the FDS tendon in the palm, is inserted through any remnants of the pulley system, and secured distally to the FDP stump with a nonabsorbable polyester suture (Fig. 3.18a, b). Usually, a 4 or 5 mm rod is employed. Pulley reconstruction is performed at stage I for the critical A2 and A4 pulleys, using either excised tendon or an ipsilateral palmaris longus tendon. The proximal end of the rod is tucked into the carpal tunnel, adjacent to the FDP and FDS to the involved digit. Both the FDP (just distal to the lumbrical) and FDS are transected in the palm, and the epitenon is carefully dissected from the proximal FDS tendon stump for 5 mm. The FDS and FDP are perfectly coapted, securing them with a 6-0 circumferential suture in the epitenon layer and a 3-0 or 4-0 core suture (Fig. 3.19). The digit is taken through a range of flexion and extension, to ensure smooth gliding of the silicone rod without impingement or dislodgement (Fig. 3.20a, b). The wound is irrigated and

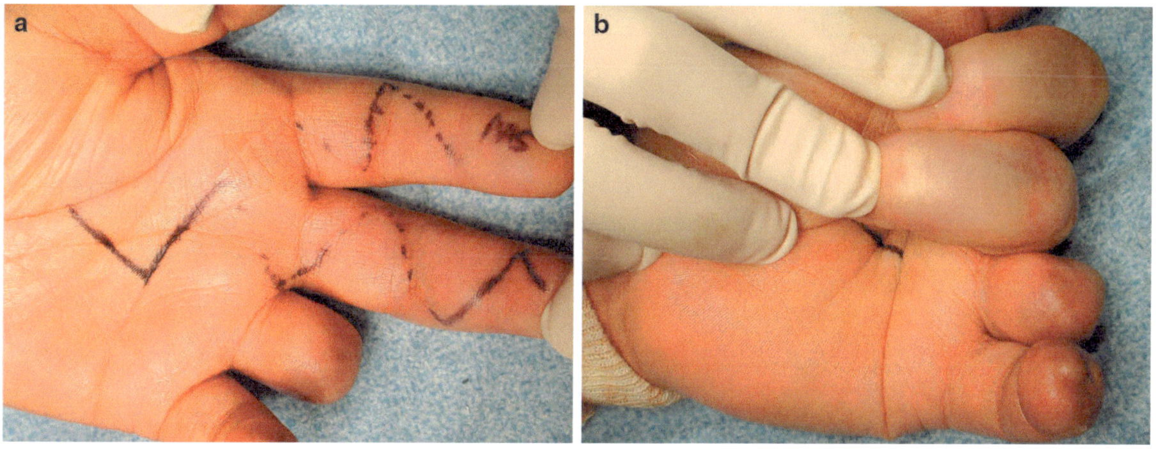

Fig. 3.16 (**a**) Surgical incision planning for the Paneva-Holevich reconstruction. Exposure of the area distal to the lumbrical origin is required. (**b**) The digit must have full passive motion

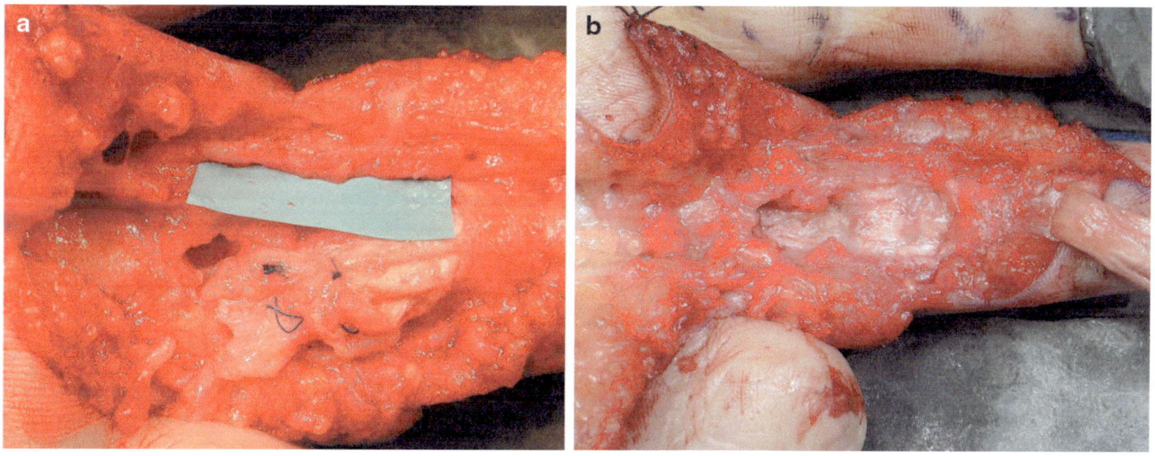

Fig. 3.17 (**a**, **b**) The scarred mass of tendons is dissected and removed from Zone II

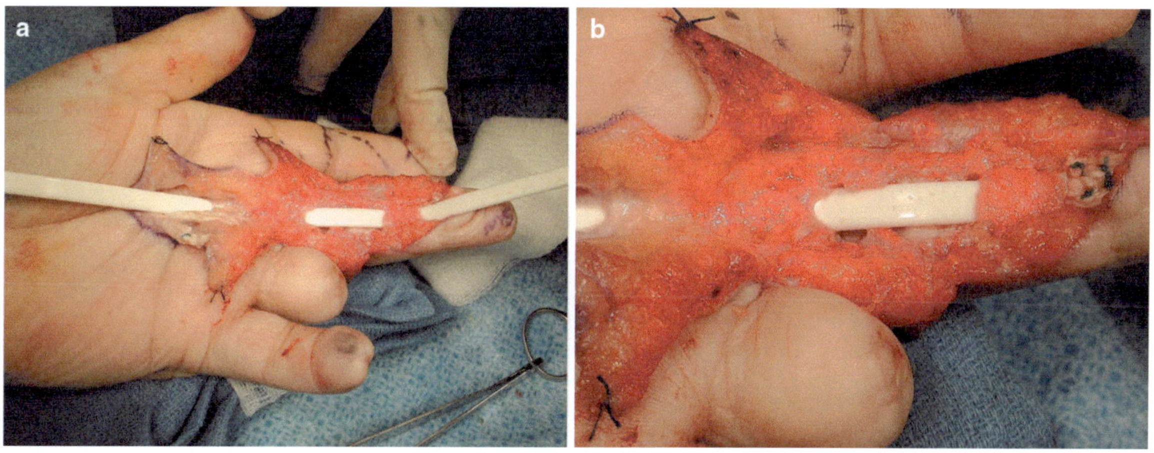

Fig. 3.18 (**a**) The silicone rod is carefully inserted through the existing pulley system, and (**b**) secured distally with nonabsorbable sutures

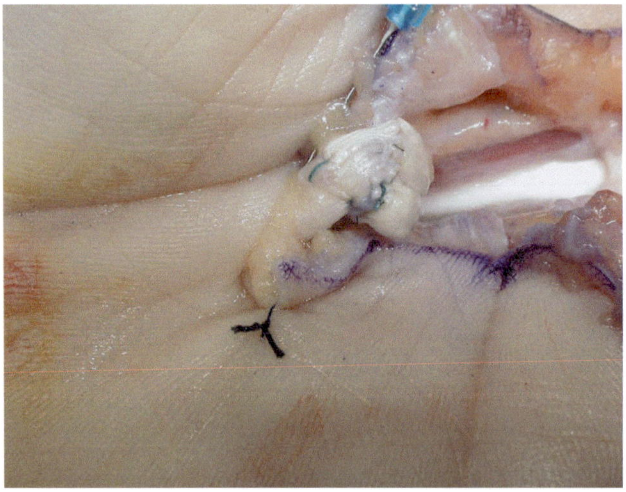

Fig. 3.19 The FDS and FDP stumps are carefully reapproximated in the palm using a core and circumferential suture

closed. Splinting is applied until the skin heals, and therapy is continued to achieve or maintain supple joints. There is no risk of gapping at the repair site because both the FDP and FDS muscles pull the junction in the same direction, thus giving it a head start at healing before any tension is placed across it. As light mechanical forces across the repair site can be beneficial to tendon repair strength, so the repair strength of this junction at Stage 2 would be expected to strengthen further with the mechanical forces applied thereafter.

Stage 2

Stage 2 is performed 2–3 months after the first stage, when the patient demonstrates full passive range of motion, and when there is no swelling or inflammatory reaction about the silicone spacer (Fig. 3.21a, b). The palmar incision is opened first, to locate the proximal end of the silicone rod (Fig. 3.22a), and the FDS-FDP junction. A 6–9 cm forearm incision is

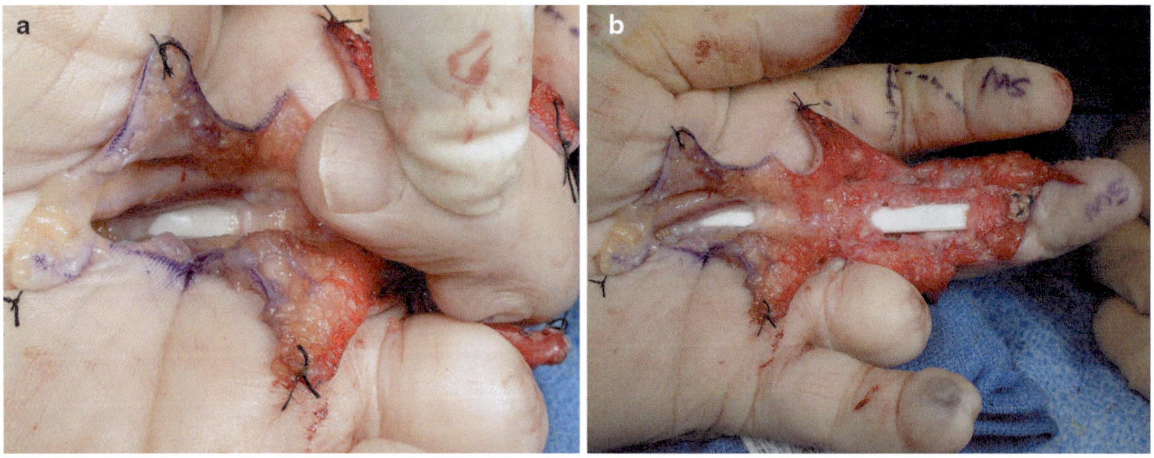

Fig. 3.20 (**a**, **b**) The digit is taken through a range of flexion and extension to ensure the silicone rod does not dislodge or impinge on neighboring structures

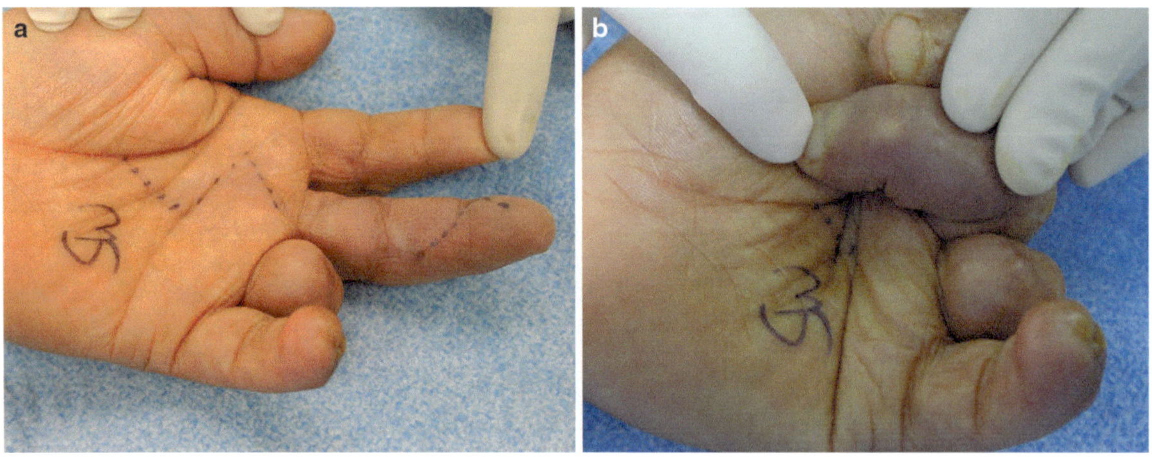

Fig. 3.21 (**a**, **b**) Prior to Stage 2, the digit should maintain its supple motion with the silicone rod in place

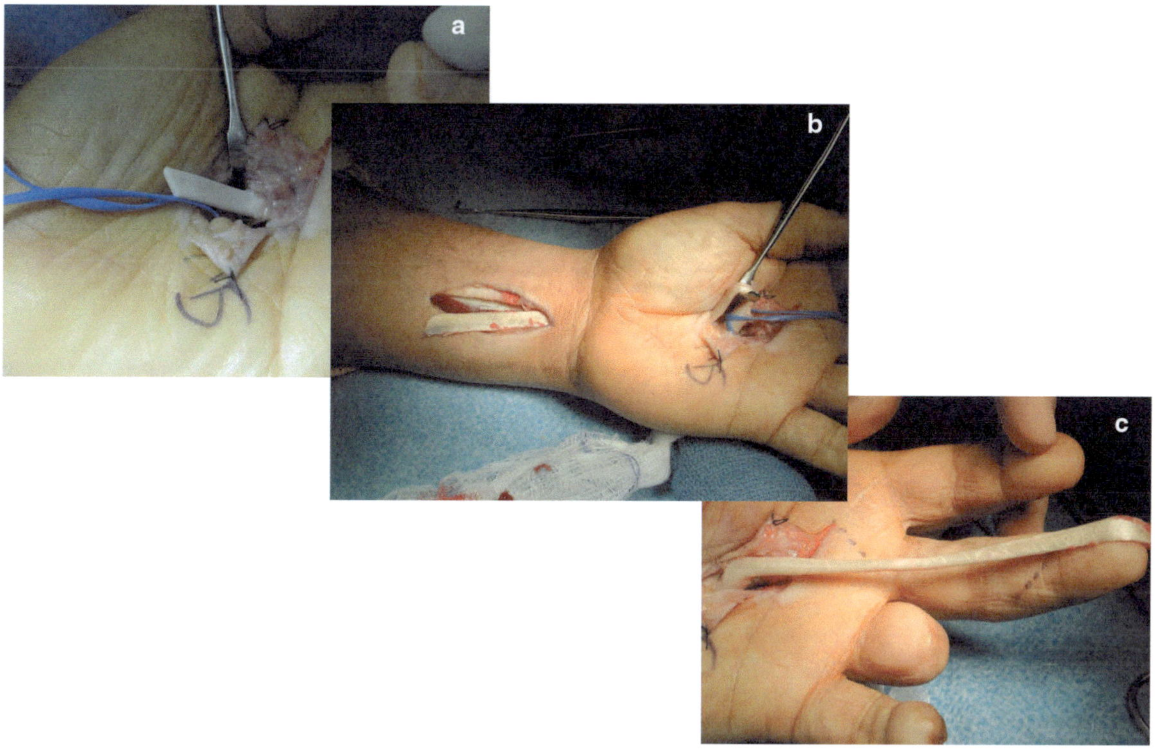

Fig. 3.22 (**a**) The palmar incision is opened first and the silicone rod and FDP–FDS anastomosis site are identified. (**b**) The forearm incision is made large enough to identify both the FDP and FDS. The FDS is truncated at the musculotendinous junction and dissected distally to prepare for reflection distally. (**c**) The FDS is gently reflected distally

made between the flexor tendons and the ulnar neurovascular bundle to accurately identify the FDS and FDP tendons. The FDS and FDP tendons to the involved digit are identified, and the FDS is freed up to its musculotendinous junction. Rarely, if significant scar tissue or adhesions are identified at this level, the forearm and palmar incisions may need to be connected. The FDS is divided at its musculotendinous junction (Fig. 3.22b) and delivered into the palmar wound as a pedicled graft, based on the muscle-tendon unit of the involved FDP (Fig. 3.22c). Mild tension can be placed across the repair site to test its strength and to encourage excursion of the FDP muscle belly.

The graft should be passed distally without exposing the flexor sheath or reconstructed pulley system: it is neither necessary nor advisable to open the Stage I incision over zone II. The incision is opened distally at the distal interphalangeal joint and the rod detached from the profundus stump. The proximal end of the FDS tendon graft is then sutured to the silicone rod in the palmar incision (Fig. 3.23a), and the rod is gently advanced distally by traction on the distal end of the rod (Fig. 3.23b). The FDS is provisionally fixed to the soft tissues with a fine-gauge needle (Fig. 3.23c) to approximate tension. The FDS is then divided and secured to the distal phalanx by a pullout wire and button at the nail plate (Fig. 3.23d). Additional sutures are placed between the graft and the FDP stump. Micro suture anchors can be placed for additional fixation, but this is not mandatory. Slight overtensioning is advised.

The skin is closed in standard fashion. If the transverse carpal ligament was transected during the approach, it must be repaired. A splint is applied with the wrist in neutral and the MP joints in flexion.

As in most flexor tendon reconstructive procedures, multiple concomitant injuries, uncooperative patients, and poor preoperative ROM are associated with poorer outcomes.

Optimizing Outcomes

- Disclose to the patient all facets of the staged procedure, including the entire duration of activity limitation (6–9 months) and the level of therapy participation required of him/her.
- Limit exposures as much as possible while maintaining safety in identifying involved tendons.
- Be cognizant of the length of silicone rod and FDS required to reach the fingertip.
- Pulleys should be tested by exerting traction on the silicone rod at Stage 1, and if pulley reconstruction or augmentation is needed, it should be performed at Stage 1.

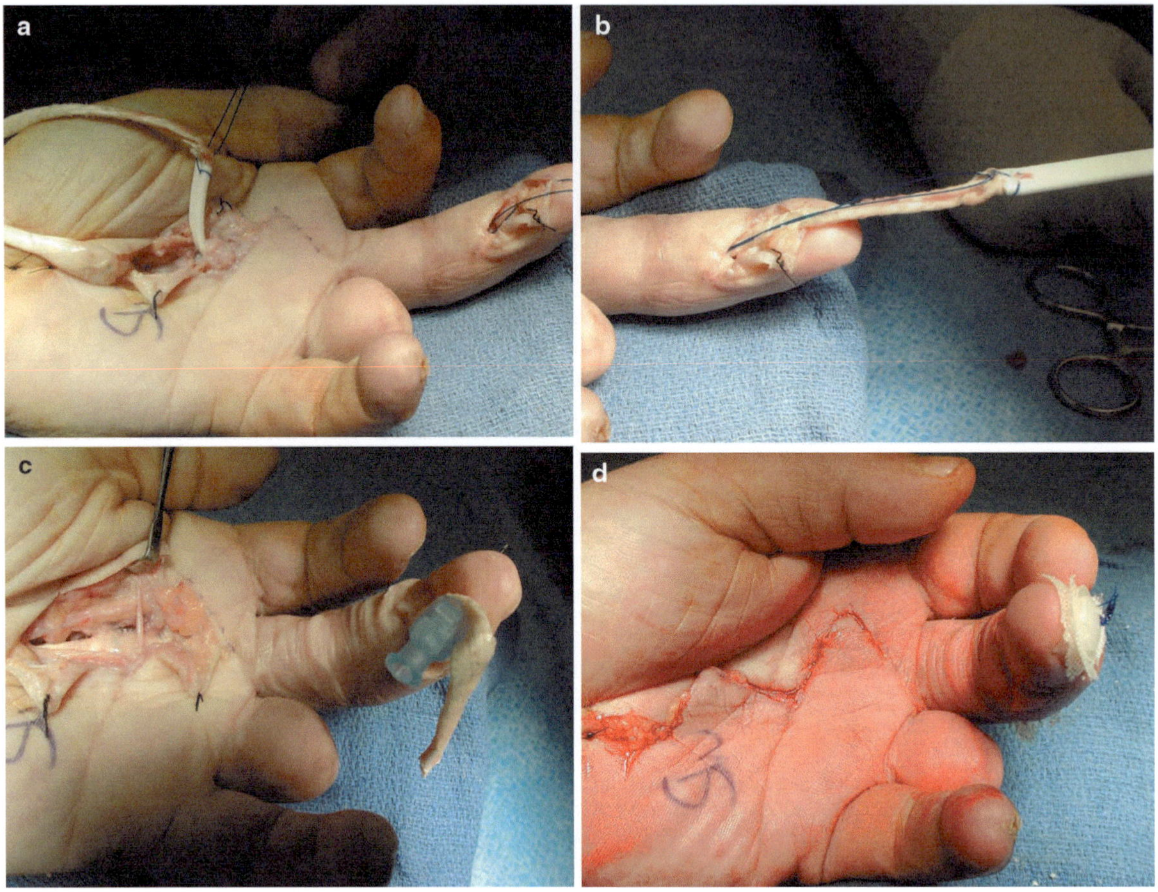

Fig. 3.23 (**a**) The FDS is sewn to the silicone rod in the palmar incision. (**b**) The silicone rod is detached from the distal stump and withdrawn distally, pulling the FDS graft through the pulley system. (**c**) A fine-gauge needle is used to approximate the tendon tension. (**d**) The graft can be secured using a pull-through technique and button, or by sewing the tendon to the residual FDP stump

- Ensure that the silicone rod is long enough that it does not dislodge with passive motion of the digit.
- Graft tensioning is critical to success.

Complications and Side Effects

Complications include adhesions, rupture of the FDS-FDP or distal junctions, dislodgement of the silicone rod, infection, Quadriga or lumbrical plus finger if the graft is too short or long, respectively, PIPJ hyperextension, flexion contracture, and synovitis.

Postoperative Care

Early motion is begun according to established protocols, protecting the repair site early in the treatment course. Theoretically, the repair site in the palm has been healing for the last 4 weeks, and primarily the FDP insertion site need be protected. In general a zone I tendon repair protocol is followed, with place and hold and tenodesis exercises. The pullout suture and button is removed at 6–8 weeks from the second stage. ROM should be advanced to include strengthening after 3 months. Sports activity is discouraged until after 6 months, if functional ROM and strength has been restored. Tenolysis may be necessary if functional range of motion is delayed and progress stalled over consecutive therapy appointments.

Zones III–V

Preoperative History and Considerations

Repair or reconstruction of acute or chronic flexor tendon injuries in this area are less technically demanding and generally have better results due to fewer adhesions than those in Zone II. However, they are more commonly associated with ulnar or median nerve lacerations, which can complicate rehabilitation and outcomes. A thorough physical examination should be performed before reoperation to assess for concomitant nerve injury.

Three techniques for reconstruction are described if a primary repair of an acute or chronic laceration cannot be carried out without undue tension. A prerequisite for reconstruction of any method is a cooperative patient with supple hand joints and a sensate hand.

Indications and Contraindications for Interposition Graft

Interposition grafts are ideal for the late repair, where several centimeters of gapping have accumulated, negating any possible primary repair without excessive tension. The difficulty with this procedure lies in determining the exact length of tendon needed. If possible, an awake patient under local anesthetic and short-acting sedation can be of assistance in determining length.

Indications

- Failure of primary repair in Zones III–V
- Chronic Zone III–V lacerations with supple hand joints and a sensate hand
- Loss of tendon tissue in Zones III–V

Contraindications

- Insensate hand
- Stiff hand joints or contractures

Operative Approach for Interposition Graft

A curvilinear incision over the distal forearm and carpal canal should be utilized, avoiding longitudinal incisions at flexor creases. An area of normal atraumatized anatomy should be identified both proximal and distal to the zone of injury, minimizing dissection of uninvolved sheath tissue. Adjacent neurovascular structures should be identified and protected. The injured tendon should be identified, and any scar or compromised tissue should be debrided from each end. If both an FDP and FDS to the same digit are injured, a segment of the injured FDS can be used to bridge the FDP repair. If only the FDP tendon is lacerated, the Palmaris longus tendon can be harvested as an interposition graft (see page 22).

A 3-0 Ethibond suture is used to perform the repair, and the authors prefer the locking cruciate stitch [27] (Fig. 3.14a, b). The suture is threaded through the graft longitudinally with a straight needle before passing into the opposite tendon stump. A 4-strand repair is ideal, but care must be taken not to damage the graft with multiple attempts to pass the sutures longitudinally through it. A 6-0 prolene epitendinous repair at each junction may help to prevent fraying or bunching of the graft with motion. The standard skin closure is performed. A dorsal blocking splint is placed with the wrist in 20–30° of flexion and the MP joints flexed to 40–50°.

Optimizing Outcomes

- Remove all devitalized tendon tissue from the wound bed
- Take the wrist through a range of motion to ensure gliding of the graft without impingement or bunching
- Begin an early active ROM protocol
- Outcomes of these injuries are often dependent on associated nerve or vascular injuries.

Complications and Side Effects

Complications are similar to those listed for Zone II reconstruction, but less frequent. These include juncture site rupture, infection, repair site attenuation, adjacent nerve irritation, adhesion formation, and finger stiffness.

Indications and Contraindications for FDS Transfer

This procedure is ideal for an isolated FDP or combined FDP/FDS laceration in Zone III with gap formation mitigating primary repair, and an uninjured adjacent digit [28].

Indications

- FDP or FDP/FDS injury in Zone III with gap formation mitigating primary repair, and with an uninjured adjacent digit

Contraindications

- Injured adjacent digits

Operative Approach for FDS Transfer

A curvilinear incision is made over the zone of injury, and the distal FDP stump of the injured digit is identified and debrided. The adjacent digit FDS is identified and transected at a point which would provide adequate length for transfer to the adjacent injured distal FDP stump with a Pulvertaft weave technique. The transfer must be passed deep to any neurovascular structures. Tensioning can be difficult, and an awake patient under local anesthetic with short-acting sedation may be helpful in gauging tension. The remaining tendon stumps can be left in the field if they do not cause any crowding or impingement. The A1 pulley of the injured digit may be opened if the weave is distal enough to cause impingement on the pulley, resulting in limitation of full digital extension. A standard skin closure is carried out, and dorsal blocking splint is applied with the wrist in neutral and MP joints in flexion.

Optimizing Outcomes

- Ensure the donor digit has an intact FDP
- Pass tendons deep to neurovascular structures
- Take the wrist and digits through a range of motion to ensure the weave bulk does not impinge or irritate adjacent structures

Complications and Side Effects

Complications include poor tensioning, transfer site rupture, finger stiffness, infection, adjacent nerve irritation, and donor digit weakness.

Indications and Contraindications for End-to-Side FDP Juncture

When the injury to the FDP occurs more proximally than Zone III, it is more amenable to end-to-side repair to an adjacent intact FDP tendon. Although it is best for use in Zones 4–5, it can be used in Zone III with careful attention to nearby neurovascular structures and the A2 pulley, which can frequently be a problem for full excursion of the repair site.

Indications

- Zones IV–V, and proximal Zone III FDP injuries with adjacent uninjured FDP

Contraindications

- Neurovascular anatomy preventing FDP transfer in distal Zone III
- Adjacent injured FDP

Operative Approach for End-to-Side FDP Juncture

A curvilinear incision is utilized and the injured distal FDP stump is identified and debrided. The adjacent digit FDP is identified. Once proper tensioning is determined, a weave technique with 4–5 weaves secured with 3-0 Ethibond suture is employed to repair the FDP to the adjacent intact FDP tendon. Full excursion must be evaluated to ensure the repair site does not catch on adjacent structures. Standard skin closure is performed and a dorsal block splint with the wrist in neutral and MP joints flexed.

Optimizing Outcomes

- Ensure that the repair site does not irritate or impinge on neurovascular structures

Complications and Side Effects

Complications include infection, juncture rupture or attenuation, poor tensioning, and digital nerve injury.

Postoperative Care

Reconstructive efforts in Zones 3–5 have similar postoperative rehabilitation protocols. A dorsal splint which is forearm-based and extends to the fingertips is recommended. The wrist should be positioned at neutral, the MP joints at 50–60°, and the remainder of the digits at a comfortable position. The splint should be maintained at all times while not undergoing therapy for the first 6 weeks. Therapy should be initiated in the first few days after surgery, with a carefully supervised active motion protocol to promote gliding of the distal FDP and maintenance of passive ROM of the MP and IP joints. Splinting is discontinued at 6 weeks and therapy is aimed at stretching and strengthening. Some lengthening of the repaired tendon can be expected, as the musculotendinous unit improves its excursion. Sports activity is discouraged until after 6 months, if functional ROM and strength has been restored.

The Thumb

Preoperative History and Considerations

Frequently an FPL laceration is amenable to primary repair in any location, for more extended periods of time (3–6 weeks) than the other four digits of the hand [28, 29], making reconstructive situations less frequent. Fortunately reconstruction of the FPL can be technically easier and fraught with less complicating factors than that of the other four digits. Restoration of motion at the IP and MP joints with a single tendon, the FPL, is the reason why it is less technically demanding, but also the reason why it is not always indicated for reconstruction [30]. Several options exist which restore excellent functionality of the thumb, including not reconstructing the tendon at all.

Indications and Contraindications for Free Tendon Graft

Ideal candidates for free tendon graft are patients who have failed primary repair and have a considerable length of compromised tendon tissue at the previous repair site. Loss of more than 1 cm mitigates against attempted primary repair or advancement, due to excessive tension and subsequent IP flexion deformity [7]. Patients must be cooperative with rehabilitation protocols and have a supple IP joint with functionally intact sensation and vascularity.

Indications

- Acute or chronic FPL laceration at any level, with gap formation mitigating against primary repair

Contraindications

- Insensate thumb
- Vascular compromise
- Stiff or painful IP joint

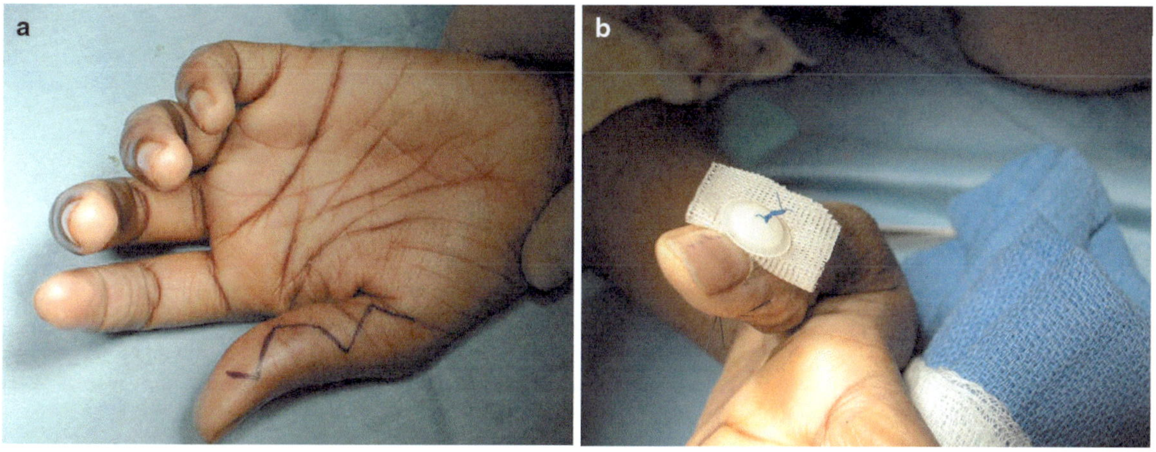

Fig. 3.24 (**a**) A volar oblique Bruner-type approach allows excellent exposure of the FPL distally. (**b**) The dorsal button can be placed more proximally in the thumb, avoiding trauma to the nail plate

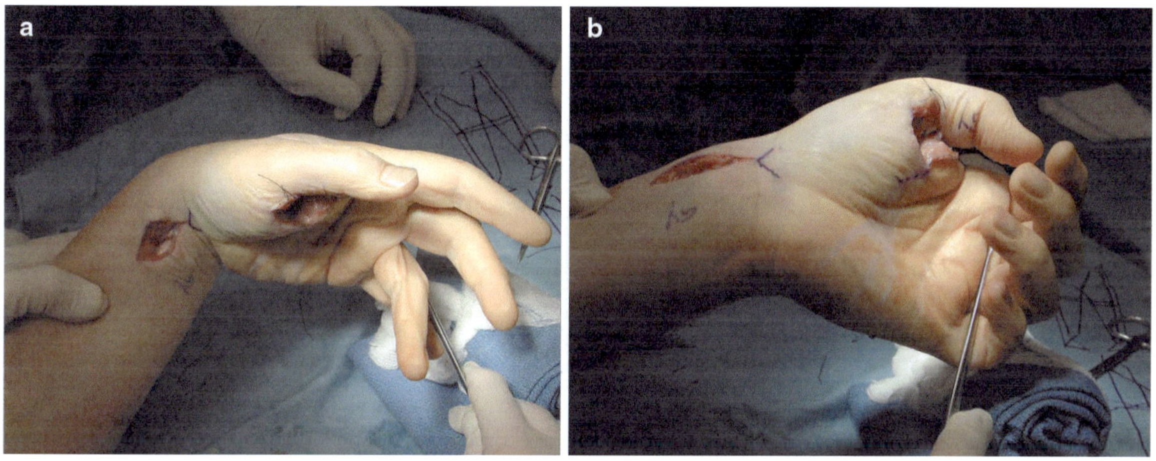

Fig. 3.25 (**a**, **b**) Tenodesis maneuvers should be performed to assess proper tensioning of the FPL graft

Operative Approach for Free Tendon Graft

A volar or volar-oblique Bruner-type incision (Fig. 3.24a) from the base of the distal phalanx to just proximal to the zone of injury is best for necessary exposure of the sheath and tendon. Careful attention to adjacent neurovascular structures must be paid, as they do cross over the tendon at the base of the thumb and may be entrapped in scar tissue. The sheath and pulleys should be minimally handled and dissected to minimize postoperative scar formation. The distal FPL tendon should be sharply excised 1 cm proximal to its insertion in the distal phalanx. A second incision should be made at the distal forearm, at the level of the FPL musculotendinous junction. A sharp transection of the tendon just distal to the musculotendinous junction will allow excision of the entire injured FPL. A prolene suture can be used to tag one end of the tendon before withdrawal, in order to easily label the FPL sheath for later blind graft passage. Harvest of the Palmaris (see page 22) or Plantaris (see page 23) tendon is performed. The authors prefer Palmaris due to its proximity to the field of operation.

The distal junction is secured first, using a pullout wire and button (Fig. 3.24b). Additional sutures or micro suture anchors can be placed to secure the graft to the residual tendon stump. The prolene suture should be secured to the opposite free end of the graft, and pulled in a retrograde direction through the sheath into the distal forearm incision to deliver the graft in an atraumatic fashion. The distal skin closure can be performed prior to tensioning. The tension should be tested with tenodesis maneuvers to ensure proper length (Fig. 3.25a, b).

Optimizing Outcomes

- Proper tensioning is critical to the success of the procedure.
- Adjacent neurovascular structures must be identified before proceeding with tendon dissection.

Complications and Side Effects

Complications include infection, juncture rupture or attenuation, poor tensioning, and digital nerve injury.

Postoperative Care

A splint is applied with the wrist in slight flexion, neutral abduction at the CMC joint, and slight flexion at the MP and IP joints. Combined active and passive motion can begin at the first postoperative visit, allowing passive flexion and active extension within the confines of the splint. Splinting can be discontinued at 6 weeks and strengthening begun at 3 months.

Indications and Contraindications for FDS Transfer

The ideal indication for an FDS transfer is a situation when the IP and MP joints remain supple, but the FPL muscle is not available as a motor. The ring finger FDS is traditionally the best donor muscle/tendon for transfer [31, 32].

Indications
- Loss of FPL as a motor, with supple IP and MP joints

Contraindications
- Insensate thumb
- Vascular compromise
- Poor FDS strength
- Stiff or painful thumb IP joint

Operative Approach for FDS Finger

A volar or volar oblique Bruner-type approach (Fig. 3.24a) is used to approach the flexor sheath of the thumb, taking care to protect any digital nerves or vessels crossing the midline. A second incision is made in a curvilinear fashion in the radial distal forearm to locate the FPL tendon proximally. The tendon is truncated 1 cm from its insertion and withdrawn proximally through the forearm incision, excised completely at this level. Harvest of the FDS is performed with a Bruner or midlateral incision at the level of the proximal phalanx, 2 cm proximal to the PIP joint. One of the tails should be tagged with a suture to facilitate manipulation and withdrawal. Once the FDS is transected, it is found in the distal forearm incision and withdrawn. A third incision may need to be made in the palm if the FDS is not easily withdrawn. The FDS is then carefully rerouted through the pulley system of the thumb and secured to the distal phalanx with a button (Fig. 3.24b), using the insertion remnant to reinforce the junction. Tensioning is critical to the success of the transfer, and it can be difficult in this situation where the only junction is the distal insertion. Tenodesis maneuvers should be performed to ensure proper tension (Fig. 3.25a, b).

Optimizing Outcomes

- Proper tensioning of the transfer is essential.
- Neurovascular structures must be identified and protected before tendon procedures are initiated.

Complications and Side Effects

Poor tensioning, infection, and nerve injury are the most common complications.

Postoperative Care

The transfer should be protected with a splint for 3–4 weeks, and focused hand therapy for training on use of the transfer should be initiated.

Indications and Contraindications for 2-Stage Tendon Reconstruction

As in the digits, 2-stage reconstruction of the thumb flexor is indicated when pulley deficiency, joint contractures, or other secondary procedures complicate the tendon reconstruction effort. This situation is best dealt with in two stages, the first to restore passive mobility and pulley function, and the second to reconstruct the flexor tendons.

Indications
- Acute or chronic FPL laceration with concomitant joint contracture or pulley deficiency

Contraindications
- Stiff or painful MP or IP joints
- Insensate thumb
- Vascular compromise

Operative Approach for 2-Stage Tendon Reconstruction

This procedure is similar to that described in the digits; however, a free tendon graft is seldom necessary because the FDS transfer for Stage II is available in this situation [32].

Optimizing Outcomes

- Appropriate tensioning is critical to success.
- Avoidance of unnecessary trauma to the tendon sheath.
- Intraoperative ROM to ensure no catching or interference of the repair sites on adjacent structures.

Indications and Contraindications for IPJ Arthrodesis

Arthrodesis should be considered as an alternative to FPL repair or reconstruction in the low-demand patient with a hyperextensile or arthritic interphalangeal joint. This procedure can provide the patient with a reasonably strong pinch when the MP and CMC joints are functioning well. Caution should be exercised in patients who have stiff of arthritic MP or CMC joints.

Indications

- FPL laceration in the presence of an arthritic or painful IP joint

Contraindications

- Stiff, painful, or arthritic MP and/or CMC joints

Operative Approach for IPJ Arthrodesis

A dorsal approach to the thumb IPJ is preferred, and there are many techniques which can be used: Kirschner wires, plates, screws, and tension band or cerclage wires. The appropriate method which accommodates the patient's bony anatomy should be used.

Optimizing Outcomes

- Minimize soft tissue trauma.

Complications and Side Effects

Infection, malunion, and nonunion are common complications of IPJ arthrodesis.

Postoperative Care

Postoperative care consists of splinting until bony union is achieved. A course of hand therapy may be required in patients who have difficulty regaining thumb CMC and MPJ motion and strength.

Conclusion

Flexor tendon reoperation remains one of the most complex and rewarding, yet unpredictable group of procedures in the hand surgeon's armamentarium. Despite adherence to the basic tenets of flexor tendon surgery, results are not universally excellent. This fact can be disappointing to both the surgeon and patient, and both should be prepared for the long journey with potential minor setbacks along the way. Focus should be kept on the end result, which is usually an improvement in function from the preoperative status. With the proper selection of motivated patients, significant improvements can be made.

We look forward to new developments in the fields of tissue engineering and biomodulation to provide the next significant jump in improvement of outcomes which appear to have plateaued with our current concepts and technology.

References

1. Khaleghian R, Tonkin LJ, De Geus JJ, Lee JP. Ultrasonic examination of the flexor tendons of the fingers. J Clin Ultrasound. 1984;12(9):547–51.
2. Lee DH, Robbin ML, Galliott R, Graveman VA. Ultrasound evaluation of flexor tendon lacerations. J Hand Surg [Am]. 2000;25(2):236–41.
3. Drape JL, Tardif-Chastenet de Gery S, Silbermann-Hoffman O, Chevrot A, Houvet P, Alnot JY, Benacerraf R. Closed ruptures of the flexor digitorum tendons: MRI evaluation. Skeletal Radiol. 1998;27(11):617–24.
4. Kumar BA, Tolat AR, Threepuraneni G, Jones B. The role of magnetic resonance imaging in late presentation of isolated injuries of the flexor digitorum profundus tendon in the finger. J Hand Surg [Br]. 2000;25(1):95–7.
5. Matloub HS, Dzwierzynski WW, Erickson S, Sanger JR, Yousif NJ, Muoneke V. Magnetic resonance imaging scanning in the diagnosis of zone II flexor tendon rupture. J Hand Surg [Am]. 1996; 21(3):451–5.
6. Sourmelis SG, McGrouther DA. Retrieval of the retracted flexor tendon. J Hand Surg [Br]. 1987;12(1):109–11.
7. Malerich MM, Baird RA, McMaster W, Erickson JM. Permissible limits of flexor digitorum profundus tendon advancement–an anatomic study. J Hand Surg [Am]. 1987;12(1):30–3.
8. Verdan C. Syndrome of the Quadriga. Surg Clin North Am. 1960;40:425–6.
9. Boyer MI, Gelberman RH, Burns ME, Dinopoulos H, Hofem R, Silva MJ. Intrasynovial flexor tendon repair. An experimental study comparing low and high levels of in vivo force during rehabilitation in canines. J Bone Joint Surg Am. 2001;83-A(6):891–9.
10. Lieber RL, Amiel D, Kaufman KR, Whitney J, Gelberman RH. Relationship between joint motion and flexor tendon force in the canine forelimb. J Hand Surg [Am]. 1996;21(6):957–62.
11. Lieber RL, Silva MJ, Amiel D, Gelberman RH. Wrist and digital joint motion produce unique flexor tendon force and excursion in the canine forelimb. J Biomech. 1999;32(2):175–81.
12. Honner R. The late management of the isolated lesion of the flexor digitorum profundus tendon. Hand. 1975;7(2):171–4.
13. Nichols HM. The dilemma of the intact superficialis tendon. Hand. 1975;7(1):85–6.
14. Robertson DC. The place of flexor tendon grafts in the repair of flexor tendon injuries to the hand. Clin Orthop. 1959;15:16–21.
15. Wilson RL. Flexor tendon grafting. Hand Clin. 1985;1(1):97–107.
16. Wehbe MA. Tendon graft donor sites. J Hand Surg [Am]. 1992;17(6):1130–2.
17. Morrison WA, Schlicht SM. The plantaris tendon as a tendo-osseous graft. Part II. Clinical studies. J Hand Surg [Br]. 1992;17(4): 471–5.
18. Tolat AR, Stanley JK. The extended palmaris longus tendon graft. J Hand Surg [Br]. 1993;18(2):239–40.
19. Thompson NW, Mockford BJ, Cran GW. Absence of the palmaris longus muscle: a population study. Ulster Med J. 2001;70(1):22–4.
20. Vastamaki M. Median nerve as free tendon graft. J Hand Surg [Br]. 1987;12(2):187–8.
21. Weber RV, Mackinnon SE. Median nerve mistaken for palmaris longus tendon: restoration of function with sensory nerve transfers. Hand. 2007;2(1):1–4.
22. Parkes A. The "lumbrical plus" finger. J Bone Joint Surg Br. 1971;53(2):236–9.
23. Pulvertaft RG. Tendon grafts for flexor tendon injuries in the fingers and thumb; a study of technique and results. J Bone Joint Surg Br. 1956;38-B(1):175–94.

24. Watson AB. Some remarks on the repair of flexor tendons in the hand, with particular reference to the technique of free grafting. Br J Surg. 1955;43(177):35–42.
25. Boyer MI, Strickland JW, Engles D, Sachar K, Leversedge FJ. Flexor tendon repair and rehabilitation: state of the art in 2002. Instr Course Lect. 2003;52:137–61.
26. Paneva-Holevich E. Two-stage tenoplasty in injury of the flexor tendons of the hand. J Bone Joint Surg Am. 1969;51(1):21–32.
27. Barrie KA, Tomak SL, Cholewicki J, Wolfe SW. The role of multiple strands and locking sutures on gap formation of flexor tendon repairs during cyclical loading. J Hand Surg [Am]. 2000; 25(4):714–20.
28. Urbaniak JR. Repair of the flexor pollicis longus. Hand Clin. 1985;1(1):69–76.
29. Urbaniak JR, Goldner JL. Laceration of the flexor pollicis longus tendon: delayed repair by advancement, free graft or direct suture. A clinical and experimental study. J Bone Joint Surg Am. 1973;55(6):1123–48.
30. Kilgore Jr ES, Newmeyer WL, Graham III WP, Brown LG. The dubiousness of grafting the dispensable flexor pollicis longus. Am J Surg. 1976;132(2):292–6.
31. Posner MA. Flexor superficialis tendon transfers to the thumb–an alternative to the free tendon graft for treatment of chronic injuries within the digital sheath. J Hand Surg [Am]. 1983;8(6): 876–81.
32. Schneider LH, Wiltshire D. Restoration of flexor pollicis longus function by flexor digitorum superficialis transfer. J Hand Surg [Am]. 1983;8(1):98–101.

Additional References

Coyle Jr MP, Leddy TP, Leddy JP. Staged flexor tendon reconstruction fingertip to palm. J Hand Surg [Am]. 2002;27(4):581–5.

Bora Jr FW. Profundus tendon grafting with unimpaired sublimus function in children. Clin Orthop Relat Res. 1970;71:118–23.

Goldner JL, Coonrad RW. Tendon grafting of the flexor profundus in the presence of a completely or partially intact flexor sublimis. J Bone Joint Surg Am. 1969;51(3):527–32.

Jaffe S, Weckesser E. Profundus tendon grafting with the sublimis intact. An end-result study of thirty patients. J Bone Joint Surg Am. 1967;49(7):1298–308.

McClinton MA, Curtis RM, Wilgis EF. One hundred tendon grafts for isolated flexor digitorum profundus injuries. J Hand Surg [Am]. 1982;7(3):224–9.

Schneider LH, Wehbe MA. Delayed repair of flexor profundus tendon in the palm (zone 3) with superficialis transfer. J Hand Surg [Am]. 1988;13(2):227–30.

Sakellarides HT, Papadopoulos G. Surgical treatment of the divided flexor digitorum profundus tendon in zone 2, delayed more than 6 weeks, by tendon grafting in 50 cases. J Hand Surg [Br]. 1996; 21(1):63–6.

Pulvertaft RG. The treatment of profundus division by the free tendon graft. J Bone Joint Surg Am. 1960;42(1):1363–71.

Ipsen T, Barfred T. Early mobilization after flexor tendon grafting for isolated profundus tendon lesions. Scand J Plast Reconstr Surg Hand Surg. 1988;22(2):163–7.

Reoperative Phalangeal and Metacarpal Fracture Management

4

Kane L. Anderson and Douglas P. Hanel

Abstract

The phalangeal or metacarpal fracture that has undergone previous surgery but resulted in nonunion, malunion, or posttraumatic arthritis can be particularly challenging. These fingers are usually stiff and sometimes painful to the patient. Besides the bone injury, there are usually soft-tissue problems that complicate the reconstructive efforts. For the PIP and MCP joints, arthroplasty and fusion remain as options for posttraumatic reconstruction. The use of osteotomies can be helpful addressing rotational or angular deformities. Hemi-hamate arthroplasty is a novel and useful technique for salvaging the failed unstable PIP fracture dislocation. Ultimately, if the digit cannot be reconstructed or if the digit becomes chronically stiff and painful, some patients will elect to have amputation as their final surgery to try and restore functionality to the hand and in order to get on with their lives.

Keywords

Phalangeal • Metacarpal • Fracture • Reoperation • Failed • Surgery

Key Points

- *Arthrodesis* eliminates the painful motion from an *unreconstructable joint*.
- Arthroplasty of the PIP joints has mediocre long-term results. Use it cautiously, especially for border digits.
- Scissoring and abutment due to either angular or rotatory deformity can be corrected with various types of osteotomies. Compensatory osteotomies proximal to the site of deformity can be performed.
- Hemi-hamate arthroplasty can be used acutely or to salvage failed ORIF/ex-fix for unstable PIP fracture dislocations with a large volar lip fragment.
- Interventions for nonunion should be pursued if there is no significant progression toward healing after 12 weeks. Persistent immobilization will lead to an increasingly stiff finger.
- Middle finger ray amputation is best addressed with subsequent index ray transposition, while ring finger ray amputation can be treated with approximation of the intermetacarpal ligaments.

K.L. Anderson, MS, MD • D.P. Hanel, MD (✉)
Section of Hand and Micro Surgery, Department of Orthopaedics and Sports Medicine, Harborview Medical Center, University of Washington, 325, 9th Avenue, Box 359798, Seattle, WA 98104, USA
e-mail: lynnande@u.washington.edu

S.F.M. Duncan (ed.), *Reoperative Hand Surgery*,
DOI 10.1007/978-1-4614-2373-7_4, © Springer Science+Business Media, LLC 2012

Introduction

Enthusiasm for reoperation in the management of phalangeal and metacarpal fractures must be tempered by the undeniable tendency for the multiply operated hand to scar and become stiff. Although the prospect of perfect radiographs is alluring, patients with deformity but good function would rarely risk that function for improved X-rays. The results of appropriate initial treatment are difficult to exceed. With this caveat, patients can derive significant benefit from appropriately chosen reoperation.

Finger deformities predominately serve to limit hand function because of pain and malposition. Pain can arise from either an incongruous joint that is becoming arthritic or from motion at the site of a delayed or nonunion. Malposition comes in several forms. Rotational malalignment limits motion by digits colliding during hand closure. Segmental bone loss and subsequent nonunion leave the digit worthlessly suspended from surrounding soft tissues. Our tools for addressing these issues are osteotomies, arthrodesis, bone grafting, amputation, and arthroplasty. Each technique, however, has its attendant drawbacks. Corrective osteotomies can be employed for early intra-articular malunion and rotational and angular deformity. Newer techniques, such as hemi-hamate arthroplasty for PIP fracture-dislocations, can also be selectively employed. To distinguish between these options, it is important to understand the relevant basic science as well as synthesize the medical literature regarding outcomes of these operations.

Understanding the basic science behind delayed/nonunions directs their treatment. Characteristic patterns of nonunion in the digits, like other long bones, are clues to assist in surgical planning. If the physiologic response at the fracture site is determined to be hypertrophic, augmented fixation will suffice. If atrophic, bone grafts need to be added as well. Similar to atrophic nonunions, segmental bone loss requires measures that either directly address the bone deficit using autografts, or allografts, or indirectly by distraction osteogenesis. Autograft therapy remains the mainstay of hand reconstruction with the role of allograft and distraction still being defined.

Proximal interphalangeal joint arthroplasty has had remarkably poor long-term results in all but the lowest demand patients. However, the constant emergence of new arthroplasty technology prompts us to continually compare these results to that of small-joint arthrodesis.

The site of corrective osteotomy is controversial. In the absence of the biology of the operative field, correcting malalignment at its source makes sense, rather than creating a compensatory correction. However, to avoid the increased difficulty of a scarred operative field, and limited motion secondary to the tendon and capsular adhesions that can ensue, osteotomies proximal to the site of malunion have been proposed.

Although considered a last resort, another reconstructive option which is often the best treatment for a hopelessly deformed and functionless digit is amputation. When an amputation involves central digits, a unique set of deformities is created that must be addressed.

This chapter reviews the present literature, recent advances, and surgical techniques in reconstruction of the hand, particularly hand joint arthrodesis, arthroplasty, and correction of malunion, nonunion, and bone loss.

Indications and Contraindications

Arthrodesis

- Unreconstructable joint (primary); arthritis (late)
- Contraindications: inadequate bone stock, active infection, insensate digit

Arthroplasty

- Controversial, especially for border digits
- Contraindications: high demand, infection

Osteotomy

- Apex dorsal metacarpal angulation: poorly tolerated in the radial metacarpals (>10–20°). Ulnar metacarpals are more tolerant secondary to greater mobility of the carpometacarpal joints.
- Apex radial/ulnar angulation and rotational malformation: (scissoring of digits).
- Intra-articular: >2-mm step-off, unicondylar depression causing angular malalignment significant enough to cause limitations in motion and digit scissoring.
- General contraindications to osteotomies: articular damage so grave that correction of alignment will not lead to functional improvement; inability to comply with demanding postoperative therapy.

Hemi-hamate arthroplasty

- Unstable comminuted palmar lip PIP fracture dislocation, lateral plateau middle phalanx fractures, instability despite prior ex-fix, or attempted ORIF/volar plate arthroplasty
- Contraindications: damage to the proximal phalanx head, arthritis, severe soft-tissue injury

Grafting

- No significant progression toward healing after 12 weeks
- Contraindications: active infection, inability to provide adequate fixation

(continued)

Amputation and adjacent digit transposition

- Salvage would leave the patient with a stiff, painful, or insensate digit. Exhausted salvage options after crush, chronic infection, or flexion contracture of the middle ray (index ray transposition after middle ray resection).
- Contraindications: injured middle metacarpal base unable to accept the transposition.

Level of Evidence

In this chapter, we have chosen to describe treatment methods found to be effective when utilized in our clinical practices. In the absence of level 1 evidence, we have relied on case cohorts presented by "experienced" surgeons to guide our judgment of best practices.

Arthrodesis

Pain, joint destruction, chronic instability, and deformity resulting from trauma or osteoarthritis continue to be indications for small-joint arthrodesis. Joints that must be stable to provide strong lateral pinch, i.e., the index and long finger proximal interphalangeal joint and the thumb metacarpophalangeal joint, are most amenable to fusion. Fusion of the joints whose contribution to hand function requires a larger range of motion results in significant disability. This is especially true of the ring and small finger proximal interphalangeal joints and to a lesser extent the carpometacarpal joint of the thumb. Until the role of vascularized joint transfer is established or more reliable prosthetic devices are developed, the treatment of choice for interphalangeal joint and thumb metacarpophalangeal joint destruction remains fusion. The question of thumb carpometacarpal arthrodesis vs. arthroplasty is not yet resolved. The contraindication to arthrodesis of the thumb CMC is pantrapezial arthrosis, which occurs in more than two-thirds of patients presenting with thumb pain [1].

In review of 171 interphalangeal joint fusions, flexion of 10–20° in the distal interphalangeal joint and 30–45° in the proximal interphalangeal joints (progressing from radial to ulnar) was felt to be most appropriate [2]. In another study based on 41 thumb metacarpophalangeal joint fusions, 15° of flexion and 10° of pronation provided optimal pinch position without compromising first web space breadth [3]. The optimal position for thumb carpometacarpal arthrodesis is 30–40° of palmar abduction, 30–35° of radial abduction, and enough pronation to maintain pulp-to-pulp pinch between the thumb, index, and long fingers [4]. The union rate for all arthrodesis procedures reported in the last 10 years is 80–100% [5–14]. Lower fusion rates have been noted in thumb carpometacarpal joints secured with Kirschner wires alone [5]. The only distinct advantage of any one fixation method over another is that more rigid fixation allows earlier mobilization. The procedure chosen should be dependent upon both the familiarity of the surgeon with the procedure and the perceived demands of the patient.

Thumb Carpometacarpal Joint

A greater than 10-year follow-up of thumb carpometacarpal arthrodesis demonstrated several trends. Normal pinch strength occurred in more than 60% of patients. Furthermore, 77% of patients were able to contract the thumb to the index, long, and ring pulp, and 70% were completely pain-free. There was a 72% decrease in the adduction/abduction arc and a 61% reduction in flexion/extension arc [6]. Despite this loss of motion, there were minimal subjective complaints and seldom any demonstrable loss of precision hand function. In both studies, less than 5% of patients developed arthritic changes in the scaphotrapezial articulation, and those who did were successfully managed with silastic or soft-tissue trapezium replacement arthroplasty. There are several techniques of arthrodesis: cup-in-cone, bone staples, sliding bone grafts, and recently plate and screw fixation (Fig. 4.1a).

Comparing arthrodesis results to a variety of arthroplasty procedures, the overall rate of satisfaction and strength could

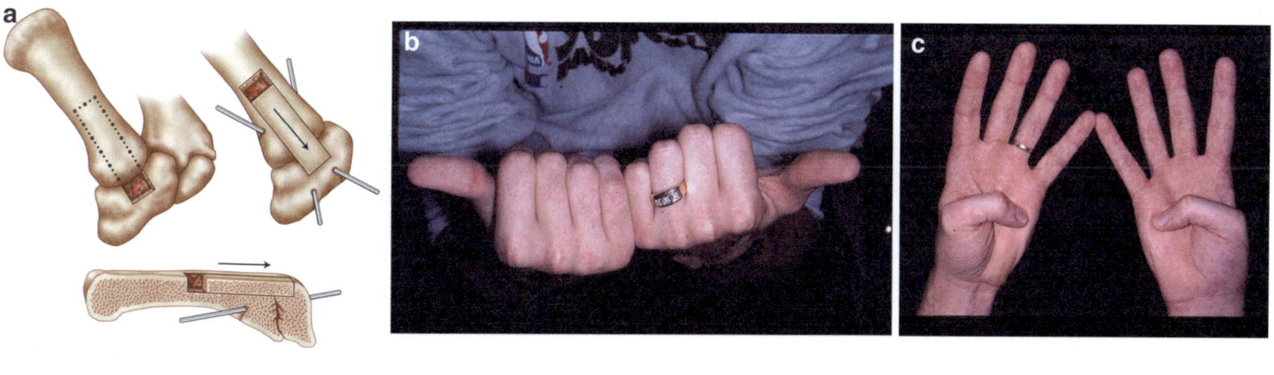

Fig. 4.1 (**a**) Sliding graft method used for trapeziometacarpal arthrodeses. (**b**, **c**) Motion after CMC fusion fixed with a blade plate (hand without ring), mild limitation of thumb retropulsion

not be correlated with the type of procedure [7]. Alternatives have been described in the literature for younger patients with moderate CMC arthrosis. These include volar beak ligament reconstruction alone, CMC arthroscopy with debridement of osteophytes, and metacarpal osteotomy to redistribute the load on the CMC joint. Carpometacarpal joint arthrodesis is the treatment of choice for patients whose vocations or avocations place high demands for stability and strength upon the thumb. The contraindications to CMC fusion are pantrapezial arthritis or a patient that cannot tolerate the subsequent restricted motion of the hand (predominately retropulsion of the thumb to flatten the hand). Though, clinically, these patients often retain excellent mobility (Fig. 4.1b, c). Relative contraindications include MCP/IP stiffness or physiologically elderly patients who usually do well with arthroplasty and who may have osteopenia that precludes stable fixation.

Thumb Metacarpophalangeal Joint

Segmuller has observed that the thumb metacarpophalangeal joint has the least motion of any digital joint, and therefore, stability of that joint should take precedence over motion. His 50 fusions, using a tension band technique, along with studies using other fixation methods portray a high fusion rate and minimal complications [3]. Fusion of the thumb MCP joint leads to a uniformly positive subjective response. Patients report increased strength, thumb ray stability, and the elimination of the painful joint. Objective measurement substantiates this claim. Postoperative thumb pinch strength was always improved when compared to preoperative strength and in a number of cases was even greater than that of the opposite thumb. There is no evidence that fusion of the MCP joint contributes to the acceleration of carpometacarpal or interphalangeal joint dysfunction. Hagan and Hastings [8] did note difficulty with fine pinch in 11 of 18 patients.

Finger Interphalangeal Joints

Biomechanical analysis of crossed Kirschner wires, intraosseous wires, and figure eight tension bands used for interphalangeal joint fusion fixation suggests that a figure-of-eight tension band is superior in anteroposterior bending and torsion [9] (Figs. 4.2 and 4.3). Each technique demonstrated the same resistance to lateral bending forces. Placing an intraosseous wire dorsal to the axis of flexion is more substantial than placing the wire on or volar to the axis of rotation. Although retrospective studies support these experimental findings with 97% union rates and infrequent postoperative infections, the advantage of this technique over other retrospectively studied fixation techniques is not established. Burton et al. [2] presented 170 successful fusions in

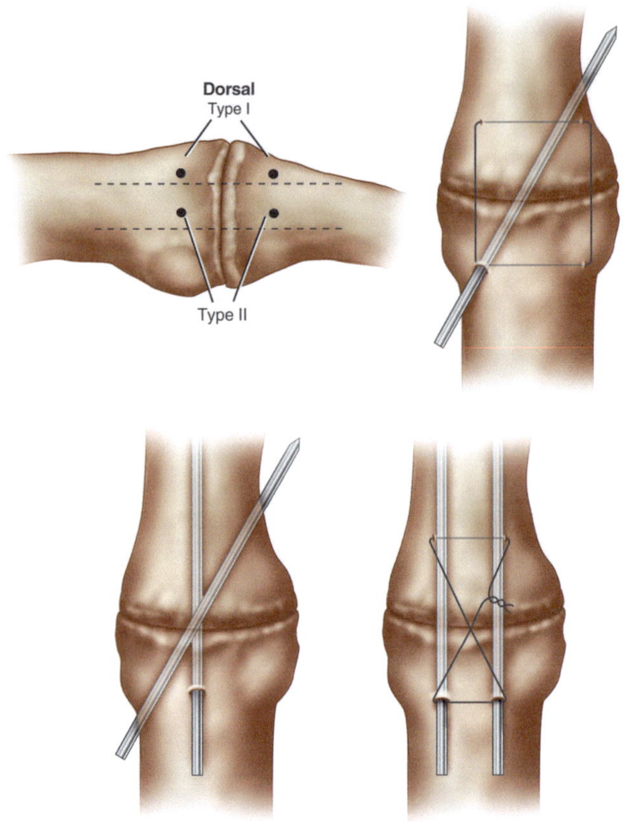

Fig. 4.2 Four methods of fixation used for arthrodesis of the proximal interphalangeal joint

171 attempts using flat osteotomies and cross K-wire technique. The success of this technique demands minimal periosteal dissection, accurate coaptation of medullary bone, circumferential contact of cortical bone, and external immobilization for 5–12 weeks. The technique can be adapted to immature bone by cutting through the secondary ossification centers, preserving the physis, coapting the bone ends, and securing fixation with diverging K-wires. Similar results have been reported using intraosseous wire techniques, cup-in-cone osteotomy with K-wire fixation, dorsal tension band, headless screw fixation, an external compression device, power-driven staples, and using a trephine to create a tenon for placement within the medullary canal of the middle phalanx [9–16] (Figs. 4.4 and 4.5). Cast or splint immobilization is recommended with each of these methods. Results are uniformly good for each arthrodesis technique.

Arthroplasty

Although reliable arthroplasties are available for the basal joint of the thumb, the available interphalangeal joint arthroplasties have tended not to provide sufficient lateral stability

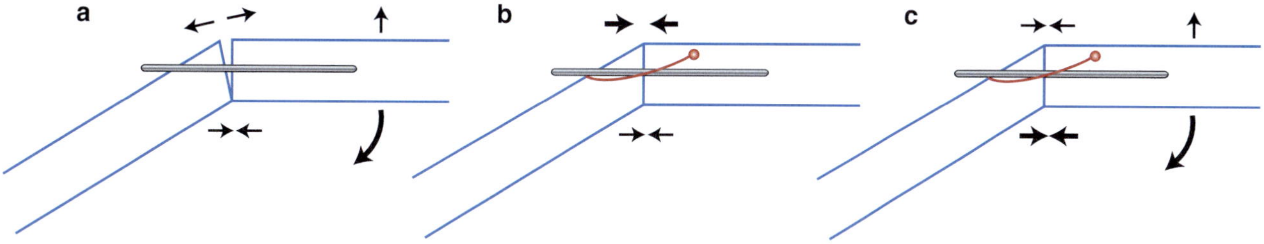

Fig. 4.3 Schematic of the mechanical advantage of tension band fixation, the addition of the tension band allows improved dorsal coaptation

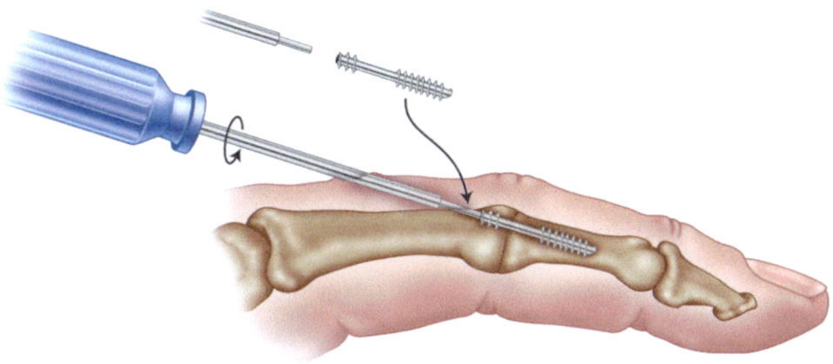

Fig. 4.4 Herbert screw small-joint arthrodesis

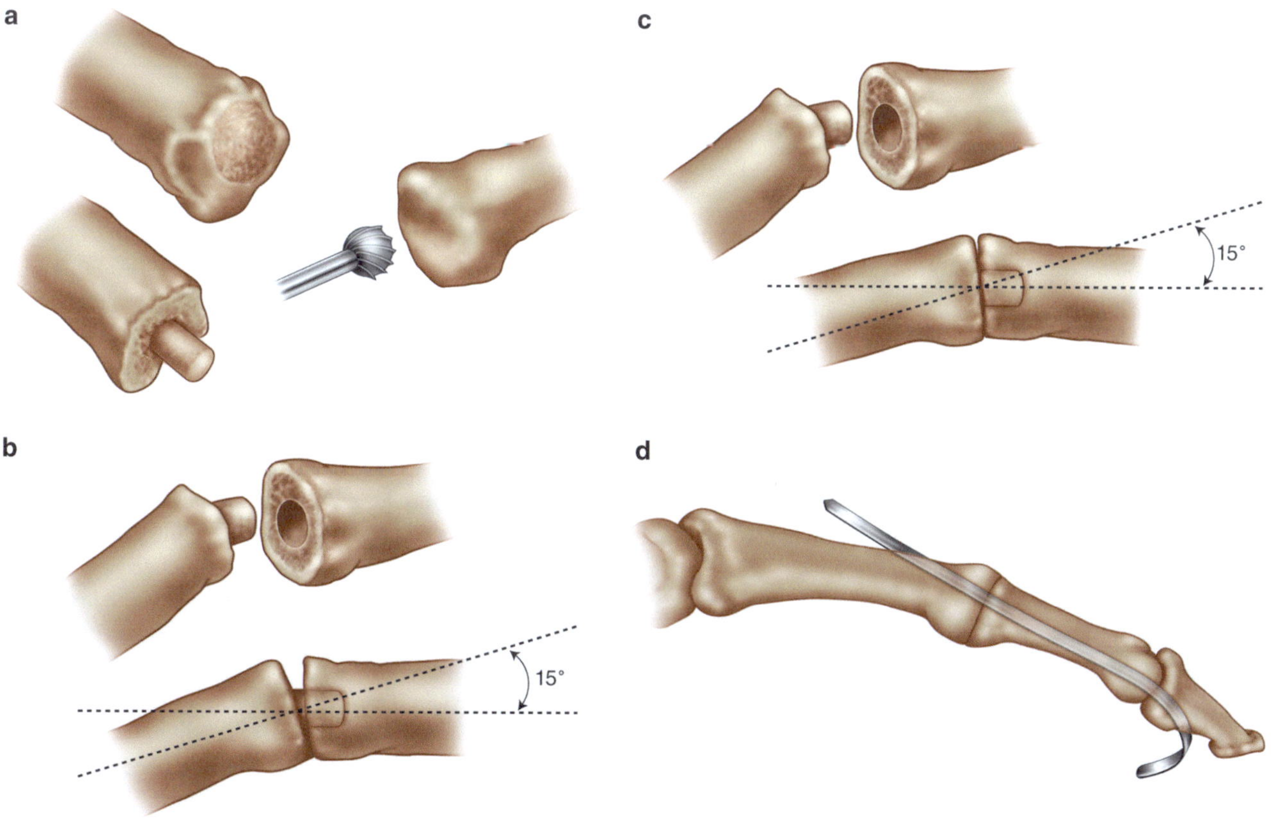

Fig. 4.5 Tenon method of small-joint fusion (**a**–**d**) construction of the tenon with subsequent fixation

after 4 years, although recent data is encouraging. The typical soft-tissue reconstruction that is employed for arthroplasty of the basal joint is well suited for the mechanics of the joint. Unfortunately, the same is not true for the interphalangeal joints. Silastic joint replacements demonstrate severe erosive changes in as many as 30% of cases, and mechanical failure occurs in all or most of the older hinged prostheses [17]. Weiss and colleagues have recently reported on an anatomically neutral silicone arthroplasty with good early functional results (84% good or excellent pain relief and ~60° ROM). They reported only one fracture and one case of osteolysis at average 4-year follow-up in 29 arthroplasties [18]. [19]. have studied results of arthroplasty with pyrolytic carbon and compared it to results of silicone arthroplasty for the PIPJ. Overall, satisfaction was high despite implant specific complications. There was slightly greater than 10% incidence of silicone implant fracture and 10% loosening rate in the pyrocarbon group at 45 months [19].

Osteotomy

There are three main types of deformity that can be addressed with osteotomy: angular, rotational, and intra-articular malalignment.

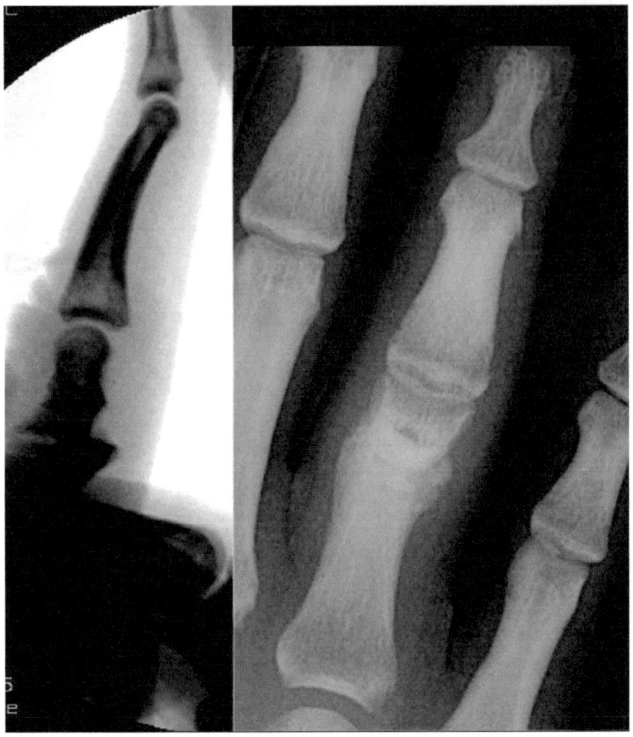

Fig. 4.6 Angular malunion of the proximal phalanx

Malunion

Angular Deformity

Angular malunion (Fig. 4.6) can cause muscle imbalance with subsequent weakness of grip or pinch and occasionally pain. Malunion of the metacarpal is treated only if there is a painful prominence of the metacarpal head in the palm, usually noted with gripping; if there is tethering of the extensor tendon over the apex of the deformity; or if there is marked clawing of the finger. Angular deformity is poorly tolerated in the radial metacarpals, and even relatively small degrees of angulation (10–20°) may create problems. The ulnar two metacarpals, because of the greater mobility of the carpometacarpal joints, are less likely to require correction of deformities. The more proximal sites of malunion within the metacarpal are more likely to create a deformity requiring treatment because the malalignment is propagated over a greater distance toward the distal aspect of the digit.

Functional limitations may result from inadequately reduced subcondylar or phalangeal neck fractures. A bony block along the volar aspect of the phalanx prevents flexion. This deformity, which represents either apex volar angulation or dorsal translation of the phalangeal head, does not remodel even in children. Three pediatric patients were treated by removal of the bony block, which resulted in gains of 25–50° of flexion. The cases were approached through palmar zigzag incisions that allowed release of the contracted volar capsule and complete visualization of the osteotomy site [20].

Rotational Deformity

Patients with rotational malunions may be subject to functional impairments of the involved and adjacent digits due to scissoring, most notable in flexion. While minor overlap or abutment can be tolerable to patients, severe impairment combined with deformity is an operative indication. Classic teaching suggests that in contrast to long bone angular deformity, rotational deformity has limited remodeling potential in children.

Although proximal metacarpal osteotomy was introduced 30 years ago, little was written about it until recently. A cadaver study has demonstrated that every 1° of metacarpal rotation corrects approximately 0.7° of phalangeal malrotation. The theoretical amount of phalangeal correction is 18–19° in the index, long, and ring and 20–30° in the small [21]. The limiting factor to additional rotational correction is the deep transverse metacarpal ligament. Releasing the transverse metacarpal ligament is not recommended because of the resultant loss of the transverse palmar arch and instability of the metacarpophalangeal joint. This procedure has been reported to be "satisfactory" in a number of small series.

In 2009, Jawa et al. [22] retrospectively reviewed 12 patients that underwent metacarpal step-cut osteotomy (Fig. 4.7a) for rotational malunion. These patients had significant improvement in total active motion from 214° preoperatively to 251° at final follow-up. Only one patient had a residual 5° deformity. In another series of 16 successfully corrected proximal phalanx malunions, 11 of the proximal phalanx

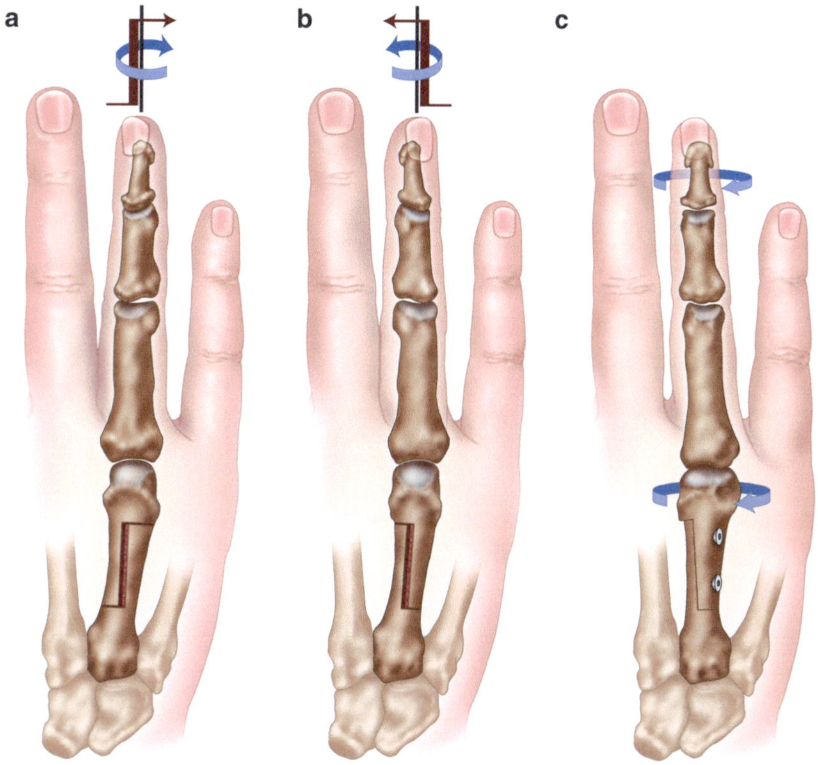

Fig. 4.7 (**a**) Principles of metacarpal derotational osteotomy. (**b**) Principle of an in situ step-cut osteotomy. (**c**) Internal fixation of the derotational osteotomy

osteotomies also underwent simultaneous extensor tenolysis and capsulotomies of adjacent joints. Scissoring was corrected in all cases, and the osteotomies healed within 8 weeks. Although increased postoperative motion was reported for most patients, several lost up to 15° [23]. The largest series of malunions corrected at the site of deformity comes from the AO center in Switzerland (Fig. 4.7b). Thirty-six cases were corrected and maintained with plate and screw fixation. Eighty-six percent of patients had satisfactory digital function. The poor results were related to chronic periarticular injury [24].

Articular Deformity

A unique malunion problem is intra-articular malalignment. This typically presents with limited motion and often angular deviation secondary to articular incongruity. With time, the incongruity leads to joint destruction manifested as crepitation, pain, increasing angular deformity, and further loss of motion and hand function. This difficult problem has been previously managed with arthroplasty, arthrodesis, or acceptance of deformity. Intra-articular realignment osteotomy has been presented as an alternative treatment. Two options are available, depending on the clinical scenario. In the setting of articular step-off, intra-articular osteotomy of various methods can be used but remains technically demanding. Unicondylar malunion, on the other hand, can be addressed by condylar advancement osteotomy, which osteotomizes the entire column to which the malunited fragment has healed [25]. This has the theoretic advantage of limiting intra-articular dissection and the ability to gain improved fixation in a larger fragment. This advancement technique is limited in its application to unicondylar impaction injuries, without deformity in the rotational plane (Fig. 4.8).

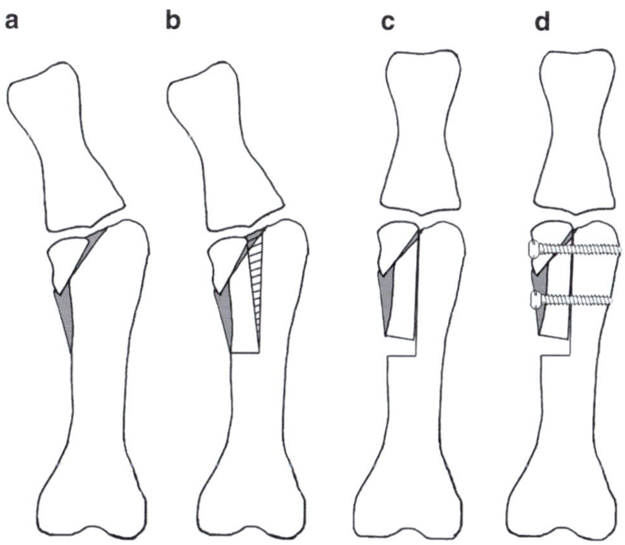

Fig. 4.8 (**a**) Malunited condyle of the proximal phalanx. Shaded areas represent fracture callus. (**b**) A longitudinal osteotomy is made down the shaft and excess bone is removed with a burr. (**c**) The bone fragment is advanced, restoring joint congruity and correcting angular deformity. (**d**) Stable fixation is achieved with screws

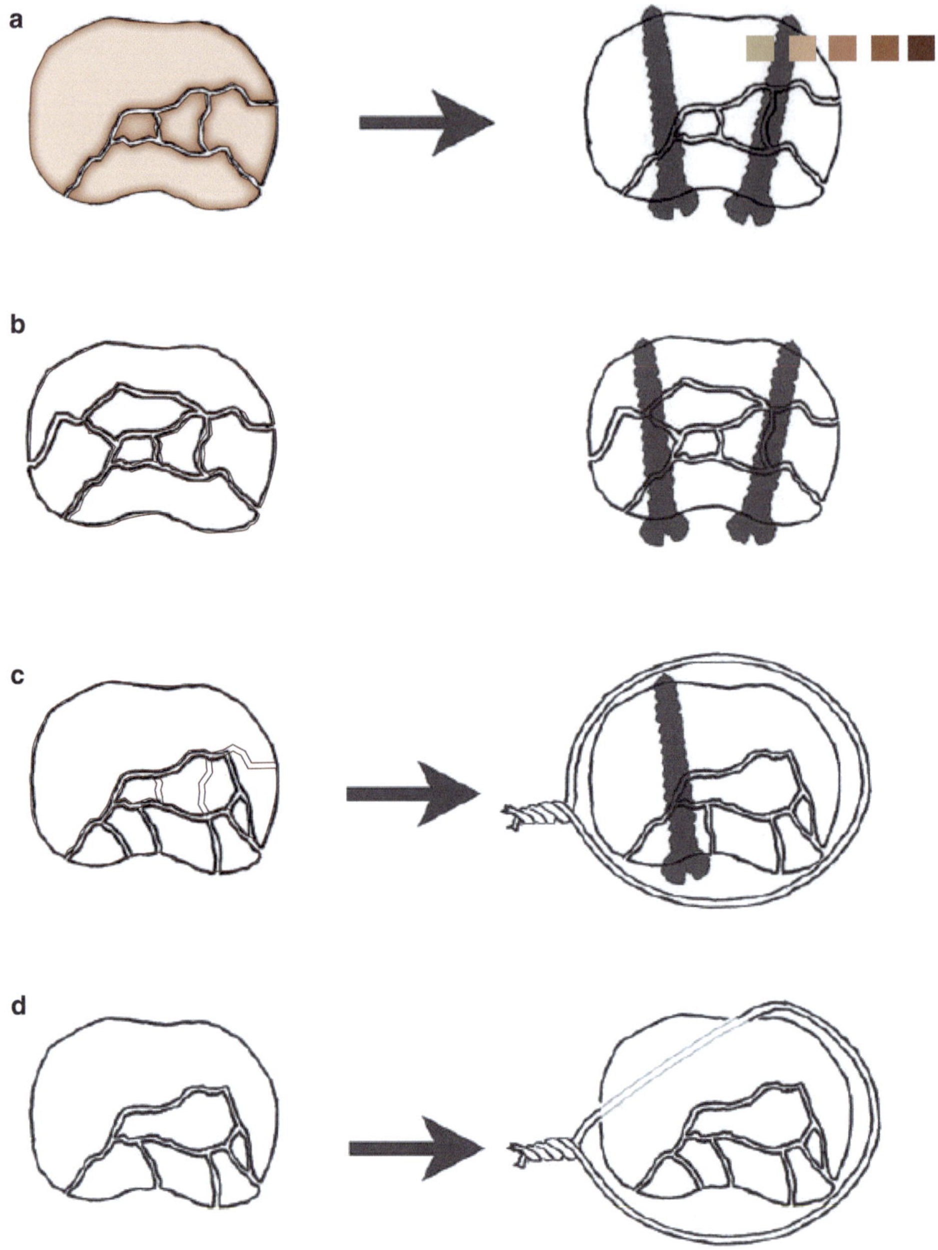

Fig. 4.9 Intra-articular phalangeal base malunions. Treatment is predicated on the comminution of the volar lip using a cerclage wire and screw fixation. (**a**–**b**) lack of volar lip comminution allows screw fixation alone. (**c**–**d**) cerclage wire fixation of the comminuted volar lip

There are several small series of published results of treating intra-articular malunion. Surgeons have presented their results of treating both head and base fractures. Del Piñal and colleagues treated middle phalangeal base fractures with intra-articular osteotomy and revision fixation, using a combination of cerclage wire with or without interfragmentary screw fixation (Fig. 4.9), and achieved good pain relief and functional range of motion in all of their patients. Nine of ten patients were reported as satisfied with the results [26]. Another series were reported in proximal phalanx condylar malunions. Five of six patients demonstrated 50–95° of improved motion after the procedure. A poor result occurred in an osteoporotic digit, which required prolonged protection and developed arthrofibrosis. Jupiter presents the argument for treating established unicondylar malunions of the phalangeal heads with extra-articular closing wedge osteotomy in his series of five patients which had marked improvement (within 1° of anatomic alignment and 50° improvement in range of motion) and which avoids the stiffness that often accompanies intra-articular surgery [27]. Although the long-term outcome of these osteotomies is not known, the procedure restores alignment, preserves bone stock, and potentially maximizes motion.

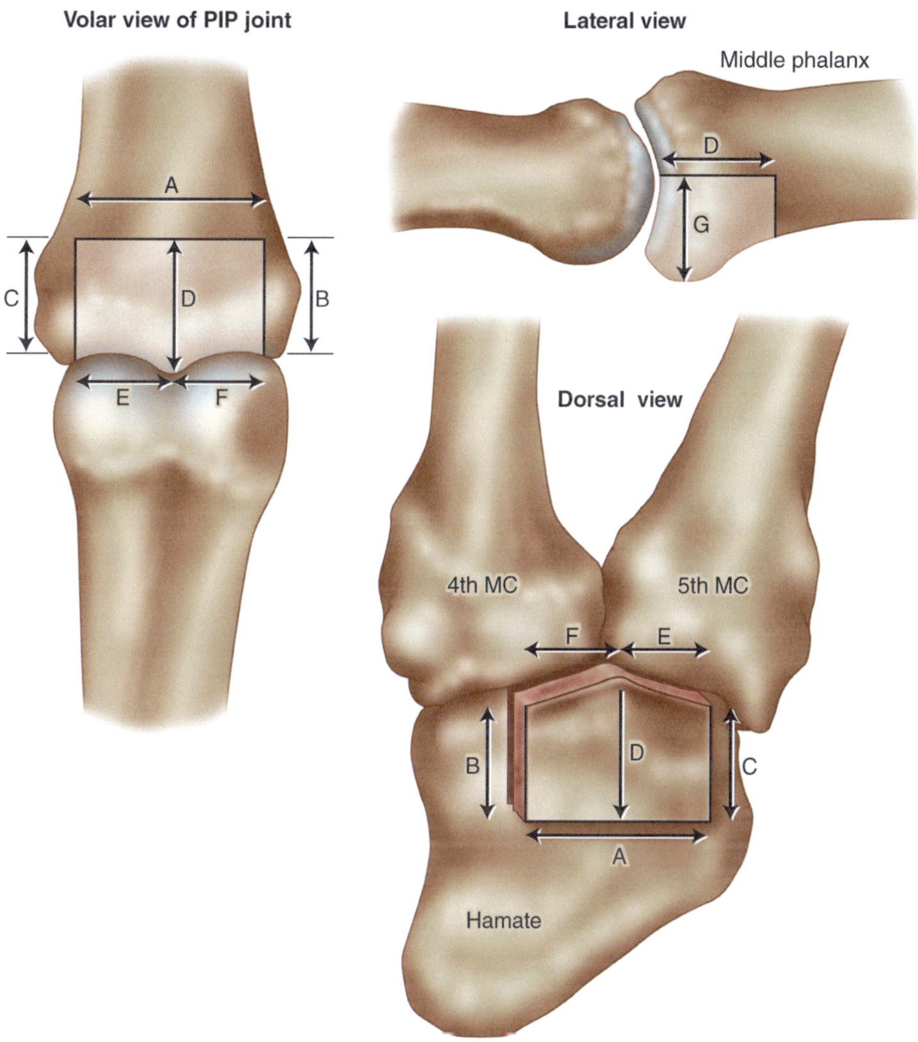

Fig. 4.10 The schematic for hemi-hamate arthroplasty for treatment of PIP fracture-dislocation. The distal hamate articulation is used as an osteochondral graft for the volar lip of the middle phalanx

Hemi-hamate Arthroplasty

A technique to specifically address dorsal fracture dislocations of the proximal interphalangeal joint, which involves a large segment of the volar lip of the middle phalanx, is hemi-hamate arthroplasty (Fig. 4.10). The indications for this technique include unstable comminuted palmar lip PIP fracture-dislocations, as well as lateral plateau middle phalanx fractures treated acutely. It can also be used in the reoperative setting for salvage of a persistently unstable PIP despite prior ex-fix or attempted ORIF/volar plate arthroplasty. Damages to the proximal phalangeal head acutely or due to arthritis are contraindications because they preclude a well functioning articulation after reconstruction.

This modification of osteochondral grafting, which was first described in 1999 by Hastings, involves transferring the distal articular surface of the hamate to the volar lip of the middle phalanx [28]. Providing a congruent joint reduces the propensity for subluxation, and the rigid fixation allows for early mobilization. Stern et al. presented the results of this technique with average 85° range of PIP motion, good pain relief, and 11 of 12 patients satisfied. Two patients were noted to have recurrent dorsal subluxation, but without functional limitations [29].

Nonunion

Metacarpal and phalangeal fractures usually heal within 3–6 weeks. Open fractures may take more time and are frequently clinically healed long before radiographic consolidation. The diagnosis of delayed union or nonunion is therefore vague. Some authors have proposed that at least 12 months must pass before a diagnosis of nonunion in a hand fracture can be

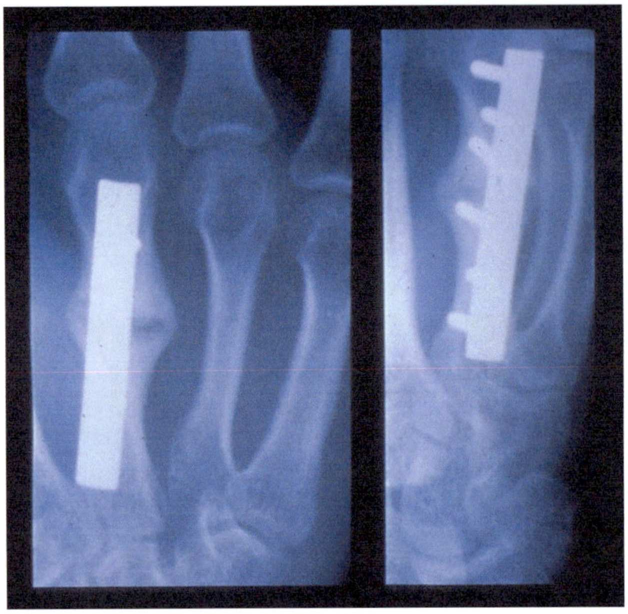

Fig. 4.11 Hypertrophic delayed union

made. Others have proposed that a functional approach is a more accurate gauge of fracture union. In practice, those fractures that have been immobilized for 12–16 weeks but continue to have pain and radiographic fracture motion or lucency are to be treated as nonunions. The basis of this approach is the clinical impression that prolonged immobilization of a finger beyond 3–4 months is associated with dramatically compromised digital function and that an aggressive approach is thus demanded. Nonunions occur more frequently in crush-type injuries and involve the proximal phalanx more often than the other phalanges or metacarpals. This is in part due to the increased frequency of proximal phalanx fractures compared to other phalangeal fractures. In addition, the fracture environment of a phalanx is less amenable to healing than the muscular bed that envelops metacarpal fractures. Although in most reported nonunions the initial fracture treatment consisted of either external splints or K-wires, the causal relationship between initial bony treatment and the subsequent failure to heal has not yet been established. It is more likely that the mechanisms of injury, rather than fixation methods, predispose a fracture to nonunion. In order to properly plan surgery, nonunion type must be assessed (Fig. 4.11). As in long bone surgery, hypertrophic nonunion presents with abundant callous and is treated with the application of rigid fixation. Atrophic unions, on the other hand, require bone grafts. In this setting, if fixation is inadequate, it is replaced. Although segmental bone loss can be managed in several ways, autografts remain the mainstay of hand reconstruction with the role of allograft, bone transfers, and distraction osteogenesis still being defined.

In a series of 25 patients with delayed union or nonunion, the recommended treatment varied from the replacement of K-wires to fixation with plates and screws [30]. The need for bone graft was defined by parameters previously described. The 25 nonunions healed within 7–16 weeks. In 9 of 14 patients, there was an improvement in digit range of motion. All patients felt that hand function improved with fracture union. By objective measure, hand strength improved in each case after the fractures were united.

Bone Loss

Most traumatic bone defects of the hand are associated with severe soft-tissue injuries. The management of these complex combined injuries requires thorough debridement, skeletal stabilization, and soft-tissue reconstruction (Fig. 4.12). The timing for each reconstructive step is becoming better defined. Recent protocols for complex injuries to the upper extremity emphasize removal of all doubtfully viable tissue, thereby creating a wound that resembles a defect after the resection of a locally aggressive tumor. These wounds are made ready for early coverage or closure. For example, a series of patients with bone defects resulting primarily from gunshot wounds were treated with plate fixation and open cancellous autograft. These ten hand injuries healed without infection, required 30 weeks to unite, and resulted in satisfactory function in all but one patient [31]. In another series, immediate corticocancellous autograft for 12 open type III fractures of the hand united within 18 weeks with no infections and total active motion at MPs and IPs of nearly 180° [32, 33]. Soft-tissue defects with exposed vessels and tendons require vascularized soft-tissue reconstruction. Negative pressure wound dressings are helpful adjuncts but are not a substitute for reconstructions that allow early mobilization.

For complex articular defects, the techniques of bone grafting and arthrodesis can be combined. Buchler and Aiken [34] reported on 18 patients with proximal interphalangeal joint osseous defects, extensor tendon loss, and soft-tissue defects that were treated with proximal interphalangeal joint arthrodesis using a solid block of iliac crest secured by plate and screws. If the distal interphalangeal joint was not destroyed, the extensor mechanism for the distal interphalangeal joint was repaired primarily using tendon grafts when necessary. These procedures require exceptionally good bone carpentry (Fig. 4.13). The value of their careful technique was the restoration of digit length, arthrodesis in a functional position, preservation of distal joint motion (when available), and infection-free healing in all but one case.

In the past, metacarpal defects have been treated with autogenous iliac crest grafts. Alternative autograft sources are presented in a series of 21 patients with hand and wrist defects secondary to either trauma or tumor resection [35].

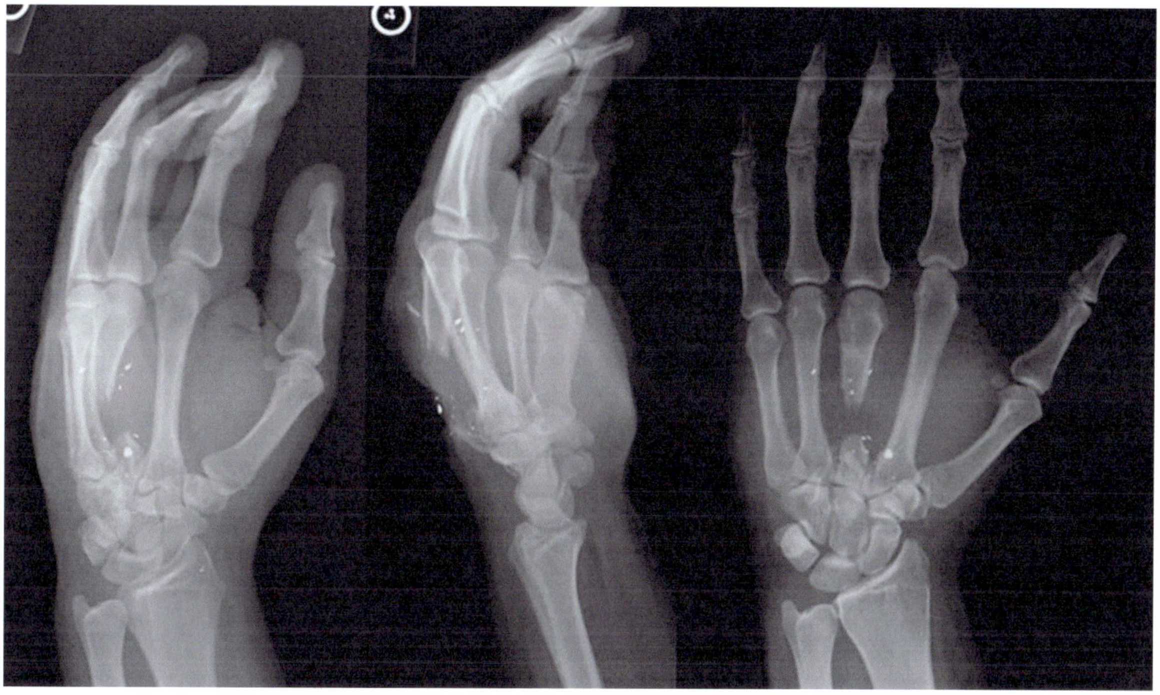

Fig. 4.12 Metacarpal bone loss after gunshot wound

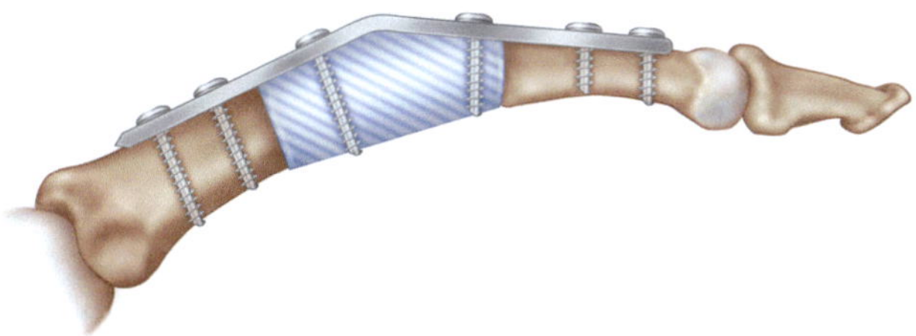

Fig. 4.13 Cortical cancellous composite graft with plate and screw for PIP arthrodesis in the setting of PIP joint destruction

Metacarpal or phalangeal defects were treated with the diaphyseal-metaphyseal metatarsal segments in 11 cases. Four cases were treated with corticocancellous segments of ulna, and three cases were treated with iliac crest. Fixation included "bone impingement" or K-wire fixation followed by prolonged immobilization. Although all the grafts were eventually incorporated, no patient gained more than 60% of digit motion, and eight had significantly less. Skeletal stabilization has also been obtained with allograft bone. There are no studies comparing the efficacy of autogenous bone graft to banked allograft or bone graft substitutes. Allograft lacks the osteogenic and osteoinductive capabilities of autograft. However, enthusiastic advocates of allograft reconstruction argue that the architectural similarity of the graft minimizes manipulation, accommodates rigid fixation, and avoids donor site morbidity as well as the need for general anesthesia. In addition, osteoarticular grafts can be used for reconstruction of joint surfaces. If the entire joint must be reconstructed, the volar plate may be split and advanced to the radial and ulnar aspects of the base to reconstruct the collateral ligaments (Fig. 4.14). Clinical examples of wrist, metacarpal head, proximal phalanx, and middle phalanx replacement have been reported. The allograft-native bone interface appears to heal without a problem. The clinical outcome is reported as being good, but no parameters for this conclusion are given [36]. The quoted rate of HIV transmission for all types of allograft is one per million. The risk is substantially less for lyophilized bone.

Distraction osteogenesis has been used to lengthen digits. There is no additional clinical information to add to the original work of Matev. In his 20 years experience, lengthenings of 3 cm will heal spontaneously in children, but more often than not require grafting in adults [37]. Finsen and Russwurm [38] were able to avoid grafting 3-cm defects by prolonged external fixation, 10 months, in their nine adult patients.

Amputation

Patients with chronic dysfunctional digits will often gain significant benefit from amputation. Motion in the remainder of the hand typically improves once unhampered by the stiff digit. Although patients typically retain 80% of pinch and grip strength following acute injuries, strength can diminish up to 50% in patients with chronic problems. Border digit amputations have less effect on the hand than central rays [39].

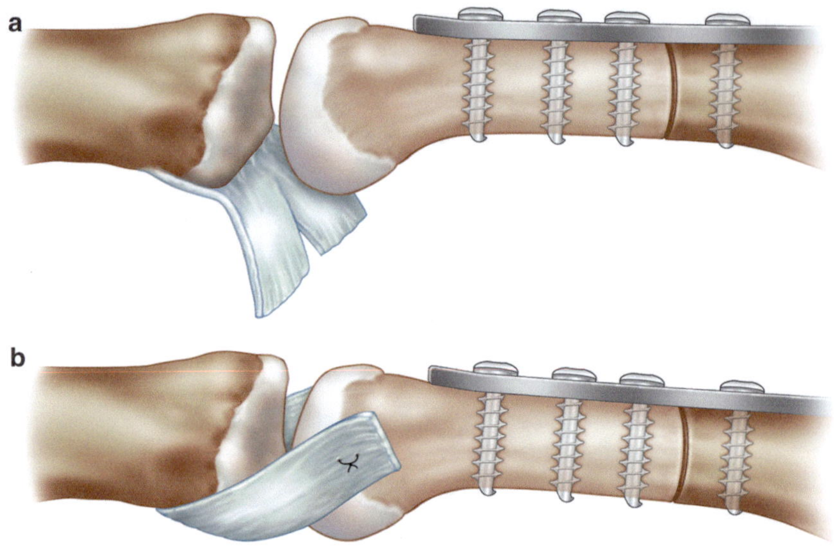

Fig. 4.14 After transfer of a composite metacarpal head and shaft allograft, ligamentous stabilization is provided by the figure split volar plate

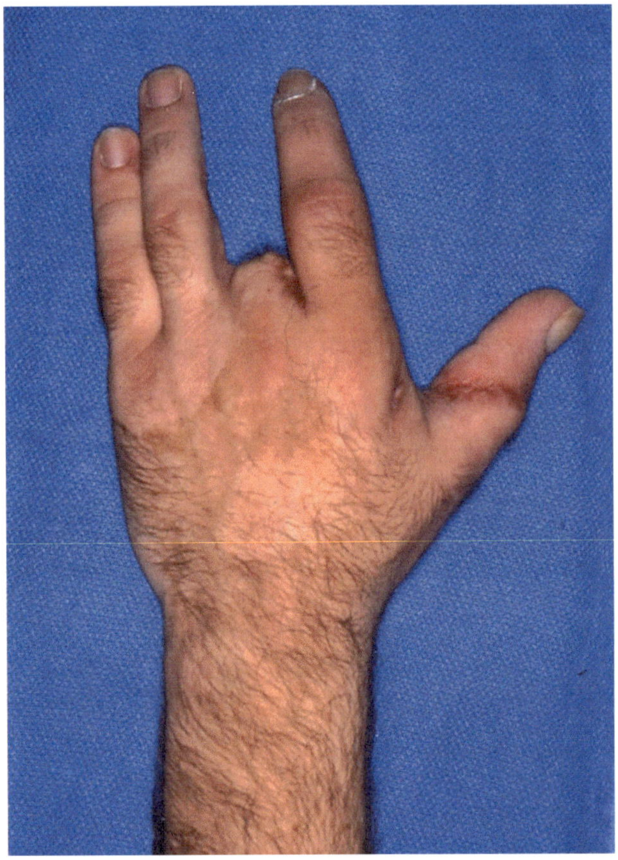

Fig. 4.15 After central ray amputation, the hand is left with a gap. The hand is unsightly and has impairment in grasping small objects (such as change)

Transposition/Amputation

Severe chronic bony deformities of the finger force the patient and physician to choose between multiple reconstructive procedures or amputation. Single digits with chronic combined injuries, especially if associated with an unreconstructable nerve loss, are best amputated. Border digit amputation is rather straightforward, especially when caution has been taken to minimize neuroma formation, and adequate skin flaps allow tension-free wound closure. Central digit amputations are unique in that the hand is rendered increasingly more unsightly and clumsy as the level of amputation approaches the metacarpal phalangeal joint (Fig. 4.15). The accepted management of this problem is ray resection. Critics have noted that ray transposition, as a means to close this gap, is frequently associated with a high incidence of malunion or nonunion and subsequent loss of hand function because of prolonged immobilization. These complications are more likely to occur with K-wire fixation and cast immobilization and can be obviated with rigid internal fixation.

Another technique for approximation of adjacent rays following amputation is carpal wedge osteotomy (Fig. 4.16). Advocates of this procedure feel that in the case of ring finger ray resections, simple approximation markedly limits carpometacarpal motion, changes the divergence of the third and fifth digits, and thereby limits the functional outcome. Wedge osteotomy of the capitate is felt to provide better results after long finger resection because it does not compromise the first web space, does not require prolonged

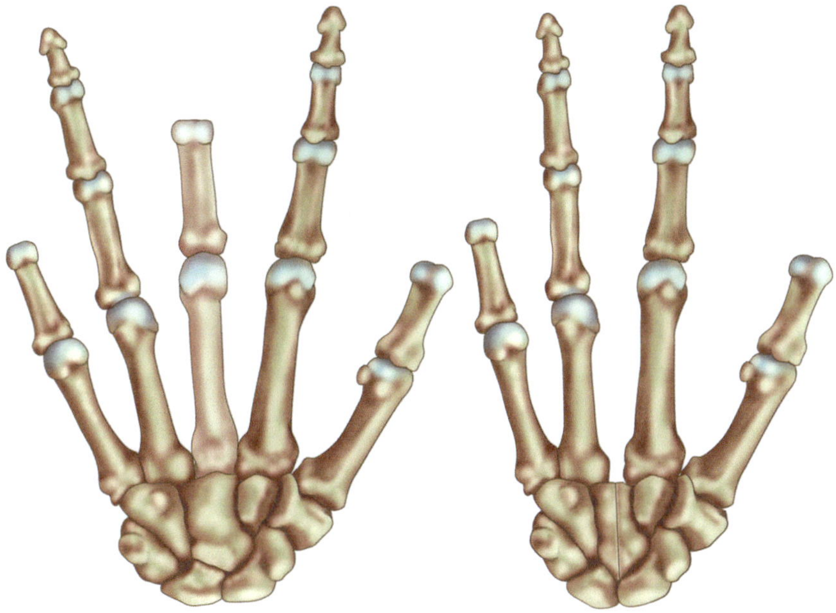

Fig. 4.16 Diagrammatic representation of amputation of third ray and V-shaped osteotomy of the capitate

immobilization, or leave a painful index metacarpal stump. However, these theoretical concerns do not appear to manifest in clinical practice. There are no long-term studies that address the effect of carpal osteotomy on intercarpal dynamics or the potential for development of intercarpal arthritis. The functional results of successful wedge osteotomy are reported to be similar to the other reported methods and cosmetically superior according to the authors [40].

Preoperative History and Considerations

Patients will typically present with a recent or remote history of trauma. The timing of the trauma and the results of treatment so far are critically important pieces of the history. Correcting nascent malunions is likely more problematic than rehabilitating an established malunion. It is imperative to maximize motion and mature the wound bed before attempting correction to avoid the cumulative insult from multiple surgeries.

A history of infection should persuade the surgeon to consider arthrodesis over arthroplasty. Furthermore, patients whose vocations or avocations place high demands on the digit may also be better candidates for fusion. Despite evolving technologies, arthroplasty has had only mediocre long-term results up to this point. It may be especially poorly suited for radial-sided digits which can develop lateral instability from pinch.

An additional portion of the history is identifying the patient's functional deficits. This lies in contrast to anatomic and radiographic abnormalities. Counseling patients on the goals of surgery will help establish patient expectations and maximize satisfaction with the outcome.

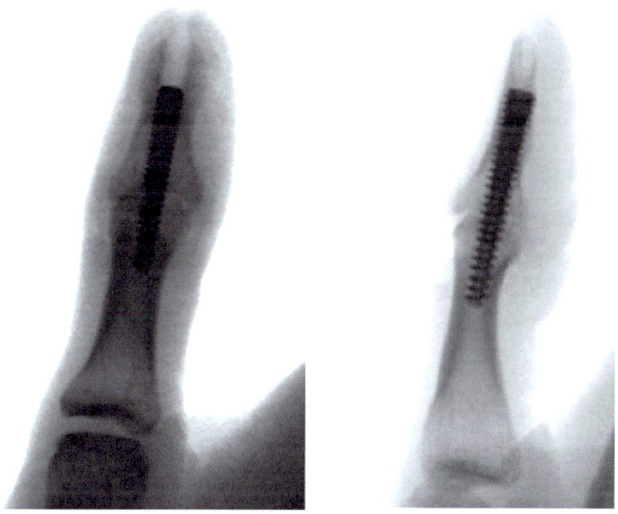

Fig. 4.17 DIP fusion and thumb IP fusion is performed from a dorsal approach with headless screw fixation

Operative Approach

Arthrodesis

There are numerous techniques for arthrodesis. Different methods of fixation are utilized, some based on preference, others unique to the fusion site. Successful arthrodesis demands minimal periosteal dissection, accurate coaptation of medullary bone, and maximizing circumferential contact of cortical bone.

For DIP arthrodesis, or thumb IP arthrodesis, we prefer a T or H-shaped dorsal incision centered over the joint with headless screw fixation (Fig. 4.17). The disadvantage of this

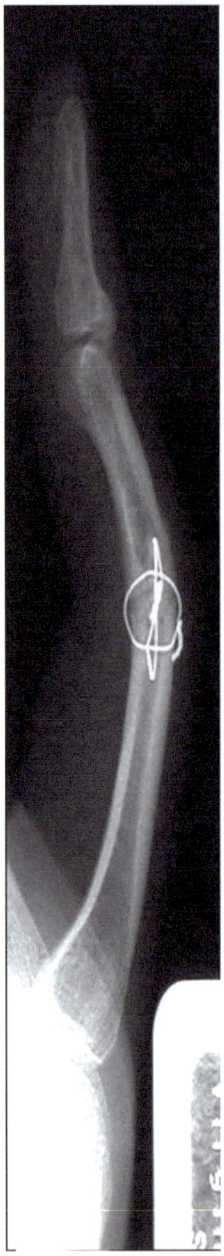

Fig. 4.18 PIP fusion with 90–90 intraosseous wiring

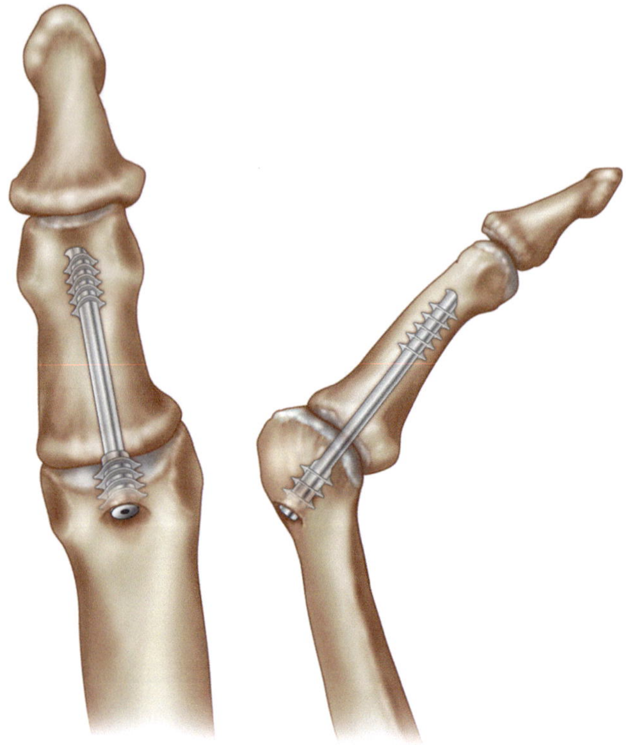

Fig. 4.19 PIP fusion with headless screw fixation

method is that it does not permit arthrodesis in flexion greater than 5°, despite slight beveling of the joint surfaces. If the patient requires greater flexion, an alternative technique is radial/ulnar intraosseous wiring with an additional stabilizing longitudinal K-wire as described by Lister [11].

For PIP arthrodesis, we approach dorsally, establish the flexion with a beveled osteotomy, and use 90–90 intraosseous wires for fixation (Fig. 4.18). We often augment this with a longitudinal K-wire. Holes for passing the 24- or 25-gauge wire can be made with either a 0.035 K-wire or a 20-gauge hollow needle with the hub removed [13]. Adequately clearing the soft tissues facilitates both passing and retrieving the wire through the lumen of the needle. Alternatively, a headless screw can be used for fixation (Fig. 4.19).

Arthrodesis of either the thumb CMC or thumb MP is accomplished using a dorsal exposure and rigid plate and screws fixation (Fig. 4.20).

The thumb CMC joint is exposed via an incision just ulnar to the EPB tendon that extends from the scaphotrapezial (ST) joint to the mid or distal one-third of the metacarpal shaft. The radial artery crossing the ST joint is identified and protected. Severely eroded CMC joints can be prepared in a cup-in-cone fashion with a burr to preserve bone that otherwise would be removed in a transverse preparation. The thumb metacarpal is positioned by placing the patients hand into a fist, resting the volar aspect of the IP joint of the thumb upon the dorsal radial aspect of the index middle phalanx. Provisional fixation with a 0.062 K-wire from either the radial or ulnar side of the metacarpal avoids interfering with plate application. Various 2.0–2.7-mm T-plates, blade plates, or newer locking plates can be used to gain rigid fixation across the arthrodesis site (Fig. 4.21). Ideally, there should be two points of fixation in the trapezium and three screws in the metacarpal shaft. Two pitfalls are failing to appreciate STT arthritis and failing to use bone graft when necessary. The first can be avoided by direct inspection of a radiographically suspicious ST joint via arthrotomy. The second pitfall can be avoided by considering using graft if there is less than 50% bony apposition at the fusion site.

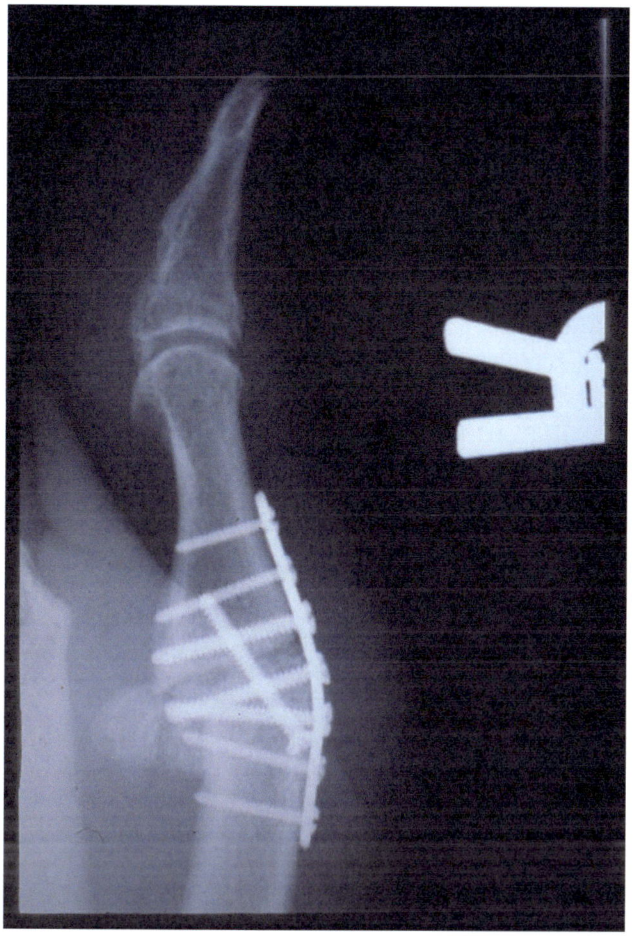

Fig. 4.20 Thumb MP fusion with plate and screws with a lag screw replacing the initial provisional K-wire. Immediate motion was imperative for this one-armed individual

The optimal position for the various joint fusions has been reinforced by a number of authors.

Distal interphalangeal 10–20° flexion[a]	
Proximal interphalangeal 30–45° flexion[a]	
Thumb interphalangeal 10–20° flexion	
Thumb metacarpophalangeal 15° flexion	
Thumb carpometacarpal 30–40° palmar abduction	
30–35° Radial abduction	
~15° Pronation	

[a]Progressing from radial to ulnar

Arthroplasty

There are three described exposures for interphalangeal joint arthroplasty: volar, dorsal, and midlateral. The advantages and disadvantages are summarized in Table 4.1 [41–43]. The authors prefer a volar exposure because it allows immediate mobilization secondary to less compromise of the extensor mechanism (Fig. 4.22).

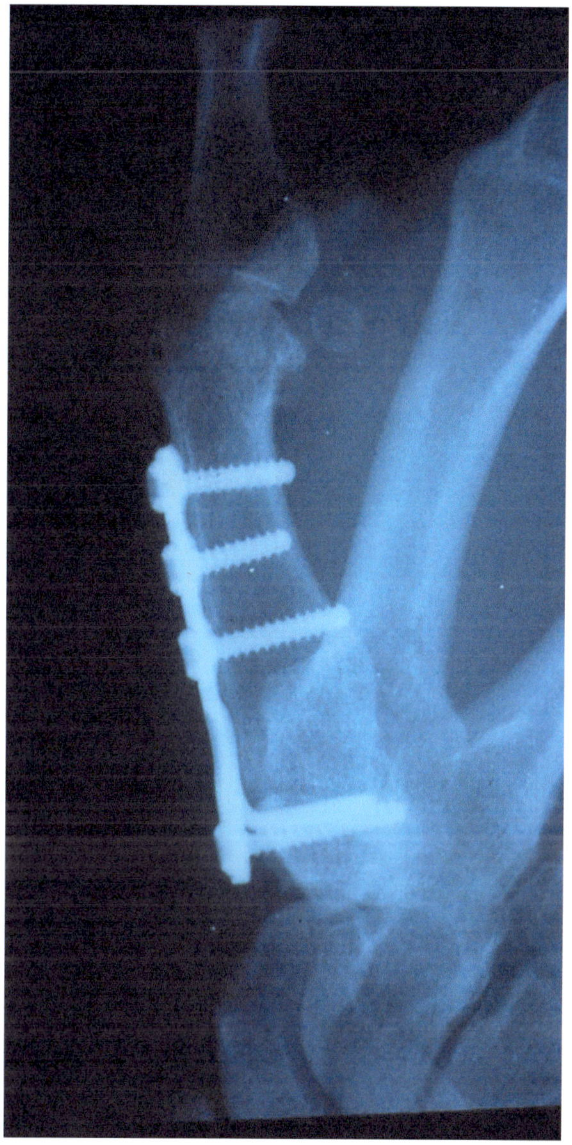

Fig. 4.21 Thumb CMC fusion with a blade plate

Osteotomy for Malunion

Angular Corrective Osteotomy

A simple angular deformity is most easily corrected with a closing wedge osteotomy. Preoperative templating is critical to avoid undercorrection of the deformity. Maintaining a partially intact opposite cortex or periosteum greatly enhances stability of the osteotomy and permits fixation with tension band or intraosseous wiring techniques. Plates and screws may also be used, but excessive soft-tissue dissection can lead to increased extensor adhesions. Radial-ulnar angular malunion can be similarly addressed (Fig. 4.23a–c).

Rotational Osteotomy

Two methods for correction of phalangeal malrotation have been advocated: osteotomy at the site of the malunion and

Table 4.1 Three exposures for interphalangeal joint arthroplasty

Approach	Advantages	Disadvantages
Volar	No disruption of extensor tendon, simplified rehabilitation	Flexion contracture, swan neck deformity
Dorsal	Simpler exposure, direct vision, easier estimation of alignment	Disruption of the extensor mechanism
Midlateral	Preservation of radial collateral ligament of index, middle, and ring fingers and ulnar collateral of small finger; preserves extensor mechanism	Difficult to estimate and correct malalignment; has historically been limited to silicone arthroplasty

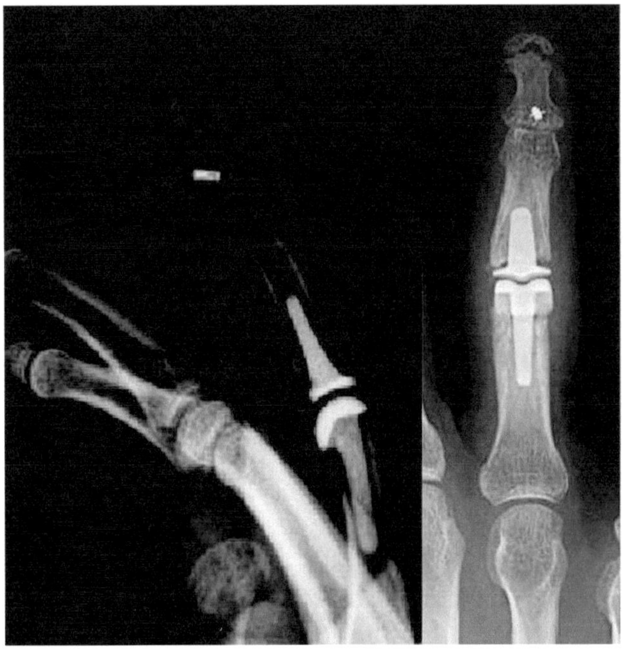

Fig. 4.22 PIP arthroplasty with pyrolytic carbon

proximal osteotomy at the level of the metacarpal. Osteotomy at the malunion site is the easiest to conceptualize and has the greatest potential for correcting the deformity. However, the adjacent flexor and extensor tendons are at greater risk of being injured and developing adhesions.

Proximal metacarpal osteotomy avoids these problems. The benefits of this method are that the longitudinal limb of the osteotomy accommodates greater adjustment and presents a larger surface area for healing. A step-cut osteotomy has been used for both metacarpal and proximal phalanx malunions. Critics of this procedure point out that although metacarpal rotational osteotomy may correct the apparent finger malrotation, there remains rotational malalignment, albeit to a lesser degree, in complete digital flexion. In addition, the digit assumes an S-shaped appearance in full extension; this is the result of two diametrically opposed angular deformities, the traumatic deformity and the correctional osteotomy, separated by 3–4 cm. If complete correction of a malunion is desired, it can only be done by addressing the malunion site. An alternative, used more extensively in the authors' practice, is pure rotational osteotomy (Fig. 4.24a–d).

Articular Malunion Procedures

Using direct visualization, the malaligned joint surface is identified, and the fracture site is taken down. In fractures that are several months old, curetting the maturing callus can reveal the fracture line. If the fracture line is not readily visible, then a radiographically assisted osteotomy is recommended. Care is taken to preserve soft-tissue attachments and to preserve the vascularity of the bone fragments. The fracture is realigned, secured with rigid fixation, and mobilized early (Fig. 4.25a–c).

A newer technique to address dorsal fracture dislocation of the proximal interphalangeal joint is hemi-hamate arthroplasty of the base of the middle phalanx. This modification of osteochondral grafting involves transferring the distal articular surface of the hamate to the volar lip of the middle phalanx (Fig. 4.26). Providing a congruent joint reduces the propensity for subluxation, and the rigid fixation allows early mobilization.

Bone Grafting and Nonunion Procedures

Most authors agree that nonunions in the metacarpals and phalanges can be addressed with nonvascularized bone grafts [44]. The use of allograft bone combined with rigid fixation is our preferred technique for bone loss less than 4 cm. It is clinically effective, eliminates donor site morbidity, and is well incorporated. Although vascularized bone transfers such as medial femoral condyle and radial metaphysis have been described for large segmental defects, the authors have limited experience with these techniques. In addition, composite grafts from the toe are an alternative when soft-tissue coverage is required, or for articular reconstruction.

Numerous authors have shown that early aggressive debridement and soft-tissue coverage followed by bone grafting and rigid fixation is safe and effective. In combined complex proximal interphalangeal joint injuries, with associated bone loss and an unreconstructable joint, a PIP arthrodesis can be accomplished with a solid block of iliac crest secured by a plate and screws. This is employed with tendon grafts to repair the extensor for the distal interphalangeal joint. Obviously, careful attention must be paid to the arthrodesis angle and restoring appropriate length.

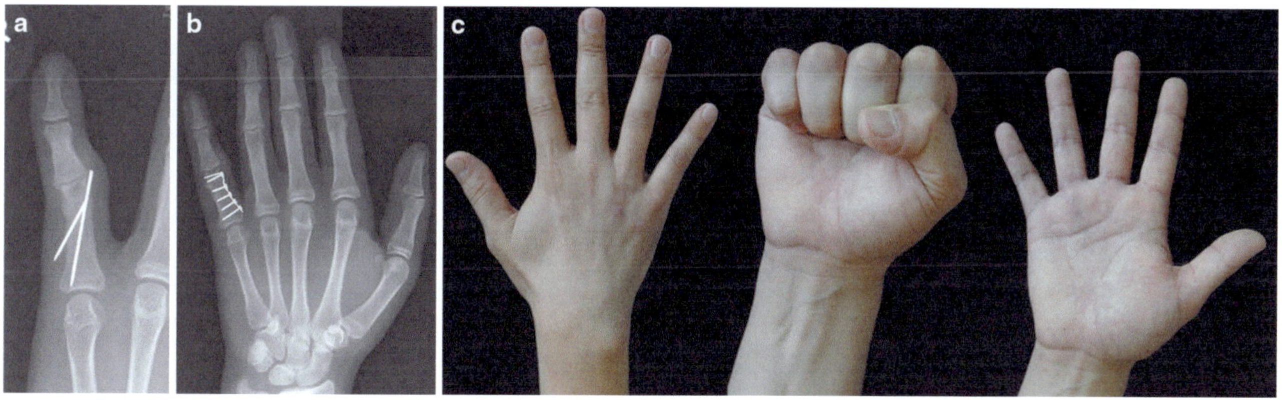

Fig. 4.23 (**a**) Angular malunion. (**b**) After corrective osteotomy of angular malunion. (**c**) Postoperative range of motion was normal

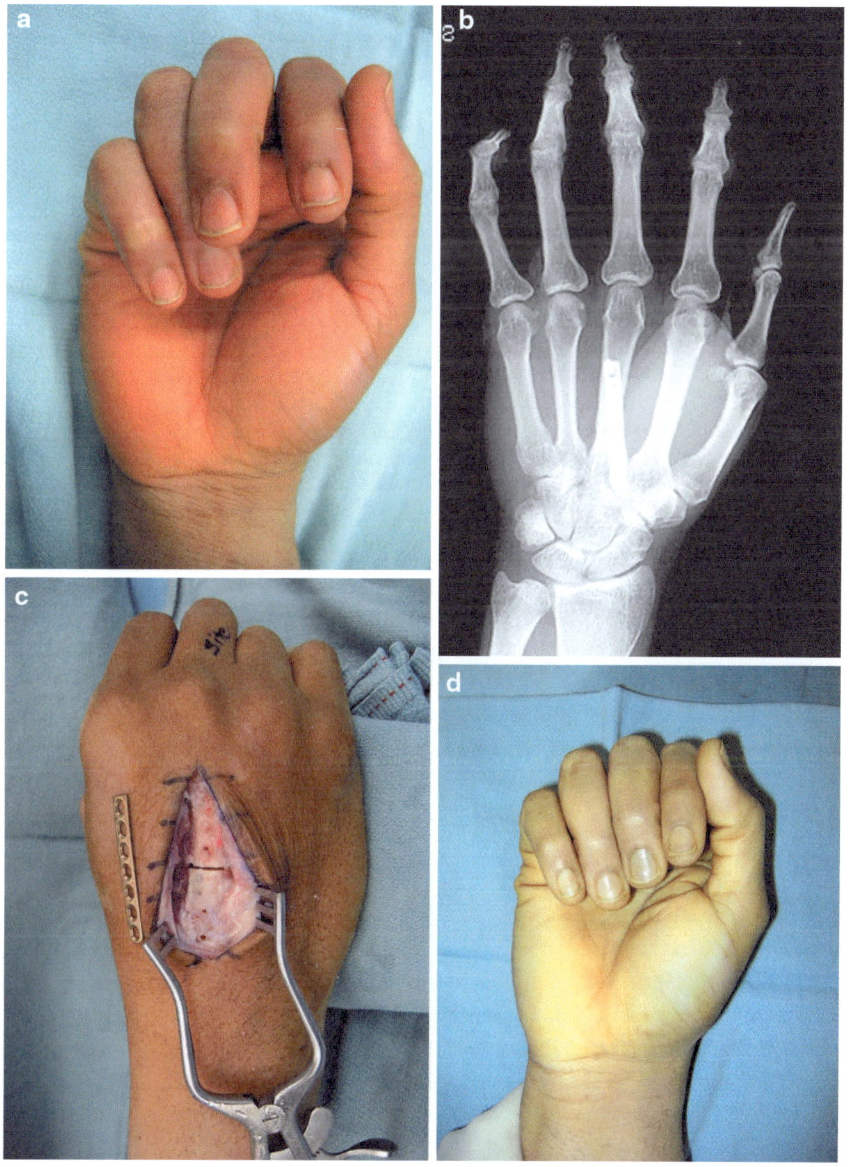

Fig. 4.24 (**a**) Initial clinical presentation reveals scissoring of the digits from rotational malunion. (**b**) Radiographs show previous ORIF in malrotated position. (**c**) Intraoperative pictures show removing the plate and the osteotomy site. (**d**) Corrected alignment after osteotomy and fixation

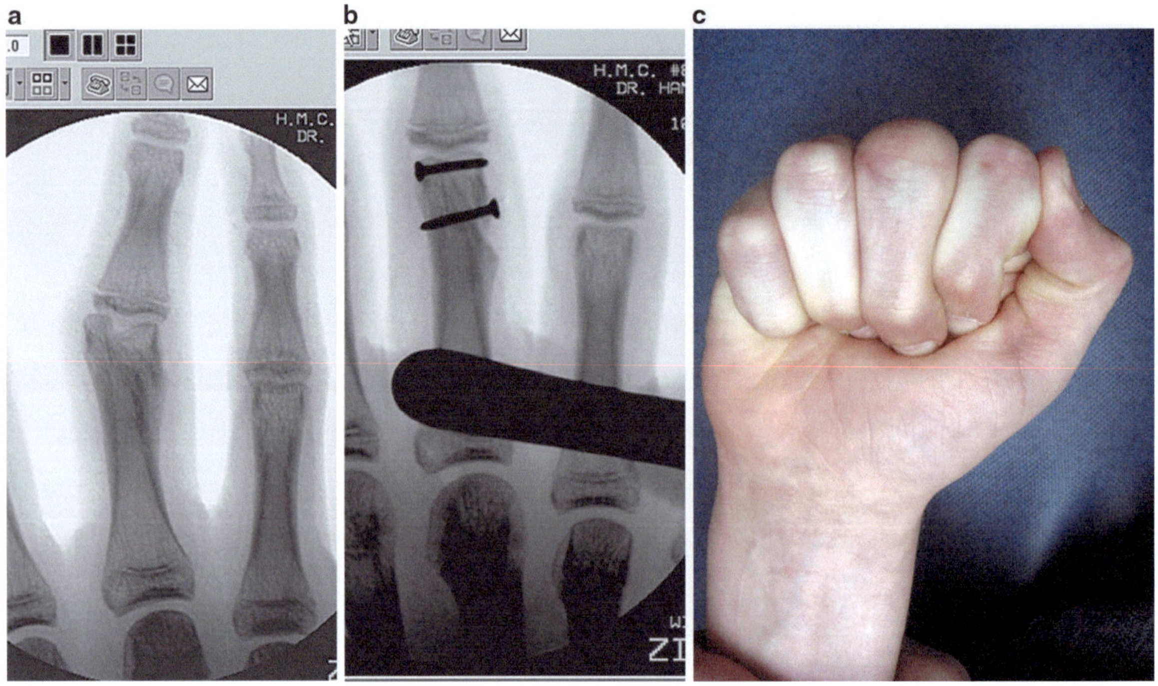

Fig. 4.25 (**a–c**) Unicondylar malunion can be addressed via intra-articular osteotomy and rigid fixation with good postoperative range of motion results

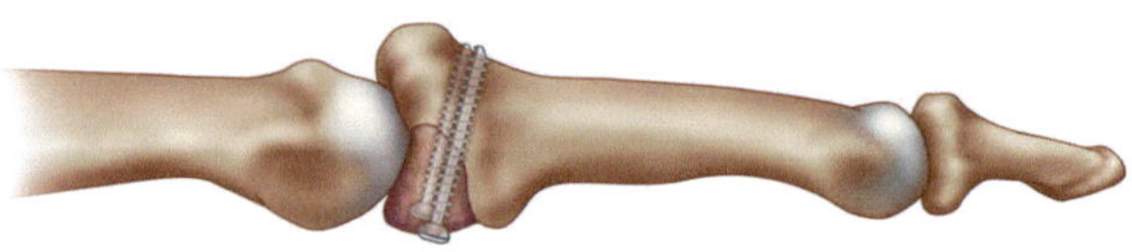

Fig. 4.26 Hemi-hamate arthroplasty. The distal hamate articulation has been harvested and transferred to the resected volar lip of the middle phalanx. The curvature of base must not be too flat in order to prevent dorsal subluxation of P2

Although metacarpal defects can be treated with the diaphyseal-metaphyseal metatarsal or ulna transfer, the authors' preference is to consider iliac crest autograft reconstruction or ray amputation for combined nonsalvageable defects. Previous failed attempts at bone grafting can be addressed with more rigid fixation, even spanning to adjacent metacarpals as needed to enhance stability (Fig. 4.27a, b). Articular nonunions can also be treated with grafting and rigid fixation (Fig. 4.28a–c).

Osteoarticular grafts (Fig. 4.29) can be used for reconstruction of joint surfaces but have not been incorporated in the authors' practice [45].

Thumb reconstruction continues to be the most common indication for bone lengthening. The authors preferred technique utilizes an external fixator and lengthening along a 0.062 longitudinal K-wire. After lengthening, the defects usually require grafting (Fig. 4.30).

Transposition

Although there are several techniques for ray resection, the authors' preferred technique following middle ray resection is index ray transposition to the middle ray position [46] (Fig. 4.31a–c). To perform the transposition, the long finger is exposed by means of palmar and dorsal zigzag incisions. The second web space is preserved from the radial or ulnar half of the long finger as further described below. The extrinsic tendons are divided, and the long finger metacarpal is dissected subperiosteally. A 2.7-mm T-shaped plate is preferred. It is placed on the proximal aspect of the long finger metacarpal. The transverse limb of the plate is fixed to the metaphyseal flare, and longitudinal limb is aligned with the diaphysis. The osteotomy site is marked between the transverse limb holes and the most proximal hole of the longitudinal limb. The osteotomy is made after the plate is removed, and the long finger is dissected free with care taken to retain the deep transverse intermetacarpal ligaments. The neurovascular structures are divided at the base of the proximal phalanx. Digital vessels are ligated. Digital nerves are sutured to each other end to end. The origin of the adductor pollicis should be tagged and subsequently reapproximated to the radial aspect of the index metacarpal once it is transposed. Once the long finger is delivered from the wound, the index finger is approached, similarly dissected and osteotomized at

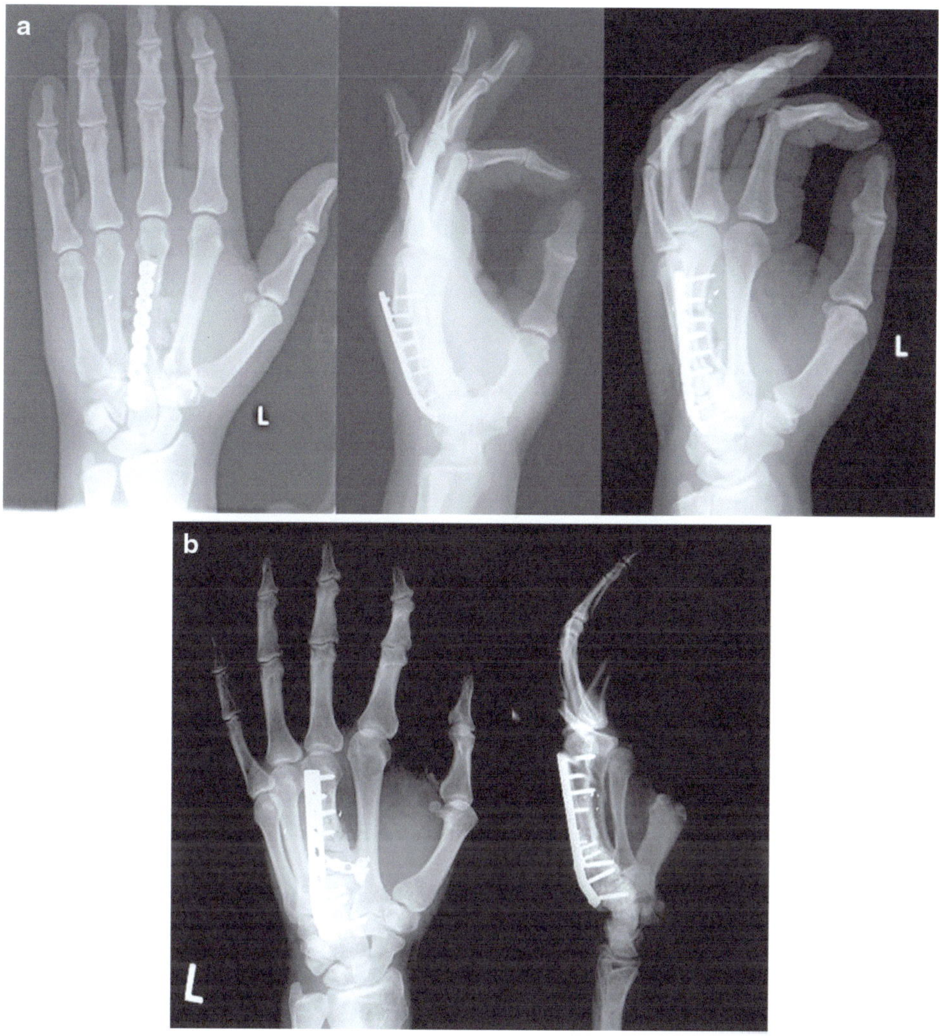

Fig. 4.27 (**a**) The patient in Fig. 4.12 was initially fixed with plate and screws and graft and went on to nonunion and hardware failure. (**b**) Revision ORIF and grafting, spanning to adjacent metacarpal to augment fixation

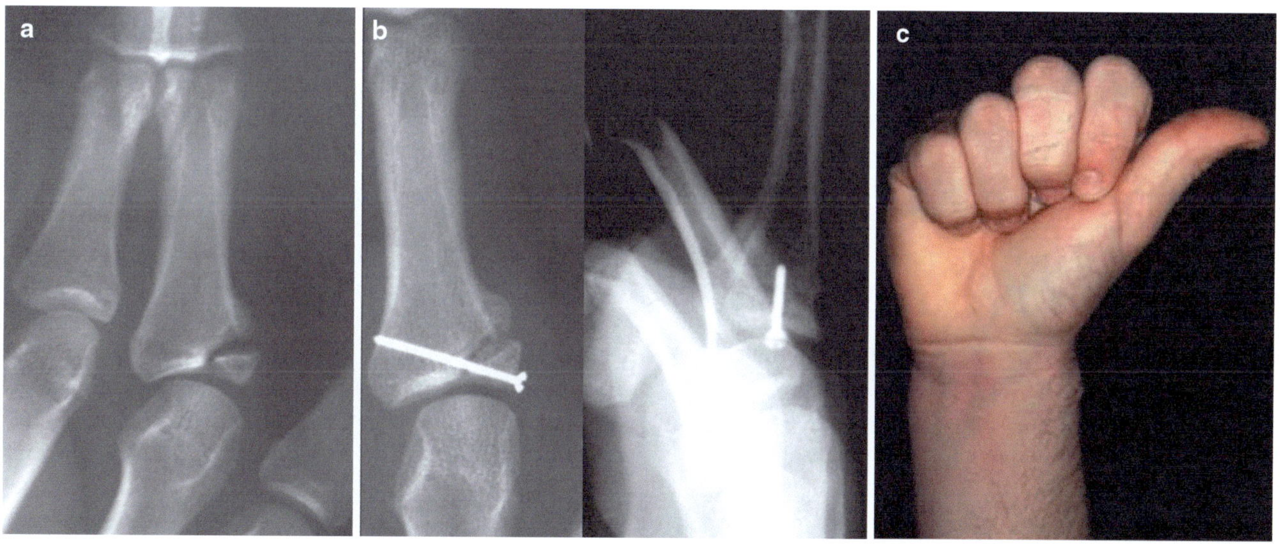

Fig. 4.28 (**a**) Symptomatic articular nonunion. (**b**) Care was taken to not over reduce the joint surface; therefore, the impacted cancellous portion was grafted followed by rigid fixation. (**c**) Postoperative range of motion

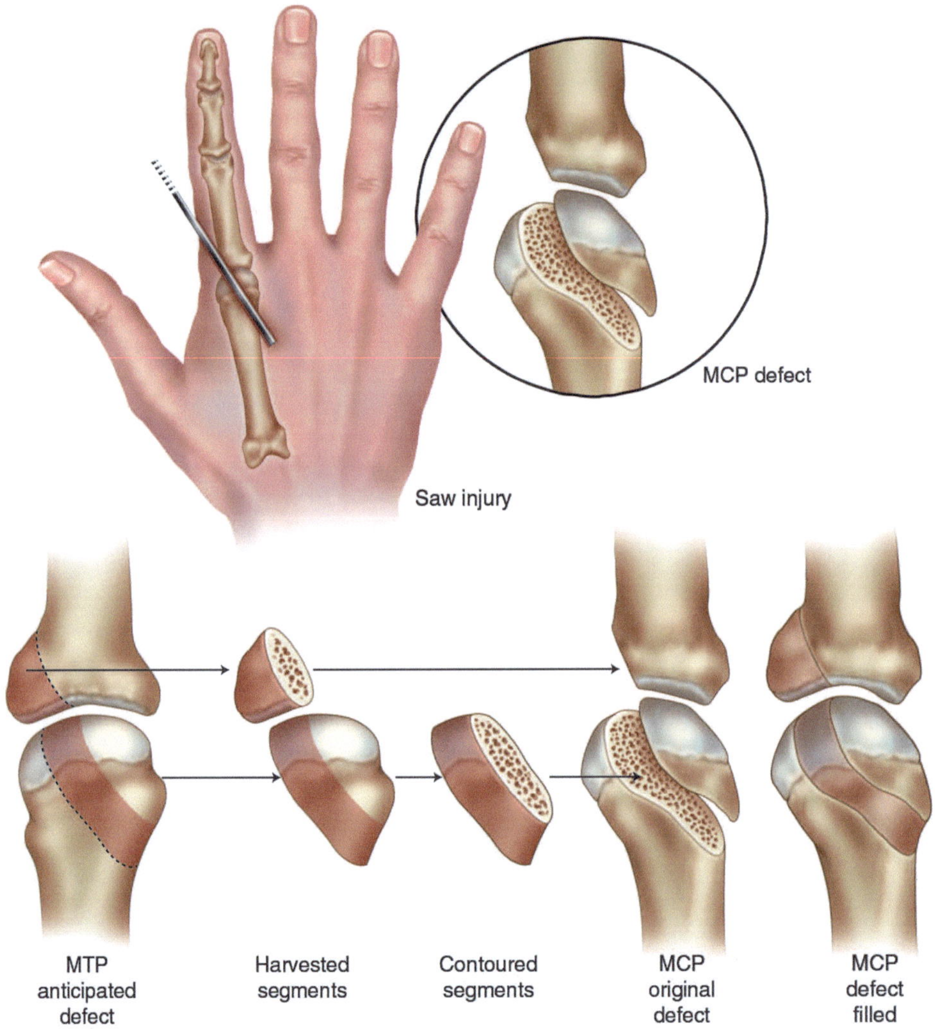

Fig. 4.29 Osteochondral autograft from the toe for segmental articular defects

the proximal metaphyseal flare. The metacarpal heads of the index and ring are aligned in height and provisionally fixed with a transverse K-wire into the ring metacarpal. Rotation is best judged with MCP joints in flexion; the fingers should point toward the scaphoid tubercle. Excess bone is then removed from the index metacarpal osteotomy site, and the osteosynthesis is accomplished in the standard fashion. Our preferred method for ring finger ray resection is complete disarticulation of the fourth CMC joint. In the setting of a damaged third metacarpal base or distal end of the capitate, a wedge resection of the capitate closes the intermetacarpal gap. In addition to closing the gap, reconstruction of central ray amputations requires preservation of the web space to assure a cosmetically attractive hand and minimizes hand dysfunction. This is best accomplished by retaining the skin from either the radial or ulnar aspect of the amputated proximal phalanx and insetting the entire web space into the adjacent digit, as presented by Plaaschaert and Hage [47]. Because of the mobility of the ring and small finger carpometacarpal joint, it has been recommended that after central ray resection, the gap between metacarpal heads can be closed by imbricating adjacent deep transverse intermetacarpal ligaments, as described by Steichen and Idler [48]. Patients with ring finger amputations are reported to have no problems following web reconstruction, digital rotation, or overall hand appearance after simple approximation and ligament imbrication. However, some patients with long finger amputations treated by this method note that the index and ring finger tend to cross as closure of the gap was completed. Although this is a potential cosmetic and functional problem, these patients were reported to be satisfied with the results of their amputation and reconstruction.

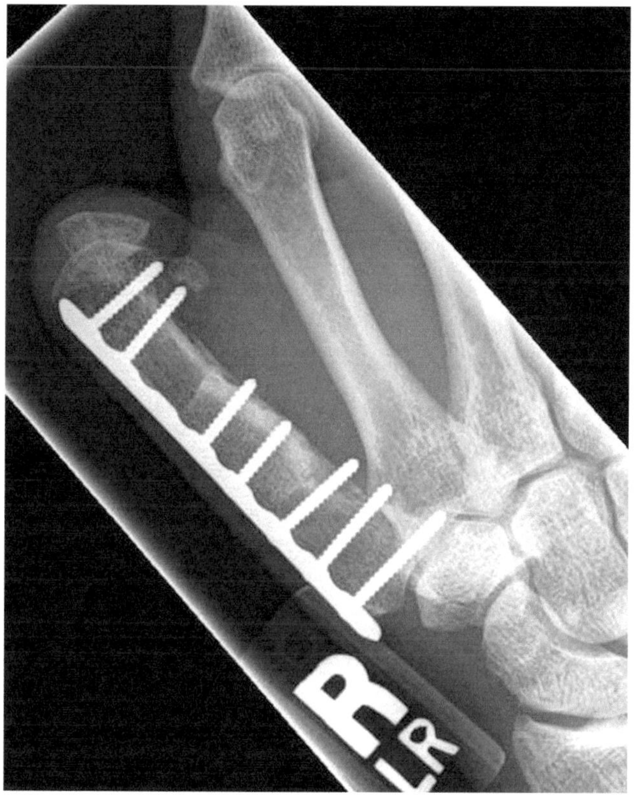

Fig. 4.30 Thumb metacarpal lengthening (with subsequent bone grafting) after amputation as an alternative to toe-to-thumb transfer. This procedure is often combined with first web space deepening

Optimizing Outcomes

Optimum outcomes are achieved by a combination of the following:

- A cooperative patient that both perceives a problem with the hand and is willing to participate in therapy before and after surgery.
- Realistic expectations from both the patient and the surgeon.
- Timing surgery to coincide with limited inflammation, edema, and maximized range of motion. This means that there has been no improvement in motion, or in fracture healing, for a period of 12 consecutive weeks. The one exception is an obvious intra-articular malalignment.

Complications and Side Effects

Stiffness

Difficulty with range of motion is common after operations on the digits. This is especially true in the case of the multiply operated hand. This is minimized by achieving rigid fixation and avoiding extensive capsular dissection. Where possible, plates are placed away from the gliding surface of the extensor tendons. With this approach, and adequate pain control, patients can fully participate in therapy. The goals of therapy are edema control, desensitization, contracture prevention via assisted range of motion, and splinting.

Residual Deformity

Undercorrection or occasionally overcorrection can occur. Careful preoperative planning, as well as the intraoperative use of K-wires and goniometers to judge actual correction, can be helpful prophylactic tools. When residual deformity occurs, it must be addressed in terms of functional deficits. Cosmesis alone will rarely be improved by further surgery.

Persistent Nonunion

As with an initial nonunion, the cause must be identified. Hypertrophic nonunions are typically treated with enhanced stabilization. Atrophic nonunions need improved vascularity to heal. This most often is derived from various grafts. In actuality, most nonunions are a mixture between these two forms, the so-called oligotrophic nonunion, and can be addressed by rigid fixation and autograft. Gapping at the site of fracture or osteotomy fixation can lead to nonunion and can respond to compression or grafting. Finally, although rare in the hand, persistent nonunion can also be caused by an indolent infection.

Infection

Superficial infection can be treated with oral antibiotics. Deep infection may require formal irrigation and debridement. In the setting of implants, this becomes more difficult as the risk of colonization, especially of an arthroplasty implant, decreases the likelihood of eradicating an infection.

Neurologic Injury

Often reoperative exposure must be more extensive in order to identify, isolate, and protect critical structures outside of the scarred bed. The best technique for prevention of neurologic injury is intimate knowledge of the surgical anatomy and safe initial dissection. Possible subsequent neurologic injury following difficult initial fixation, or anticipated hardware removal, can be assisted by marking key neurologic structures with adjacent small vessel clips as well as thorough

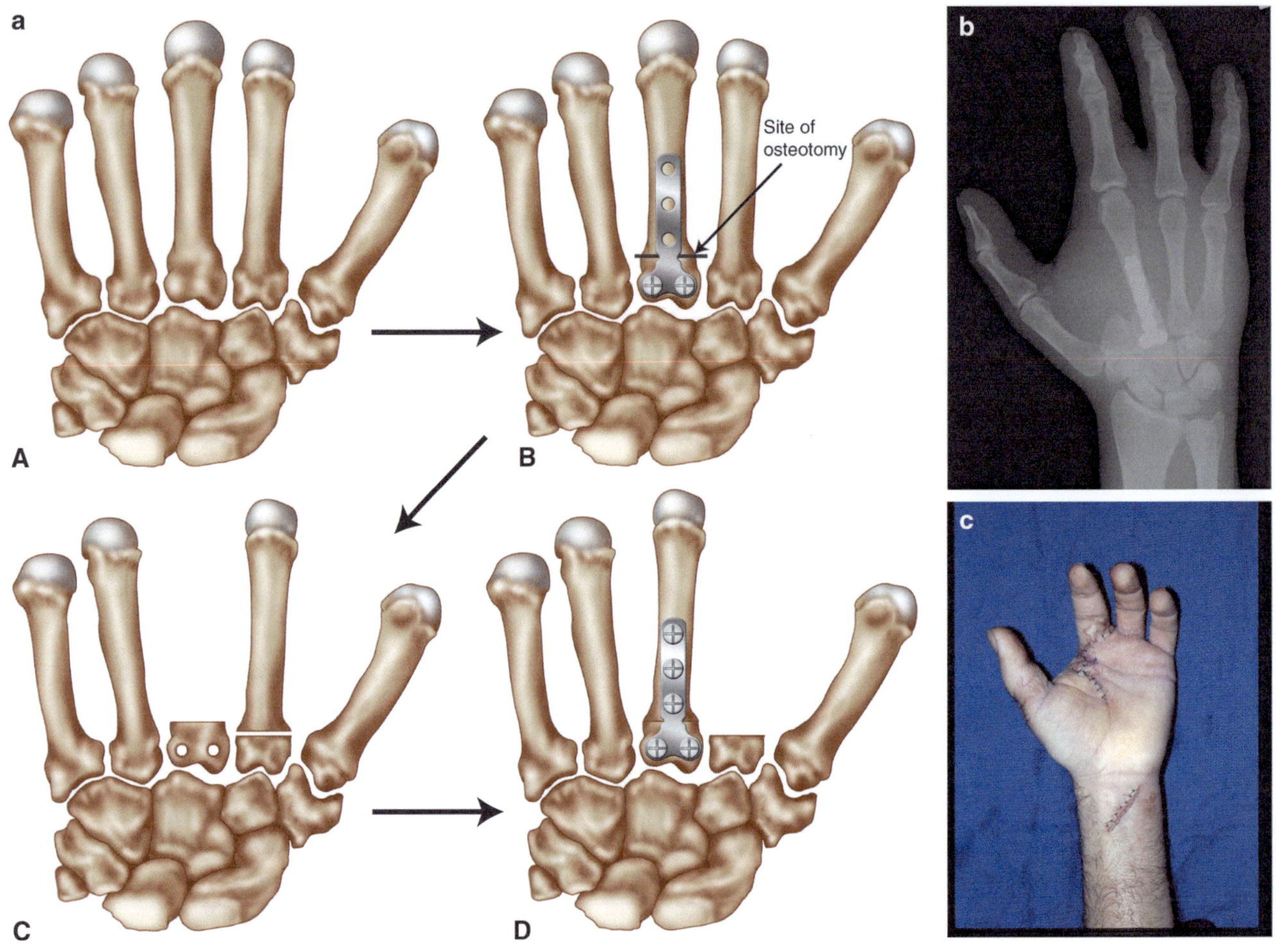

Fig. 4.31 (**a**) Schematic for index ray transposition following middle finger ray amputation. (**b**) Radiographs following index transposition with T-plate. (**c**) Postoperative appearance of patient in Fig. 4.15

description in the operative record of the relationship of nerves to the surgical approach.

Arthritis

Arthritis inevitably complicates articular injuries. Even some injuries with near anatomic articular reduction have sustained chondral injuries that can lead to arthritis. Careful attention to initial reduction is the best preventive tool. Arthrodesis and arthroplasty are the surgical techniques to address the unremitting painful arthritic joint.

Complications Specific to Lengthening

Similar to long bone transport, the most common problems arise from pin tract infections and angulation of the lengthened segment after premature removal of the distraction device. The first problem can be avoided if fixation pins remain firm; the second problem is avoided by postponing removal of the distractor until there is evidence of consolidation along the full length and width of the bone. A third possible problem, angulation while distracting the digit, can be addressed by passing a K-wire down the axis of the finger being lengthened. This may be accompanied by release or Z-plasty techniques for contractures, which may tether the digit as it is lengthened.

Postoperative Care

The basis for therapy is deciding how soon mobilization can begin. The best tool for making this decision is assessing the rigidity of the fixation and documenting this with intraoperative radiographs that can be shared with the therapist and compared to subsequent films. Confirmation of bony consolidation is confirmed with radiographs every 4–6 weeks. In general, our basic approach to reconstructive procedures in the fingers is dictated by the rigidity of the fixation. The more rigid the fixation, the earlier mobilization. A 48–72-h period to allow for acute swelling is essential. In the setting of tenolysis, we mobilize patients sooner with supervised therapy. We closely communicate with the therapists to construct individual plans for patients to include splints for resting posture, timing of progression from active assisted range of motion to unlimited active motion.

As mentioned previously, consideration for revision and/or tenolysis is not made before a patient who has been compliant with therapy has made no improvements for at least 12 consecutive weeks.

Conclusion

There are three things that must be present in the reoperative management of metacarpal and phalangeal fractures to have a successful outcome: a *definable* problem appreciated by the patient and the surgeon, a cooperative patient, and a problem with a surgical solution. Patients should be counseled by their surgeons that the desire to correct a hand deformity must be balanced with the poor tolerance of the hand for multiple operations. However, in the appropriate setting, reoperation can be rewarding for both parties: significantly improving function, decreasing pain, and possibly slowing or preventing the onset of arthritic changes. Because amputation is often reserved for the unsalvageable digit, it is erroneously connoted as a failure. It should, however, be considered reconstructive, as a complement to osteotomy, grafting, arthrodesis, and arthroplasty.

References

1. Carroll RE. Arthrodesis of the carpometacarpal joint of the thumb. A review of patients with a long postoperative period. Clin Orthop. 1987;220:106–10.
2. Burton RL, et al. Small joint arthrodesis in the hand. J Hand Surg. 1986;11A:678–82.
3. Steiger VR, Segmuller G. [Arthrodesis of the metacarpophalangeal joint of the thumb]. Handchir Mikrochir Plast Chir. 1989;21:18–22.
4. Saldana MJ, Clark EN, Aulicino PL. The optimal position for arthrodesis of the metacarpophalangeal joint of the thumb: a clinical study. J Hand Surg. 1987;12B:256–9.
5. Ijsselstein CB, van Egmond DG, Hovius SER, van der Meulen IC. Results of small joint arthrodesis. Comparison of Kirschner wire fixation with tension band wire technique. J Hand Surg. 1992;17A:952–6.
6. Bamberger BH, Stern PI, Kiefhaber TR, McDonough JJ, Cantor RM. Trapeziometacarpal joint arthrodesis: a functional evaluation. J Hand Surg. 1992;17A:605–11.
7. Hartigan B, Stern P, Kiefhaber T. Thumb carpometacarpal osteoarthritis: arthrodesis compared with ligament reconstruction and tendon interposition. J Bone Joint Surg Am. 2001;83A:1470–8.
8. Hagan HJ, Hastings II H. Fusion of the thumb metacarpophalangeal joint to treat posttraumatic arthritis. J Hand Surg Am. 1988;13(5):750–3.
9. Kovach IC, Wemer FW, Palmer AK, Greenkey S, Murphy DI. Biomechanical analysis of internal fixation techniques for proximal interphalangeal joint arthrodesis. J Hand Surg. 1986;11A:562–6.
10. Lewis RC, Nordyke MD, Tenny JR. The tenon method of small joint arthrodesis in the hand. J Hand Surg. 1986;11A:567–9.
11. Lister GD. Intraosseous wiring of the digital skeleton. J Hand Surg. 1978;3:427–35.
12. Pellegrini Jr VD, Burton RI. Osteoarthritis of the proximal interphalangeal joint of the hand: arthroplasty or fusion? J Hand Surg. 1990;15A:194–209.
13. Scheker LR. A technique to facilitate drilling and passing intraosseous wiring in the hand. J Hand Surg Am. 1982;7(6):629–30.
14. Uhl RL, Schneider LH. Tension band arthrodesis of finger joints: a retrospective review of 76 consecutive cases. J Hand Surg. 1992;17A:518–22.
15. Vanik RK. The comparative strengths of internal fixation techniques. J Hand Surg Am. 1984;9(2):216–21.
16. Williams RM, Kiefhaber TR, Sommerkamp TG, Stern PJ. Treatment of unstable dorsal proximal interphalangeal fracture/dislocations using a hemi-hamate autograft. J Hand Surg Am. 2003;28(5):856–65.
17. Takigawa S, Meletiou S, Sauerbier M, Cooney WP. Long-term assessment of Swanson implant arthroplasty in the proximal interphalangeal joint of the hand. J Hand Surg Am. 2004;29(5):785–95.
18. Namdari S, Weiss AP. Anatomically neutral silicone small joint arthroplasty for osteoarthritis. J Hand Surg Am. 2009;34(2):292–300.
19. Branam BR, Tuttle HG, Stern PJ, Levin L. Resurfacing arthroplasty versus silicone arthroplasty for proximal interphalangeal joint osteoarthritis. J Hand Surg Am. 2007;32(6):775–88.
20. Simmons B, Peters T. Subchondylar fossa reconstruction for malunion of fractures of the proximal phalanx in children. J Hand Surg. 1987;12A:1079–82.
21. Gross M, Gelberman R. Metacarpal rotational osteotomy. J Hand Surg. 1985;10A:105–8.
22. Jawa A, Zucchini M, Lauri G, Jupiter J. Modified step-cut osteotomy for metacarpal and phalangeal rotational deformity. J Hand Surg Am. 2009;34(2):335–40.
23. Pichora DR, Meyer R, Masear VR. Rotational step-cut osteotomy for treatment of metacarpal and phalangeal malunion. J Hand Surg. 1991;16A:551–5.
24. Lucas GL, Pfeiffer CM. Osteotomy of the metacarpals and phalanges stabilized by AO plates and screws. Ann Chir Main. 1989;8(1):30–8.
25. Teoh LC. Condylar advancement osteotomy for correcting condylar malunion of the finger. J Hand Surg Br. 2002;27(1):31–5.
26. Del Piñal F. Results of osteotomy, open reduction, and internal fixation for late-presenting malunited intra-articular fractures of the base of the middle phalanx. J Hand Surg Am. 2005;30(5):1039.e1–1039.e14.
27. Harness NG, Chen A, Jupiter JB. Extra-articular osteotomy for malunited unicondylar fractures of the proximal phalanx. J Hand Surg Am. 2005;30(3):566–72.
28. Williams RM, Hastings II H, Kiefhaber TR. PIP fracture/dislocation treatment technique: use of a hemi-hamate resurfacing arthroplasty. Tech Hand Up Extrem Surg. 2002;6(4):185–92.
29. Williams RM, Kiefhaber TR, Sommerkamp TG, Stern PJ. Treatment of unstable dorsal proximal interphalangeal fracture/dislocations using a hemi-hamate autograft. J Hand Surg Am. 2003;28(5):856–65.
30. Jupiter JB, Koniuch MP, Smith RJ. The management of delayed union and nonunion of the metacarpals and phalanges. J Hand Surg. 1985;10A:457–66.
31. Calkins MS, Burkhalter WE, Reyes F. Traumatic segmental bone defects in the upper extremity: treatment with exposed grafts of corticocancellous bone. J Bone Joint Surg. 1987;9A:19–27.

32. Saint-Cyr M, Miranda D, Gonzalez R, Gupta A. Immediate cortico-cancellous bone autografting in segmental bone defects of the hand. J Hand Surg Br. 2006;31(2):168–77.
33. Freeland AE, Jabaley ME, Burkhalter WE, Chaves A. Delayed primary bone grafting in the hand and wrist after traumatic bone loss. J Hand Surg. 1984;9A:22–7.
34. Buchler U, Aiken AA. Arthrodesis of the proximal interphalangeal joint by solid bone grafting and plate fixation in extensive injuries to the dorsal aspect of the finger. J Hand Surg Am. 1988; 13A:589–94.
35. Rinaldi E. Autografts in the treatment of osseus defects in the forearm and hand. J Hand Surg. 1987;12A:282–6.
36. Trumble TE, Freidlaender GE. Use of allogenic bone in hand injuries. Tech Orthop. 1986;1:79–83.
37. Matev IE. The bone-lengthening method in hand reconstruction: twenty years' experience. J Hand Surg. 1989;14A:376–8.
38. Finsen V, Russwurm H. Metacarpal lengthening after traumatic amputation of the thumb. J Bone Joint Surg Br. 1996;78(1):133–6.
39. Melikyan EY, Beg MS, Woodbridge S, Burke FD. The functional results of ray amputation. Hand Surg. 2003;8(1):47–51.
40. Iselin F, Peze W. Ray centralization without bone fixation for amputation of the middle finger. J Hand Surg. 1988;13B:97–9.
41. Segalman KA. Lateral approach to proximal interphalangeal joint implant arthroplasty. J Hand Surg Am. 2007;32(6):905–8.
42. Bickel KD. The dorsal approach to silicone implant arthroplasty of the proximal interphalangeal joint. J Hand Surg Am. 2007;32(6):909–13.
43. Duncan SF, Merritt MV, Kakinoki R. The volar approach to proximal interphalangeal joint arthroplasty. Tech Hand Up Extrem Surg. 2009;13(1):47–53.
44. del Piñal F, Innocenti M. Evolving concepts in the management of the bone gap in the upper limb. Long and small defects. J Plast Reconstr Aesthet Surg. 2007;60(7):776–92.
45. Boulas HJ. Autograft replacement of small joint defects in the hand. Clin Orthop Relat Res. 1996;327:63–71.
46. Hanel DP, Lederman ES. Index transposition after long finger ray resection. J Hand Surg. 1993;18A:271–7.
47. Plasschaert MJ, Hage JJ. A web-saving skin incision for amputation of the third or fourth ray of the hand. J Hand Surg Br. 1988;13(3):340–1.
48. Steichen JB, Idler RS. Results of central ray resection without bony transposition. J Hand Surg. 1986;I1A:466–74.

Surgical Options for Failed Thumb Basal Joint Arthroplasty

5

Scott A. Mitchell and Roy A. Meals

Abstract

Failed basal joint arthroplasty can be a very challenging condition to treat. There can be multiple potential sources for continued pain about the base of the thumb. These sources can be neurogenic in nature, but can also represent continued arthritic problems in some of the other small joints of the wrist. In some cases, there may be carpal instability present that is contributing to continued symptoms. In other cases, there may be frank failure of the previous procedure. The reoperative hand surgeon must carefully weight potential treatment options which will depend on what the previous procedure was and what is believed to be causing the symptoms. If the true source of the patient's continued pain can be identified, frequent improvement in the patient's symptoms can be achieved with further surgical intervention. However, these patients should be counseled that it is rare for them to ever achieve complete pain relief, but that the surgical goal is improvement in their symptoms.

Keywords

Thumb • Basal • Joint • Arthroplasty • Revision • Failure

Key Points

- Despite the success of a diverse array of primary trapeziometacarpal arthroplasty procedures, treatment failures inevitably occur.
- Numerous potential causes of failure have been described—identifying the subset patients who may benefit from revision surgery represents a key step in achieving successful outcomes.
- Neurogenic pain is best treated nonoperatively. Care should be taken to identify those patients with pain attributable to sensory nerves.
- Mechanical causes of failure represent the best indications for revision surgery.
- Properly selected patients can be salvaged using the same technical principles described for the primary treatment of CMC arthritis.
- Selection of revision procedures depends upon both the cause of failure of the index surgery as well as the technique utilized. No single surgical technique will be applicable to all revisions.
- Failed arthrodesis, implant arthroplasty, and most soft tissue arthroplasty procedures may be reliably converted to a hematoma distraction arthroplasty.
- All potential regions of bony impingement around the thumb metacarpal base must be adequately decompressed including the scaphotrapezoid articulation.

(continued)

S.A. Mitchell, MD, MPH • R.A. Meals, MD (✉)
Department of Orthopedic Surgery,
University of California, Los Angeles,
100 UCLA Medical Plaza #305, Los Angeles, CA 90024, USA
e-mail: rmeals@ucla.edu

S.F.M. Duncan (ed.), *Reoperative Hand Surgery*,
DOI 10.1007/978-1-4614-2373-7_5, © Springer Science+Business Media, LLC 2012

- Ligament reconstruction is not routinely required. When necessary, options include transferring all or portions of the flexor carpi radialis, abductor pollicis longus, or extensor carpi radialis brevis tendons.
- Coexisting laxity of the thumb metacarpophalangeal joint should be routinely addressed during revision procedures.

Indications and Contra-indications
Mechanical causes of failure comprise the prime indications for revision surgery. For failed implant arthroplasties, this includes implant loosening, breakage, or peritrapezial arthritis. Arthrodesis procedures most commonly require revision due to either progressive peritrapezial arthritis or failure to achieve a solid fusion. For soft tissue arthroplasty procedures, mechanical problems result primarily from painful bony impingement around the first metacarpal base secondary to either instability, inadequate decompression, or an overly tight ligament reconstruction. Relative contraindications to revision surgery include neurogenic pain secondary to sensory nerve irritation or complex regional pain syndrome

Introduction

Numerous surgical techniques have been described for the treatment of symptomatic arthritis of the basal joint of the thumb. Though diverse in their methods, most have met with considerable long-term success [1–3]. Trapezial excision arthroplasty in particular, with or without ligament reconstruction or soft tissue interposition, has been shown to reliably relieve pain and restore function [4]. Although most patients remain quite satisfied with their surgical outcomes, treatment failures inevitably occur. In such situations, the surgeon is faced with the formidable task of determining whether relief of symptoms can be achieved with a revision procedure. Unfortunately, literature focusing specifically upon failures following primary basal joint arthroplasty procedures remains scarce. Most complications and unsatisfactory outcomes are discussed only briefly within the context of studies reporting overall good results with specific surgical techniques. The etiology of failures in these series often remains speculative or undetermined. There is even less data in the literature to guide the management of a patient following failed primary surgery or the selection of revision or salvage procedures. For these reasons, treatment of the patient with persistent disability following trapeziometacarpal arthroplasty often presents a challenging clinical problem. However, careful patient selection combined with an adaptive application of revision techniques will optimize outcomes in these difficult cases.

Table 5.1 Trapeziometacarpal arthroplasty: potential causes of failure

All procedures
Infection
Sensory nerve injury/neuroma
Reflex sympathetic dystrophy
Metacarpophalangeal joint hyperextension laxity
Scaphotrapezoidal arthritis
Soft tissue arthroplasty (trapeziectomy ± ligament reconstruction/tendon interposition)
Incomplete trapezial excision
Instability of the first metacarpal base
Scaphoid-first metacarpal impingement
Dislocation of interpositional material
Rupture of ligament reconstruction
First to second metacarpal impingement
First metacarpal-trapezoid impingement
Implant arthroplasty
Aseptic loosening
Dislocation/subluxation
Peritrapezial arthritis
Implant fragmentation, foreign body reaction
Trapeziometacarpal arthrodesis
Nonunion
Peritrapezial arthritis
Metacarpophalangeal instability or arthritis
Hardware impingement, migration

Evaluation and Patient Selection

Patient selection represents a critical step towards achieving successful outcomes in the revision setting. This process begins with a search to determine the cause of persistent symptoms. Numerous etiologies have been reported or at least speculated as potential causes of failure in the literature [5] (Table 5.1). A distinction should be made between mechanical and nonmechanical causes of failure. Unfortunately, reports of pain and weakness are common in both of these categories and diligence is required to differentiate between them. Evaluation in these cases must include a careful history and physical examination, supplemented in selected cases by imaging studies. It is important to note that while studies have demonstrated high success rates in terms of pain relief following basal joint arthroplasty procedures, pain in the first 3–6 months postoperatively is quite common. Reassurance that healing is still underway in this setting is recommended, regardless of the X-ray appearance which at times may erroneously forecast doom. Avoidance of repetitive forceful pinch activities will likely result in a satisfactory result in a few more months.

Pain that extends beyond 6 months, however, requires further investigation.

It is helpful to first determine if persistent pain is secondary to neurogenic factors. In the majority of reported series, problems attributable to the sensory nerves overlying the basal joint of the thumb are the most common source of residual pain. As most surgical approaches to the trapeziometacarpal joint involve mobilization of the branches of the radial sensory nerve and lateral antebrachial cutaneous nerve of the forearm, damage or irritation of these sensory nerves may occur even in the absence of direct laceration. Complaints of burning pain or hypersensitivity in the region of the incision should direct the examination towards a tender surgical scar, painful neuroma, or even complex regional pain syndrome. In these cases, early desensitization therapy and pain management intervention are recommended as first-line treatment. Any surgical intervention should be pursued with caution. However, should nonoperative measures fail and examination confirm the presence of discrete neuroma, surgery to repair injured branches or bury the neuroma in deeper tissues may be considered. Selective nerve blocks before revision surgery usually help identify the specific offending nerve branches.

Perhaps most pivotal in the evaluation of the patient with persistent symptoms is to discern mechanical factors from other potential causes of failure, as mechanical pain is arguably the best indication for revision surgery. The identification of patients with mechanical causes of failure following trapeziometacarpal arthrodesis or implant arthroplasty procedures may be relatively straightforward in cases of obvious nonunion or implant loosening, breakage, or instability (Figs. 5.1–5.3). However, progression of peritrapezial arthritis must always be suspected as a contributing factor. Determining the cause of failure of a soft tissue arthroplasty procedure often presents a more challenging task. Mechanical causes of failure should be suspected when complaints of deep pain are accompanied by reports of grinding or a feeling of instability of the thumb with pinch or grip. Examination in these cases will typically reveal crepitation around the base of the first metacarpal accompanied by pain with joint loading or grinding maneuvers. Symptoms typically arise from regions of painful bony impingement around the first metacarpal base. Impingement may result from either instability or overconstraint of the metacarpal base following the primary surgical procedure. Several potential sources of impingement have been described. Proximal migration of the first metacarpal with or without overt instability may lead to abutment between the scaphoid and the metacarpal base. Though there is considerable debate in the literature regarding the clinical significance of postoperative subsidence detected radiographically, excessive proximal migration will ultimately lead to either overt dislocation of the metacarpal base or abutment against the scaphoid. Subsidence may reflect insufficiency or even rupture of a suspensionplasty or

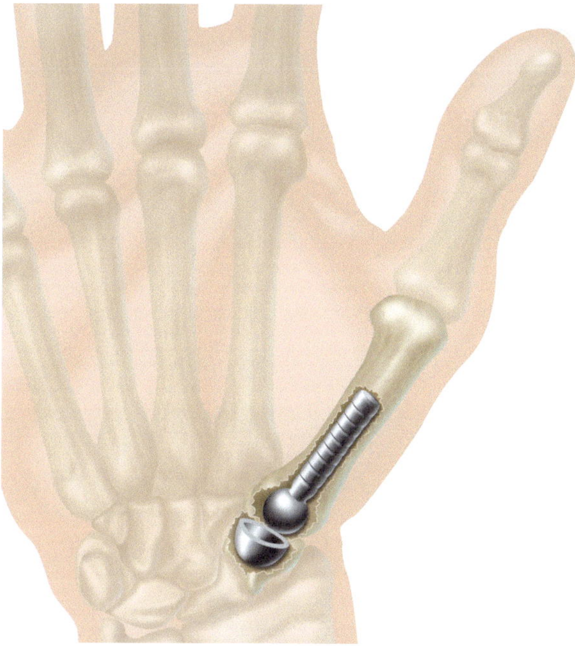

Fig. 5.1 Failed implant arthroplasty. Note the extensive periprosthetic radiolucencies and erosion of the metacarpal diaphysis at the tip of the loosened stem

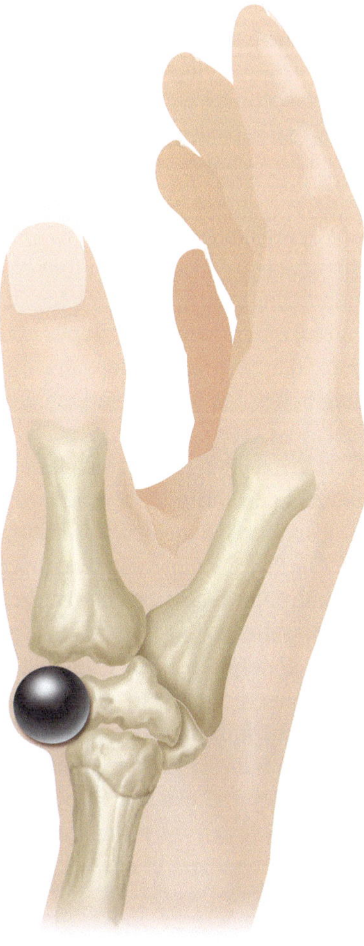

Fig. 5.2 Implant dislocation

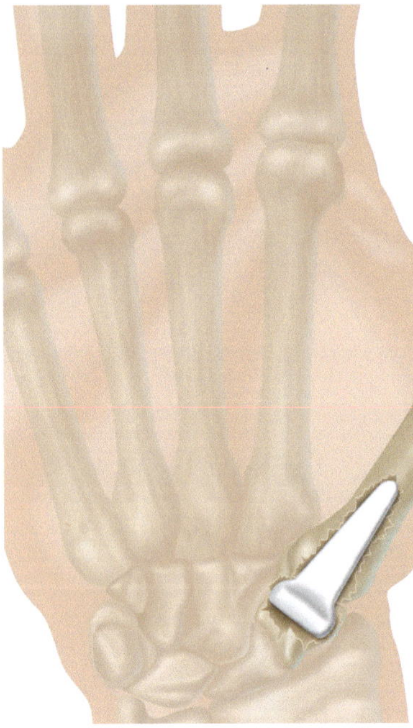

Fig. 5.3 Extensive peritrapezial synovitis following silastic arthroplasty. Note the diffuse intraosseous cysts in the distal radius, scaphoid, trapezoid, capitate, and proximal metacarpals

ligament reconstruction or may result from inadequate distraction or immobilization following trapezial excision alone. Similarly, in patients who have undergone a partial trapeziectomy, first metacarpal subsidence in combination with inadequate bony resection may lead to early painful impingement. Stress views obtained during forceful key pinch may aid in the diagnosis of symptomatic subsidence. It should be cautioned, however, that subsidence is best treated according to symptoms rather than purely radiographic findings. One must also be careful interpreting radiographs of this obliquely oriented anatomical area, because mere shadow overlapping of the remaining bones can be misinterpreted as actual contact and impingement.

Conversely *over*tightening of a reconstructed ligament may lead to abutment and arthritic degeneration between the bases of the first and second metacarpal or between the first metacarpal and trapezoid. A ligament that is pulled too tight may also contribute to an abduction contracture of the thumb in these cases and patients may complain of an inability to lay the palm flat. Careful physical examination will often localize areas of tenderness due to these mechanical problems. Carefully placed injections of small quantities of local anesthetic, on different days in different places as necessary, may also help identify the exact area of pain generation. Radiographs may also be helpful, but again caution is advised because mere shadow overlap can easily be misconstrued as impingement.

Preoperative Considerations

It is important to remember that persistent symptoms may also result from failure during an otherwise successful primary procedure to address coexisting pathology. Unrecognized scaphotrapezoidal arthritis may lead to persistent pain following trapeziometacarpal arthroplasty. Examination may reveal tenderness over the scaphotrapezoid joint, though crepitation may be minimal or absent. It may be helpful to test these joints by axially loading the index metacarpal against the trapezoid and scaphoid. Similarly, unrecognized or progressive peritrapezial arthritis may lead to recurrent mechanical pain following either trapeziometacarpal arthrodesis or implant arthroplasty. Radiographs will typically confirm the presence of arthrosis and selective injections can be used to determine the extent to which these findings are clinically symptomatic.

Another common source of residual symptoms is failure to adequately address the hyperextension deformity of the metacarpophalangeal joint that often develops in concert with basal joint arthritis. Progressive laxity of this joint, particularly following procedures that limit motion around the basal joint, may lead to reports of weakness or instability of the thumb. Dorsal instability at the metacarpal base may also develop secondary to the swan neck deformity driven by metacarpophalangeal hyperextension. Treatment of metacarpophalangeal joint hyperextension is based primarily upon extent of laxity, thus it is important to quantify the degree of passive hyperextension on clinical examination. Associated insufficiency of the collateral ligaments leading to multidirectional instability should be elicited as well. The presence of pain or crepitation with metacarpophalangeal motion suggests arthritic degeneration, predicting the need for an arthrodesis procedure rather than soft tissue reconstruction. Again, testing with local anesthetic in the joint helps localize the source of symptoms.

Revision Surgical Procedures

Selection of appropriate revision procedures depends upon both the presumed cause of failure of the primary surgery as well as the specific technique used for the original procedure. Considering the diversity in primary arthroplasty procedures themselves as well as the ways in which they may fail, it becomes apparent that no single surgical technique is applicable to all revision situations. Treatment must be tailored to specific clinic scenarios, and flexibility is required to customize surgical technique to the pathology encountered intraoperatively.

Revision options for failed trapeziometacarpal arthroplasty include soft tissue procedures such as tissue interposition and ligament reconstruction as well as further bony resection of the trapezium, trapezoid, and/or first metacarpal with or without interposition and ligament reconstruction. Cooney et al. suggest that satisfactory outcomes with revision procedures can be achieved utilizing the standard techniques as described for primary soft tissue arthroplasty procedures [6]. Other options include arthrodesis or implant arthroplasty procedures. Although revision of an ununited trapeziometacarpal arthrodesis may at time be a reasonable option, arthrodesis of the first metacarpal to the scaphoid following trapezial excision has met with near universally poor results [7, 8] and is not recommended in this setting. Implant arthroplasty remains a quite controversial choice for both primary and revision procedures. Prior generations of silicone and ceramic implants have suffered from high complication and revision rates, whereas long-term data for the newer generations of metallic, fabric mesh, and pyrolytic carbon prostheses remain lacking. Though acknowledging that there is some historical support for the use of silicone implants for revision following failed trapeziectomy [7], we do not recommend the use of prosthetic implants in the revision setting.

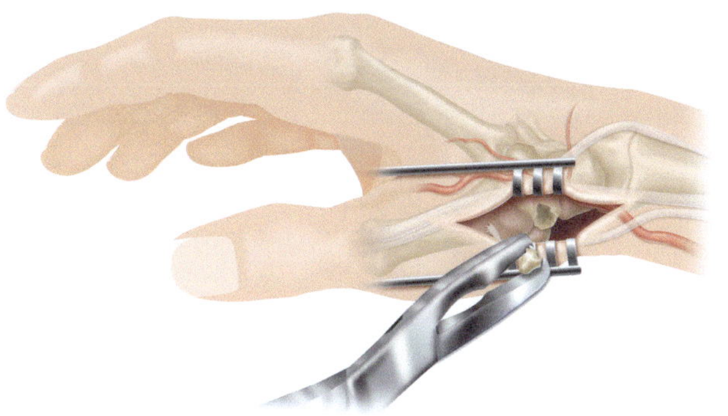

Fig. 5.4 Meals preferred approach to the basal joint

Preferred Technique

Our preferred technique for revision of failed trapeziometacarpal implant arthroplasty, arthrodesis, and most soft tissue arthroplasty procedures is the hematoma distraction arthroplasty as described by Meals and Kuhns [9]. We have not found use of interpositional material necessary as long as the trapezial void is maintained in a distracted position for enough time to allow organization of the postoperative hematoma. Although ligamentous reconstruction or suspensionplasty procedures are occasionally required to achieve stability of the metacarpal base, they are not routinely incorporated.

The patient is placed in the supine position with the arm supported by the hand table. Regional anesthesia is preferred. A tourniquet is placed around the proximal arm and routine sterile preparation and draping is performed. A long-acting local anesthetic is placed adjacent to the posterior and anterior interosseous nerves, the superficial radial nerve, and the palmar cutaneous branch of the median nerve to aid in postoperative pain control. The patient's surgical scar is incorporated into the surgical incision, acknowledging that more extensile exposure may be required. Great care must be taken to protect branches of the dorsal radial nerve and lateral antebrachial cutaneous nerve that invariably course through or adjacent to the surgical exposure. Blunt longitudinal scissor dissection in the subcutaneous tissues is used. Occasionally, formal neurolysis of nerve branches may be required. The extensor pollicis longus, extensor pollicis brevis, and abductor pollicis longus tendons are identified and gently retracted to reveal the underlying first metacarpal base and capsule in the anatomical snuffbox (Fig. 5.4). The radial artery is identified coursing obliquely across the operative field and gently retracted proximally. The dorsal capsule is then incised longitudinally and elevated from the base of the first metacarpal. At this point, the surgical procedure must be tailored to accommodate the patient's prior surgical procedure as well as the presumed etiology of persistent symptoms.

Failed Trapeziometacarpal Arthrodesis

The primary mechanical reasons for failure of a trapeziometacarpal arthrodesis are nonunion and progressive peritrapezial arthritis. Our surgical approach to these cases involves conversion to a hematoma distraction arthroplasty. The residual trapezium and arthrodesis site are exposed by sharp reflection of the remaining capsule from the metacarpal base proximally to the scaphotrapezial and scaphotrapezoidal joints. The arthrodesis site is cut and the residual trapezium is then fractured longitudinally into multiple pieces using an osteotome. The fragments are then removed using a rongeur. It is helpful to maneuver the deeper bone fragments with a Key elevator in order to deliver them into the wound and release palmar capsular attachments. Care must be taken to avoid injury to the flexor carpi radialis tendon coursing obliquely across the depths of the trapezial void. The scaphotrapezoid joint is then carefully inspected, and if evidence of arthritic changes is present, the articulation is decompressed by excision of a wedge of the proximal, radial portion of the trapezoid. The wound is then irrigated and inspected and palpated to ensure that all major bony fragments have been removed. Longitudinal traction is then

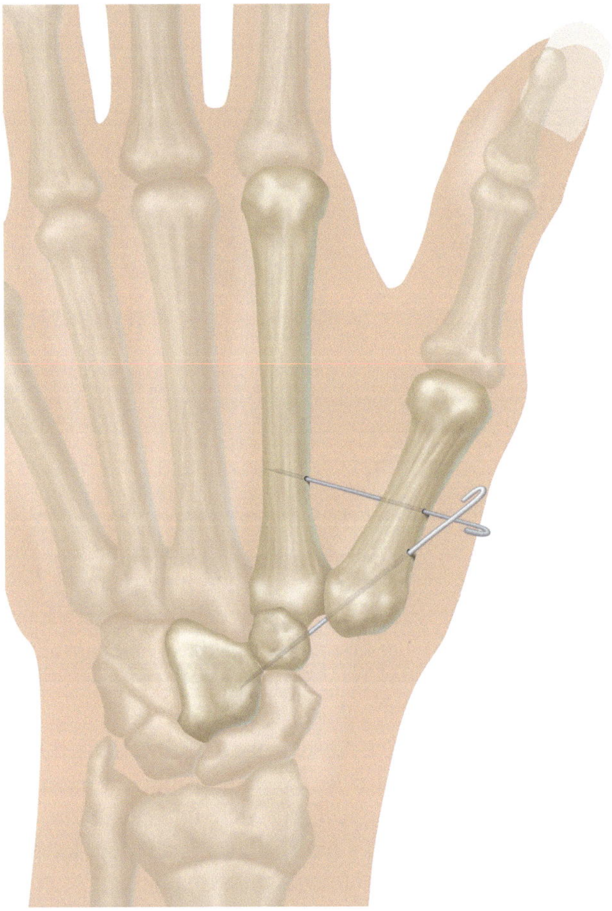

Fig. 5.5 Treatment option for failed trapeziometacarpal arthrodesis

applied to the thumb and it is then held in a position of slight distraction and opposition. Two 0.062 in. Kirschner wires are then driven through the base of the thumb metacarpal. The first is aimed in a dorsoulnar direction and driven into the base of the second metacarpal. A second wire may be placed in similar fashion or may be driven from the base of the first metacarpal across the trapezial void into the distal scaphoid (Fig. 5.5). Thumb positioning and K-wire placement is a critical step, and the thumb must be carefully inspected to ensure that the metacarpal base is indeed supported in a distracted and opposed position. Avoid overpenetration of the second metacarpal with the K-wires, as prominent tips may contribute to dorsal skin irritation postoperatively. The wires are then cut short, but allowed to protrude through the skin for ease of later removal. If tension on the skin around the Kirshner wires is evident, it should be released sharply to avoid skin necrosis and reduce the risk of pin track infection. The wound is then irrigated and the capsular remnants are reapproximated with sutures. Following skin closure, a short arm thumb spica splint is placed leaving the thumb pulp exposed.

Failed Implant Arthroplasty

Salvage of a failed implant arthroplasty begins with implant removal through a longitudinal capsular incision. While removal of silicone implants or loosened cemented prostheses may be accomplished readily, removal of an osteointegrated or otherwise well-fixed stem from the metacarpal canal may be quite difficult. In these cases, the interface between the implant and bone must be disrupted using either a stout elevator or fine osteotome. Care must be taken to avoid fracturing the metacarpal during attempts to reach the distal extent of the stem. Following stem removal, the canal should be curetted to remove any remaining membranous tissue. Any remaining portions of the trapezium are then fragmented using a 10-mm osteotome and excised as described previously. The scaphotrapezoid articulation should be inspected and decompressed if necessary. It is not necessary to excise the entire pseudocapsule that has developed around the prosthetic articulation, but its inner surface layer should be roughened with a curette or rongeur to ensure adequate postoperative hematoma and subsequent fibrous formation in the void left by implant removal. The thumb is then secured in a distracted and opposed position using Kirshner wires as previously described followed by capsular closure.

Failed Soft Tissue Arthroplasty

Revision of a failed ligament reconstruction or suspensionplasty procedure must be directed towards the source of mechanical pain. If impingement between the first and second metacarpal bases has developed, our surgical approach first entails release of the reconstructed ligament from the base of the first metacarpal. It is generally not necessary to excise all scar tissue or previously utilized interpositional material that now fills the trapezial void; however, sharp release of the capsular and fibrous attachments to the metacarpal base should be performed to allow mobilization into a position of slight distraction. Exposure is carried dorsoulnarly over the metacarpal base to the region of impingement between the first and second metacarpals. Any remaining osteophytes on the metacarpal bases should be excised along with loose bodies which may occupy this space. It may be necessary to excise a portion of the ulnar margin of the first metacarpal base to achieve adequate decompression of this interval. Some authors have advocated placement of interpositional material using local tissue or distant tendon which may be considered at this point. Longitudinal traction is applied to the thumb at this point and it is held in a position of slight distraction and opposition to allow placement of two Kirschner wires as previously described (Fig. 5.6). Thumb position is confirmed and the first-second metacarpal interval is inspected to ensure that no regions of impingement persist.

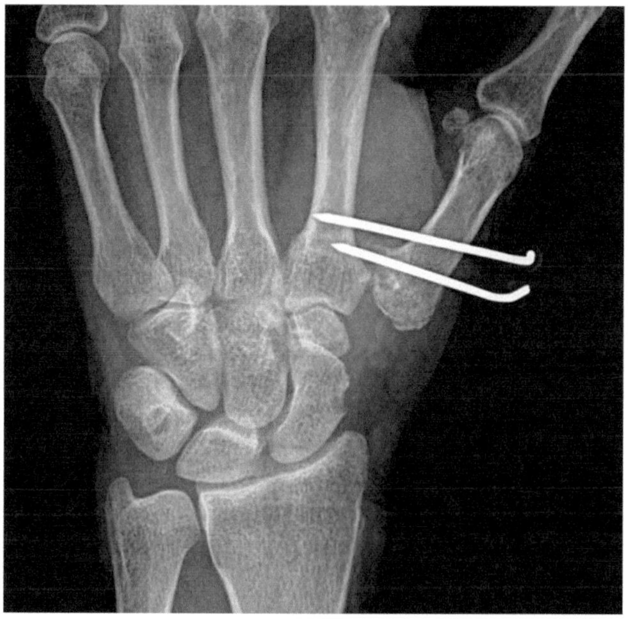

Fig. 5.6 Postoperative radiograph following hematoma distraction arthroplasty. The first metacarpal base has been suspended in slight distraction following decompression of the trapezial space

Excessive subsidence of the first metacarpal resulting in proximal impingement, particularly when associated with dorsal subluxation, may require some form of ligamentous reconstruction or suspension procedure. Reconstruction may also be considered if there is a sense that the patient is a poor scar former. Although we have not needed to resort to ligament reconstruction in revision cases, we offer the following suggestions. Graft selection will depend on the nature of the primary procedure and remaining tendons available for harvest. Choices include all or part of the flexor carpi radialis, abductor pollicis longus, and extensor carpi radialis longus or brevis. Capsular attachments are released sharply from the metacarpal base and any impinging osteophytes are removed using the rongeur. Any remaining fibrous tissue is then excised from the trapezial void, with care taken to preserve the flexor carpi radialis tendon, if remaining. Our preference for ligamentous reconstruction would be to use the flexor carpi radialis tendon as described by Eaton and Littler [10]. A distally based slip of this tendon is harvested through a small transverse incision in the forearm at the musculotendinous junction. The tendon is then delivered distally into the wound. If not performed during the primary procedure, a tunnel is created in the base of the metacarpal from the dorsal metaphysis to exit proximally using either a drill or curette. The tendon is then passed from palmar to dorsal through this tunnel and wrapped around the insertion of the abductor pollicis longus tendon. Delivery of the tendon graft through the bony tunnel may be facilitated by the use of loop of monofilament suture or wire. Tension is then applied to the tendon while the thumb is held in slight distraction and the tendon is the sutured back to itself at the metacarpal base (Fig. 5.7). The bases of the first and second metacarpals should rest at approximately the same level once the suspension is secured. Care must be taken to avoid placing excessive tension on the tendon during this step, as this may contribute to impingement between the first and second metacarpal bases as well as a palmar abduction contracture of the thumb. A slight amount of buoyancy upon gentle axial loading should be present, though no proximal impingement should occur. Once adequate suspension is confirmed, gentle traction is applied to the metacarpal and it is secured in a position of slight distraction and opposition using two Kirschner wires. In some cases, it may be advisable to position and pin the thumb metacarpal *before* tendon tensioning to avoid overtightening. Prior to closure, the interval between the first and second metacarpal bases should be again inspected to confirm the absence of impingement.

If the flexor carpi radialis tendon has been previously harvested or otherwise not available for ligamentous reconstruction, one of several alternative suspension procedures may be used. A distally based slip of the abductor pollicis longus as described by Thompson [11] may be routed from radiopalmar to dorsoulnar through a hole drilled across the second metacarpal base. The starting point for this tunnel should be the trapezial facet of the second metacarpal or slightly distal in the meta-diaphysis as modified by Diao [12] to exit the dorsoulnar aspect of the metacarpal. The tendon is then sutured to itself or woven into the insertion of the extensor carpi radialis brevis tendon (Fig. 5.8). Alternatively, a distally based slip of the extensor carpi radialis longus tendon may be harvested. The tendon is passed through a hole in the first metacarpal base and sutured to itself (Fig. 5.9). Suspensionplasty using the extensor carpi radialis brevis may also be performed. A distally based slip is passed from dorsal to palmar through the second-third intermetacarpal space, woven beneath the abductor pollicis longus insertion and sutured back upon itself.

If the soft tissue options have been exhausted, then a fusion of the thumb to index metacarpal can be considered. This procedure is technically quite challenging. A dorsal approach is utilized with care being taken to protect the sensory nerves. An iliac crest cortico-cancellous graft is ideal. The bone surfaces of the index and thumb metacarpals are then roughened at their bases to expose bleeding bone. The bone graft wedge is then trimmed to meet the position requirements. A 2.4-mm plate (other types can be utilized as well) is bent to bridge the thumb metacarpal—bone graft—index metacarpal construct. It is then secured with several screws. Please see Fig. 5.10 for an illustration of the technique.

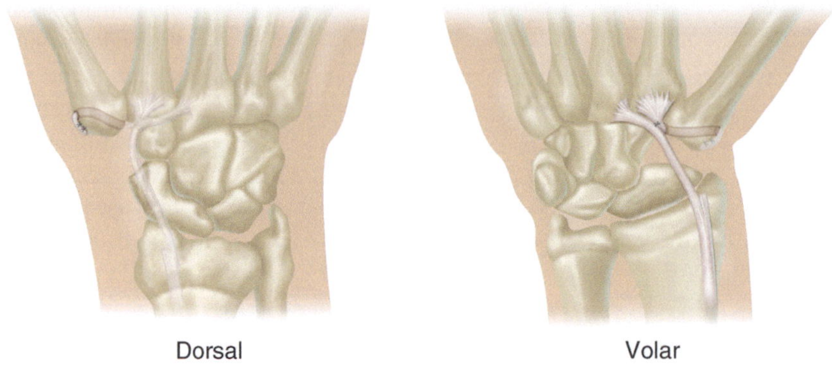

Fig. 5.7 Eaton and Littler ligamentous reconstruction using the flexor carpi radialis tendon

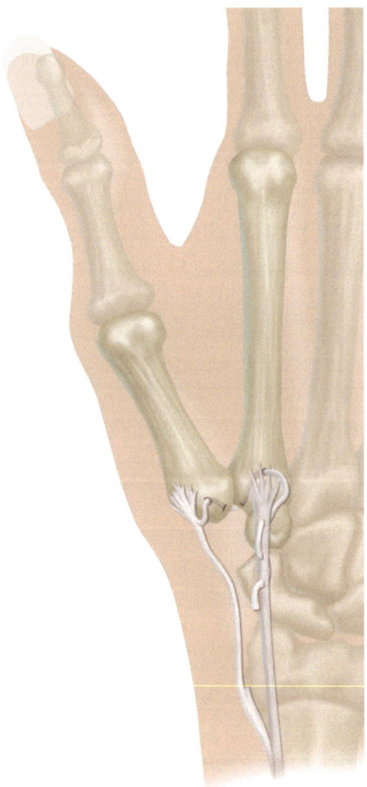

Fig. 5.8 Thompson's procedure if the FCR is no longer present or viable

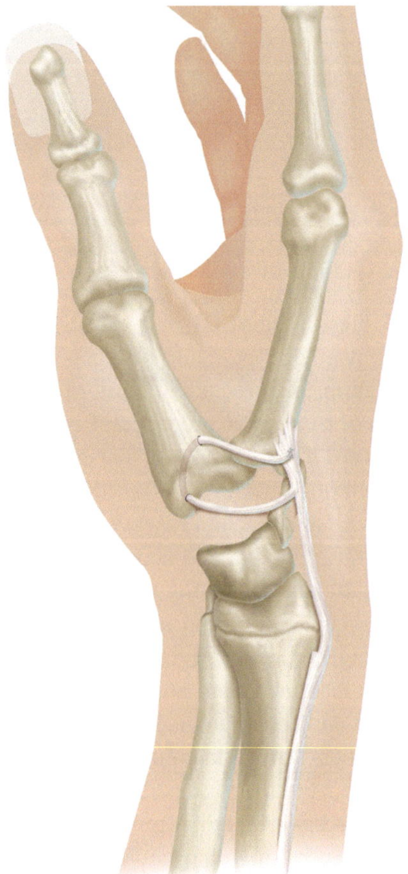

Fig. 5.9 Alternate suspensionplasty using a slip of the ECRL tendon

Metacarpophalangeal Joint Laxity

Laxity of the metacarpophalangeal joint may contribute to both thumb weakness and instability of the metacarpal base. Its presence must be considered at least a contributing factor to failure of the primary procedure and should be addressed routinely at the time of revision. Treatment is based primarily upon the degree of instability noted on physical examination. If hyperextension is 30° or less, options include volar plate capsulodesis or extensor pollicis brevis transfer. Following either procedure, the metacarpophalangeal joint is pinned in slight flexion for a period of 4 weeks. For more severe hyper-extension, either volar plate capsulodesis or arthrodesis of the metacarpophalangeal joint is recommended. The latter is

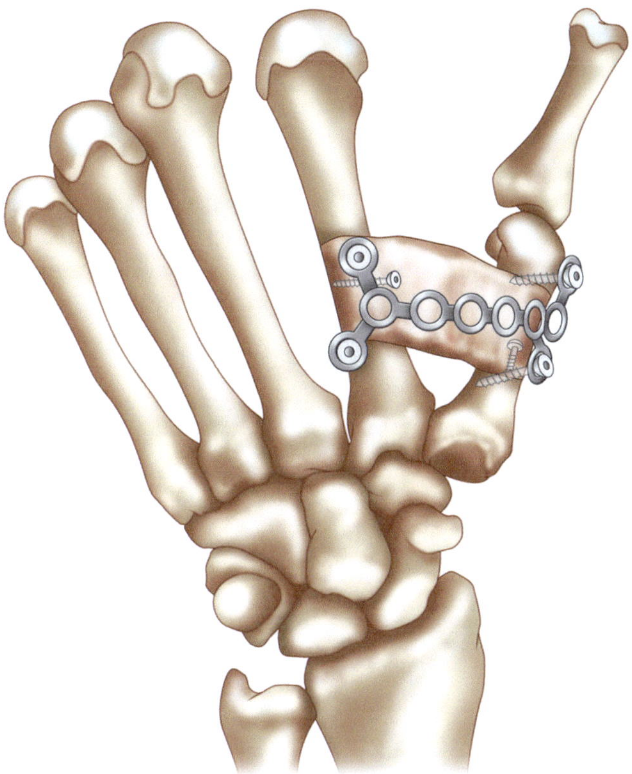

Fig. 5.10 Salvage technique for fusing index to thumb metacarpal

preferred in joints with minimal passive flexion, advanced arthrosis, or evidence of more global instability with associated coronal plane laxity.

Optimizing Outcomes

- A thorough preoperative discussion is essential. Patients must be prepared to participate in aftercare including at least 3–6 months convalescence. Expectations regarding outcomes must also be tempered. The possible need for job adjustment to minimize requirements for extensive forceful pinch activities should be addressed.
- Identify and protect branches of the dorsal radial nerve and lateral antebrachial cutaneous nerve that invariably course through the surgical exposure. Blunt longitudinal scissor dissection in the subcutaneous tissues is recommended.
- The trapezial void and first-second metacarpal intervals should be inspected following K-wire placement to confirm adequate decompression and absence of any loose bony debris.
- Thumb positioning and K-wire placement is a critical step: the thumb must be carefully assessed to ensure that the metacarpal base is indeed supported in a distracted and opposed position.
- Avoiding problems with Kirshner wires:
  - Dot the intended entry and exit points.
  - Look out of your loupes while aiming to obtain a global view.
  - Run driver slowly—a single pass will maximize bone-K-wire interference fit.
  - Avoid overpenetration of the second metacarpal with the K-wires, as prominent tips may contribute to dorsal skin irritation postoperatively.
- Proper tensioning during ligament reconstruction. The bases of the first and second metacarpals should rest at approximately the same level once the suspension is secured. Consider positioning and pinning the thumb metacarpal *before* tendon tensioning to avoid overtightening.
- Laxity of the metacarpophalangeal joint may contribute to both thumb weakness and instability of the metacarpal base and should be addressed routinely at the time of revision.
- Postoperative immobilization. Consider extending the splint to the tip of the thumb at the conclusion of surgery. This will preclude functional use of the thumb during immobilization and minimize the risk of Kirschner wire loosening and metacarpal subsidence. Particularly in the revision situation, a somewhat stiff, painless, well-positioned thumb is to be valued over one that is unstable and painful.

Complications and Side Effects

There are numerous potential complications that must be considered when performing revision surgery. Though these complications are not unique to revision procedures, at least one report suggests they are more common in this setting [8]. Injury to the dorsal sensory nerves remains a great concern, particularly during dissection through a scarred surgical bed. Caution must be employed during the initial exposure to avoid this difficult problem. Recurrent bony impingement around the first metacarpal base may also develop postoperatively from failure to address all potential sites, including the scaphotrapezoid, scaphoid-first metacarpal, and first-second metacarpal intervals. Instability of the first metacarpal base may contribute to this, particularly if postoperative distraction/immobilization is inadequate. Kirshner wire loosening and/or migration intermittently arise, although loss of distraction is minimized by securing the thumb metacarpal with two divergent pins. If ligament reconstruction is deemed necessary during revision, care must also be taken to avoid overtightening during ligament reconstruction, particularly when using an APL suspensionplasty, as this may lead to stiffness and first-second metacarpal abutment. Progressive laxity of the metacarpophalangeal joint may also develop with reconstructions that further limit motion around the basal joint.

Postoperative Rehabilitation

Patients are placed in a short arm thumb spica splint extending to the tip of the thumb at the conclusion of surgery. This will preclude functional use of the thumb during immobilization and minimize the risk of Kirschner wire loosening and metacarpal subsidence. Particularly in the revision situation, a somewhat stiff, painless, well-positioned thumb is to be valued over one that is unstable and painful. The splint is removed between 10 and 14 days postoperatively allowing the surgical wound and pin sites to be inspected and sutures removed. A short arm thumb spica cast is then applied with care taken to provide adequate padding around the pin sites to prevent irritation or loosening. Again, we advise extending the cast to the tip of the thumb to preclude functional use of the thumb. The patient must be advised preoperatively that covering the thumb entirely will create some additional disability compared to the index surgery where we routinely leave the pulp of the thumb free for light pinch activities, but this additional protection will optimize the opportunity for a good result from the revision surgery. The cast and Kirshner wires are removed between 5 and 6 weeks postoperatively and range of motion exercises are begun. The pins are left 7–8 weeks in patients on steroids or in those sensed to be poor scar formers. An elastic wrap for comfort may be helpful for the first several days after cast and Kirschner wire removal. Patients are instructed to perform warm water soaks with thumb range of motion exercises for the first 2 weeks after cast removal, following which they are again evaluated. Those who are not able to place their palm flat on the table or oppose the thumb to the base of the small finger are referred to a hand therapist. At 3 months, unrestricted activity is permitted. Formal strengthening exercises are avoided since overzealous activity may allow excessive remodeling of the supporting connective tissue. Rather, the patient is advised to expect strength to naturally improve over the following 12–18 months through routine daily use.

Literature Review

Cooney et al. reported on 17 revision procedures performed out of a cohort of 654 primary trapeziometacarpal arthroplasty procedures over a 12-year interval [6]. All revision procedures were performed for the treatment of mechanical pain related to instability and/or bony impingement. An array of revision procedures were used, including further bony resection from the first metacarpal base, trapezial remnants, and lateral aspect of the trapezoid, followed by interposition of soft tissues with or without ligamentous reconstruction. Satisfactory outcomes were seen in 75% of patients and did not seem to be influenced by the particular method of soft tissue reconstruction. The authors conclude that mechanical pain resulting in failure may be effectively treated using the same types of soft tissue arthroplasty procedures utilized for primary trapeziometacarpal arthritis.

Conolly and Rath described revision procedures used in a series of patients with complications after primary trapeziometacarpal arthroplasty [7]. Four patients in this series underwent revision for failed trapeziectomy with proximal migration of the first metacarpal and scaphometacarpal abutment. Three were treated by silicone interpositional arthroplasty and the fourth, given a history of postoperative infection, underwent scaphoid-first metacarpal arthrodesis. Eleven patients in this series underwent revision surgery for complications following silicone implant arthroplasty—ten of these patients had painful subluxation or dislocation of the trapezium implant and the remaining two had persistent pain and stiffness. Eight patients were treated with implant removal and soft tissue interposition—good results were seen in four patients, fair results in three, and poor results in one of this subset of patients. Two patients were treated by relocation of the implant with ligament reconstruction; both ultimately failed with recurrent instability ultimately requiring implant removal and soft tissue arthroplasty. The final patient underwent implant removal with bone grafting between the bases of the first and second metacarpals for gross instability of the first ray. This result was poor with persistent pain due to instability and osteoarthrosis of the metacarpophalangeal joint.

Renfree and Dell reported functional outcomes in 12 patients who underwent revision procedures for failed trapeziometacarpal arthroplasty [8]. Patients were treated with a variety of techniques, most commonly suspensionplasty with the APL or FCR tendons. Attempted scaphometacarpal arthrodesis failed in all instances (seven patients) prompting the authors to recommended alternate salvage techniques. While 9 out of 12 patients were ultimately satisfied with their outcomes in terms of strength and degree of pain relief, the overall complication rate in this series was 27%, most notably due to iatrogenic sensory nerve injuries. The authors also note that multiple procedures were commonly required, averaging four per patient. While they do not advocate a specific surgical technique for revision, caution is recommended in approaching patients with painful trapeziometacarpal arthroplasties given the significant risks involved with revision surgery and the potential need for multiple procedures.

Conclusions

Successful revision of a failed trapeziometacarpal arthroplasty is a complex task that begins with careful assessment and selection of surgical candidates. Given the diversity of primary procedures commonly performed as well as their mechanisms of failure, treatment must be tailored to specific clinic scenarios. Mechanical causes of failure represent the best indication for revision surgery and most can be salvaged using the same technical principles described for the primary treatment of CMC arthritis. Flexibility is required to customize these techniques based on the nature of the primary procedure as well as the pathology encountered at the time of surgery. Although challenging in its application, this approach will optimize outcomes in these difficult cases.

References

1. Burton RI, Pellegrini Jr VD. Surgical management of basal joint arthritis of the thumb. Part II. Ligament reconstruction with tendon interposition arthroplasty. J Hand Surg Am. 1986;11(3):324–32.
2. Eaton RG, Glickel SZ, Littler JW. Tendon interposition arthroplasty for degenerative arthritis of the trapeziometacarpal joint of the thumb. J Hand Surg Am. 1985;10(5):645–54.
3. Tomaino MM, Pellegrini Jr VD, Burton RI. Arthroplasty of the basal joint of the thumb. Long-term follow-up after ligament reconstruction with tendon interposition. J Bone Joint Surg Am. 1995;77(3):346–55.
4. Gray KV, Meals RA, Gray KV, Meals RA. Hematoma and distraction arthroplasty for thumb basal joint osteoarthritis: minimum 6.5-year follow-up evaluation. J Hand Surg Am. 2007;32(1):23–9.
5. Wagner W. Why ligament reconstruction, tendon interposition arthroplasty failes, and salvaging failed ligament reconstruciton, tendon interposition arthroplasty. Curr Opin Orthop. 2006;17:288–94.
6. Cooney 3rd WP, Leddy TP, Larson DR. Revision of thumb trapeziometacarpal arthroplasty. J Hand Surg Am. 2006;31(2):219–27.
7. Conolly WB, Rath S. Revision procedures for complications of surgery for osteoarthritis of the carpometacarpal joint of the thumb. J Hand Surg Br. 1993;18(4):533–9.
8. Renfree KJ, Dell PC. Functional outcome following salvage of failed trapeziometacarpal joint arthroplasty. J Hand Surg Br. 2002;27(1):96–100.
9. Kuhns CA, Emerson ET, Meals RA. Hematoma and distraction arthroplasty for thumb basal joint osteoarthritis: a prospective, single-surgeon study including outcomes measures. J Hand Surg Am. 2003;28(3):381–9.
10. Eaton RG, Littler JW. Ligament reconstruction for the painful thumb carpometacarpal joint. J Bone Joint Surg Am. 1973;55(8):1655–66.
11. Thompson JS. Complications and salvage of trapeziometacarpal arthroplasties. Instr Course Lect. 1989;38:3–13.
12. Diao E. Trapezio-metacarpal arthritis. Trapezium excision and ligament reconstruction not including the LRTI arthroplasty. Hand Clin. 2001;17(2):223–36; ix.

Surgical Options for the Failed Wrist Arthrodesis

6

Nathan A. Hoekzema and Jose A. Ortiz, Jr.

Abstract

Failed wrist fusions fortunately are an infrequent problem for the hand surgeon to deal with. However, when it does occur, the surgeon may be faced with a multitude of problems relating to poor bone quality, bone loss, as well as copious scar tissue. Reconstructive options include autologous bone grafting, bone morphogenic protein, and external and/or internal bone stimulators. If the hardware has truly failed, the hardware may need to be changed out, but if there has been any windshield wiper effect to the bone, bony struts may have to be used. In the presence of previous infection, one can consider vascularized fibular bone graft. More recently, some wrist fusions that have failed to unite are being replaced with joint arthroplasty of the wrist. Ultimately, the surgeon has several options available in order to treat this clinical problem, which can leave the patient functionally impaired, secondary to the wrist deformity and pain. Ultimately, if satisfactory fusion or joint replacement can be obtained, improved but not total pain relief can be expected.

Keywords

Arthrodesis • Failed • Wrist • Fusion • Surgical • Reconstruction

Introduction

Wrist arthrodesis has long been considered the gold standard in the treatment of unstable or severely arthritic wrists. Using a variety of surgical techniques, total wrist fusion is a time-tested salvage procedure used when other options to treat wrist pathology have failed [1–9].

Methods of Fusion

1. Kirschner wires
2. Mannerfelt technique
3. Gill technique
4. AO plate fixation
5. Staples

With modern AO technique, fusion rates in most series have been reported to be as high as 100% [10–12]. Even with the significant success reported with this technique, some authors have reported rates of nonunion up to 7% [13, 14]. When a nonunion is seen, it is most commonly present at the third carpometacarpal joint.

Complete pain relief after arthrodesis has been reported to range from 25% [15] upward to 100% [10]. The majority of studies generally report favorable results supporting wrist arthrodesis.

Strength after fusion has been generally reported to be functional. Actual grip strengths have been noted to improve up to 1 year from surgery. Grip strengths can be as high as up to 72% of normal [14, 16].

As with many procedures performed around the wrist, wrist arthrodesis is not without risks or complications. Specific risks vary with the surgical technique used [17]. Here, we

N.A. Hoekzema, MD • J.A. Ortiz, Jr., MD (✉)
Orthopedic Center, Mayo Clinic Health System,
1400 Bellinger Street, Eau Claire, WI 54702, USA
e-mail: Ortiz.jose@mayo.edu

S.F.M. Duncan (ed.), *Reoperative Hand Surgery*,
DOI 10.1007/978-1-4614-2373-7_6, © Springer Science+Business Media, LLC 2012

Complications of Wrist Arthrodesis

1. Nonunion
2. Ulnar abutment
3. Failed hardware
4. Symptomatic hardware
5. Infection
6. Neuroma
7. Chronic regional pain syndrome
8. Carpal tunnel syndrome
9. DRUJ arthritis
10. Transient nerve palsy

discuss the surgical management of one of the most serious causes of wrist arthrodesis failure, namely, nonunion.

Indications/Contraindications

The indications for a revision surgical procedure in total wrist arthrodesis are varied. Potential complications of index surgery are numerous. These can be categorized as nonunion, malunion, symptomatic hardware, progressive arthrosis, infection, and carpal tunnel syndrome. Additionally, other potential adverse conditions can be seen such as neuromas and complex regional pain syndrome. Not all of these conditions necessitate surgical intervention.

Complications such as carpal tunnel syndrome, neuromas, DRUJ arthrosis, or symptomatic hardware may require limited surgical management. These complications each have their respective surgical solutions. However, these conditions will not be addressed here. Our focus is to discuss the patient with failed arthrodesis secondary to nonunion, hardware failure, or progressive intercarpal or carpometacarpal arthrosis.

There are multiple techniques available for primary arthrodesis of the wrist. Procedures vary depending on underlying pathology, prior surgeries, patients' bone stock, and surgeons experience and preferences. It has been our experience, as well as shown in the literature, that the AO/ASIF fusion technique provides a reliable result. We use the titanium low-contact dynamic compression plate designed by the AO group and manufactured by Synthes (Paoli, PA). In addition, we recommend bone grafting with meticulous attention to detail.

Regarding contraindications, careful patient screening is paramount to a successful outcome. Patients who present with elusive symptoms or nonorganically based pain profiles are risky prospects who may not obtain the results desired. Likewise, clear patient expectation is critical to determining whether to proceed with surgery or not. If a patient's understanding of outcome is not in line with what is truly achievable, that should be seen as a red flag, and consideration should be given to exploring other treatment options.

The prime indication for revision surgery is pain. It is imperative that there is a clear understanding of the source of that pain. If the source of the pain cannot predictably be addressed with revision fusion, like in the case of a neuroma, alternative treatments should be sought. Revision wrist fusion can help to address pain that results from nonunion, from failed hardware, from malunion, infection, or from progressive arthrosis.

Indications for Revision Wrist Arthrodesis

1. Nonunion
2. Failed hardware
3. Malunion
   (a) Rotational
   (b) Deviation
4. Infection
5. Progressive arthrosis

Preoperative Evaluation

Any patient with a "failed operation" being considered for revision surgery requires a thorough history and examination. Just as with any proper patient evaluation, a complete history is paramount. Many important patient characteristics can be learned, which can help with discovering the reason for the failure and ways to prevent a failed revision operation. Pain patterns, rest or night pain, a history of prior postoperative infection, or poor wound healing, as well as current systemic symptoms such as fevers, chills, and malaise are helpful. One should understand the course of the patient's disease and prior treatments. Every effort should be made to acquire a complete medical record if another physician attempted the initial fusion. A social history is also of utmost importance; hand dominance, occupation, and tobacco use can change outcomes.

The physical examination should be complete and include the neck and both upper extremities. Specifically with a failed wrist fusion, one should pay special attention to the following:

1. Areas of tenderness and swelling
2. Condition of the incision (erythema, drainage, warmth)
3. Motion at both fused and nonfused joints
4. Sensation and strength
5. Clinical alignment
6. Carpal tunnel syndrome tests (carpal tunnel compression and Phalen's tests, Tinel's signs, nerve conduction studies if warranted)

Initial imaging studies must include current wrist radiographs in three views (anterior-posterior, lateral, and oblique).

Occasionally, theses images will show progressive arthrosis, hardware failure, ulnar impaction, gross malalignment, and an obvious nonunion and would be sufficient for diagnosis and preoperative planning.

Examination of the wrist under fluoroscopy can assess for gross motion as well as ulnar impaction. The dynamic views may be helpful when clinical examination or radiographs are inconclusive.

Often a wrist CT scan will add more information during the prerevision workup. The study may add valuable information on the location and quality of the fusion, as well as a possible sequestrum. Metallic implants may compromise the images, and this has to be taken into consideration. Unless there is a blatant area of nonunion, a CT is recommended as component of a nonunion evaluation.

Magnetic resonance imaging may be helpful for evaluation of ulnar impaction as well as areas of abscess or osteomyelitis. MRI is not one of the most useful of adjunctive imaging due to its poor resolution of bony detail and the likely presence of metallic artifact.

Technetium bone scan may be helpful in a patient whose symptoms and/or exam is clinically vague. The technetium scan will highlight areas of increased bone activity. Its nonspecific nature, especially in an area of early arthrodesis where increased bone activity is desired, can be less helpful. It may be more beneficial in working up a painful wrist that is several years removed from the surgical arthrodesis to evaluate for progressive arthrosis or occult pseudarthrosis.

Selective diagnostic injections using local anesthetic can be very informative in locating the exact area of the pain generator and likelihood of improvement with revision surgery. The addition of fluoroscopic guidance with the injection can improve physician confidence and patient response.

Postoperative infection is a major cause for revision arthrodesis, and infection should be considered in all cases of failed wrist arthrodesis. A C-reactive protein (CRP), erythrocyte sedimentation rate (ESR), and a white blood cell count with differential should be obtained for infection screening. If an occult infection is suspected, a radionuclide and indium-labeled white blood cell scan can be an informative imaging modality.

Before undertaking a revision wrist arthrodesis, one needs to have a clear understanding of why the index surgery failed. It is imperative to treat or avoid the original problems in order to increase the likelihood of a stable, pain-free wrist.

Operative Approach

Surgical Anatomy

Our preferred approach is a straight dorsal exposure. The anatomy encountered is essentially that of the dorsal wrist. Keep in mind that the native anatomy is now somewhat distorted due to prior surgery. Being mindful of the likely transposed extensor pollicis longus (EPL) tendon prevents injury to this structure. Likewise, prior modifications to the extensor retinaculum for hardware coverage should also be kept in mind (Fig. 6.1). Respect of the superficial radial and ulnar nerves is critical in the prevention of additional complications.

If not performed during the index surgery, we advocate division of the posterior interosseous nerve. This may provide some added pain relief postoperatively.

Patient Position

As with most upper extremity surgery, the patient is maintained supine on the operating table. Their arm is abducted 90° onto an arm board. The procedure is performed under tourniquet control, under an axillary or supraclavicular block. Care is taken to make sure all bony prominences are well padded. Traction over the end of the table can be an asset during decortication of the carpus and placement of bone graft (Fig. 6.2).

Surgical Exposure

A straight dorsal approach affords the best exposure to the relevant anatomy. One tries to incorporate the original incision, extending the new excision past the borders of the first. It is helpful to incise into new tissue at both poles of the incision to facilitate the dissection (Fig. 6.3).

If the EPL was not transposed initially, it is done so at this time. Once a dorsal incision has been made, creating full thickness radial and ulnar flaps, a midline approach to the carpus is preferred (Fig. 6.4). Identifying and tagging the radial and ulnar superficial nerves can be helpful in preventing iatrogenic injury to these structures (Fig. 6.5).

A subperiosteal approach through the third compartment affords an excellent exposure to the carpus. Creating thick retinacular/capsular flaps radially and ulnarly allows for optimal plate coverage upon closure. Alternatively, one can elevate the extensor retinaculum radially and ulnarly, separate from the capsule. Upon closure, the extensor retinaculum can be split using half to cover the plate and the other half to function as the extensor retinaculum (Fig. 6.6). Regardless of which option is chosen, maximum soft tissue coverage of the plate is the desired goal.

Decortication

It is particularly critical to pay attention to this step in the procedure in order to obtain the highest possible success with fusion. Areas to be decorticated include all joints

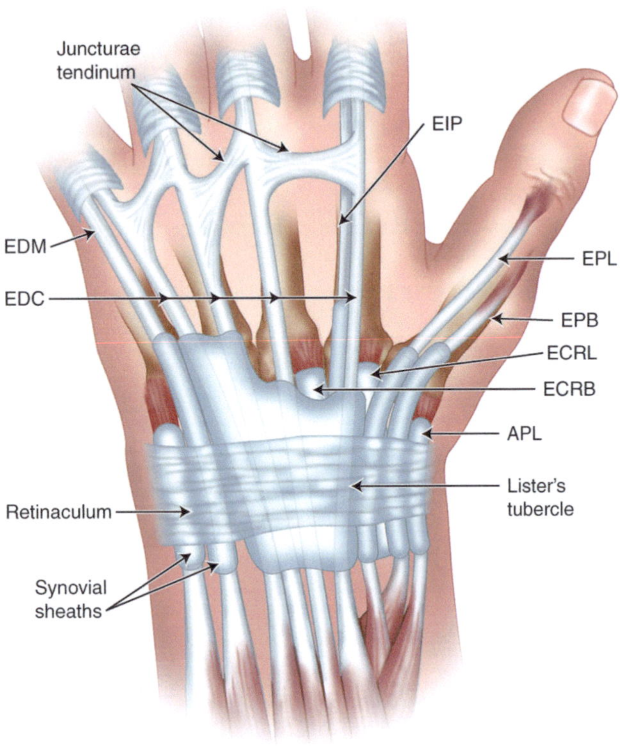

Fig. 6.1 Dorsal anatomy—be mindful of altered anatomy on approach. Review of prior operative reports is critical

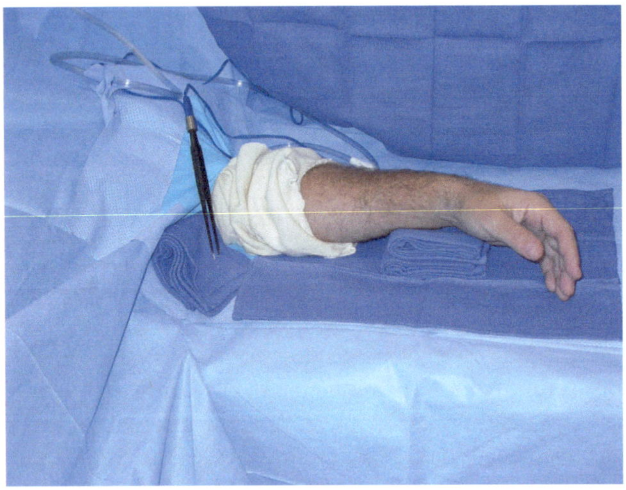

Fig. 6.2 Patient's arm is abducted 90° onto an arm board. Consider the use of traction

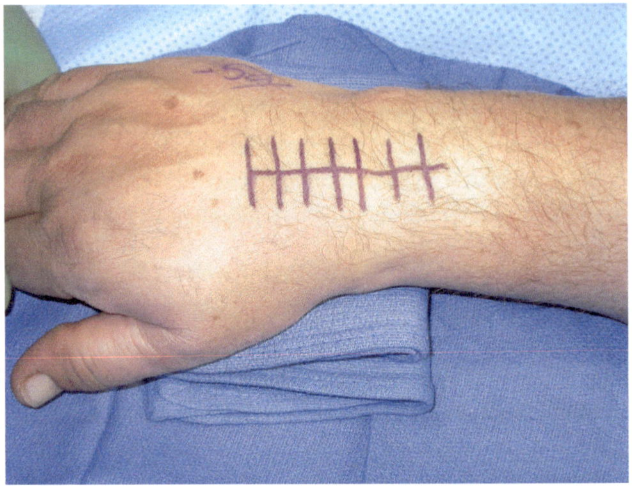

Fig. 6.3 Incision—extending the incision on each pole of the original incision can aid in identifying the correct planes to dissect through

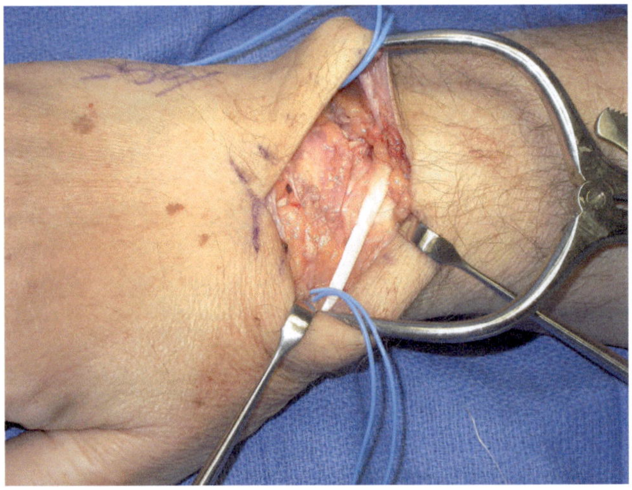

Fig. 6.4 If not done in a prior procedure, consider transposition of the extensor pollicis longus upon closure

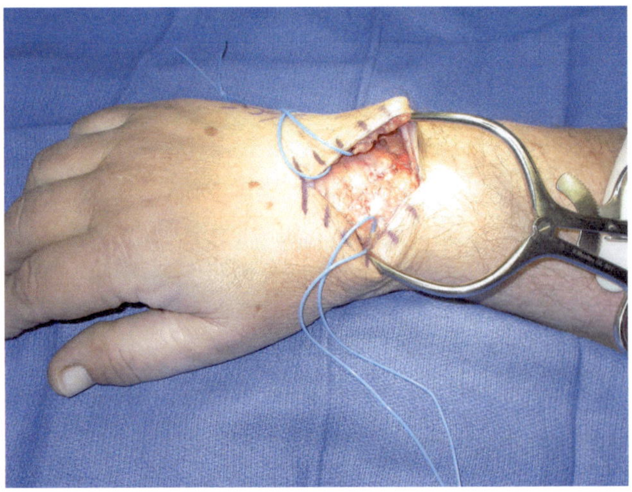

Fig. 6.5 Identifying and tagging the superficial radial and ulnar nerves during the approach can help serve as a reminder of the nerves location and can be helpful in preventing iatrogenic injury to these structures

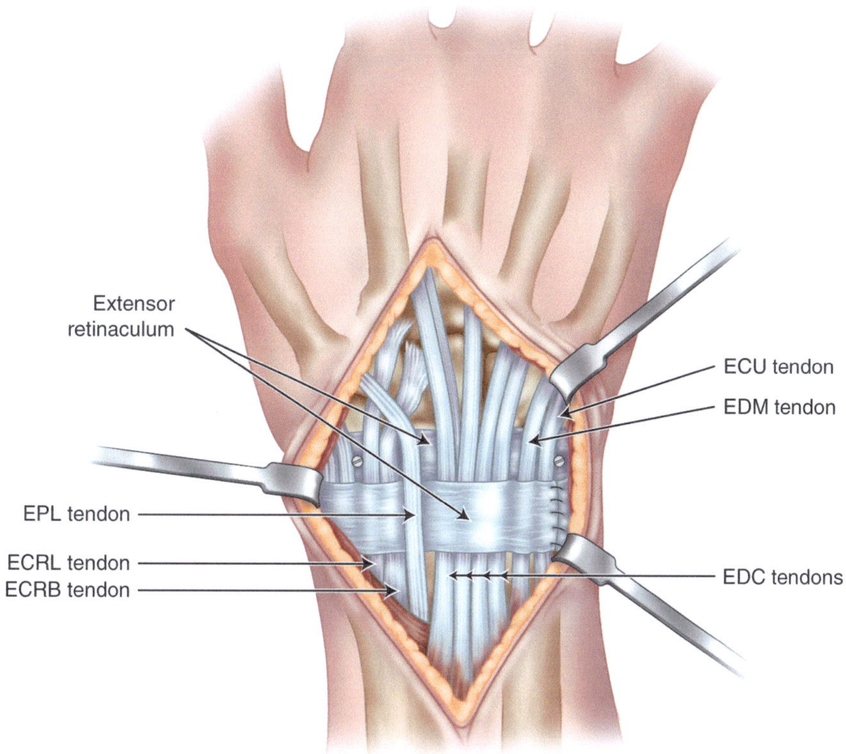

Fig. 6.6 The extensor retinaculum can be split using half to cover the plate and the other half to function as the extensor retinaculum preventing bow stringing of the extensor tendons

typically decorticated with the initial fusion. These include the radioscaphoid, radiolunate, scapholunate, scaphocapitate, lunocapitate, as well as the capitate third metacarpal joint. In addition, although optional with primary arthrodesis, we feel that the lunotriquetral, triquetralhamate, and capitohamate should also be decorticated with revision arthrodesis (Fig. 6.7). If the patient had a prior proximal row carpectomy, we also advocate inserting bone graft in the radiotrapeziotrapezoidal area to increase surface area, promoting greater carpal union (Fig. 6.8).

Technique for decortication is a combination of bony curettes, rongeurs, and judicious use of a high-speed burr. The goal is to decorticate while maintaining maximum bone stock for fusion. Again, it is critical that meticulous attention to detail is applied in this step of the procedure. It is also suggested to use a K-wire, or small diameter drill, to create a channel into the radius/carpal bones to facilitate vascular in growth.

Bone Graft

There are many choices for bone grafting. With revision arthrodesis, we feel that autograft is the best option. To obtain sufficient bone, we suggest utilizing the iliac crest. This can be supplemented with other products, such as cancellous allograft, to increase yield. Bone morphogenic protein, in any of its marketed forms, can also be used to promote fusion, but has not been extensively studied in this scenario.

Plate Selection

Our preference is to use the titanium low-contact dynamic compression wrist fusion plate designed by the AO group and manufactured by Synthes (Paoli, PA). If this plate was used with the index procedure, one option with the revision surgery is to use the Synthes LCP plate with locking screw technology. The holes on this plate are slightly offset from the holes of the nonlocked plate. This allows for the placement of screws in solid bone, avoiding falling into the original screw holes. The locked technology may also aid the outcome by providing increased stability, although that has not been demonstrated in the literature as of yet (Fig. 6.9).

Arthrodesis

The ideal position of the wrist in fusion remains controversial. Some authors report the ideal position to be 10–15° of

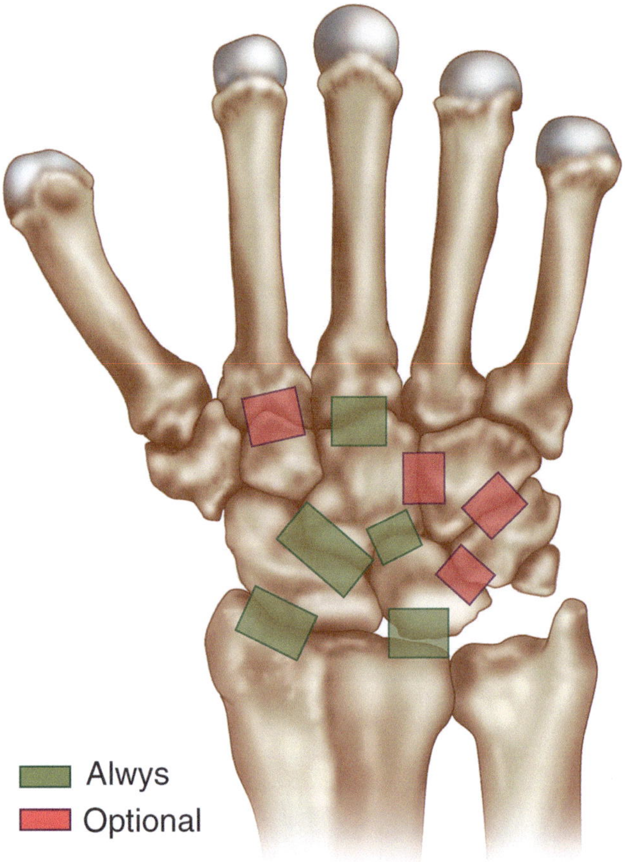

Fig. 6.7 Areas to fuse include the radioscaphoid, radiolunate, scapholunate, scaphocapitate, lunocapitate, as well as second and third carpometacarpal joints. In addition, although optional with primary arthrodesis, we feel that the lunotriquetral, triquetralhamate, and capitohamate should also be decorticated with revision arthrodesis

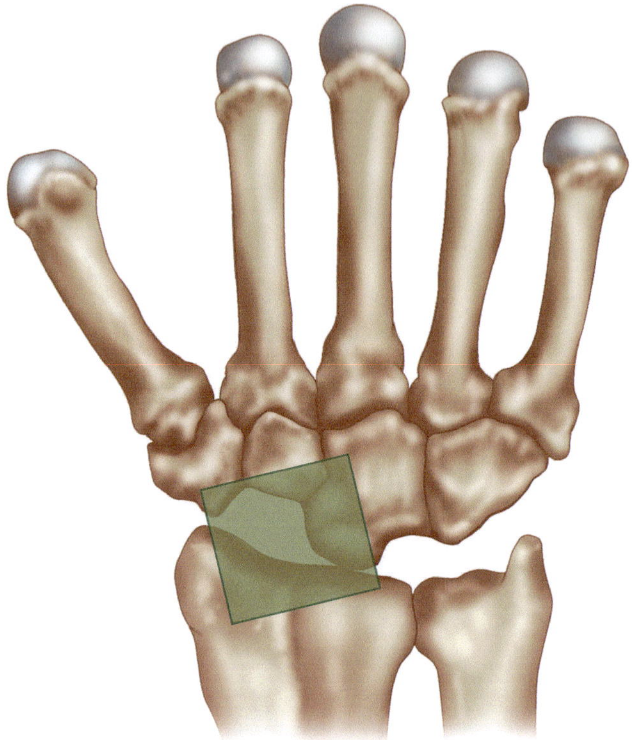

Fig. 6.8 In patients with a prior proximal row carpectomy, we advocate inserting bone graft in the radiotrapeziotrapezoidal area to increase surface area, promoting greater carpal union

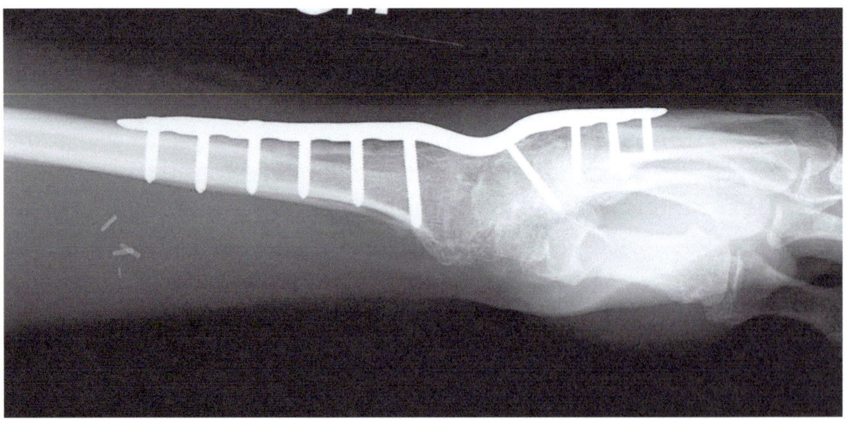

Fig. 6.9 In revision surgery, consideration can be given to using the locking AO plate. The holes on this plate are slightly offset from the holes of the nonlocked plate, allowing for the placement of screws in new bone

extension [10]. Others have reported that 15° of extension and 15° of ulnar deviation yield superior results to neutral fusion in both planes [18]. There is the contralateral wrist to take into consideration. In situations of bilateral fusion, it is suggested to fuse one wrist in slight extension and the other in flexion for better hygiene.

Our preference is to use the Synthes precontoured AO wrist fusion plate (Fig. 6.10). This puts the wrist in a position of 10° of extension and in neutral deviation. Additionally, there is the option of using the straight plate, placing the wrist in neutral flexion/extension, or custom bending it to a desired alignment.

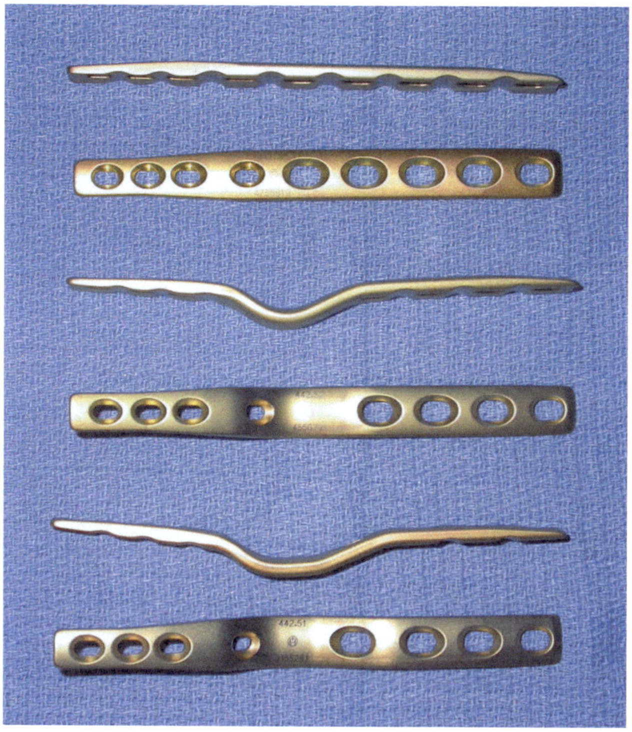

Fig. 6.10 Preferred plates are the synthesis AO plate. Shown are the titanium nonlocking plates. From top to bottom, we see the straight, the 10° extension option for prior PRC patients, and the 10° extension for non-PRC patients

Optimizing Outcomes

The key to a successful "refusion" is paying close attention to detail. This includes appropriate patient selection, meticulous surgical management, appropriate bone grafting, and postoperative management.

A thorough preoperative assessment is mandatory. This includes ruling out other possible causes of ongoing concern which may not improve with fusion. Conditions such as carpal tunnel syndrome and ulnar abutment need to be ruled out, as well as any possible contribution from superficial radial or ulnar nerve neuromas.

It is strongly recommended that all hardware be removed and that particular attention is paid to performing a thorough decortication. This increases the predictability of a successful fusion. To that end, it is also important to use adequate amount of bone graft to fill the carpus completely. Again, our recommendation is to use autograft, which can be supplemented with cancellous allograft. Careful attention to filling all of the possible spaces is strongly suggested.

Using fluoroscopy to ensure optimal placement of hardware (as well as overall wrist alignment) is instrumental to revision surgery. If bone quality is poor, strong consideration should be given to using a locking plate that may provide for new purchase of the bone. Incorporation of the third CMC joint into the fusion is also highly recommended.

Postoperatively, elevation with aggressive maintenance of digital range of motion, with antiedema measures, is critical for a well-functioning terminal unit. Postoperative immobilization must be strictly adhered to with maximal patient compliance in this regard. Consideration to early use of bone stimulation may be warranted in select individuals.

Areas to exercise caution include appropriate handling of the soft tissues ensuring no crushing or other injury. This includes the dorsal wound flaps, as well as the superficial radial and ulnar nerves.

Clinical Pearls

1. Thorough preoperative assessment including evaluation for carpal tunnel syndrome and ulnar abutment.
2. Complete hardware removal and decortication.
3. Bone graft as indicated with preference for autogenous graft.
4. Intraoperative radiographic assessment to ensure hardware placement and alignment.
5. Using locking plates may allow for new screw hole placement.
6. Incorporate the third CMC joint into fusion.
7. Aggressive post-op maintenance of digital ROM.
8. Judicious postoperative immobilization.
9. Consideration of postoperative external bone growth stimulator.

Ensuring proper placement of all screws is also of great concern, as is prevention of prominent hardware. This would include prevention of rotational malalignment and maintenance of neutral deviation.

Pitfalls

1. Inadequate debridement between bones
2. Superficial radial/ulnar nerve neuroma
3. High-speed burr damage
4. Failure to completely denude cartilage
5. Failure to drill into bones to promote fusion
6. Rotational malalignment
7. Prominent hardware

Complications

The complications of total wrist arthrodesis, both in the primary and revision setting, can be generally divided into short-term and long-term complications.

The short-term complications include conditions that can be encountered after any surgical procedure, such as hematoma, edema and skin blistering, wound dehiscence or infection, and transient paresthesias. It is imperative to avoid these acute complications in order to maximize early patient digital motion and avoid a return trip to the operating room.

The long-term potential concerns include infection, stiffness, pseudarthrosis, perifusion fractures, and progressive perifusion mass arthrosis [11].

Whereas the acute complications are more routinely encountered by the surgeon, the decision process tends to be more straightforward. One must be vigilant and quick to act on the early signs of these unwanted outcomes. Without adequate treatment, a "simple" postoperative infection can evolve into a chronic infected nonunion.

It is the authors' opinion that the problems encountered after the acute postoperative period (typically greater than 3 months out) pose increased diagnostic and treatment difficulties. Consistent postoperative follow-up, as well as aggressive patient education, promotes early detection of any of these conditions.

Postoperative Care

The wrist is kept in the postoperative volar splint full time for the first 2 weeks after surgery. Elevation and finger range of motion are encouraged. The patient is seen back in clinic 2 weeks after surgery for splint removal, X-rays, and suture removal. At this same visit, the hand therapist fabricates a static, volar, forearm-based wrist splint. The patient also begins working with active and passive digital motion, as well as supination and pronation. The patient is allowed to shower and use the hand for lifting no greater than 2 lb. The splint is worn full time except for when performing hygiene.

The patient is seen back 6 weeks after surgery for X-rays and evaluation. Splint use is discontinued, and therapy is increased to involve gentle strengthening.

Complications

Short term

1. Hematoma formation
2. Edema
3. Wound dehiscence
4. Blistering
5. Wound infection
6. Transient paresthesia

Long term

1. MCP stiffness
2. Painful hardware
3. Radius fracture
4. Metacarpal fracture
5. STT arthritis
6. DRUJ arthritis
7. DRUJ instability
8. Infection
9. Pseudarthrosis
10. Ulnar impaction
11. Carpal tunnel syndrome
12. Tendinous adhesions

At the 12-week postoperative visit, X-rays are taken to verify continuing fusion. Activity restrictions are lifted, and the patient may return to full-duty work.

Other Less Utilized Options

Muramatsu et al. have described utilizing a free vascularized fibular transfer in order to reconstruct the wrist following tumor resection [19]. They have noted that this could also work for failed wrist fusions. In their small series, they were able to achieve fibuloscapholunate fusion that provided wrist stability and functional finger range of motion about the fingers and forearm. Chin et al. have described utilizing a vascularized fibula autograft to achieve successful fusion in the case of trying to obtain fusion after wrist sepsis [20]. In their case, they had complete incorporation of the graft. Germann et al. described a new technique for wrist fusion utilizing a vascularized bone graft [21]. They use a reverse segmental pedicled ulna transfer as a salvage procedure for failed wrist fusion. This distally based pedicled segment of the distal ulna is nourished by the ulnar artery or the distally based palmar branch of the anterior interosseous artery. After this procedure, the forearm is essentially converted to a situation that is similar to a wide distal ulna resection. In their small case series, all fusions healed uneventfully. The authors of that technique believe it is useful in cases where vascularized bone graft is required, but microsurgical techniques are either not appropriate and cannot be technically performed, or the idea of a vascularized fibula is rejected by the patient (Fig. 6.11).

Another option for the failed wrist fusion attempt is wrist arthroplasty. Enough bone stock must be present both in the distal aspect of the wrist as well as the proximal aspect (radius). In some cases, a custom wrist implant may need to be requested from the manufacturer. These types of cases obviously are uncommon, but certainly are an option for the

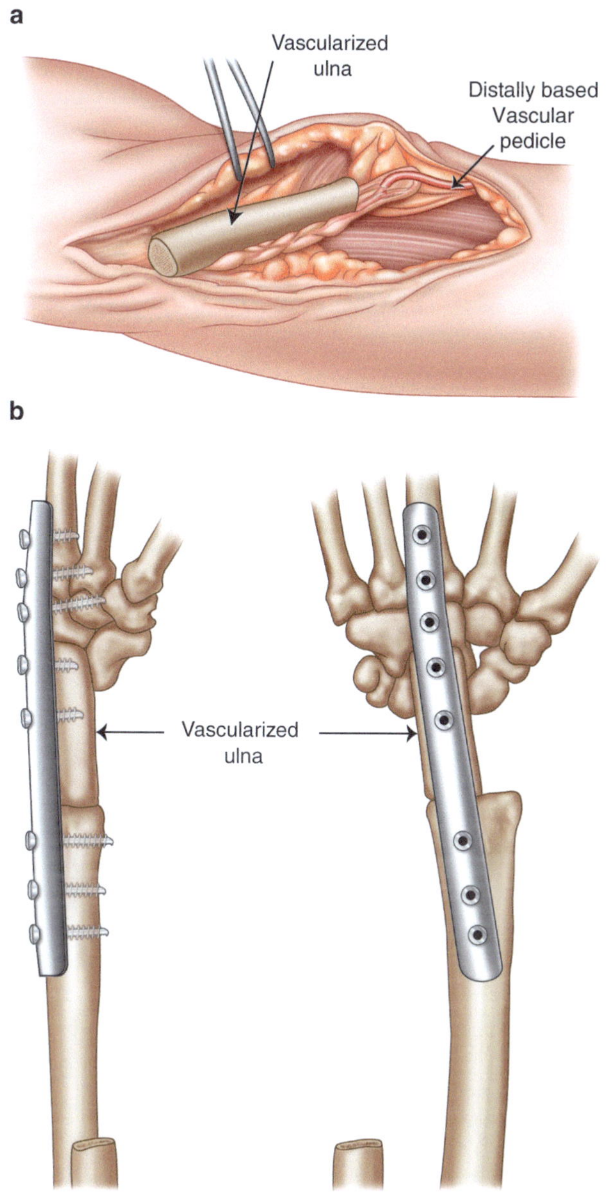

Fig. 6.11 (**a**) Ulnar-vascularized bone graft. (**b**) Ulnar-vascularized bone graft interposed between radius and carpus, secured by plate

patient whose wrist does not fuse and has adequate bone stock to support such an implant. Obviously, in a patient with previous infection, this could be a risky proposition. Other concerns would include compromised soft tissue envelope, poor bone quality, inadequate bone quality, and a patient on wound-healing modifying medications. Revision surgery from fusion nonunion to total wrist arthroplasty has been discussed in hand surgery circles, but there are no large or even small series published to date. However, this should remain an option for the hand surgeon faced with such a challenging clinical problem.

Conclusion

Total wrist arthrodesis remains a mainstay in the salvage treatment of many wrist conditions. It is a reliable, safe operation, with reported union rates from 93% to 100%, and patient satisfaction rates up to 100%. When a wrist fusion fails to unite or give adequate pain relief, it may be a difficult condition to manage. A careful history and physical exam, a thorough preoperative evaluation, and a critical surgeon can lead to a correct diagnosis and, potentially, a successful revision operation. One must keep in mind, however, that not all unsatisfied patients are candidates for surgery. Patients who ultimately come to a pan-wrist fusion operation often have had multiple surgeries, over years of treatment. Treatments should be individualized for each patient, with anatomic considerations to achieve stable union, minimize pain, correct alignment, eradicate infection, and maximize function.

References

1. Millender LH, Nalebuff EA. Arthrodesis of the rheumatoid wrist. J Bone and Joint. 1973;55A:1026–34.
2. Wood MB. Wrist arthrodesis using dorsal radial bone graft. J Hand Surg. 1987;12A:208–12.
3. Tannenbaum DA, Louis DS. The Stein and Gill technique for wrist arthrodesis. Tech Hand Up Extrem Surg. 1999;3(3):181–4.
4. Minami A, Kato H, et al. Total wrist arthrodesis using bowed crossed K-wires. J Hand Surg. 1999;24B:410–5.
5. Voutilainen N, Juutilainen T, et al. Arthrodesis of the wrist with bioabsorbable fixation in patients with rheumatoid arthritis. J Hand Surg. 2002;27B:563–7.
6. Hartigan B, Nagle DJ. Wrist arthrodesis with excision of the proximal carpal bones using the AO/ASIF wrist fusion plate and local bone graft. J Hand Surg. 2001;26B:247–51.
7. Meads BM, Scougall PJ, et al. Wrist arthrodesis using a Synthes wrist fusion plate. J Hand Surg. 2003;28B:571–4.
8. Nagy L, Buchler U. AO-wrist arthrodesis: with and without arthrodesis of the third carpometacarpal joint. J Hand Surg. 2002;27A:940–7.
9. Kumar K, Cox QGN. Pin arthrodesis of the wrist—a modified technique. J Hand Surg. 2005;30B:461–3.
10. Weiss A-P, Hastings H. Wrist arthrodesis for traumatic conditions: a study of plate and local bone graft application. J Hand Surg. 1995;20A:50–6.
11. Zachary SV, Stern PJ. Complications following AO/ASIF wrist arthrodesis. J Hand Surg [Am]. 1995;20(2):339–44.
12. Larsson SE. Compression arthrodesis of the wrist: a consecutive series of 23 cases. Clinical Orthop. 1974;99:146–53.
13. Wright CS, McMurtry RY. Arthrodesis in the hand. J Hand Surg [Am]. 1983;8:932–5.
14. Leighton RK, Petri D. Arthrodesis of the wrist. Can J Surg. 1987;30:115–6.
15. Gaisne E, Dap F, Bour C, Merle M. Arthrodesis of the wrist in manual workers. Apropos of 36 cases. Rev Chir Orthop Reparatrice Appar Mot. 1991;77(8):537–44.
16. Hastings H. Arthrodesis of the osteoarthritic wrist. In: Gelberman RH, editor. Master Techniques in Orthopaedic Surgery. The Wrist. New York: Raven; 1994. p. 345–50.

17. Hastings II H, Weiss APC, Quenzer D, et al. Arthrodesis of the wrist for post-traumatic disorders. J Bone Joint Surg. 1996;78(6):897–902.
18. Hayden RJ, Jebson PJ. Wrist arthrodesis. Hand Clin. 2005;21(4): 631–40.
19. Muramatsu K, Ihara K, Azuma E, Orui R, Goto Y, Shigetomi M, Doi K. Free vascularized fibula grafting for reconstruction of the wrist following wide tumor excision. Microsurgery. 2005; 25(2):101–6.
20. Chin KR, Spak JI, Jupiter JB. Septic arthritis and osteomyelitis of the wrist: reconstruction with a vascularized fibular graft. J Hand Surg Am. 1999;24(2):243–8.
21. Germann G, Sauerbier M, Steinau HU, Wood MB. Reverse segmental pedicled ulna transfer as a salvage procedure in wrist fusion. J Hand Surg Br. 2001;26(6):589–92.

Reoperative Indications in Vascular Disorders of the Hand

7

William C. Pederson

Abstract

Fortunately in most cases of vascular or microvascular intervention, once the vessels have healed, the chances of needing repair are small. However, in some cases such as traumatic events, the vessels may thrombose or otherwise fail in the postoperative period. In these cases, reoperation is sometimes needed and is usually done in a very expeditious manner. Other cases relate to chronic vascular disease. In these cases, sympathetectomy sometimes may be of benefit. In other cases, a vascular access procedure may be stealing or shunting blood away from the hand resulting in ischemia. In these cases, revision options are sometimes needed in order to help the patient with their symptoms. Microvascular surgery requires not only a steady hand but also a steady mind, and these cases can be quite challenging.

Keywords

Vascular • Injury • Ischemia • Disease • Access

Introduction

The indications for reoperative intervention on patients with vascular injury of the hand are uncommon, as in most cases vascular repairs and bypasses remain patent for the life of the patient. This is certainly true in most cases of vascular injury and repair, but there are instances where thrombosis occurs and intervention may be necessary. The appropriateness of reoperative management of individuals with vascular disease in the upper extremity is more likely to present itself, however, and surgery may become necessary to salvage these limbs. This chapter discusses the indications and techniques utilized in these cases.

W.C. Pederson, MD, FACS (✉)
The Hand Center of San Antonio, The University of Texas Health Science Center at San Antonio,
21 Spurs Lane, Suite 310, San Antonio, TX 78240, USA
e-mail: micro1@ix.netcom.com

Traumatic Vascular Injury

Penetrating Vascular Injury

Vascular injury to the upper extremity from penetrating trauma or cutting/avulsion injury is fairly common. While injury to one of the arteries of the forearm, or hand, may or may not require repair (for the purposes of adequate distal blood flow), brachial artery injuries almost always need repair or reconstruction. Depending on the mechanism of injury, these vessels may be primarily repaired or vein grafted (using saphenous or upper extremity veins as a conduit). The early results of brachial arterial repair are quite good, with many studies attesting to the excellent patency rate in these patients. Even 30 years ago, in reports from the 1980s, patency rates after vascular repair and/or grafting in the upper extremity were high with limb salvage rates near 100% [1]. One report from that time period noted a 93% rate of palpable pulses at follow-up in upper extremities undergoing vascular repair and/or bypass [2]. Reports on the results of repair

S.F.M. Duncan (ed.), *Reoperative Hand Surgery*,
DOI 10.1007/978-1-4614-2373-7_7, © Springer Science+Business Media, LLC 2012

of forearm vessels have been less optimistic, with Gelberman reporting only a 54% patency rate after arterial repair of the ulnar and/or radial arteries in the forearm [3]. However, these patients apparently remained asymptomatic after thrombosis of their repairs. Nonetheless, patients with critical ischemia from thrombosis of a forearm vessel repair can certainly become symptomatic.

The primary causes of vascular thrombosis after repair of traumatic injury would have to be technical, and thus the management of these is surgical. In the later postoperative period, infection can certainly lead to blow-out of an otherwise technically adequate anastomosis which can present as a surgical emergency. Other factors which can lead to late failure of an anastomosis or vein graft are irradiation of the vessels or presence of a foreign body (i.e., a drain in proximity to the anastomosis or vessel). While thrombolysis of clotted vessels with various thrombolytics has been reported [4], thrombosis of an arterial repair or vein graft has to be assumed to be due to some sort of technical problem and thus must be dealt with surgically. In the case of a thrombosed primary repair, the initial repair should be taken down and almost always managed with an interposition vein graft rather than attempting to re-repair the thrombosed artery. While the search for a suitable substitute for autogenous vein graft is ongoing, at present no graft material under 6–8 mm exists which does not have unacceptable rates of thrombosis. This includes polytetraflouroethylene (PTFE) and cadaveric allograft saphenous vein grafts [5, 6]. Thus, one must utilize autologous vein, either from the upper or lower extremity. While some prefer the saphenous over arm veins, I have utilized arm veins for bypass in the upper extremity on many occasions with no significant problems.

One must be aware of the potential for embolization of thrombus down the distal vessel. This must be managed with either local removal of clot under direct vision, or embolectomy with the appropriate Fogarty catheter. In the forearm or hand, this is usually a very small catheter, i.e., a number 2 or 3 French size. The balloon should only be inflated with air, as water or saline is less distensible and can cause potential damage to the vessel wall. The catheter is carefully placed down the distal vessel and the balloon is then inflated using a tuberculin syringe (with air). This is done with the surgeon feeling the pressure on the syringe to avoid overinflation and resulting intimal damage to the vessel. Once the balloon is inflated, the catheter is gently withdrawn until the balloon reaches the site of repair. Clots should be expressed just at the balloon reaches the site of injury. Passage of the Fogarty catheter should probably be performed both proximal and distally, unless there is brisk arterial flow from the proximal end of the vessel (see Fig. 7.4).

Once the vessel has been thrombectomized, heparinized saline in the dosage of 100 U/mL should be irrigated both proximally and distally in the vessel prior to placing vascular clamps to decrease the likelihood of re-thrombosis while the anastomosis is revised. Once this is done, the vessel edges are carefully trimmed back so that no further damage (from either the inciting trauma or initial repair) is evident. At this point, a vein graft is harvested from either the arm or leg, and reversed for anastomosis. I prefer to perform the proximal anastomosis first, which allows the vein graft to "unwind" and also gives a better idea of what length will be appropriate. This graft is irrigated with heparinized saline as well, once the proximal clamp is removed. Once trimmed to the appropriate length, the distal anastomosis is then performed in standard fashion.

The other issue with late failure of vein bypass grafts involves the presence of foreign material in proximity to the graft (i.e., a drain) or infection at the site of anastomosis. A drain should never be left in close proximity to either a vascular anastomosis or a vein graft, as it can cause ingress of bacteria in and can cause a "blowout" of the anastomosis or vessel graft if it inadvertently comes in contact with the vessel. An abscess around a vascular anastomosis is also a problem, as this can lead to thrombosis of the anastomosis and/or blowout of the artery as well. While arterial blowout in the upper extremity is a dramatic and life-threatening complication, it can usually be managed successfully by application of a pneumatic tourniquet (or in fact a blood pressure cuff) to the upper arm until proximal and distal control of the involved vessel can be obtained. In any case, thrombosis or dehiscence of an anastomosis will have to be managed by a vein graft, and in the case of severe infection and abscess formation, one should consider taking an extra-long segment of vein graft and routing it around the area of infection (an "extra-anatomic" bypass).

Closed Vascular Trauma

This category covers primarily patients with ulnar artery thrombosis due to "hypothenar hammer syndrome" [2, 7, 8]; however, radial artery thrombosis is also fairly common [9, 10]. If the patient presents with significant symptoms of pain and ischemia, Koman's group has shown that bypass grafting is of benefit [11, 12]. Most large series of these patients who have a true traumatic etiology of their arterial thrombosis have shown a very good long-term patency of these grafts, in the range of 75–80% [7, 8, 11, 13]. My own experience with ulnar artery bypass has been that patients without other systemic reasons for thrombosis (i.e., collagen vascular disease) have a 2-year patency rate of around 88%. Nonetheless, these bypass grafts can thrombose, and this is often due to patients returning to prior habits of hand use (using the hand as a hammer). My approach to these patients is based on the severity of their symptoms. Those patients who present with clear symptoms such as a white cold finger,

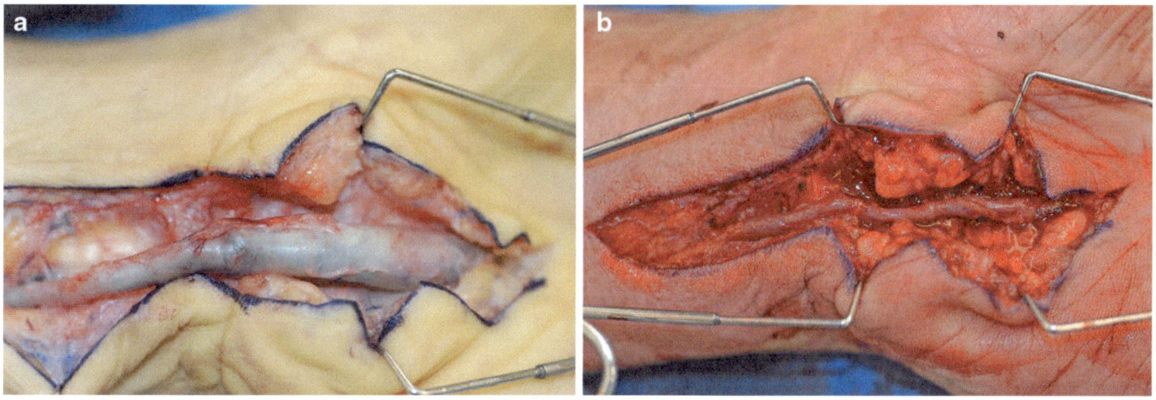

Fig. 7.1 (**a**) View of cephalic vein graft placed 9 years previously for hypothenar hammer syndrome. Patient recently became symptomatic again after banging his hand on a screwdriver. Graft is thrombosed and dilated with clot. (**b**) View of hand after revision of the bypass with a portion of saphenous vein. Fortunately, in this patient clot had not propagated beyond the original length of the graft

but without severe pain and/or gangrene and ulceration, can probably be watched, at least for a period of time. The mere loss of flow through the ulnar artery (or a bypass graft) does not necessarily dictate surgical intervention; however, the development of severe ischemic pain or tissue necrosis usually leads to re-do of the bypass.

Going back into a hand after failure of a bypass graft is certainly not as easy as the primary operation. The primary goal of the surgeon should be to avoid further injury to the existing vessels which are still patent and supplying flow to the hand. Thus, the clotted graft must be dissected out very carefully, and it is often found that thrombus extends well beyond the level of the first bypass graft. Vessels will clot back to a site where there is outflow, which generally is the first available branch. Primary hypothenar hammer syndrome patients will usually have thrombus back to the deep branch of the ulnar artery (which accompanies the deep branch of the ulnar nerve) or more commonly to the dorsal branch of the ulnar vessel which takes off about 3–4 cm proximal to the pisiform. On the superficial palmar arch side, the vessel is almost always patent at the site where the common digital artery to the fourth webspace comes off the arch. In the case of re-thrombosis of the graft, the clot may well extend beyond these levels, thus necessitating a longer graft (Fig. 7.1). If there is more clot distally in the palmar arch, revision grafting may necessitate multiple anastomoses to revascularize the common digital arteries to the third and fourth webspaces, while providing flow to the arch with the graft as well. Some have suggested that arterial grafts have a superior patency rate to that of vein grafts. The use of the thoracodorsal [14] and deep inferior epigastric vessels [15] has been proposed as an alternative to vein grafts. These vessels have the advantage that they have multiple distal branches which can be utilized to anastomose to the common digital vessels (Fig. 7.2). I have experience in one patient who was revised utilizing the descending branch of the lateral femoral circumflex artery, which also was of appropriate proximal and distal diameter and had appropriate branches for anastomosis to the common digital vessels. The use of these arterial grafts may have a role in revisional surgery in patients with recurrent hypothenar hammer syndrome; however, there is not enough data to prove arterial grafts' superiority.

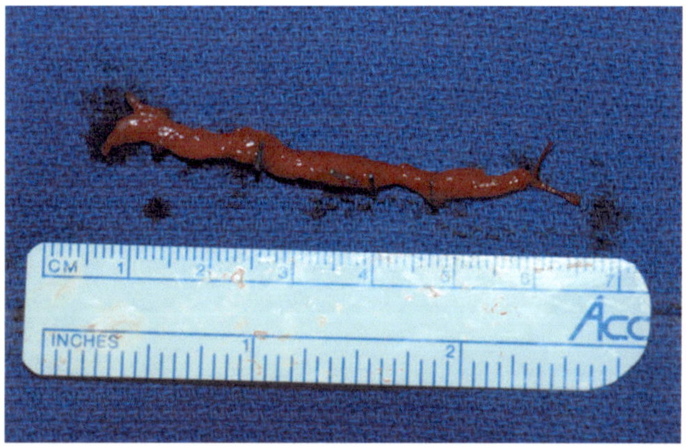

Fig. 7.2 Thoracodorsal artery which has been harvested to repair a re thrombosed ulnar artery vein graft. Note small branches to the left which can be utilized to sew into the common digital arteries of the hand beyond the arch

Another potential problem with vein grafting of arterial lesions is the potential for aneurismal dilatation of the vein graft. This has been reported in the upper extremity, while it is actually fairly uncommon based on personal experience with many vein graft reconstructions in the hand [16, 17]. Nonetheless, if the patient presents with a pulsatile swelling along the course of the previously placed vein graft, there should be a high index of suspicion of the presence of aneurismal change in the graft. This can be evaluated with an arteriogram or CT angiogram, but color-flow Doppler imaging is noninvasive and can also be utilized to evaluate the

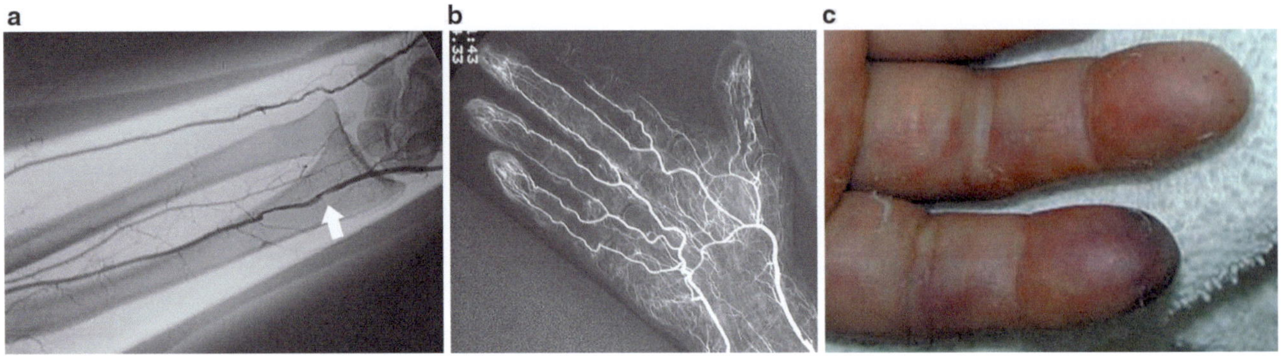

Fig. 7.3 (**a**) Arteriogram of patient whose hand became ischemic after placement of a radial arterial line. *Arrow* points to site of intimal flap in radial artery. (**b**) Note lack of flow to index finger due to embolization of clot. (**c**) Index finger of patient

graft. If aneurismal dilatation of the graft is confirmed, it should be revised with a new graft (either artery or vein).

Iatrogenic Injury

Iatrogenic arterial injury in the upper extremity is limited, but has certainly been reported with arthroscopy [18, 19] and can occur with other open procedures as well. Many times an injured vessel in the forearm or hand can be simply tied off without major sequelae. This is certainly true of the radial artery in the anatomic snuffbox, which can be injured with improper portal placement in wrist arthroscopy [20, 21]. The more proximal the injury, the more likely it will need repair, at least in the upper extremity. The usual rules apply to repair of injured vessels in this setting as in any other, most injuries will require vein grafting but on occasion the vessel can be freed up enough to allow for excision of the damaged segment and primary repair. If any question exists, however, the damaged segment should be repaired with a vein graft.

Symptomatic thrombosis of the radial artery after cannulation for arterial pressure monitoring is fortunately uncommon. A recent review quotes an incidence of permanent ischemic complications of 0.09% in radial arterial cannulation [22]. Another prospective study of patients undergoing radial artery catheterization for monitoring found that 28% developed abnormal flow in the radial artery by Doppler ultrasound studies, and a full 10% lost their radial pulse. None of these patients, however, became symptomatic [23]. Patients who develop ischemia of the fingers or hand after cannulation of the radial artery usually shower emboli to the involved digits, making repair of the injured segment less likely to improve flow [24] (Fig. 7.3). It would also appear from published reports that patients on vasopressors are also more at risk to develop ischemic complications from radial arterial monitoring [25]. One report utilized patch angioplasty at the site of injury, and noted that 75% of their angioplasties had thrombosed within the first 24 h [24]. They also failed to note improvement in distal circulation as compared to patients they treated without surgery; however, they only performed one excision and vein grafting at the site of injury. I have seen two hands lost due to gangrene after radial artery catheterization who did not have surgical intervention, and thus my bias is to explore these patients, perform thrombectomy, and place a vein graft in the area of damage to the radial artery. This again involves using a small Fogarty embolectomy catheter placed into the distal circulation which can be hazardous, but is necessary to make sure that there is not an ongoing blockage to flow which can be corrected (Fig. 7.4). It is not feasible, however, to perform embolectomy on the digital vessels without significant risk to the involved vessel. It may be possible to manage some of these patients with thrombolytic therapy [26, 27], but my experience has not been good in this area, as the radiologists are often reluctant to perform this in the face of an otherwise potentially unstable patient.

Ischemic Disease of the Hand

Chronic Ischemia Related to Vascular Disease

Vascular disease leading to ischemia of the upper extremity is rather uncommon. However, it is becoming more prevalent in longer-surviving patients on chronic renal dialysis and those who are post major organ transplantation. It has been reported that only 4–18% of vascular surgical interventions are in the upper extremity [28]. These patients can develop multilevel vascular disease, and may have a particularly virulent form of calcific arthritis. This entity can be very difficult and frustrating to manage, as these patients frequently end up with major amputations despite our best efforts. Ischemia is often associated with dialysis access procedures, in the face of underlying multilevel vascular disease [28, 29]. Arterial bypass in the upper extremity is usually highly successful, with 3-year patency rates in the 85% range [30]. However,

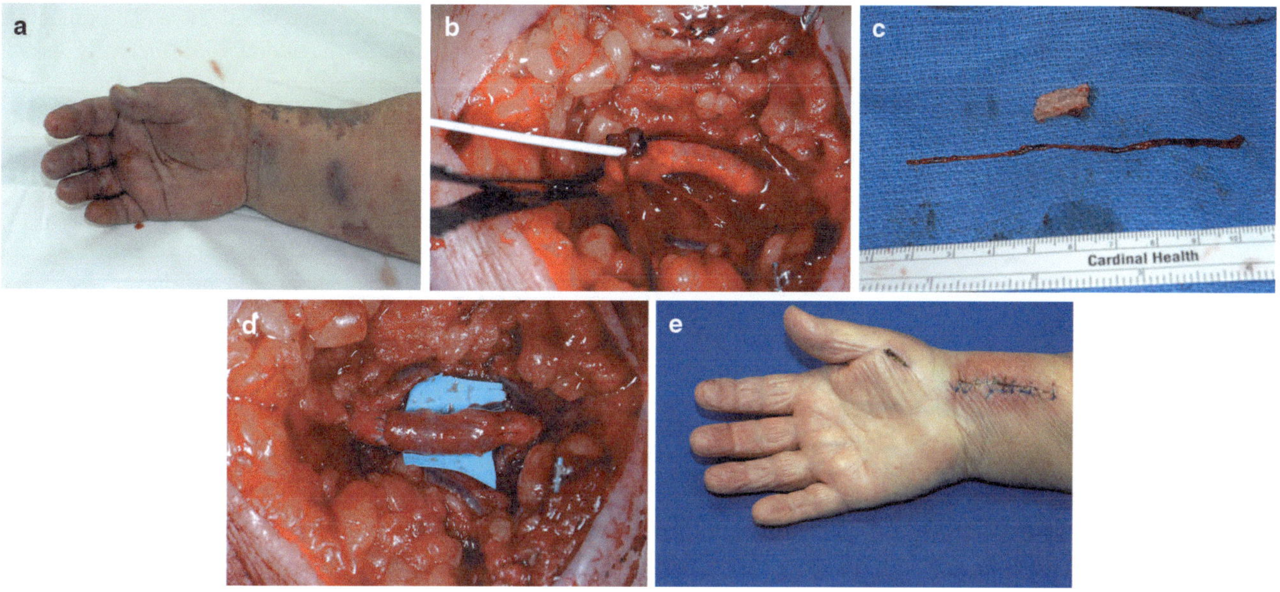

Fig. 7.4 (**a**) View of patient's hand which became ischemic after attempted placement of a radial arterial line. (**b**) Removing distal clot from radial artery with #3 French Fogarty catheter (**c**) 10 cm thrombus removed with balloon catheter. Note damaged segment of vessel wall above. (**d**) Segment of saphenous vein utilized to repair damaged segment of artery. (**e**) Hand at 2 weeks with good pulses and no tissue loss

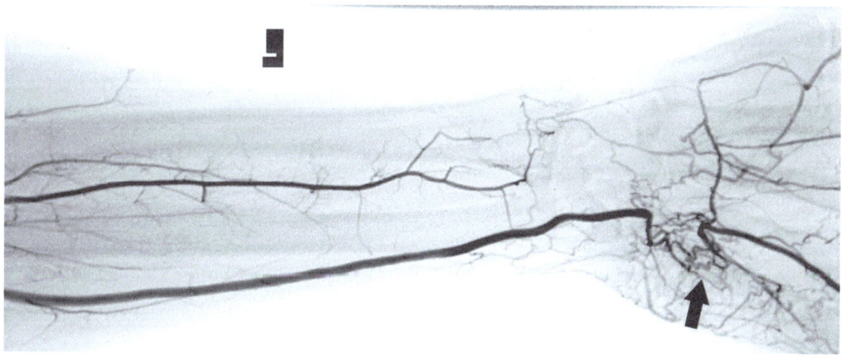

Fig. 7.5 Arteriogram of a 34-year-old male who is a heavy smoker. *Arrow* points to "corkscrew" collateral vessels around area of ulnar artery thrombosis indicating Buerger's disease. Note that patient also has occlusion of radial artery

thrombosis of a bypass to the distal extremity in the severe vasculopath usually portends major amputation in my experience [31]. Because of poor outflow, a vein graft that suffers thrombosis is usually not salvageable.

Another form of ischemia in the upper extremity which is much less common is Buerger's Disease (thromboangiitis obliterans). This problem is infrequently seen today with the decrease in smoking, but can still present significant problems in management. Cessation of smoking is key in the management of these patients, but it is often impossible for the patient to comply. While I have a fair number of patients referred with this diagnosis, it is distinctly uncommon in my experience. The hallmark of this disease is "corkscrew" collateral vessels seen in the extremity on an arteriogram, which are infrequently seen (Fig. 7.5). Initial management consists of treatment of digital and hand ulcers with wound care. Bypass is appropriate in some patients. Long-term patency rates in this setting are not very good, however, and other options may be needed to avoid limb loss in these patients [32]. Novel approaches such as vascularized omental transfer [33] may be of benefit in some instances, and has proven to be a useful technique in some patients [34] (see below). Nonsurgical management of these patients with stem cell infusion has shown some benefit [35, 36] and may become a useful adjuvant in the future.

One option for restoration of flow in the patient with a failed bypass or lack of adequate outflow vessels is arterialization of the venous system. In this procedure, the venous system is utilized as a conduit for arterial blood to reach the hand. This can be done with a proximal anastomosis to the arterial system (usually end-to-side to the brachial artery), but the valves in the veins must be removed to the level of the wrist. The valves in the hand do not need to be removed in my experience, as the arterial pressure apparently renders

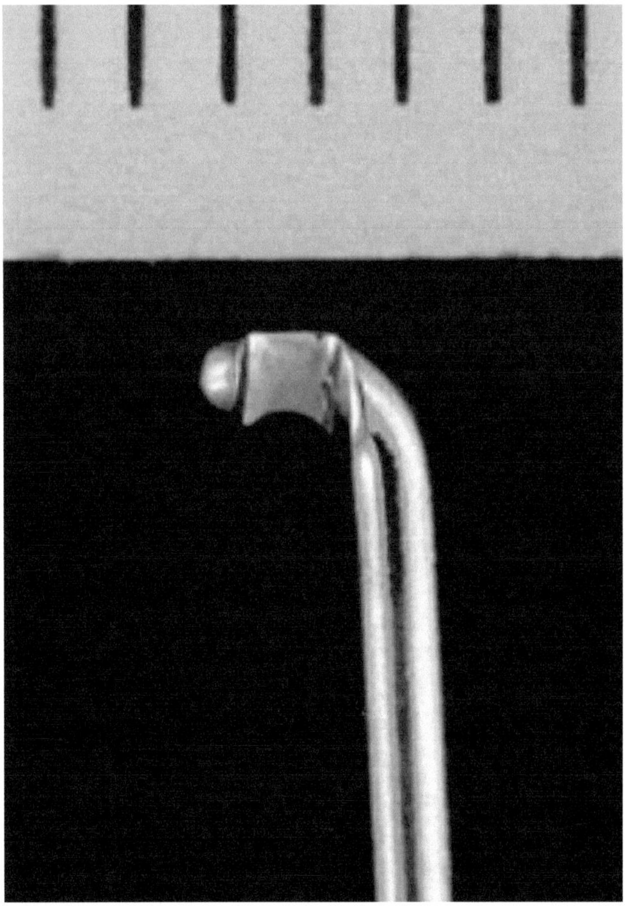

Fig. 7.6 End of Leather-Mills valvulotome utilized to remove valves in veins prior to bypass

them incompetent [37]. The valves in the cephalic or basilic vein are removed with a valvulotome via a side branch (Fig. 7.6). All side branches to the level of the wrist are tied off to prevent the development of significant arteriovenous fistulae in the forearm. Once this is done, an end-to-side anastomosis is performed between the vein and the brachial artery (Fig. 7.7). The arteriovenous anastomosis can be performed more distally; however, in most of these patients there is not adequate distal flow to allow for this. This procedure should not be performed in the face of active infection, as I have had two patients who developed severe swelling and required hand amputation in this setting. Nonetheless, this procedure can offer long-term improvement in blood flow and quality of life [38], and symptoms of pain and ulceration usually resolve [39, 40].

Another option in the face of failed bypass is vascularized free tissue transfer to the ischemic limb. While free flap transfer has been proposed to aid in the revascularization of distal tissue [41], the omentum has been shown to have ideal characteristics in this regard. It can be harvested with a long vascular pedicle and can easily be made to reach the hand with an anastomosis in the antecubital fossa. The omentum has been utilized primarily in patients with Buerger's disease [33, 34], and has proven efficacy in these patients. I have also utilized vascularized omental transfer in patients with severe vascular disease related to long-term immunosuppression after cardiac or renal transplantation. In this technique, the omentum is harvested from the abdomen on the gastoduodenal vessels. These vessels are then utilized for anastomosis in the proximal forearm or antecubital fossa. The omentum is then placed along the arm, either in pockets or in incisions made along the forearm and dorsal hand. If the omentum is left without cover, a split-thickness skin graft is placed over it. Maximum contact area between the transferred omentum and the forearm and/or hand allows for better revascularization of the ischemic limb. Improvement in pain and ulcerations is usually seen by 6–8 weeks, and I have even seen return of a Doppler signal to the vessels in the palm about 3 months after omental transfer (Fig. 7.8). This procedure certainly has benefits to prevent loss of the hand in younger patients with advanced arterial disease.

While some have advocated periarterial sympathectomy for the management of digital ulcers from arteriosclerotic disease, I have not found this useful, particularly in patients with severe calcific arterial disease (as is seen in diabetics and patients after transplant). Studies of the efficacy of this procedure have confirmed that it is not generally of significant benefit in individuals with arteriosclerosis as a basis for their digital ulcerations [42].

Vascular Access Procedures and Hand Ischemia

Patients with chronic renal failure and on dialysis present a number of issues in terms of the vascular supply to the hand. They often suffer from severe calcific arterial disease, which may lead to thrombosis and ischemia. In addition, they frequently have had one or more vascular access procedures in the forearm and upper extremity, and this can compound their other vascular issues. The renal physicians and particularly the vascular surgeons are usually unable or unwilling to revise a forearm shunt if it provides good access for dialysis. The patients' symptoms may range from pain and/or numbness (due to ischemia of the median nerve) to gangrene and tissue loss. The likelihood of a forearm fistula causing symptomatic steal syndrome is estimated to be about 1%, and about 5–10 times higher if the shunt involves the brachial artery [43]. Definitive diagnosis is usually made on arteriogram, and at the time of the study the fistula should be occluded at one point to see if flow improves into the distal hand.

If the fistula is large, the first option is to simply band the vessel to reduce flow somewhat. This is usually done with a

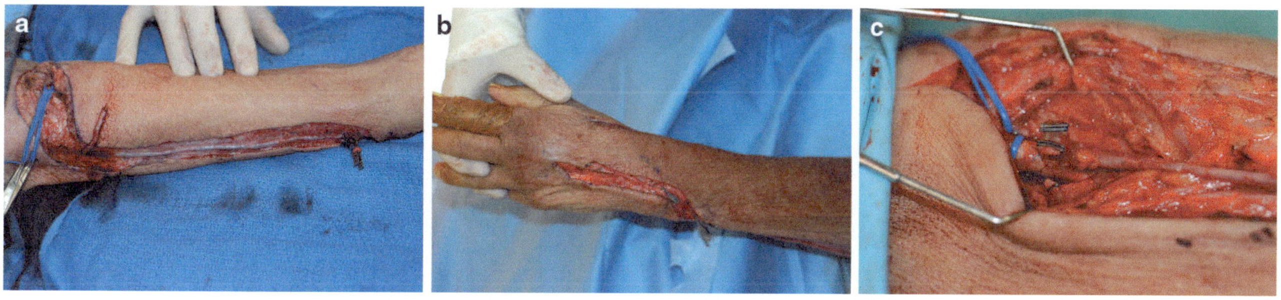

Fig. 7.7 (**a**) Basilic vein dissected out and branches ligated for arterialization of the venous system. (**b**) View of dorsal hand with distal connection to basilic dissected out. (**c**) Proximal end-to-side anastomosis between basilic vein and brachial artery

Fig. 7.8 (**a**) View of 32-year-old male's hand who is 18 years post renal transplant. He has already had an arterialization of the venous system which thrombosed 2 years postop when an I.V. was placed in the vein. He now has recurrent ischemic symptoms and ulceration of the middle finger. (**b**) Patient's omentum at time of harvest. (**c**) Hand at 6 months postop with healing of ulcer and no ischemic symptoms. Note bulge in dorsal hand where omentum was placed in pocket under the skin. Proximal anastomosis was to the brachial artery at the elbow

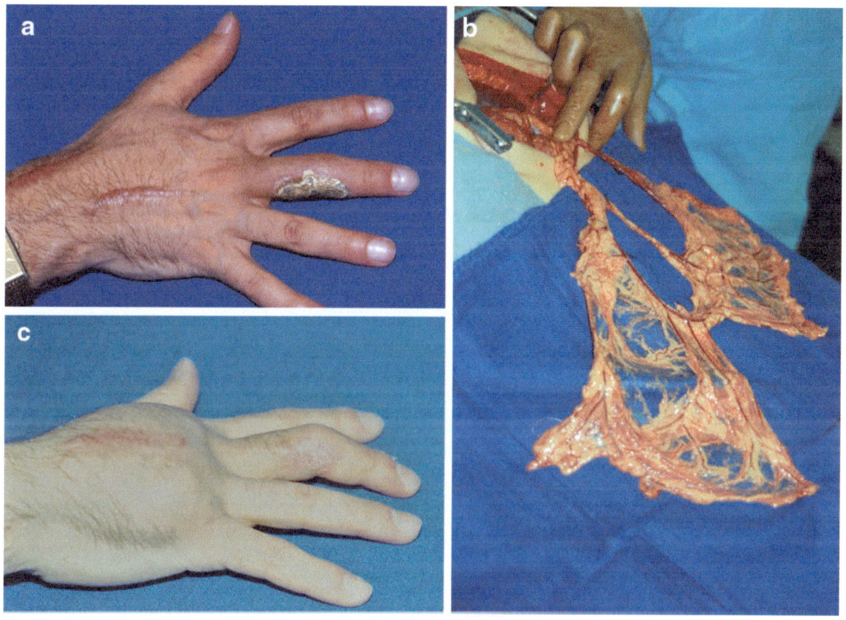

piece of PTFE vascular graft which is placed around the draining vein of the fistula. The PTFE is tightened down until better flow is noted in the distal circulation while on the operating table. At this point, the PTFE is sutured in place as a "flow restrictor." If the patient has severe ischemic symptoms and impending tissue loss, the shunt may simply be ligated. Preferably, a "distal revascularization interval ligation" (or DRIL) procedure may be performed. This procedure allows maintenance of the fistula while improving distal flow. The DRIL procedure consists of vein grafting from the proximal artery (above the fistula) to the distal native artery (beyond the fistula). Once this is done, the artery is ligated just distal to the arteriovenous fistula, and thus flow is maintained through the fistula, but now the "steal" is from above this level via the vein graft to the distal limb (Fig. 7.9). This procedure can be quite effective in managing ischemia in the hand [44, 45], and it allows continued use of the fistula for dialysis access.

Vasospastic Disease

The surgical management of patients with vasospastic disease, or Raynaud's and digital ischemia and ulceration, usually involves periarterial sympathectomy of the distal forearm vessels, palmar arch, and common digital vessels. In patients with occlusion of one of the major vessels to the hand bypass may be indicated as well. The failure rate of arterial bypass in patients with collagen vascular disease is higher than that in patients with traumatic occlusion in the hand, and thus patients can present with recurrence of symptoms [46]. Periarterial sympathectomy has been well shown to be of benefit in patients with vasospastic problems due to collagen vascular disease [42, 47, 48] as well as after vascular trauma and/or ulnar artery thrombosis [49, 50]. Studies with follow-up to the range of 8 years have shown benefit from this procedure [51]; yet, there is no question that recurrence of ischemia and ulceration can be a significant issue in patients

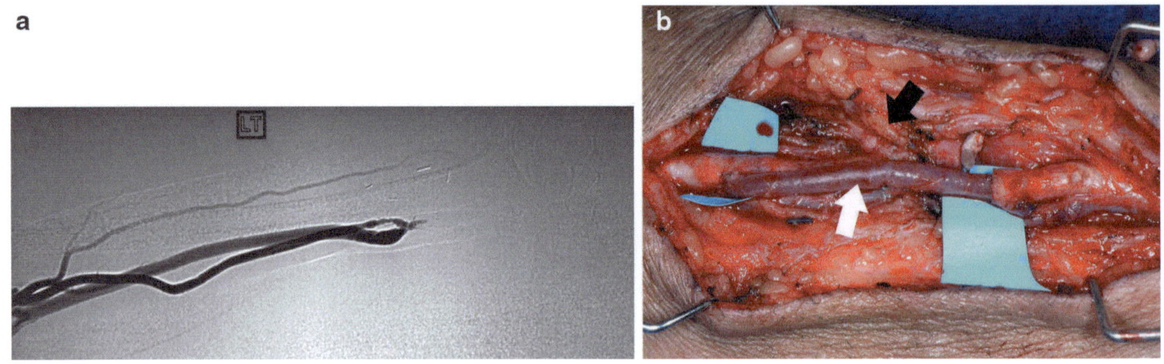

Fig. 7.9 (**a**) Arteriogram of patient showing near complete "steal" of flow from distal forearm radial artery-cephalic vein fistula. (**b**) View after distal bypass interval ligation (DRIL) procedure. *Light arrow* points to site of fistula, *dark arrow* points out vein graft from proximal radial artery end-to-side to distal radial artery end-to-end

who have previously undergone periarterial sympathectomy. There is very little data on the management of recurrent vasospastic symptoms after surgical sympathectomy; however, Dorafshar reviewed three patients who had recurrent symptoms after surgery and eventually had reoperation. They noted that these patients had remained asymptomatic for a period of 2–8 years after their original procedure. Likewise, these three individuals had a period of recurrent symptoms averaging 41 months prior to re-do of their surgical sympathectomy. Symptoms improved in all of these patients and ulcers on 15 fingers healed after the second procedure with a 1-year follow-up [51]. From my own personal experience and this brief report, it would appear that repeat surgical periarterial sympathectomy is a worthwhile procedure.

There is little data on the management of patients with thrombosis of a bypass graft under these circumstances, but in my experience they can benefit from reoperation. As noted above, patency rates of arterial bypass in patients with collagen vascular disease are well below those patients who simply suffer from traumatic occlusion of the ulnar or radial arteries. In my experience, many patients who thrombose their vein grafts in the first year will remain asymptomatic, presumably from the sympathectomy effect of excision of the involved artery (a so-called "Leriche sympathectomy" [52, 53]). Patients who have later thrombosis of their bypass grafts may become symptomatic, probably due to the loss of the sympathectomy effect of the prior surgery. This is probably the reason that periarterial sympathectomy eventually fails as well, most likely due to regeneration of the sympathetic nerves to the involved vessels.

Based on personal experience with a few patients, revision of the clotted vein graft bypass with a new graft does improve these patients' symptoms. This surgery can be difficult, due to scarring around the vessels and also propagation of thrombus above the anastomosis between the original graft and the native artery. Collateral vascular development [54] in collagen vascular disease patients is usually poor, and thus their hand may rely fairly heavily on the bypass graft for critical perfusion. Successful revascularization of these patients usually requires a longer vein graft and resection of at least a portion of the proximal and distal "normal" vessel to allow for successful restoration of flow to the hand and fingers. This may not be problematic in the forearm, but can present problems at the level of the arch and/or digital vessels. If the first graft was anastomosed to the arch (which is almost always possible at the first surgery in these patients), thrombosis may make revision anastomosis to the arch impossible. In order to successfully restore flow to the digits, the surgeon must be prepared to perform the distal anastomoses at the level of the digital vessels. This will require either multiple end-to-side anastomoses between the digital arteries and the vein graft, or conversely one can harvest either a vein graft with multiple branches or an arterial graft as discussed above [14, 15]. Veins from the dorsal foot may be quite useful in this regard, as they will often have multiple small branches. The thoracodorsal, deep inferior epigastric, and descending branch of the lateral femoral circumflex arteries have all been proposed or utilized for reconstruction of the palmar arch. While one should carefully measure the in situ length of the defect and match the graft to this, I prefer to perform the proximal anastomosis first in all instances. After the proximal anastomosis is complete, clamps are removed and the vein or artery graft is allowed to fill with blood, stretch out, and un-kink. This technique gives a much better idea of how to site the distal anastomoses on the graft. Once the graft is filled with blood, distal clamp(s) can be placed, and after appropriate trimming, the distal anastomoses can be performed. Patients who suffer from re-thrombosis of a vein graft may benefit from systemic oral antiplatelet therapy (in the form of Plavix) or even systemic oral anticoagulation, depending on the severity of their ischemic symptoms at the time of re-thrombosis.

Another approach to the patient suffering from recurrent symptoms after periarterial sympathectomy and/or bypass is the use of local botulinum toxin. Injection of this substance in the periarterial areas of the palm has been shown to be of some benefit in patients with vasospastic disease [55–57], although long-term controlled studies are lacking. Further study may delineate the indications for this form of management.

References

1. Pasch AR, Bishara RA, Lim LT, Meyer JP, Schuler JJ, Flanigan DP. Optimal limb salvage in penetrating civilian vascular trauma. J Vasc Surg. 1986;3:189–95.
2. Borman KR, Snyder III WH, Weigelt JA. Civilian arterial trauma of the upper extremity. An 11 year experience in 267 patients. Am J Surg. 1984;148:796–9.
3. Gelberman RH, Nunley JA, Koman LA, Gould JS, Hergenroeder PT, MacClean CR, Urbaniak JR. The results of radial and ulnar arterial repair in the forearm. Experience in three medical centers. J Bone Joint Surg Am. 1982;64:383–7.
4. Wheatley MJ, Swift R. Successful hand revascularization with urokinase following a crush injury. Ann Plast Surg. 1997;39:94–6.
5. Harris RW, Schneider PA, Andros G, Oblath RW, Salles-Cunha S, Dulawa L. Allograft vein bypass: is it an acceptable alternative for infrapopliteal revascularization? J Vasc Surg. 1993;18:553–9.
6. Lauterbach SR, Torres GA, Andros G, Oblath RW. Infragenicular polytetrafluoroethylene bypass with distal vein cuffs for limb salvage: a contemporary series. Arch Surg. 2005;140:487–93.
7. De MD, Fritsche E, Rigoni G, Schlunke S, Von WU. Hypothenar hammer syndrome. Retrospective study of nine cases. J Hand Surg Br. 1999;24:731–4.
8. Troum SJ, Floyd III WE, Sapp J. Ulnar artery thrombosis: a 6-year experience. J South Orthop Assoc. 2001;10:147–54.
9. McNamara MG, Butler TE, Sanders WE, Pederson WC. Ischaemia of the index finger and thumb secondary to thrombosis of the radial artery in the anatomical snuffbox. J Hand Surg Br. 1998;23:28–32.
10. Richards RR, Urbaniak JR. Spontaneous retrocarpal radial artery thrombosis: a report of two cases. J Hand Surg Am. 1984;9:823–7.
11. Chloros GD, Lucas RM, Li Z, Holden MB, Koman LA. Post-traumatic ulnar artery thrombosis: outcome of arterial reconstruction using reverse interpositional vein grafting at 2 years minimum follow-up. J Hand Surg Am. 2008;33:932–40.
12. Fitridge RA, Raptis S, Miller JH, Faris I. Upper extremity arterial injuries: experience at the Royal Adelaide Hospital, 1969 to 1991. J Vasc Surg. 1994;20:941–6.
13. Ruch DS, Aldridge M, Holden M, Smith TL, Koman LA, Smith BP. Arterial reconstruction for radial artery occlusion. J Hand Surg Am. 2000;25:282–90.
14. Dethmers RS, Houpt P. Surgical management of hypothenar and thenar hammer syndromes: a retrospective study of 31 instances in 28 patients. J Hand Surg Br. 2005;30:419–23.
15. Smith HE, Dirks M, Patterson RB. Hypothenar hammer syndrome: distal ulnar artery reconstruction with autologous inferior epigastric artery. J Vasc Surg. 2004;40:1238–42.
16. Dorweiler B, Neufang A, Schmiedt W, Hessmann MH, Rudig L, Rommens PM, Oelert H. Limb trauma with arterial injury: long-term performance of venous interposition grafts. Thorac Cardiovasc Surg. 2003;51:67–72.
17. Higgs PE, Weeks PM. Traumatic pseudoaneurysm in an ulnar artery vein graft. Plast Reconstr Surg. 1993;91:726–8.
18. Culp RW. Complications of wrist arthroscopy. Hand Clin. 1999; 15:529–35; x.
19. Marecek GS, Saltzman MD, Johnson DL. Complications in shoulder arthroscopy. Orthopedics. 2010;33:492–7.
20. De SL. Pitfalls in wrist arthroscopy. Acta Orthop Belg. 2002; 68:325–9.
21. Rocchi L, Canal A, Pelaez J, Fanfani F, Catalano F. Results and complications in dorsal and volar wrist Ganglia arthroscopic resection. Hand Surg. 2006;11:21–6.
22. Brzezinski M, Luisetti T, London MJ. Radial artery cannulation: a comprehensive review of recent anatomic and physiologic investigations. Anesth Analg. 2009;109:1763–81.
23. Sfeir R, Khoury S, Khoury G, Rustum J, Ghabash M. Ischaemia of the hand after radial artery monitoring. Cardiovasc Surg. 1996;4: 456–8.
24. Valentine RJ, Modrall JG, Clagett GP. Hand ischemia after radial artery cannulation. J Am Coll Surg. 2005;201:18–22.
25. Wallach SG. Cannulation injury of the radial artery: diagnosis and treatment algorithm. Am J Crit Care. 2004;13:315–9.
26. Wheatley MJ, Marx MV. The use of intra-arterial urokinase in the management of hand ischemia secondary to palmar and digital arterial occlusion. Ann Plast Surg. 1996;37:356–62.
27. Witz M, Sagiv P, Lehmann JM. Fibrinolytic treatment of acute arterial occlusion distal to the wrist in two cases. J Hand Surg Eur Vol. 2008;33:342–4.
28. Warren JA, Agarwal G, Wynn JJ. Arterial revascularization for upper extremity ischemia in patients with chronic kidney disease. Am Surg. 2009;75:848–52.
29. Chang BB, Roddy SP, Darling III RC, Maharaj D, Paty PS, Kreienberg PB, Ozsvath KJ, Mehta M, Shah DM. Upper extremity bypass grafting for limb salvage in end-stage renal failure. J Vasc Surg. 2003;38:1313–5.
30. Hughes K, Hamdan A, Schermerhorn M, Giordano A, Scovell S, Pomposelli Jr F. Bypass for chronic ischemia of the upper extremity: results in 20 patients. J Vasc Surg. 2007;46:303–7.
31. Pederson WC. Management of end-stage ischemia of the arm. Clin Plast Surg. 1997;24:107–20.
32. Bozkurt AK, Besirli K, Koksal C, Sirin G, Yuceyar L, Tuzun H, Sayin AG. Surgical treatment of Buerger's disease. Vascular. 2004;12:192–7.
33. Bhat MA, Zaroo MI, Darzi MA. Omental transplantation for critical limb ischemia in Buerger's disease. Plast Reconstr Surg. 2007;119:1979–80.
34. Agarwal VK. Long-term results of omental transplantation in chronic occlusive arterial disease (Buerger's disease). Int Surg. 2005;90:167–74.
35. Matoba S, Tatsumi T, Murohara T, Imaizumi T, Katsuda Y, Ito M, Saito Y, Uemura S, Suzuki H, Fukumoto S, Yamamoto Y, Onodera R, Teramukai S, Fukushima M, Matsubara H. Long-term clinical outcome after intramuscular implantation of bone marrow mononuclear cells (therapeutic angiogenesis by cell transplantation [TACT] trial) in patients with chronic limb ischemia. Am Heart J. 2008;156:1010–8.
36. Motukuru V, Suresh KR, Vivekanand V, Raj S, Girija KR. Therapeutic angiogenesis in Buerger's disease (thromboangiitis obliterans) patients with critical limb ischemia by autologous transplantation of bone marrow mononuclear cells. J Vasc Surg. 2008;48:53S–60S.
37. Pederson WC. Surgical techniques for revascularization in the chronically ischemic hand. Tech Hand Upper Extrem Surg. 1997;1:103–15.
38. Chloros GD, Li Z, Koman LA. Long-term successful outcome of severe hand ischemia using arterialization with reversal of venous flow: case report. J Hand Surg Am. 2008;33:1048–51.
39. Kind GM. Arterialization of the venous system of the hand. Plast Reconstr Surg. 2006;118:421–8.
40. King TA, Marks J, Berrettoni BA, Seitz WH. Arteriovenous reversal for limb salvage in unreconstructible upper extremity arterial occlusive disease. J Vasc Surg. 1993;17:924–32.

41. Sasajima T, Azuma N, Uchida H, Asada H, Inaba M, Akasaka N. Combined distal venous arterialization and free flap for patients with extensive tissue loss. Ann Vasc Surg. 2010;24:373–81.
42. Hartzell TL, Makhni EC, Sampson C. Long-term results of periarterial sympathectomy. J Hand Surg Am. 2009;34:1454–60.
43. Malik J, Tuka V, Kasalova Z, Chytilova E, Slavikova M, Clagett P, Davidson I, Dolmatch B, Nichols D, Gallieni M. Understanding the dialysis access steal syndrome. A review of the etiologies, diagnosis, prevention and treatment strategies. J Vasc Access. 2008; 9:155–66.
44. Berman SS, Gentile AT, Glickman MH, Mills JL, Hurwitz RL, Westerband A, Marek JM, Hunter GC, McEnroe CS, Fogle MA, Stokes GK. Distal revascularization-interval ligation for limb salvage and maintenance of dialysis access in ischemic steal syndrome. J Vasc Surg. 1997;26:393–402.
45. Knox RC, Berman SS, Hughes JD, Gentile AT, Mills JL. Distal revascularization-interval ligation: a durable and effective treatment for ischemic steal syndrome after hemodialysis access. J Vasc Surg. 2002;36:250–5.
46. Jones NF. Ischemia of the hand in systemic disease. The potential role of microsurgical revascularization and digital sympathectomy. Clin Plast Surg. 1989;16:547–56.
47. Balogh B, Mayer W, Vesely M, Partsch H, Piza-Katzer H. Periarterial sympathectomy of the radial and ulnar arteries in Raynaud's phenomenon—a preliminary study. Handchir Mikrochir Plast Chir. 2002;34:374–80.
48. Li Z, Smith BP, Holden M, Koman LA. Periarterial sympathectomy of the foot for the treatment of necrotizing Raynaud's phenomena. J Reconstr Microsurg. 2009;25:133–7.
49. el-Gammal TA, Blair WF. Digital periarterial sympathectomy for ischaemic digital pain and ulcers. J Hand Surg Br. 1991;16:382–5.
50. Henry M, Levaro F, Masson M. Periarterial sympathectomy salvage of the acutely ischemic hand. J Reconstr Microsurg. 2003;19:7–10.
51. Dorafshar AH, Seitz IA, Zachary L. Reoperative digital sympathectomy in refractory Raynaud's phenomenon. Plast Reconstr Surg. 2009;123:36e–8e.
52. Leriche R. Sympathetic effect in vascular diseases of the extremities. Dia Med. 1957;29:3031–3.
53. Zook EG, Kleinert HE, Van Beek AL. Treatment of the ischemic finger secondary to digital artery occlusion. Plast Reconstr Surg. 1978;62:229–34.
54. Haerle M, Tonagel F, Schaller HE. Collateral arterial pathways in the forearm. Surg Radiol Anat. 2004;26:208–11.
55. Fregene A, Ditmars D, Siddiqui A. Botulinum toxin type A: a treatment option for digital ischemia in patients with Raynaud's phenomenon. J Hand Surg Am. 2009;34:446–52.
56. Neumeister MW, Chambers CB, Herron MS, Webb K, Wietfeldt J, Gillespie JN, Bueno Jr RA, Cooney CM. Botox therapy for ischemic digits. Plast Reconstr Surg. 2009;124:191–201.
57. Sycha T, Graninger M, Auff E, Schnider P. Botulinum toxin in the treatment of Raynaud's phenomenon: a pilot study. Eur J Clin Invest. 2004;34:312–3.

Reoperative Conditions Following Distal Radius Fractures

8

Amy L. Ladd and Kristen Fleager

Abstract

Distal radius fractures are a very routine case for both the orthopedic and hand surgeon. However, these injuries can be difficult to treat when severe comminution, poor bone quality, and marked displacement occur. Sometimes in these circumstances, the initial fixation may fail. This then requires reoperative intervention to try and restore articular congruity and bony alignment as best as possible within the given constraints of the tissue and bone quality, as well as the configuration of the fracture. There are a variety of options that can be utilized from external fixators to bridge plating. There are dorsal and volar plates to help try and reconstruct the articular surface. Also, autologous bone graft is the gold standard, but there are numerous other bone graft substitutes that can be utilized to reduce the morbidity from autologous grafting. Finally, soft tissues must be taken into account and these include the tendons which may be gliding over the plate as well as the carpal canal which can sometimes become tight after significant displacement and/or swelling. Even with optimum treatment, many of these patients with severe injuries will have outcomes that result in a stiff wrist but, hopefully, functional hand and extremity.

Keywords

Distal • Radius • Fracture • Reoperation • Malunion

Key Points

- Comprehend the history of the patient's injury and prior intervention.
- Understand patient's functional level and needs, hand dominance, and symptoms.
- Perform a thorough physical exam, including strength testing and upper limb motion.
- Perform new radiographic studies: plain radiographs of the contralateral wrist, possibly computed tomography.
- Study prior radiographs to understand cause(s) for failure.
- Set realistic goals and expectations preoperatively.
- Prepare to have multiple types of fixation and systems available in the OR such as: volar/dorsal/fragment specific plates, arthrodesis plate, external fixation, Kirschner (K)-wires, Rush rods, and autogenous bone graft harvest.
- Primary anatomic goals: restore articular surface, restore length/tilt/inclination.
- Careful attention to soft tissues—consider extensor retinacular lengthening, brachioradialis release, carpal tunnel release.
- When all else fails, consider limited or partial fusion.

A.L. Ladd, MD (✉) • K. Fleager, MD
Department of Orthopaedic Surgery, Stanford Hospitals and Clinics, 450 Broadway, M/C 6342, Redwood City, CA 94063, USA
e-mail: alad@stanford.edu

S.F.M. Duncan (ed.), *Reoperative Hand Surgery*,
DOI 10.1007/978-1-4614-2373-7_8, © Springer Science+Business Media, LLC 2012

Introduction

Treatment of distal radius fracture has evolved with time, and surgical intervention has become more common. While open treatment affords the opportunity to surgically reduce the fracture, malreductions and malunions are unfortunate complications. Patients may present with a significant deformity, pain, decreased range of motion or grip strength, infection, soft tissue defects, complex regional pain syndrome, or cosmetic concerns.

The causes of fixation failure are multifaceted. The patient may have underlying biology which delays healing or is not adequate to support fixation until union occurs. Patients may advance their activity ahead of indications or have subsequent trauma causing loss of reduction. Patients may have received inadequate fixation, due to a lack of appreciation of the complexity of the initial injury, such as using Kirschner (K)-wires for an unstable injury when a plate would have provided more stability. Comprehending the original injury and previous treatment(s), therefore, is paramount in the evaluation of the reoperative distal radius fracture.

Basic knowledge of the wrist anatomy and function is vital to a successful operation and outcome. It is known that the distal radius has a radial tilt of 11–12° volar, radial inclination of 22–23°, and radial length of 11–12 mm [1–4] (Fig. 8.1). Ulnar variance is best measured by comparison to the contralateral side, with symmetry as the goal. Contralateral radiographs are an important adjunct to reoperative treatment. Graham's review article supported acceptable limits of deformity as: greater than 15° of radial inclination, radial tilt between 15° dorsal and 20° volar, 2 mm of articular step-off or less, and radial shortening less than 5 mm at the distal radial ulnar joint compared to the contralateral wrist [5] (Table 8.1).

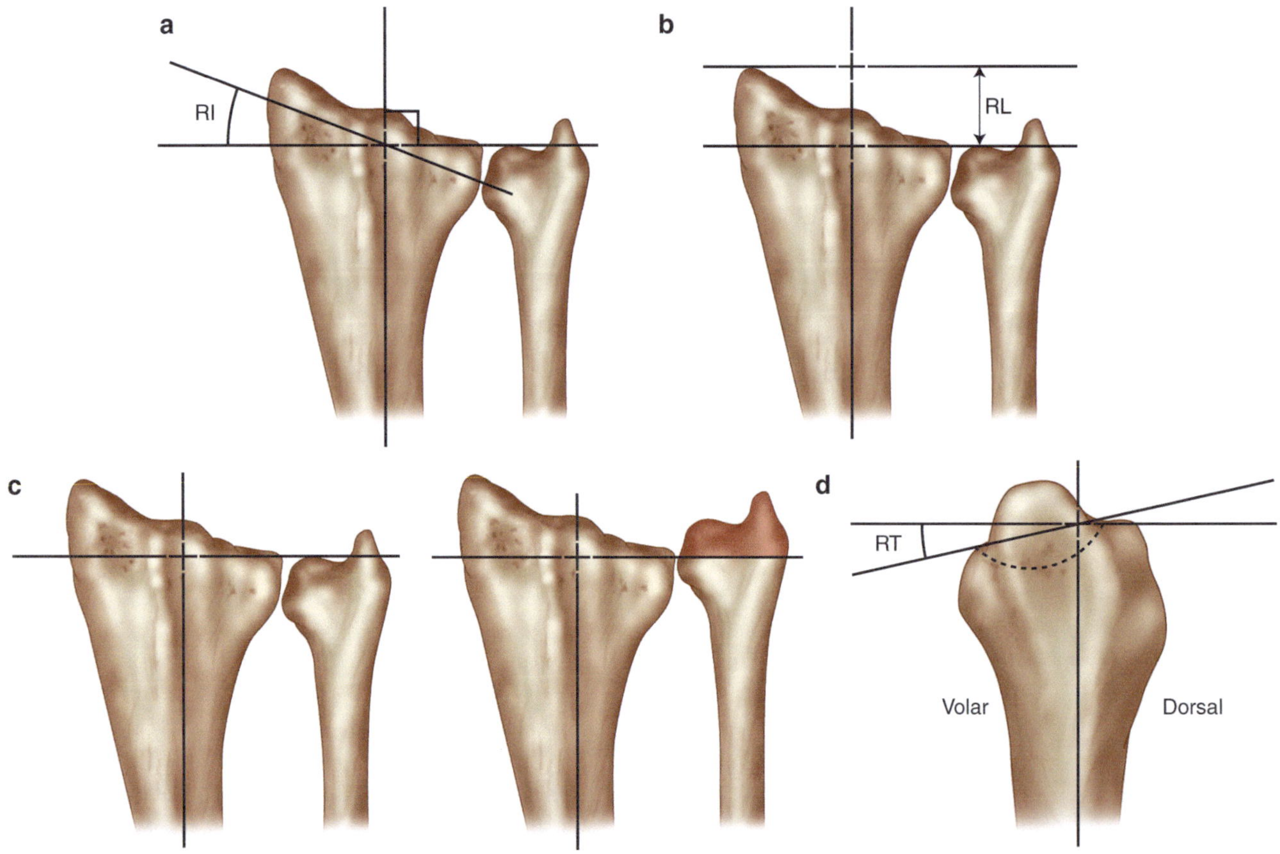

Fig. 8.1 Radiographic measurements of the distal radius. (**a**) Radial inclination (RI): angle formed by a line perpendicular to the long axis of the radius, and a line along the articular surface of the radius. (**b**) Radial length (RL): distance between tangential lines at the radial styloid and ulnar pole, perpendicular to the long axis. (**c**) Ulnar variance: axial distance between the ulnar pole and ulnarmost aspect of the distal radius. On *left*, neutral; on *right*, positive ulnar variance. (**d**) Radial tilt (RT): angle between radius articular surface and a line drawn perpendicular to the shaft

Table 8.1 Radiographic parameters of the distal radius: averages of normal and accepted postreduction limits of deformity

Radiographic criterion	Acceptable measurement
Radioulnar length	Radial shortening of <5 mm at DRUJ compared with contralateral wrist
Radial inclination	Inclination on PA film ≥15°
Radial tilt	Sagittal tilt on lateral projection between 15° dorsal tilt and 20° volar tilt
Articular incongruity	Incongruity of intra-articular fracture is ≤2 mm at radiocarpal joint

Reprinted with permission from Graham [5]

Distal radius fracture malunion may significantly alter the kinematics of the wrist. Dorsal angulation has been shown to increase ulnar load and instability of the distal radial ulnar joint [6–8]. It may also lead to a painful dorsal intercalary segment instability (DISI) type deformity, which results from compensatory flexing at the midcarpal level [4, 9–11]. This deformity may be classified into *adaptive* (type I) and *fixed* (type II) deformities (Fig. 8.2). Adaptive deformities will correct if the wrist is placed in the same amount of dorsal angulation as the distal radius malunion. This type of deformity may benefit from a corrective distal radius osteotomy, which will restore carpal alignment. Fixed type deformities, on the other hand, will not correct and may require fusion [12].

Radial shortening may lead to triangular fibrocartilage complex (TFCC) impingement, disruption of the distal radial ulnar joint, and ulnar impingement on the triquetrum or lunate [13, 14]. Significant pain and loss of supination and pronation may ensue [15, 16]. A change in radial inclination may affect the position of the carpal tunnel, which may lead to weaker grip strength. Decreased radial inclination also leads to mechanical difficulty with ulnar deviation and an increased loading of the lunate facet [16–18].

Malunion of the intra-articular distal radius must also be considered. Involvement of greater than 1–2 mm step-off of the articular surface has been shown to lead to poor results with increased arthritis [19–24]. In addition, collapse of the lunate facet may eventually lead to volar intercalary segment instability (VISI) [9]. If there is any concern for an intra-articular involvement, a CT scan is helpful to adequately assess the joint surface congruity. Restoring articular congruity is believed to lessen predisposition of posttraumatic arthritis by preserving cartilage. Intra-articular fractures, however, may cause injury to the cartilage even in relatively nondisplaced setting, and thus the development or severity of arthritis cannot be predicted on articular restoration alone.

Nonunion of the distal radius is uncommon, but may occur. Most commonly, they are associated with multiple extensive surgeries, smoking, and open injuries with diaphyseal extension. Delayed union is defined as no radiographic signs of bridging trabeculae at 4 months, while nonunion is defined at 6 months duration. The cause of a nonunion is yet to be elucidated, though several studies suggest a higher prevalence with concomitant ulnar fracture or dislocation [25, 26]. The majority of nonunions are synovial, unstable, and painful. [27, 28].

Indications and Contraindications

Indications and contraindications for distal radius revision

Indications	Contraindications
Motivated, active, compliant patient with clear, correctable etiology	Patients with poor general health or significant medical comorbidities
Infection	Repeated noncompliance
Malunion, deformity, or mechanical alterations that cause	Nonfocal pain, or associated with complex regional pain syndrome
Dysfunction	Able to perform activities of daily living with mild pain or impairment
Weakness	Advanced posttraumatic arthritis of radiocarpal or intercarpal joints
Stiffness	Severe osteoporosis
Pain	Severely comminuted articular surface, difficult to reconstruct
Dislocated or subluxated joint(s)	
Unacceptable hardware failure	

The decision for operative vs. nonoperative intervention should focus primarily on the patient's symptoms and function, and not solely radiographic parameters. Distal radius malunions fitting descriptions above may be asymptomatic [29–31].

The ideal patient is a motivated, compliant, healthy individual with a clear, correctable deformity. Patients who experience significant pain, significant decreased range of motion, or a disabling loss of grip strength will benefit the most from distal radius revision [5, 29, 32, 33]. Other patients may present without symptoms, but have a deformity so severe that future pain or dysfunction is predictable [33]. These patients may be considered reasonable operative candidates.

Patients with only mild pain or small changes in their functional activity level may not improve significantly after a repeat operation. Pain that is secondary to complex regional pain syndrome, radiocarpal or intercarpal degenerative disease, or soft tissue injury is also unlikely to improve. Severe comminution of the articular surface may be difficult to reconstruct, and therefore, may be more appropriate for fusion. As with any surgical procedure, poor general health or nutritional deficiencies are relative contraindications to operative intervention [5, 29–33].

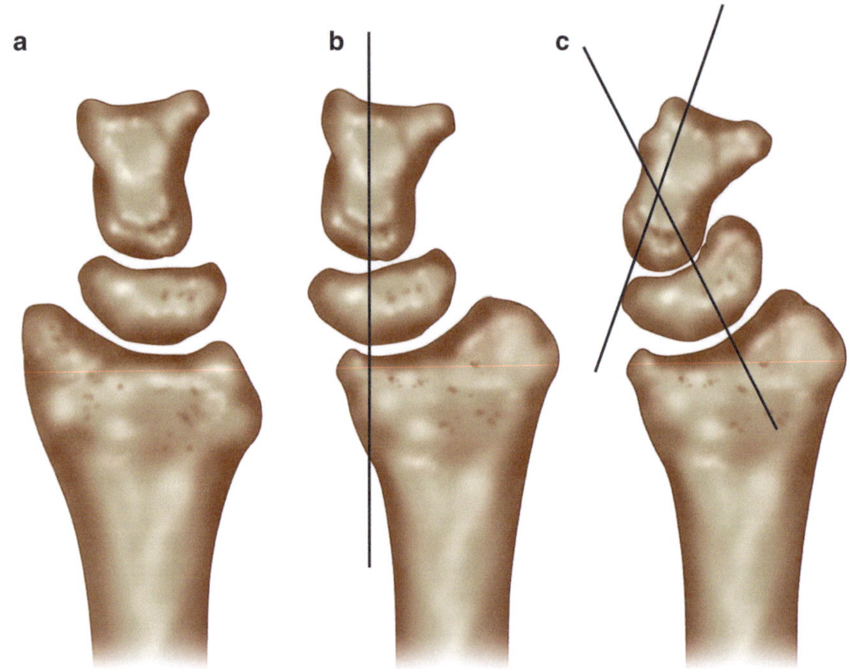

Fig. 8.2 Example of normal anatomy (**a**), fixed deformity (**b**), and adaptive deformity (**c**). Adaptive deformities may correct with a corrective distal radius osteotomy, while fixed deformities will not and may require fusion

Preoperative History and Considerations

The preoperative history, physical, and radiographic analysis are vital to a successful operative outcome. When taking the history, a general timeline of the patient's disease, outcomes, and previous interventions should be well understood. In addition, special attention must be paid to the mechanism of the initial injury. High-energy trauma with a high angle of impact is more likely to have associated ligament, nerve, and other soft tissue injury. The patient's overall health and nutritional status, tobacco use, and compliance may lend clues to the etiology of the failure. Symptoms of carpal tunnel syndrome and complex regional pain syndrome (pain out of proportion, swelling, and vasomotor instability such as changes in color/temperature/perspiration) should be discussed. Finally, the patient's primary complaint, activity level, hand dominance, and expectations will help guide treatment.

The physical exam should focus on the condition of the soft tissues, level of pain with range of motion of the hand and wrist, and overall functional status and preoperative demands of the upper limb. Pronation, supination, flexion, extension, and grip strength should be measured and compared to the contralateral limb. Median nerve function may be tested with monofilament testing, typically by a hand therapist. The vascular status may be assessed with the Allen text, capillary refill, and overall perfusion of the hand.

Although original injury films may be critical to best understanding future treatment and failure, they may be difficult to obtain. If possible, discussion with the operating/referring physician is advised to understand the background of the problem.

General themes for fixation failure include inadequate reduction and recognition, inadequate fixation (Fig. 8.3), unrecognized carpal or ulnar column involvement (including ulnar styloid, TFCC, DRUJ, or ulnar shaft) (Fig. 8.4), osteopenia/osteoporosis, and patient factors such as smoking, diabetes, other metabolic diseases, nutritional deficiencies, and smoking.

Specific pitfalls to external fixation and percutaneous pin fixation include a failure to recognize intra-articular, carpal, or diaphyseal involvement. Volar plate fixation may fail to address dorsal segments; diaphyseal and shear involvement may similarly remain unaddressed; or dorsal plating may inadequately capture vital volar fragments (Fig. 8.5). Poor screw placement, typically too long, may prevail.

During the preoperative visit, obtain new radiographs. Radiographs of the contralateral wrist allow the surgeon to assess the patient's normal anatomic parameters. Complex fractures may be evaluated with fine-cut CT scan, typically 1 mm cuts obtained axial, sagittal, and coronal planes. Reformatting into 3D projection is especially helpful when assessing for intra-articular malunions. CT angiography may be added if there is concern for vascular injury or if possible local flap coverage is anticipated.

Timing of reoperation requires careful consideration. Patients with few symptoms, limited needs, and expectations may be best served with nonoperative treatment.

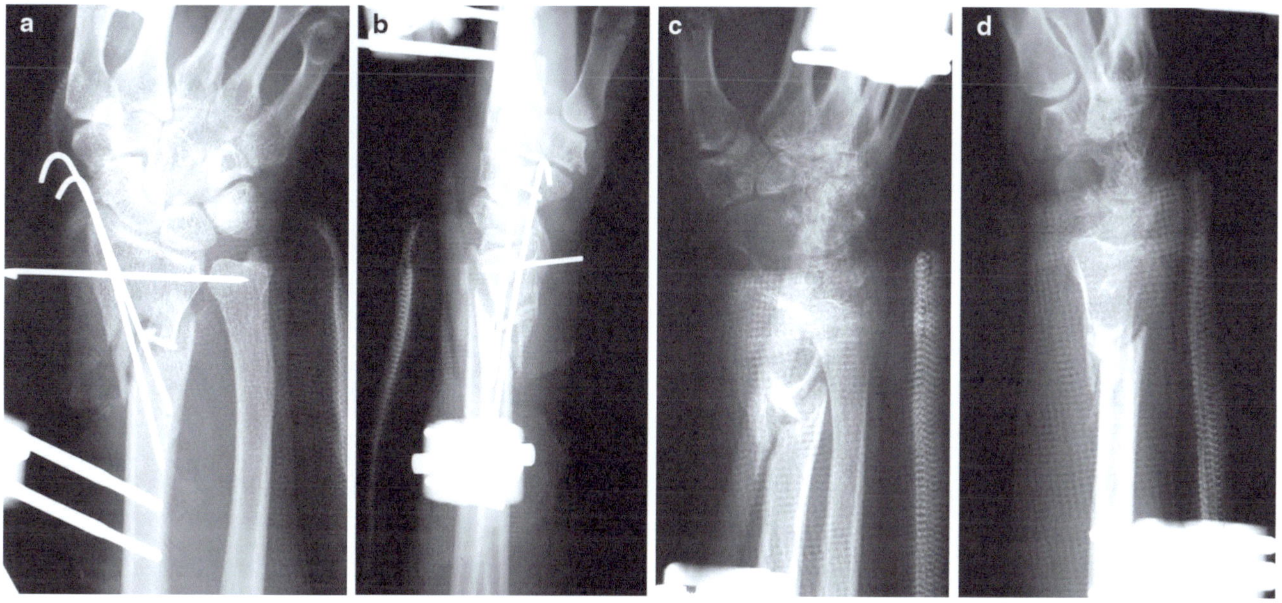

Fig. 8.3 Radiographic example of inadequate fixation using external fixation and pinning for a distal radius fracture with diaphyseal involvement (**a, b**), resulting in inadequate healing and loss of reduction (**c, d**)

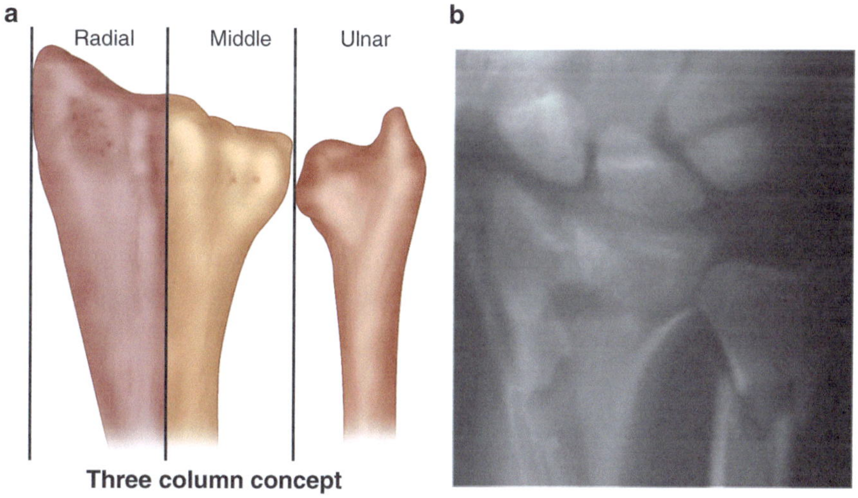

Fig. 8.4 (**a**) The "Three Column Concept" includes the radial (lateral radius with scaphoid fossa and styloid process), middle (medial radius, lunate fossa, and sigmoid notch), and ulnar (distal ulna, TFCC, and DRUJ) columns. (**b**) A radiographic example of involvement of all three columns

Soft tissue and bone quality in the early stages may be challenging. In the early inflammatory stage (first 1–4 weeks), the inflammatory state of the soft tissue may complicate closure and increase the risk of infection.

Early intervention, however, may promote earlier return to work, and thus early osteotomy is recommended in patient with high functional demand [34]. For some patients, it may be preferable to wait for healing to progress to a malunion, anticipating delayed surgical correction. This is often driven by a "wait and see" position from the patient. The advantage of a relatively low inflammatory state is balanced by the challenges of soft tissue contractures in the delayed setting.

Possible accessory procedures should be explained as part of the surgical consent. Carpal tunnel release, bone grafting from local or remote sites, or the use of synthetic or allograft bone should be discussed. In severe cases, soft tissue coverage options should be anticipated. The patient may also be consented for possible external fixation, osteotomy, or fusion.

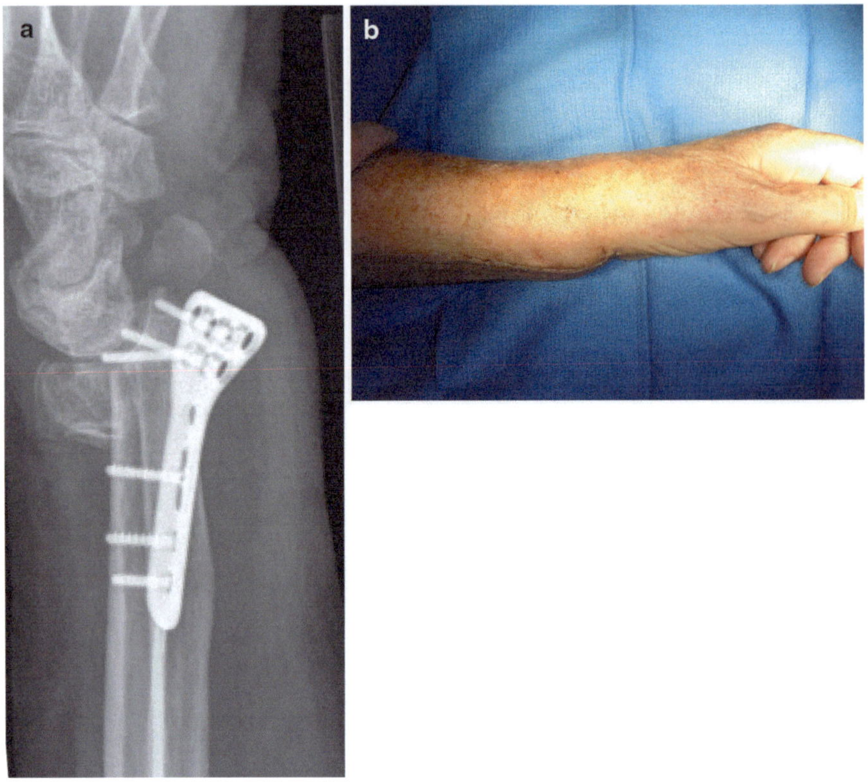

Fig. 8.5 Example of volar distal radius plate that failed to capture the dorsal fragments, resulting in loss of reduction. (**a**) demonstrates the loss of reduction, (**b**) the clinical deformity at time of reoperation. (photo courtesy of Dr. Amy Ladd, MD)

The clinical scenario will dictate the probability of such procedures.

Most importantly, realistic expectations should be set with surgical counseling. Not every patient should undergo another attempt at surgical treatment. The risks of a complication, including complex regional pain syndrome, infection, and nonunion, are amplified in the reoperative distal radius fracture. Realistic expectations as to achieving preinjury status should be discussed [9, 12, 29–33].

Operative Approach

Reoperation often occurs in the setting of inflammation, scar tissue, and distorted anatomy. While using an old incision will often be the best approach, it is worthwhile to think beyond the constraints of the previous incision: this may allow access to key pathology inaccessible at the index operation. An alternate approach through native tissue may be more straightforward or provide exposure to nerves at risk, or fragments previously ignored. A different approach, however, may require circumferential stripping, devascularization, and further complicate healing.

Volar Approach [35–37]

An Allen test should be performed preoperatively. Typically the site of the previous surgical approach, additional caution should be taken with handling the radial artery, which is often in scar.

A Henry approach between the flexor carpi radialis (FCR) and radial artery may be used, either dissecting through the FCR sheath, as commonly performed in primary volar distal radius procedures, or alongside the structure. The Henry approach allows for proximal extension of the incision and dissection if necessary (Fig. 8.6).

The deep dissection continues down to the pronator quadratus. In the reoperative setting, this typically consists of more scar tissue than muscle. Plate removal ensues, obtaining adequate exposure. Elevation of the scar tissue should be taken distally to the edge of the plate or to the region of the proximal wrist capsule. Great care should be taken to preserve and not violate the wrist capsule. The dissection should be carried ulnarly to visualize the subchondral bone beneath the lunate facet of the distal radius, sparing the distal radio ulnar joint. Proximally, the intramuscular plane can be taken as far as is necessary, releasing the distal

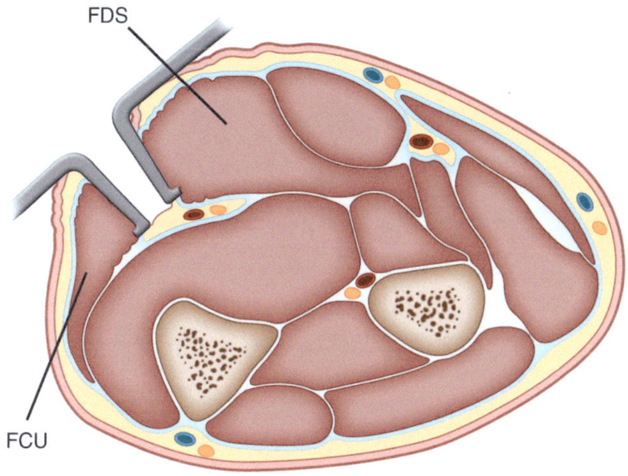

Fig. 8.6 The Henry approach to the volar aspects of the forearm

fibers of the flexor pollicis longus on the bone. Fasciotomy about the distal flexor mass also ensures proximal visualization of the radius. Distally, the brachioradialis insertion will be encountered just proximal to the radial styloid. It has a broad insertion, which permits partial release, or a full tenotomy if needed for manipulation and reduction. The radial styloid itself and the first dorsal compartment may be approached through the distal most aspect of this wound, or with a separate dorsal exposure.

With the exposure completed, and the hardware removed, the bone should be evaluated and compared visually and radiographically with what was obtained from preoperative imaging studies. Often rotational deformity of the distal radius may alter the radial column, and thus the position of the brachioradialis and first dorsal compartment. In cases where a carpal tunnel release is indicated, a separate incision in the palm is recommended, rather than with a distal extensile approach.

Dorsal Approach [38]

The dorsal approach may be selected for fractures or malunions involving displaced dorsal lunate facet, especially as it articulates with the distal radial ulnar joint, and very distal metaphyseal or articular fragments. Dorsal opening wedge osteotomy is readily achieved from this approach as well. The incision is longitudinal and centered just ulnar to Lister's tubercle. The retinaculum is divided, with a slight oblique angle to permit a relaxing incision for later closure, between the third and fourth extensor compartments. The retinacular flaps are temporarily sutured to the skin transposing the extensor pollicus longus (EPL) superficial to the retinaculum radially and the digital extensors superficial to the retinaculum ulnarly. This wide exposure allows subperiosteal access to the entire surface of the dorsal distal radius, dorsal radial styloid, distal radial ulnar joint, and dorsal ulna. The posterior interosseous nerve (PIN) innervates the dorsal wrist capsule and is encountered just beneath the muscle belly of the extensor indicis proprius (EIP), the distal most muscle belly in the fourth compartment. The PIN may be transected and avulsed, cauterizing the accompanying small branch of the posterior interosseous artery, if believed to be a source of pain and a reason for its removal.

Operative Choices

The injury, previous surgery, ability to restore anatomy, or correct malalignment determine the reoperative treatment. Revision fracture fixation, shortening or resecting a prominent distal ulna, and corrective osteotomy are commonly performed procedures. A few are highlighted below.

Osteotomy Techniques

An opening wedge osteotomy is useful for malunited volarly or dorsally displaced fractures of the distal radius, which typically represent extra-articular fractures, or with a relatively nondisplaced intra-articular component [9, 39] (Fig. 8.7). The primary indications for this technique include functional limitations and pain, rather than radiographic angle. The common complaint with both types of malunion includes distal ulna and rotational symptoms. This procedure is not recommended in patients with articular incongruity or osteoarthritis of the radiocarpal joint, diffuse pain without specific functional limitations, and complex regional pain syndrome. Relative contraindications include severe osteopenia/osteoporosis, with the understanding that bone fixation may be challenging. Other systemic diseases and patient variables may influence the relative indication for surgery.

The techniques for the volar and dorsal opening wedge osteotomies are similar. Typically, a plate or 90–90 plate configuration is chosen for fixation, along with provisional or permanent K-wires.

Dorsal osteotomy for a dorsal malunion hinges off the volar cortex. The prominence which typically includes Lister's tubercle or its healed, displaced remnant is removed with a saw or rongeur to provide a flat surface for the anticipated plate. A 0.062 or 0.045 K-wire is first inserted dorsally, proximal to the proposed osteotomy, and perpendicular to the long axis of the radius. Another wire may be passed tangential to the distal articular surface to judge the orientation of the distal radius. A third wire is then inserted distal to the osteotomy site, at the angle of the articular deformity. This process may be repeated for correction in the coronal plane, with two additional wires. The osteotomy is then completed with a sagittal saw, attempting to preserve the volar periosteum to enhance stability if significant distraction is not needed.

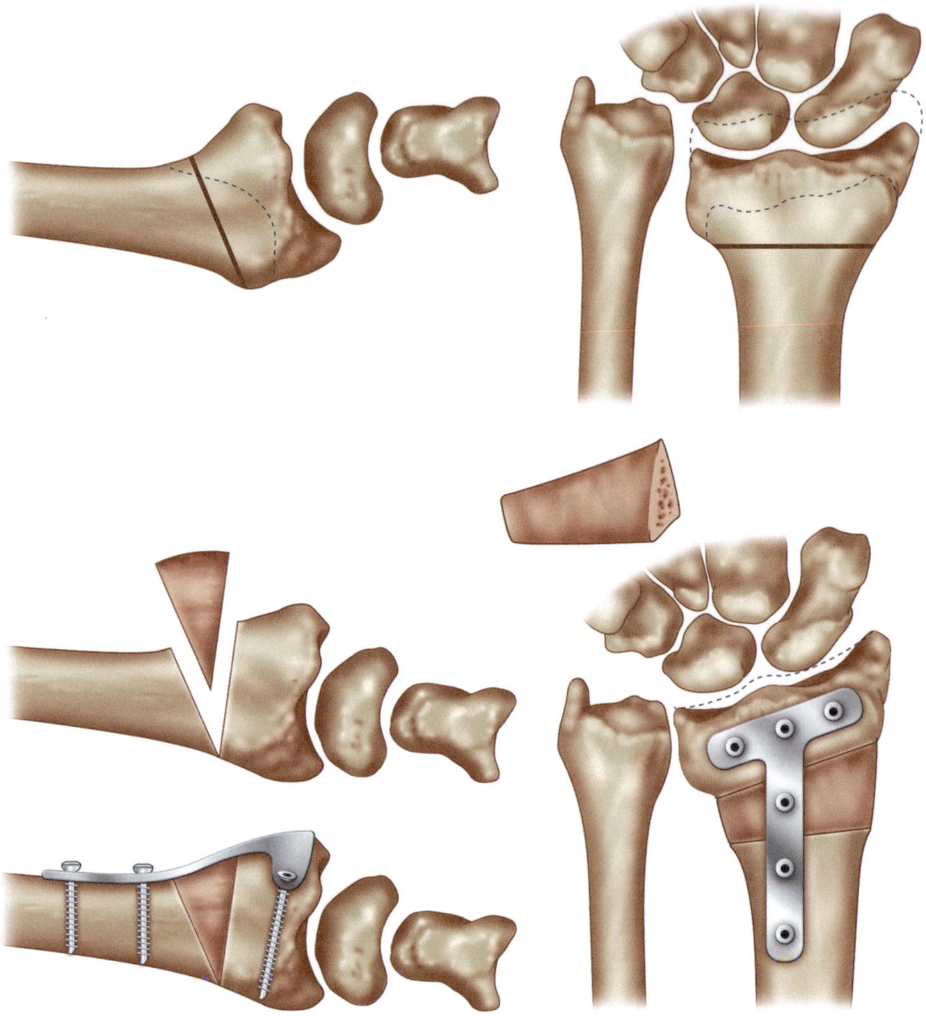

Fig. 8.7 Diagram of opening wedge osteotomy performed for correction of distal radius malunion

Distraction may be achieved with a laminar spreader; we prefer inserting a Cobb of desired width to "dial" in the distraction, radial inclination, and volar tilt without needing to overdistract as when seating a laminar spreader. The pin pairs are made parallel, and the correction is held in place with one to two K-wires placed obliquely through the radial styloid, or with an external fixation device [5, 9, 25, 30–33, 39] (Fig. 8.8). The void is filled with a variety of means: (1) a tri-cortical cortico-cancellous iliac crest bone graft placed before the K-wire placement, in a trapezoidal shape, to fit the defect; (2) Calcium phosphate cement fixation, around the inserted K-wires; and (3) allograft bone of varying shapes and types. The authors have no experience with the latter, or the absence of graft, although reported by some with good success [40–42]. Typical fixation is achieved using a T- or H-shaped plate with two to three screws in both the distal and proximal fragments. Locking construct is not necessary if the graft lends sufficient cortical reconstitution. Typically, periosteal division and tenotomy or Z-lengthening of the brachioradialis is required for distractions that require large distraction of the radial column and total lengthening.

A *volar* opening wedge osteotomy for a malunited volarly displaced fracture is similar to that described above with a few caveats in addition to the approach [43]. Patients with this malunion often complain bitterly of ulnar-sided wrist pain and often have subluxated if not dislocated distal radial ulnar joint. Care then must be taken to assure reduction of the distal radial ulnar joint when the malunion is corrected. Bone graft may not be necessary as volar comminution is less problematic in this fracture. Volar plating ensues. Another reported technique involves a sliding osteotomy with an oblique cut that recreates the original fracture; the distal fragment is then slid into the appropriate position and fixed with K-wires [44]. The authors have no experience with this potentially useful technique (Fig. 8.9).

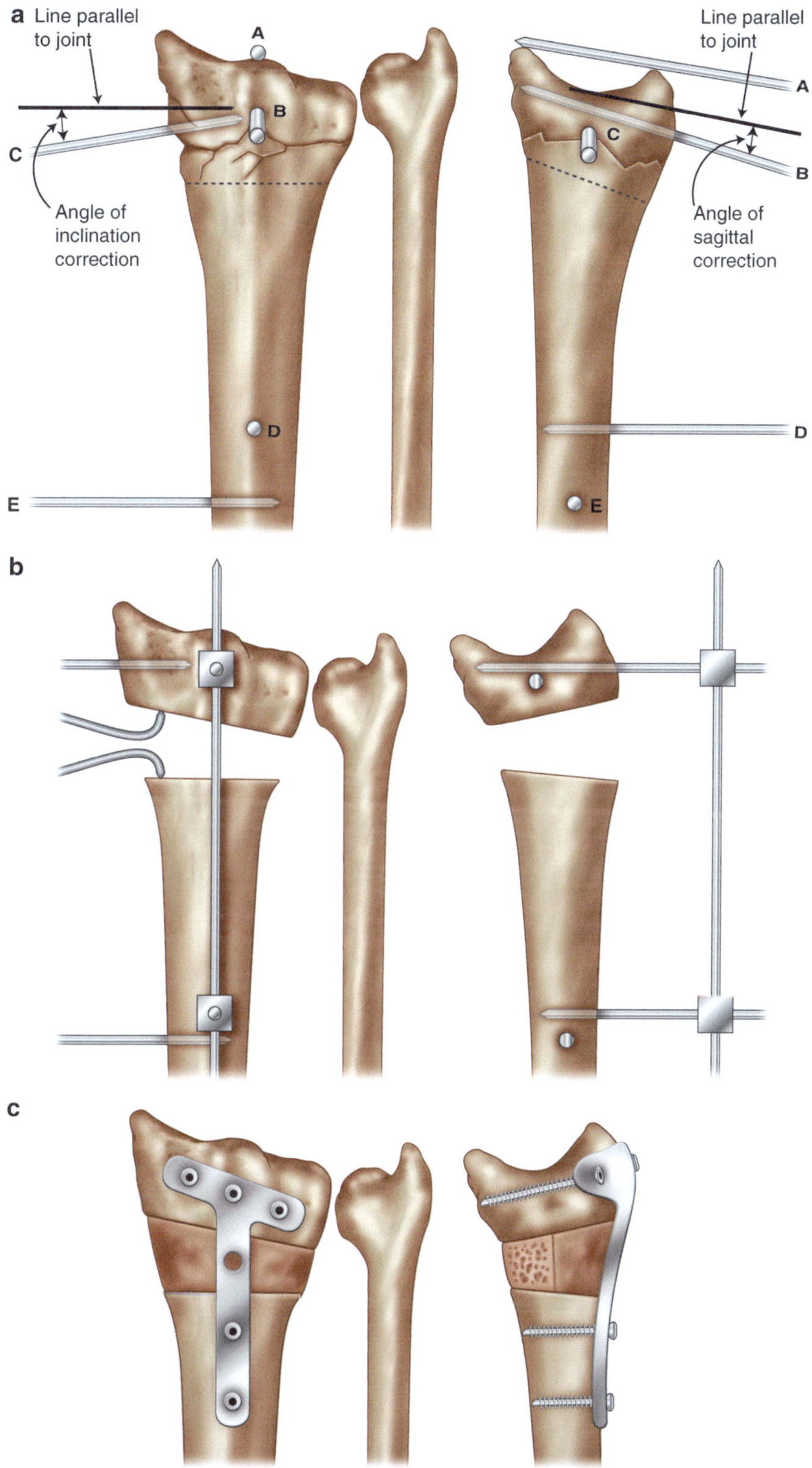

Fig. 8.8 (**a**) Pin A is inserted dorsally to judge the angle of the articular surface in the sagittal plane. Pin B diverges from being parallel to pin A by the angle of desired sagittal correction. Pin D is the companion pin to pin B and is placed perpendicular to the axis of the radius from the dorsal side. Pin C is used for correction in the frontal plane; it diverges from being parallel to the joint by the angle of desired correction. Pin E is the companion pin to pin C and is perpendicular to the axis in the radial ulnar direction. (**b**) The osteotomy is performed, and the pin pairs (B/D and C/E) are made parallel, restoring the anatomical alignment of the radius. Temporary fixation may include external fixation (as shown) or additional K-wires. (**c**) Final plate fixation with bone graft fixation

Closing wedge osteotomy of the radius, which eliminates the need for bone graft, is an alternative to the opening wedge osteotomy [45] (Fig. 8.10). This technique may be more appropriate in older, inactive patients, or in patients with osteopenia/osteoporosis. Young active adults are probably better served with radial lengthening osteotomy to restore anatomic length and architecture for anticipated best functional return [46].

Regardless of the osteotomy chosen, ulnar shortening procedures may be warranted if ulnar prominence or distal

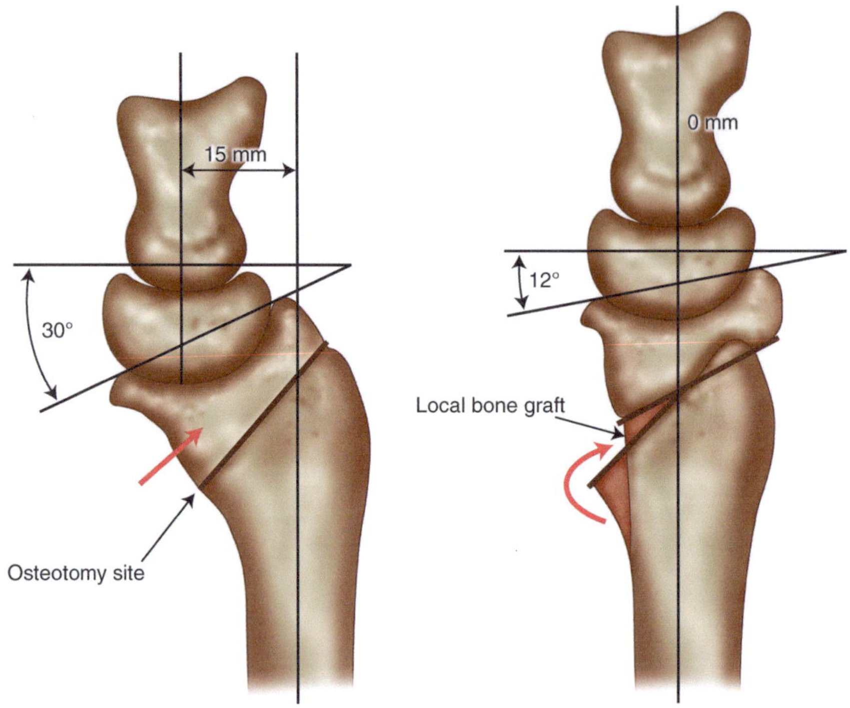

Fig. 8.9 Example of sliding osteotomy for a distal radius malunion with significant volar angulation and translational deformity. The distal fragment is repositioned in an anatomic position, and the local bone graft may be used volarly

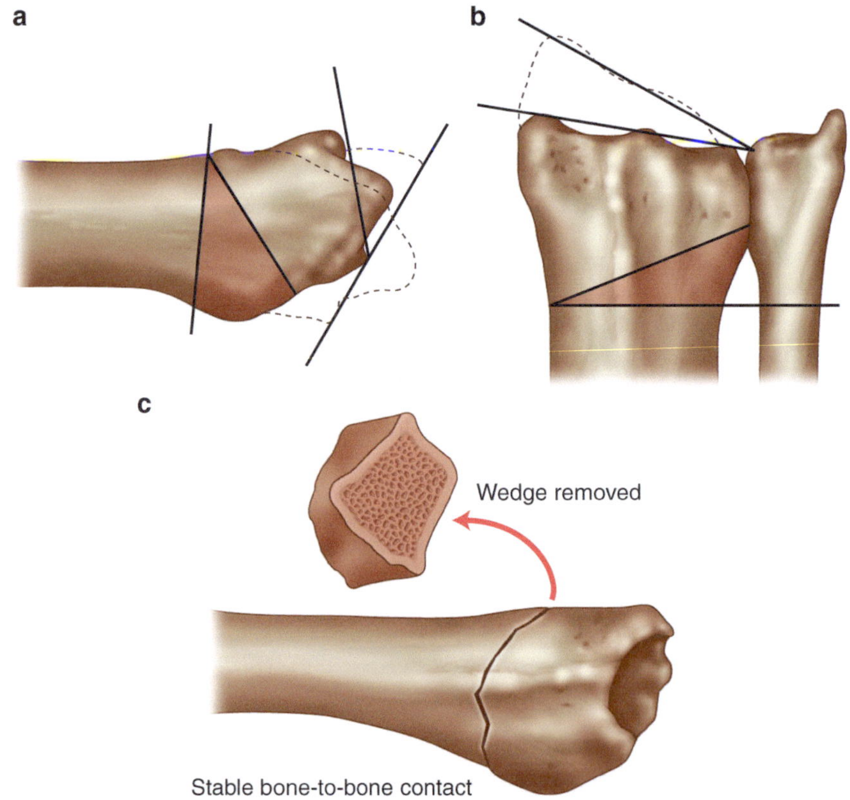

Fig. 8.10 Biplanar closing wedge osteotomy involving the frontal and sagittal planes, resulting in stable bone-to-bone contact without the need for bone graft

radial ulnar joint problems persist. A concomitant ulnar shortening osteotomy may be required especially in younger patients with mechanical aberrations of the distal radial ulnar joint amenable to relocation by shortening [46, 47]. The ulnar shortening osteotomy should be completed before final fixation of the radial components, or the ulna will act as a strut and prevent appropriate alignment of the radius. Shortening or leveling operations, especially in older patients or those with distal radial ulnar joint arthritis, include a Darrach, Sauve–Kapandji, or hemiresection arthroplasty [48–51].

A recent trend has included the use of volar fixed-angle plates for fixation of both dorsal and volar fractures. Because of the strength of the fixed-angle construct, cancellous bone graft, rather than cortical graft, may be used. Cancellous bone graft—either autograft, allograft, or porous synthetic calcium phosphate graft—may be chosen, packing the defect. A plate reduction technique is a good option, which first begins with predrilling the distal holes (Fig. 8.11). The osteotomy is then completed, and the distal aspect of the plate is fixated to the distal fragment. The proximal aspect of the plate is then reduced down to the proximal bone, which should restore anatomic alignment. The proximal, sliding screw is placed first, to allow for minor adjustments. Once the reduction is satisfactory, the remaining screw holes are filled, and bone graft is placed [52].

An *intra-articular* osteotomy can be selected only in cases where the articular incongruity is straightforward and understood, and in the absence of posttraumatic arthritis. The approach to an intra-articular osteotomy is from the side of greatest displacement. During a volar approach, the articular surface is visualized through the osteotomy, leaving the volar radiocarpal ligaments intact. A dorsal approach allows direct visualization through a dorsal osteotomy, with fluoroscopic assistance permitting real time correction. A combined dorsal and volar approach may be necessary in particularly difficult malunions. An osteotome is used along the original fracture line, followed by debridement of the fibrocartilage. The reduction is then performed and secured with K-wires. Definitive fixation may be performed with K-wires, screws, or a plate(s). If the articular surface is unsalvageable, arthrodesis of the radiolunate or radioscapholunate are alternative options [34, 53, 54].

Disorders of the Distal Radioulnar Joint

Distal radius malunion often causes distal radial ulnar joint incongruity, which can affect forearm rotation and cause significant pain. Multiple procedures have been described to address derangement of the distal radioulnar joint, which include the Darrach procedure, hemiresection arthroplasty, the Sauve–Kapandji procedure, prosthetic replacement of the distal radial ulnar joint, and ulnar head replacement.

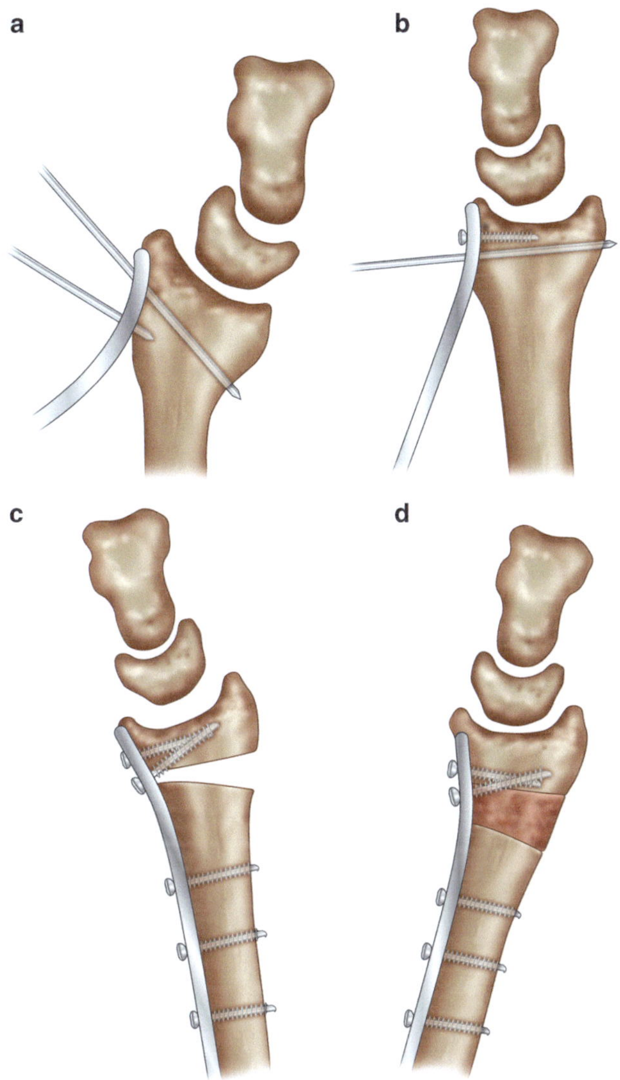

Fig. 8.11 Plate reduction technique. The distal holes are predrilled, using a volar plate with a K-wire guide hole that directs the wire parallel to the joint surface. The osteotomy is completed and the distal aspect of the plate is fixated to the distal fragment. The proximal aspect of the plate is reduced down to proximal bone, restoring anatomic alignment. The proximal sliding screw is placed first, followed by remaining screw holes and bone graft

The Darrach procedure involves total resection of the ulnar head, removing approximately 2 cm [48]. It may be well tolerated in the low-demand, elderly population with severe degenerative changes of the distal radial ulnar joint. Author's preferred technique includes preserving the periosteum from the removed stump and passing it over the ulnar stump by suturing it into the shaft with a 4-0 braided suture. This helps prevent "piano keying" of the ulna and minimize associations including ulnar impingement, decreased grip strength, and radioulnar instability. Improved results have been reported in patients who have an ulnar stump that resides within the sigmoid notch cavity, patients who have a

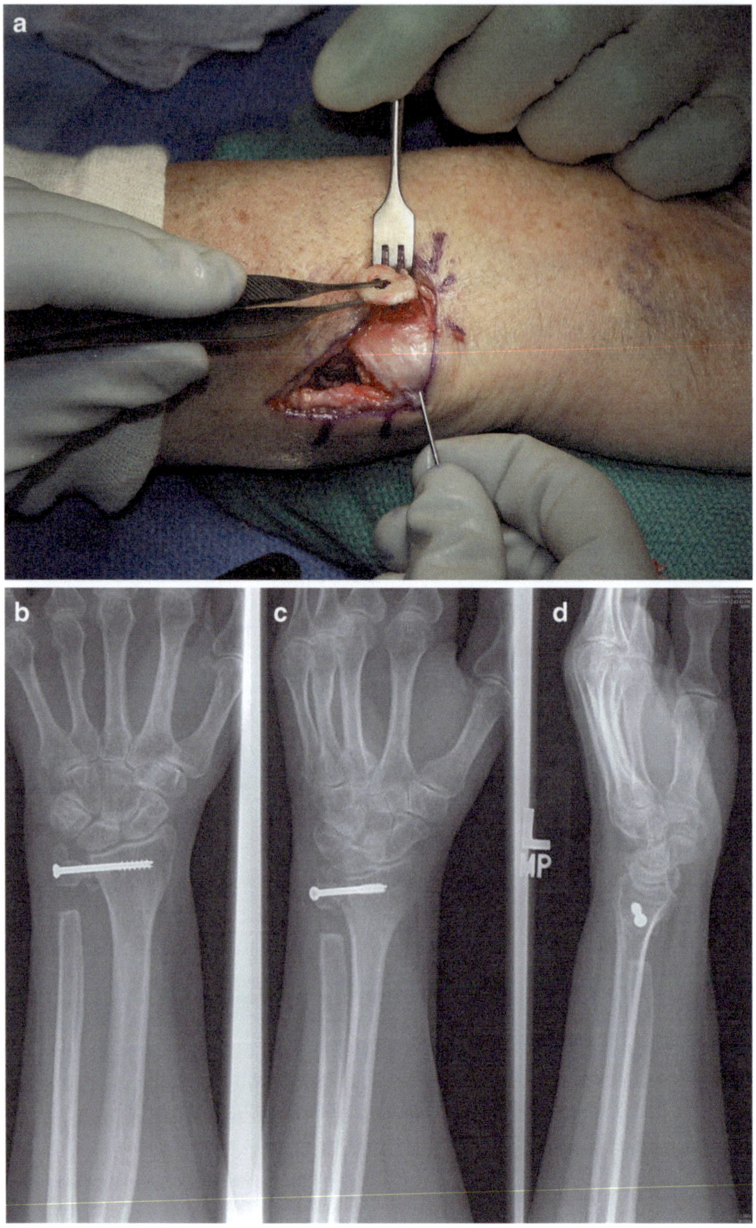

Fig. 8.12 The Sauve–Kapandji Procedure. The articular surfaces of the DRUJ are removed and the distal cut is made, approximately 2 mm proximal to the sigmoid notch, and the periosteum elevated to the level of the proximal cut, which is typically 12–15 mm. A 2-mm wafer, which is cut from the resected ulna, is inserted between the decorticated surfaces of the DRUJ (**a**). A permanent K-wire or screw, crossing the ulnar stump, wafer, and radial surface, serves at the definitive fixation, as seen on the PA, oblique, and lateral x-rays (**b, c, d**) (images courtesy of Dr. Amy Ladd, MD)

rounded or tapered stump, and those with complete closure of the extensor carpi ulnaris tendon—to prevent dorsal subluxation of the ulna [55–57].

A Bower's hemiresection arthroplasty, or partial resection of the ulnar head, is reserved for low-demand patients [51]. An ulnar shortening procedure may need to be completed in conjunction with the hemiresection arthroplasty, to prevent ulnar styloid impingement.

We prefer the Sauve–Kapandji procedure for severe distal radial ulnar joint incongruity, arthritis, or ulnar prominence [49, 58] (Fig. 8.12). This fuses the distal radial ulnar joint with creation of a proximal ulnar pseudoarticulation Advantages of this procedure include preservation of the TFCC and ulnocarpal ligaments and maintenance of the physiologic load transmission of the hand and carpus, through the supporting arch of the radius and ulna, and dispersed in the forearm. This procedure is best used in young, active patients with high demands on the upper extremity [59–61]. Disadvantages of the procedure include painful clicking or instability of the ulnar stump [58, 61, 62]; suturing of the periosteum similar to that described in the Darrach procedure helps minimize this complication.

Our technique is as follows. We begin with a dorsal "hockey stick" incision over the distal radial ulnar joint and ulnar head, continuing straight ulnar on its distal shaft. The dorsal branch of the ulnar nerve is protected, if identified.

The distal radial ulnar joint is approached through the interval of the fourth and fifth extensor compartments, where the articular surfaces are removed with a rongeur. The distal ulnar shaft is identified between the extensor carpi ulnaris and flexor carpi ulnaris. A 0.045 K-wire is passed through the distal ulna in a radial direction to provide a rotational reference once the osteotomy is made, removing a segment of ulna so that the final defect, correcting for any desired shortening, should be approximately 12–15 mm total. The distal cut is made first, corresponding to 2 mm proximal to the sigmoid notch to minimize scoring the distal radial ulnar joint. Once the distal cut is made, the periosteum from this cut is elevated proximally and circumferentially to the level of the proposed proximal cut, and thus developed as a tethering flap to suture to the proximal stump. The section of ulna is removed with a towel clip, and an additional wafer cut from this approximately 2 mm in height inserted as a "doughnut" between the decorticated surfaces of the distal radial ulnar joint. Occasionally, cancellous bone may be removed from the shaft to serve as additional graft. Either a provisional guide wire or a permanent 0.062 K-wire is passed through the ulnar stump, the doughnut, and the radial surface. A cannulated screw, sometimes two, is preferable for good bone; typically one or two K-wires are used for osteoporotic bone.

The periosteal flap, if adequately preserved, is used to suture to the proximal ulnar stump, passing through the bone with a 2-0 braided mattress suture through two holes made with a 0.045 K-wire. Fascia of the pronator quadratus may also be used. Bone from the resected segment can be used to bone graft the distal radial ulnar joint. The extensor retinaculum over the distal radial ulnar joint is closed if necessary. Patients are initially immobilized to include the elbow for 3–4 weeks, and then a short-arm cast for an additional 3–4 weeks, permitting light rotation at this time. It's debated whether radiographic healing of the distal radial ulnar joint is necessary, but is preferred in our hands.

Isolated ulnocarpal impaction may be managed with an ulnar shortening osteotomy if distal radial ulnar joint congruity can be anticipated, or with an arthroscopic partial ulnar head resection (wafer procedure) [63]. The amount of appropriate ulnar resection is determined with radiographs of the patient's unaffected contralateral side. Typically, ulnar variance that is greater than 2 mm is managed with an ulnar shortening osteotomy, while variance less than 2 mm is managed with an arthoscopic wafer procedure [64].

Fusion Options

Radioscapholunate Arthodesis [65]

Comminuted intra-articular distal radius fractures may lead to violation of and significant pain at the radioscaphoid (RS) and radiolunate (RL) joints. A "fossa-lateral" and volar tilt AP radiograph may be taken to best assess the radioscapholunate (RSL) joint. A RSL arthrodesis may provide substantial relief in these circumstances. Indications include young patients who require midcarpal joint motion. It should not be performed in patients with degeneration of the midcarpal joint.

Technique follows: the most important facet is reduction of the scapholunate articulation in a restored status with the radius, in order to preserve the midcarpal articulation. A longitudinal, dorsal incision is made over Lister's tubercle, and the extensor pollicis longus is retracted radially. Distal to Lister's tubercle, the capsule is incised; this exposes the distal scaphoid and triquetrum. The second dorsal compartment and its tendons are elevated subperiosteally and retracted radially, and the fourth compartment and tendons are elevated and retracted ulnarly.

The distal 40% of the scaphoid is then excised, using a saw and rongeur, making an effort to preserve the radial and volar ligaments. The lunotriquetral ligament is divided, and the triquetrum removed. Cartilage and subchondral bone from the radioscaphoid and radiolunate joints are removed. The lunate is then fixed to the radius in neutral flexion with two K-wires inserted from the dorsal radius. The scaphoid is then fixed with two K-wires reducing the radioscaphoid angle. They should lie radial to the repositioned second dorsal compartment and ulnar to the fourth compartment. Either the K-wires are then bent, cut, and tamped into the dorsal aspect of the radius, or a plate may be used (Fig. 8.13). The capsule is closed, and the third dorsal compartment retinaculum is sutured together, followed by skin closure.

A thumb-spica cast is applied at the 2-week follow-up, which is removed at 6 weeks for active range of motion. Full progressive use is allowed after radiographic healing, typically 8–10 weeks.

Radiolunate Arthrodesis [65]

Intra-articular die punch distal radius fractures often disrupt the cartilaginous surface of the lunate fossa, leading to deformity. Arthrodesis of the radiolunate joint is one solution to the resultant pain and altered kinematics that develops from such an injury. It should not be performed if the surrounding joints (particularly the midcarpal joint) are abnormal.

Our preferred technique is as follows. A longitudinal incision is made over Lister's tubercle, and the third dorsal compartment is opened. EPL is retracted radially, and the capsule between the third and fourth compartments is longitudinally incised. The fourth dorsal compartment is then elevated subperiosteally and reflected ulnarly. The cartilage and subchondral bone of the lunate fossa and radius are removed and prepared for fusion. Bone graft is interpositioned between the radius and lunate to preserve normal height of the lunate. This prevents excessive pressure on the radioscaphoid joint and ulnocarpal joint.

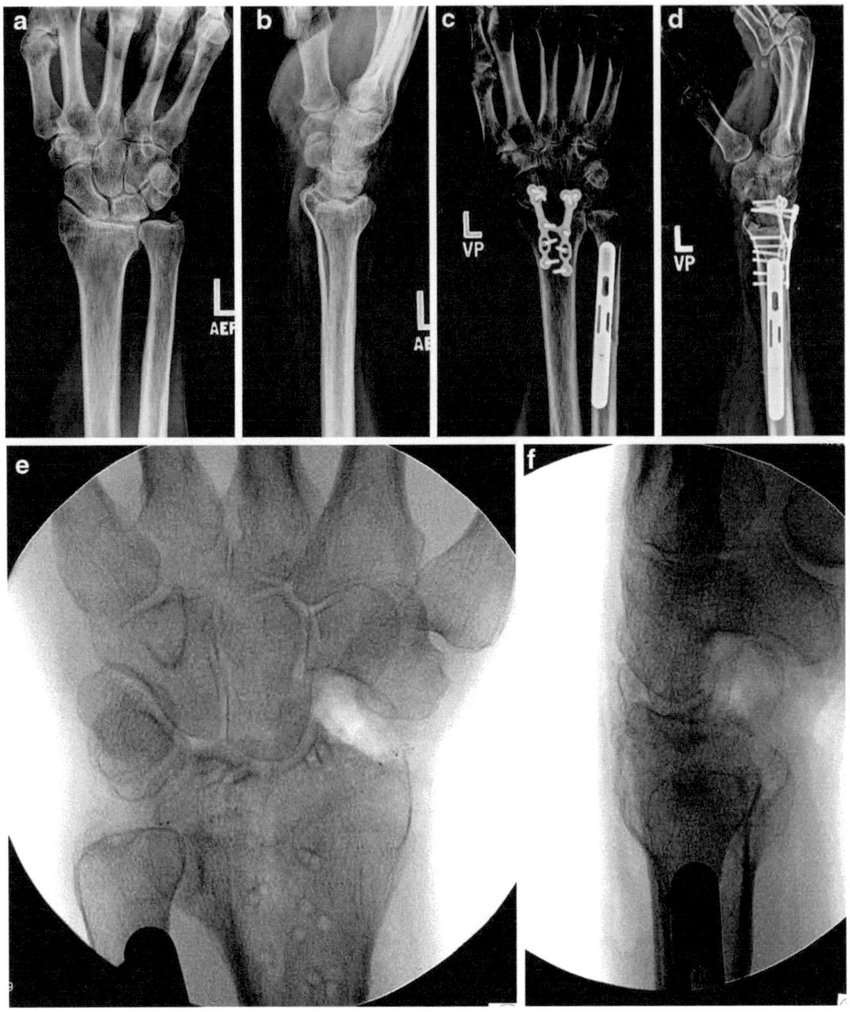

Fig. 8.13 Radioscapholunate (RSL) fusion using a dorsal plate. (**a**, **b**) Preoperative X-rays showing radial carpal arthritis and malreduced position, confirmed arthroscopically with a preserved midcarpal joint. (**c**, **d**) RSL fusion performed at same time of ulnar shortening. (**e**, **f**) Inadequate distal pole excision was performed at index procedure, completed with plate removal for tendon irritation

A K-wire may be inserted into the dorsal lunate, to use as a "joystick," and the lunate is aligned with the radius and temporarily fixed with a K-wire, from the ulnar dorsal lunate into the volar radius. A second K-wire is then inserted from the area of Lister's tubercle to the volar distal lunate. It is important to avoid penetration into the capitolunate joint. The K-wires are then bent and cut flush with the surface of the radius. Fixation may be supplemented with staples. Alternate fixation includes a fixed-angle blade plate or combi plate. The third dorsal compartment is then closed, followed by the skin.

Postoperatively, a short thumb-spica cast is placed, and 12 weeks of healing is allowed before return to full activity. It is important to avoid radioulnar deviation postoperatively, as these motions may allow flexion of the lunate with wrist radial deviation and flexion to the triquetrum with ulnar deviation.

Total Wrist Arthodesis [65]

Indications for total wrist arthrodesis are multiple. In the setting of a revision distal radius fracture, these may include: (a) posttraumatic pancarpal arthritis of the radiocarpal and midcarpal joints, (b) reconstruction after infection or segmental bone loss of the distal radius or carpus, and (c) after a failed, previous arthrodesis. A concomitant carpal tunnel release may be required, if symptomatic (Fig. 8.14).

Our preferred technique follows the recommendations of the AO Hand Study Group [66]. A straight longitudinal incision is made between the second and third metacarpals and passes over Lister's tubercle, ending just proximal to the muscle belly of the APL. A radial flap, which contains the superficial branch of the radial nerve, is raised off of the dorsal retinaculum. The third compartment is then opened, and the EPL is transposed radially.

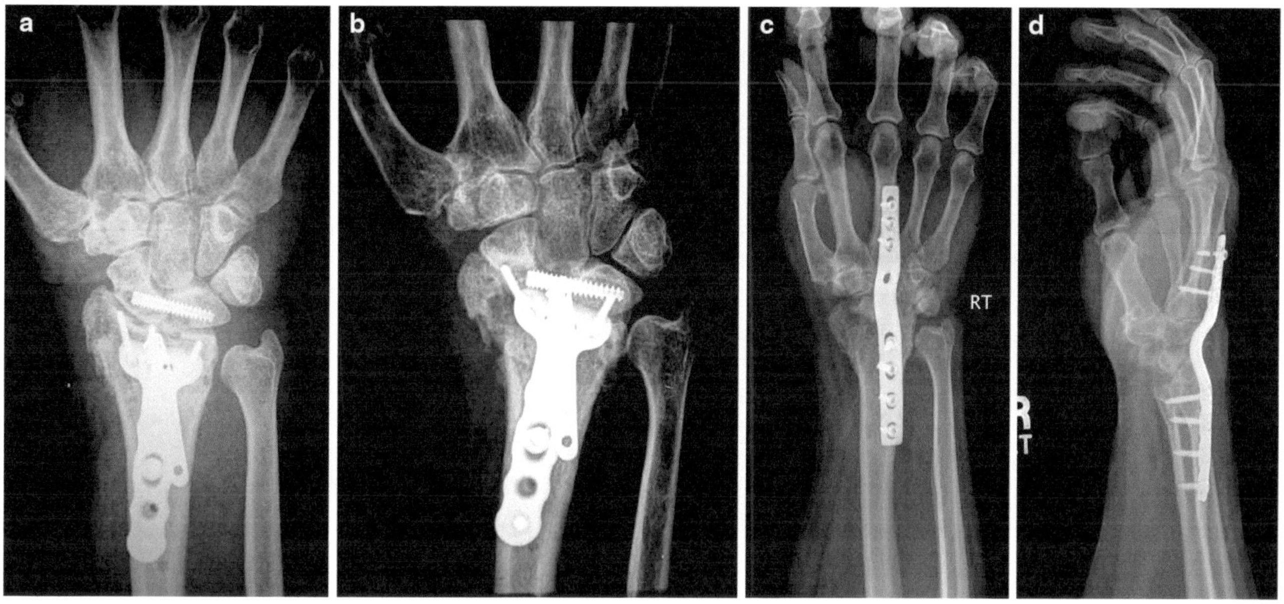

Fig. 8.14 Example of total wrist arthrodesis, completed after failure of previous arthrodesis and loss of reduction. (**a**) early postoperative image; (**b**) demonstrating lucency and loss of reduction consistent with infection at 6-months; (**c, d**) ultimate surgery with fusion (photos courtesy of Dr. Amy Ladd, MD)

A longitudinal incision is then made from the radial base of the third metacarpal, through the capsule, and proximally—exposing the distal radius subperiosteally. The extensor carpi radialis brevis insertion is elevated subperiosteally and reflected radially. An incision is then made on the radial aspect of the third metacarpal, and the dorsal surface of the third metacarpal is exposed. Using a scalpel, two flaps of the capsule are elevated from the carpus.

The second and fourth dorsal compartments are elevated subperiosteally and reflected radially and ulnarly, respectively. These compartments should not be opened. Lister's tubercle and the dorsal cortices of the third metacarpal base and carpal bones are then removed with an osteotome or ronguer. A proximal row carpectomy (PRC) is then performed, which minimizes the need for graft and avoids potential ulnocarpal impingement. These bones are then morselized for bone graft. The cartilage and subchondral bone are then removed from the distal radius, capitate, proximal hamate, and the dorsal 80% of the third CMC joint. The dorsal distal radius should also be removed to allow the plate to fit.

The precontoured Synthes titanium low-contact dynamic compression plate is our implant of choice. Plate size will depend on the size of the individual. Prior to plate fixation, cancellous bone is packed into the third CMC joint and the fusion site. The plate is then positioned so that three screws may be placed in the third metacarpal. The most distal hole of the plate is marked, and the plate is removed. A 2.0-mm drill hole is then made under direct vision, ensuring central placement in the narrow metacarpal. Failure to drill the metacarpal hole in the sagittal plane will lead to a metacarpal rotational deformity. With the plate repositioned, a 2.7-mm cortical screw of appropriate length is inserted. The most proximal metacarpal screw should be inserted next, followed by the central metacarpal screw. A 2.7-mm cancellous screw is then placed in the capitate. It is important that the capitate screw is of appropriate length; a long screw will protrude into the carpal tunnel.

The capitate is then compressed into the distal radius, and the hand aligned with the forearm. A radial screw, preferably one that lies in cortical bone, is then inserted after drilling. The remaining radius screw holes are then inserted with cortical screws. A small suction drain is inserted, and the capsule is closed using the radial and ulnar leaves of the third compartment. The EPL is left transposed radially. Postoperatively, a bulky dressing is applied for 10 days, followed by a removable short-arm splint for 6 weeks. Strengthening begins at 8 weeks, and full use allowed at 10 weeks.

Other Salvage Procedures

Proximal Row Carpectomy

There are few indications for a PRC following failed distal radius fixation. As this is a procedure primarily indicated for a wrist with a scapholunate advanced collapse pattern (SLAC) and a preserved cartilage of the capitate articulation and lunate facet, then in the face of a previous distal radius fracture it will most likely be for an unrecognized scapholunate dissociation at the time of injury.

The exposure for a PRC is similar to that listed above. Once down to the wrist capsule, a longitudinal incision is made along the third metacarpal axis. The lunate and triquetrum are removed, as well as the proximal two thirds of the scaphoid. Attachment of the distal third of the scaphoid to the trapezium and trapezoid help support the thumb ray. The proximal aspect of the capitate is then approximated with the lunate cavity of the distal radius, and a temporary K-wire may be placed. The pisiform is kept in place. After closure, a bulky dressing is applied, followed by a short-arm cast for 4–6 weeks. Motion may begin after cast removal.

Optimizing Outcomes

- Select patients carefully—agreed expectations for surgeon and patient alike.
- Functional demands and limitations understood.
- Detailed exam—compare ROM and grip strength to the contralateral side.
- Obtain accurate radiographs of both wrists, additional imaging if helpful.
- Injury films valuable to understand mechanism and stability.
- Operative reports and postoperative images helpful in understanding loss of reduction.
- Check carpal involvement, often overlooked.
- Check ulnar column involvement (styloid, TFCC, DRUJ, shaft) as potentially unstable contributions.
- Osteoporosis from metabolic disease or secondary surgery—beware! Hardware fixation can be challenging.
- Prepare for alternative, extended, or salvage treatment intra-operatively: external fixation, volar/dorsal plates, bone graft/substitute, arthrodesis plate, ulnar-sided procedures.
- Prepare the patient in the OR for bone grafting.
- Lengthen or cut brachioradialis in volar approach if necessary for exposure.
- Carpal tunnel release if prolonged surgery or preoperative symptoms.
- Restore articular surface, radial length/tilt/inclination if technically feasible.
- Wound closure—consider drain to minimize hematoma; staples in friable skin.
- When all else fails, fuse (PRC, RS, RSL, or total).
- Ensure adequate postoperative immobilization.

Complications and Side Effects

In the reoperative setting, the patient is at greater risk for postoperative complications when compared to a primary distal radius fracture. Soft tissue infection, localized or imprecise pain, persistent malunion, nerve compression, stiffness and complex regional pain syndrome all are possibilities. Multiple procedures and poor blood flow impair the body's innate immunological response to surgery, alters the local environment, and inhibits the delivery of antibiotics to the site. Bone and soft tissue devascularization may occur from multiple surgical incisions about a complex injury site. Nonunion, rare in the primary setting, occasionally is seen, and autologous bone grafting is recommended in this scenario. Smoking cessation is mandatory. The risk of infection also increases with revision surgery. In cases with significant soft tissue injury, flap coverage may be required.

If revision surgery leads to a malunion or nonunion, repeat ORIF vs. arthrodesis are considerations. This decision depends on the desires of the patient and their circumstances. Progressive severe degenerative disease is typically best treated with a fusion of the involved joint. Finally, symptomatic hardware is best treated with hardware removal.

Postoperative Care

Close, short-term follow-up is important in the reoperative distal radius fracture. Early complications such as wound breakdown and infection must be monitored. Depending on style of fixation and the state of the soft tissue, this may mean weekly cast/bandage changes under close supervision. A balance must be struck between immobilization and activity. The extremity must be immobilized adequately to allow healing, while mobilizing early enough to prevent stiffness. Revision patients are especially at risk of soft tissue contractures and joint stiffness.

The immobilization for revision surgery about the distal radius varies, but in general the arm is placed in a bulky dressing and splint for 2 weeks, then changed to a cast or custom orthosis for an additional 2–4 weeks. Whether the elbow is immobilized in the initial and subsequent immobilization primarily depends on the involvement of the distal radial ulnar joint in the reconstruction—and if so, would typically require a long arm or Muenster cast or splint.

Conclusion

Distal radius reoperation represents complex, multifaceted procedures requiring sufficient planning. The patient's symptoms, functional impairments, goals, and expectations must complement the surgeon's understanding and capabilities. Healthy active patients with functional disability and localizing pain associated with deformity stand to benefit the most from revision. A thorough examination of the patient and preoperative radiographs will optimize outcome. Having a variety of implants available in the operating room, including bone graft material, is wise. Tendon lengthening and/or carpal tunnel release may also be required. The authors prefer to complete a Fernandez osteotomy, with a concomitant Suave–Kapandji procedure for distal radial ulnar joint involvement. When all else fails, fusion may be the best option.

References

1. Gartland Jr JJ, Werley CW. Evaluation of healed Colles' fractures. J Bone Joint Surg Am. 1951;33:895–907.
2. Dowling JJ, Sawyer B. Comminuted Colles' fractures: evaluation of method of treatment. J Bone Joint Surg Am. 1961;43:657–68.
3. Friberg S, Lundstrom B. Radiographic measurements of the radiocarpal joint in normal adults. Acta Radiol Diagn (Stockh). 1976;17(2):249–56.
4. Taleisnik J, Watson HK. Midcarpal instability caused by malunited fractures of the distal radius. J Hand Surg Am. 1984;9:350–7.
5. Graham T. Surgical correction of malunited fractures of the distal radius. J Am Acad Orthop Surg. 1997;5(5):270–81.
6. Short Wh, Palmer AK, Werner FW, et al. A biomechanical study of distal radius fractures. J Hand Surg Am. 1987;12:529–34.
7. Hirahara H, Neale PG, Lin YT, et al. Kinematic and torque-related effects of dorsally angulated distal radius fractures and the distal radial ulnar joint. J Hand Surg Am. 2003;28:614–21.
8. Kihara H, Palmer AK, Werner FW, et al. The effect of dorsally angulated distal radius fractures on the distal radioulnar joint congruency and forearm rotation. J Hand Surg Am. 1996;21:40–7.
9. Fernandez DL. Malunion of the distal radius: current approach to management. Instr Course Lect. 1993;42:99–113.
10. Linscheid RL. Kinematic considerations of the carpal joint. Clin Orthop. 1986;202:27–39.
11. Taleisnik J. Post-traumatic carpal instability. Clin Orthop. 1980; 149:73–82.
12. Amadio PC, Botte MJ. Treatment of malunion of the distal radius. Hand Clin. 1987;3(4):541–61.
13. Adams BD. Effects of the radial deformity on distal radioulnar joint mechanics. J Hand Surg Am. 1993;18:492–8.
14. Poque DJ, Viegas SF, Patterson RM, et al. Effects of distal radius fracture malunion on wrist joint kinematics. J Hand Surg Am. 1990;15:721–7.
15. Bronstein AJ, Trumble TE, Tencer AF. The effects of distal radius fracture malalignment on forearm rotation: a cadaveric study. J Hand Surg Am. 1997;22:258–62.
16. Jenkins NH, Mintowt-Czyz WJ. Mal-union and dysfunction in Colles' fracture. J Hand Surg Br. 1988;13:291–3.
17. Fernandez DL, Capo JT, Gonzalez E. Corrective osteotomy for symptomatic increased ulnar tilt of the distal end of the radius. J Hand Surg Am. 2001;26:722–32.
18. Tang JB, Ruy J, Omokawa S, et al. Biomechanical evaluation of wrist motor tendons after fractures of the distal radius. J Hand Surg Am. 1999;24:121–32.
19. Kreder HJ, Hanel DP, Agel J, et al. Indirect reduction and percutaneous fixation versus open reduction and internal fixation for displaced intra-articular fractures of the distal radius: a randomized, controlled trial. J Bone Joint Surg Br. 2005;87(6):829–36.
20. Hastings H, Leibovic SJ. Indications and techniques of open reduction. Orthop Clin North Am. 1993;24:309–26.
21. Bradway JK, Amadio PC, Cooney WP. Open reduction and internal fixation of displaced, comminuted intra-articular fractures of the distal end of the radius. J Bone Joint Surg Am. 1989;71:839–47.
22. Fernandez DL, Geissler WB. Treatment of displaced articular fractures of the radius. J Hand Surg Am. 1991;16:375–84.
23. Knirk JL, Jupiter JB. Intra-articular fractures of the distal end of the radius in young adults. J Bone Joint Surg Am. 1986;68:647–59.
24. Trumble TE, Schimitt SR, Vedder NB. Factors affecting functional outcome of displaced intra-articular distal radius fractures. J Hand Surg Am. 1994;19:325–40.
25. Fernandez DL, Ring D, Jupiter JB. Surgical management of delayed union and nonunion of distal radius fractures. J Hand Surg Am. 2001;26A:201–9.
26. McKee MD, Waddell JP, Yoo D, Richards RR. Nonunion of distal radial fractures associated with distal ulnar shaft fractures: a report of four cases. J Orthop Trauma. 1997;11:49–53.
27. Ring D. Nonunion of the distal radius. Hand Clin. 2005;21: 443–7.
28. Segalman KA, Clark GL. Un-united fractures of the distal radius: a report of 12 cases. J Hand Surg Am. 1998;23A:914–9.
29. Ring D. Treatment of the neglected distal radius fracture. Clin Orthop. 2005;431:85–92.
30. Fernandez DL. Reconstructive procedures for malunion and traumatic arthritis. Orthop Clin North Am. 1993;24(2):341–63.
31. Jupiter JB, Fernandez DL. Complications following distal radius fractures. Instr Course Lect. 2002;51:203–19.
32. Bushnell B, Bynum D. Malunion of the distal radius. J Am Acad Orthop Surg. 2007;15:27–40.
33. Slagel B, Luenam S, Pichora D. Management of post-traumatic malunion of fractures of the distal radius. Orthop Clin North Am. 2007;38:203–16.
34. Jupiter JB, Ring D. A comparison of early and late reconstruction of malunited fractures of the distal end of the radius. J Bone Joint Surg Am. 1996;78:739–48.
35. Henry AK. Extensile exposure. 2nd ed. New York: Churchill Livingstone; 1973.
36. Protopsaltis TS, Ruch D. Volar approach to distal radius fractures. J Hand Surg Am. 2008;33(6):958–65.
37. Henry MH, Griggs SM, Levaro F, Clifton J, Masson MV. Volar approach to dorsal displaced fractures of the distal radius. Tech Hand Up Extrem Surg. 2001;5(1):31–41.
38. Tavakolian JD, Jupiter JB. Dorsal plating for distal radius fractures. Hand Clin. 2005;21(3):341–6.
39. Fernandez DL. Correction of post-traumatic wrist deformity in adults by osteotomy, bone-grafting, and internal fixation. J Bone Joint Surg Am. 1982;64:1164–78.
40. Ladd AL, Huene DS. Reconstructive osteotomy for malunion of the distal radius. Clin Orthop Relat Res. 1996;327:158–71.
41. Ring D, Reberge C, Morgan T, Jupiter JB. Osteotomy for malunited fractures of distal radius: a comparison of structural and nonstructural autogenous bone grafts. J Hand Surg Am. 2002;27: 216–22.
42. Luchetti R. Corrective osteotomy of malunited distal radius fractures using carbonated hydroxyapatite as an alternative to autogenous bone grafting. J Hand Surg Am. 2004;29(5):825–34.
43. Shea K, Boston DL, Fernandez DL, et al. Corrective osteotomy for malunited, volarly displaced fractures of the distal end of the radius. J Bone Joint Surg Am. 1997;79:1816–26.
44. Thivaios GC, McKee MD. Sliding osteotomy for deformity correction following malunion of volarly displaced distal radial fractures. J Orthop Trauma. 2003;17(5):326–33.
45. Posner MA, Ambrose L. Malunited Colles' fractures: correction with a biplanar closing wedge osteotomy. J Hand Surg Am. 1991;16:1017–26.
46. Wada T, Tsuji H, Iba K, et al. Simultaneous radial closing wedge and ulnar shortening osteotomy for distal radius malunion. J Hand Surg Am. 2004;29:264–72.
47. Oskam J, Bongers KM, Karthaus AJM, et al. Corrective osteotomy for malunion of the distal radius—the effect of concomitant ulnar shortening osteotomy. Arch Orthop Trauma Surg. 1996;115:219–22.
48. Darrach W. Partial excision of lower shaft of ulna for deformity following Colles's fracture. Ann Surg. 1913;57:764–5.

49. Sauve L, Kapandji M. Nouvelle technique de traitement chirurgical des luxations recidivantes isolees de l'extremite inferieure du cubitus. J Chirurg. 1936;47:589–94.
50. Bower WH. Distal radioulnar joint arthroplasty: the hemiresection-interposition technique. J Hand Surg Am. 1985;10A:169–78.
51. Dingman PVC. Resection of the distal end of the ulna (Darrach operation). An end-result study of twenty-four cases. J Bone JointSurg Am. 1952;34:893–900.
52. Malone KJ, Magnell T, Freeman DC, et al. Surgical correction of dorsally angulated distal radius malunions with fixed angle volar plating: a case series. J Hand Surg Am. 2006;31:366–72.
53. Ring D, Prommersberger KJ, Del Pino JG, et al. Corrective osteotomy for intra-articular malunion of the distal part of the radius. J Bone Joint Surg Am. 2005;87:1503–9.
54. Marx RG, Axelrod TS. Intraarticular osteotomy of distal radius malunions. Clin Orthop. 1996;327:152–7.
55. McKee MD, Richards RR. Dynamic radio-ulnar convergence after the Darrach procedure. J Bone Joint Surg Br. 1996;78:413–8.
56. DiBenedetto MR, Lubbers LM, Coleman CR. Long-term results of the minimal resection Darrach procedure. J Hand Surg Am. 1991;16:445–50.
57. Field J, Majkowski RJ, Leslie IJ. Poor results of Darrach's procedure after wrist injuries. J Bone Joint Surg Br. 1993;75:53–7.
58. Taleisnik J. The Sauve-Kapandji procedure. Clin Orthop. 1992;275:110–23.
59. Millroy P, Coleman S, Ivers R. The Sauve-Kapandji operation: technique and results. J Hand Surg Br. 1992;17:411–4.
60. Lichtman DM, Ganocy TK, Kim DC. The indications for and techniques and outcomes of ablative procedures of the distal ulna: the Darrach resection, hemiresection, matched resection and Sauve-Kapandji procedure. Hand Clin. 1988;14:265–77.
61. Sanders RA, Frederick HA, Hontas RB. The Sauve-Kapandji procedure: a salvage operation for the distal radioulnar joint. J Hand Surg Am. 1991;16:1125–9.
62. Mikkelsen SS, Lindblad BE, Larsen ER, et al. Sauve-Kapandji operation for disorders of the distal radioulnar joint after Colles' fracture. Acta Orthop Scand. 1997;68:64–6.
63. Feldon P, Terrono AL, Belsky MR. The wafer procedure. Partial distal ulnar resection. Clin Orthop. 1992;275:124–9.
64. Lindau T. Treatment of injuries to the ulnar side of the wrist occurring with distal radial fractures. Hand Clin. 2005;21:417–25.
65. Green DP, Hotchkiss RN, Pederson WC, Wolfe SW. (eds.). Operative hand surgery. 5th ed. New York: Churchill Livingstone; 2004.
66. Scott WW, Robert NH, William CP, and Scott HK (eds.). Operative hand surgery. 6th ed. New York: Churchill Livingstone; 2010.

Reoperative Issues Following Carpal Bone Fracture Surgery

9

Vipul P. Patel and Jesse B. Jupiter

Abstract

The carpal bones can be fraught with difficulties in trying to obtain union in these bones that have large articular surfaces. Of these bones, the scaphoid is the most notorious because of its unique blood supply. However, the lunate is well known for its predilection to develop avascular necrosis. Furthermore, even the hook of the hamate despite its rich muscular attachments and blood supply usually does better with simple excision than attempts to provide internal fixation. There exist options to try and correct the nonunion or malunion in the scaphoid. However, ultimately, if the carpal bones do not heal, the patient is potentially looking at a partial wrist fusion or complete wrist fusion, depending on which bones are involved and how much degeneration involves the proximal and midcarpal rows. The goal in most of these patients is to try to improve their pain. In counseling patients, they should have the reconstructive ladder discussed with them so that they can participate in the decision making process as some patients may prefer to go straight to a partial fusion or total fusion rather than subject themselves to a sequence of multiple surgeries.

Keywords

Scaphoid • Carpal • Nonunion • Malunion • Hamate • Fracture

Reoperative Issues Following Scaphoid Surgery (Table 9.1)

Substantial improvements have been made in both diagnostic evaluation and the surgical treatment of scaphoid fractures yet failure to gain union remains a well-recognized problem [1]. Reasons for this may be multifactorial but tend to fall into either technical problems related to the surgical realignment and internal fixation or biological problems.

The timing for and type of reoperation will also depend upon a number of relevant factors. Among these include the age of the patient, duration of time since the initial surgical procedure, characteristics and location of both the scaphoid fracture and nonunion, associated carpal problems, and sequelae following prior attempts at internal fixation. In this chapter, we will identify the indications and surgical options for the management of scaphoid fractures as well as other carpal trauma that have failed to unite following surgical intervention. The problems will be divided into timing issues, technical pitfalls and pearls, and alternative treatment. A recognition of a technical problem such as misplaced Kirschner wire or screw fixation and/or a malalignment at the fracture site which is recognized within weeks following the initial surgery should prompt the surgeon to consider

V.P. Patel, MD
Department of Orthopedic Surgery, Crystal Run Healthcare, Middletown, NY, USA

J.B. Jupiter, MD (✉)
Department of Orthopedic Surgery, Harvard Medical School and Massachusetts General Hospital, Yawkey Center, Suite 2100, 55 Fruit Street, Boston, MA, USA
e-mail: jjupiter1@partners.org

S.F.M. Duncan (ed.), *Reoperative Hand Surgery*,
DOI 10.1007/978-1-4614-2373-7_9, © Springer Science+Business Media, LLC 2012

Table 9.1 Reoperative issues following scaphoid surgery

Scaphoid nonunion options	Indications	Contraindications
Percutaneous or minimally invasive management of scaphoid nonunion	Early scaphoid nonunion without deformity Minimal bone resorption Minimal collapse Vascular proximal pole	Carpal malalignment Humpback deformity Avascular necrosis Arthritic changes Significant bone loss—void from previous fixation with screw
Open anterior wedge bone grafting and internal fixation—palmar approach	Scaphoid waist or distal third nonunion	Avascular proximal pole
± Radial styloidectomy in early SNAC changes	Viable proximal fragment Minimal periscaphoid arthritic changes Humpback deformity	Advanced periscaphoid arthritic changes Avascular necrosis
Dorsal approach with internal fixation	Proximal pole fracture Viable proximal fragment	Scaphoid waist nonunions Advanced arthritic changes Avascular nonunion
1,2 ICSRA 2,3 ICSRA	Scaphoid waist or proximal pole nonunion with an avascular fragment	Viable proximal pole
Vascular bundle implantation with corticocancellous graft Second metacarpal vascularized corticocancellous wedge graft	Mild to moderate humpback deformity	Advanced arthritic changes

reoperation given the real risk of later failure to unite the scaphoid fracture.

Reoperative surgery of the scaphoid requires a complex understanding of scaphoid anatomy, vascularity, and carpal kinematics and evaluation of deformity. The scaphoid plays an integral role in carpal biomechanics by linking the proximal and distal carpal row. The entire proximal, distal, medial, and half of the lateral surface of the scaphoid (encompassing 80%) is covered with articular cartilage. The scaphoid tuberosity on the volar radial aspect of the wrist serves as an attachment for radioscaphocapitate and scaphotrapezial-trapezoid ligaments and the dorsal scaphotriquetral ligament attaches to the dorsal surface of the scaphoid [2]. The nonarticular dorsal ridge of the scaphoid serves as an attachment for the dorsal wrist capsule and perforating branches of the radial artery. The scaphoid has a well-defined blood supply with 70–80% of its contribution from the radial artery entering via the dorsal ridge of the scaphoid and its dorsal branches supply all of the proximal pole via interosseous circulation. The distal pole has abundant blood supply from the volar branches of the radial artery which comprise the rest of the 20–30% of the scaphoid's circulation [3].

Scaphoid alignment is determined by measuring scaphoid length, intrascaphoid angle, carpal ratio, and normal angular relationships of the scaphoid with surrounding carpal bones. Sagittal cuts on a thinly sliced CT scan of the scaphoid allows for determination of location of fracture or deformity, intrascaphoid angle, and carpal collapse. The AP and lateral intrascaphoid angles are formed by the angle between two lines drawn perpendicular to the diameters of the proximal and distal pole of the scaphoid. A lateral scaphoid angle greater than 45° is associated with an increased incidence of arthrosis secondary to a humpback deformity despite bony union. Normally, the lateral intrascaphoid angle varies between 15° and 34° and the AP intrascaphoid angle between 32° and 46° [4]. Bain et al. have suggested that a more reliable measurement of carpal collapse or humpback deformity is the height-to-length ratio; this is measured by drawing a line along the volar aspect of the scaphoid as a baseline, and the length is measured along the baseline from the tip of the proximal and distal pole while the height is measured perpendicular to the baseline. A height-to-length ratio above 0.65 is considered abnormal [5]. Measuring radiographic relationships such has scapholunate, radiolunate, radiolunate-capitate angles enables the determination of the degree of carpal malalignment. If avascular necrosis of the proximal scaphoid is suspected, it should be confirmed with an MRI to choose the appropriate intervention. Proximal fragments with an absence of T1 marrow signal should be suspicious for avascular necrosis.

If recognized at this early stage in the presence of malalignment and without bony or cartilage destruction from an eccentrically placed screw, consideration is justified for implant removal, percutaneous realignment of the fracture site with or without arthroscopic guidance, and percutaneous screw or Kirschner wire placement in a more anatomic central location (see Case 9.1).

Preoperative Considerations

Minimally invasive scaphoid nonunion surgery is indicated in patients with early scaphoid nonunion without any significant cystic bone resorption, with minimal to no collapse of scaphoid architecture, and without any objective findings of avascular necrosis. These patients should have a normal scapholunate angle and no evidence of a humpback deformity. If any doubt exists, a CT scan or arthroscopy can confirm if there is any collapse present. Evidence of avascular necrosis, intrascaphoid deformity, carpal malalignment, arthritic changes, or collapse should be considered as contraindications to this technique.

Percutaneous Technique for Scaphoid Nonunion [6]

Essentially, volar and dorsal percutaneous or minimally invasive methods for scaphoid nonunion surgery rely on stable rigid fixation with compression for nonunion healing. The volar and dorsal screw placement technique is the same as standard scaphoid fracture treatment. If fracture malalignment is noted preoperatively from radiologic studies or intraoperatively, reduction maneuvers with percutaneously placed K-wires in the proximal and distal fragment can act as joysticks for reduction. Wrist arthroscopy is performed to assess the adequacy of reduction and the nonunion site for peripheral fibrocartilaginous tissue, ensure absence of arthritic changes, and check for associated bony or soft tissue injuries. However, in patients with minimal cystic changes or fibrous unions, compression alone may be needed for union. If bone grafting is required, cancellous bone graft can be obtained from the distal radius using a cannulated trephine. The nonunion site can be debrided from the proximal scaphoid drill site using a small neurosurgical curette and packed with the cancellous graft from the same entry site. Furthermore, the proximal pole can be assessed for viability by placing a 1.9-mm angle scope through the reamer path.

Management of a Well-Defined Nonunion Associated with Failed Internal Fixation

In the assessment and management of a well-defined nonunion following prior surgical intervention, a number of factors must be considered. These also include the location and duration of the nonunion, presence or absence of adequate vascularity, characteristics and alignment at the nonunion site, the deleterious impact of the prior internal fixation with regard to bone resorption or articular cartilage damage, and importantly, the number of prior attempts to gain union. Each one of these will have a major impact on management decisions. For example, a nonunion involving the proximal pole especially after failed screw fixation may be characterized by a combination of poor vascularity, limited residual bone stock, resorption around the screw, and radiocarpal articular damage from a protruding screw thread (Case 9.2). A nonunion at the scaphoid waist can be additionally complicated by a fixed malalignment of the bony fragments, a synovial lined cavity, and/or prior screw fixation that has created interval bony resorption around the entire axis of the screw (Case 9.3). Lastly, a scaphoid nonunion following two or more prior surgical procedures and/or present for over 5 years offers a much less favorable chance at union following yet another procedure.

Scaphoid Waist or Distal Third Nonunion with a Viable Proximal Segment

Preoperative Considerations

An ideal patient considered for anterior wedge bone grafting and internal fixation for a scaphoid nonunion would have a waist or distal third nonunion, viable proximal fragment, and absence of degenerative changes around the scaphoid or midcarpal joint. Some early degenerative changes around the styloid are acceptable and addressed with a radial styloidectomy during the procedure [7]. An incidentally diagnosed nonunion with minimal symptoms warrants a thorough discussion with the patient regarding the natural history of scaphoid nonunion advanced collapse (SNAC) and associated risks. Patients with advanced degenerative changes are candidates for a salvage procedure as fixation of their nonunion will not give symptom relief. The goal of the surgery is to maintain the intact blood supply to the scaphoid while correcting the intrascaphoid angle, scaphoid length, and carpal alignment with a stable well-placed internal fixation device.

Preoperatively, careful tracing of the radiographic findings in the PA and lateral views of both the injured and uninjured wrists will allow the determination of the amount of angular deformity, scaphoid length, carpal collapse, and scapholunate and capitolunate angles. If there is gross motion at the nonunion site, a PA in maximal ulnar deviation will open up the nonunion gap and allow for measurement of the amount of interposition graft that is required. However, a CT scan with three-dimensional formats will allow for more exact determination of the above parameters. One should note that the graft measurement preoperatively may change as the nonunion sclerotic edges are burred to healthy cancellous bone, and an intraoperative measurement of the required graft size is most reliable.

Surgical Technique

The palmar approach of Russe allows for the best exposure for scaphoid waist and distal third nonunions and correction of a humpback deformity [8]. The patient is placed supine and general anesthesia is required. A nonsterile tourniquet can be used and a rolled sheet placed under the ipsilateral hip will bring the iliac crest into prominence. First, identify and palpate the prominent scaphoid tubercle. Identify the flexor carpi radialis (FCR) in the distal forearm as it courses into the wrist. The intersection of the wrist crease and FCR tendon marks the waist of the scaphoid. A 5-cm incision is centered over the wrist crease. The proximal limb of the incision courses along the FCR and distal limb is directed radially toward the base of the thumb. After skin incision, terminal branches of the lateral antebrachial cutaneous nerve should be preserved and protected radially. At the wrist crease, the palmar branch of the radial artery crossing in a radial to ulnar fashion should be either retracted or ligated. Proximally, incising the FCR sheath on its radial aspect will allow the tendon to be retracted radially; distally, the musculature of the thenar muscles in split along its fibers and its fibrous origin is sharply incised. A self-retaining retractor is placed. The anterior capsule and volar radiocarpal ligaments are incised in-line with the scaphoid starting at the scaphoid tubercle and exposing distally up to the scaphotrapezial joint. Caution must be exercised when exposing the palmar-radial corner of the distal scaphoid to avoid injury to its vascular supply. Directing the cutting edge of the scalpel upward will protect the scaphoid articular surface and the scapholunate interosseous ligament. Proximally, it should be extended as much as needed for adequate exposure of the nonunion site. It is important to preserve as much of the radiocarpal ligament as possible because the ligament contains the proximal pole of the scaphoid and prevents it from subluxating volarly. The capsular flaps with the stout radiocarpal ligaments are held open with stay sutures to allow for its anatomic closure later on.

The scaphoid is better visualized by longitudinal traction of the thumb and ulnar deviation of the wrist. Often, identifying the nonunion site is not an easy task as it may be enveloped in fibrous tissue and the distal fragment markedly flexed. Placing a needle at the presumed nonunion site and confirming with fluoroscopy often helps if no gross motion is present. The nonunion site is plied open using a freer or a thin osteotome to reveal the fibrous tissue and sclerotic edges. The nonunion site is rongeured and resected using a small oscillating saw in small increments until healthy cancellous bone is encountered. Care must be taken not to disrupt the dorsal cortex of the scaphoid as it may disrupt the remaining blood supply to the proximal segment. The flexion deformity and shortening of the scaphoid is corrected by extending the wrist over a rolled towel or by placing a small spreader clamp distracting the palmar radial side. Additionally, the dorsal rotation of the lunate is also corrected at the same time using a fine bone spike or a volarly placed K-wire as a joystick. Several authors have recommended an alternative technique for correcting lunate extension [9]. The wrist is passively flexed to bring the lunate into neutral alignment, and a K-wire is placed percutaneously from the radius to the lunate from a radial to ulnar direction to maintain lunate correction. The wrist is then extended and the nonunion site opens up since the proximal segment is pinned, which allows for measurement of the graft needed. Ulnar deviation views are not done with the pin in place; thus, the radiolunate pin should be removed before screw placement to ensure accurate imaging of the scaphoid and guide wire. Cystic defects within the scaphoid should be curetted and filled with autogenous cancellous graft. Based on the preoperative and intraoperative measurements, a tricortical trapezoidal graft with cancellous bone on either side is obtained from the iliac crest. The graft should be oversized by approximately 2 mm in order to obtain a compressive fit. The goal is to place the cancellous surface of the graft against the cut edges of the scaphoid, and the graft is usually wider than the scaphoid and may require a small tamp and mallet for insertion. It is aligned along the scaphocapitate surface and may protrude over the palmar and radial surfaces of the scaphoid which is later trimmed with a burr if necessary.

The scaphotrapezial joint is identified with a hypodermic needle and a transverse capsulotomy is made to expose the distal pole of the scaphoid. Central screw placement is essential for adequate stability: this is more likely to enhance union and avoid hardware failure. The extra-articular foot process of the trapezium needs to be removed to ensure a central screw placement; if this is not done, the screw may penetrate the dorsal cortex in the proximal fragment. If the flexion deformity is not corrected, the screw may lie palmar. A K-wire is placed from distal to proximal fragment in central location. Its central placement and the correct alignment of the scaphoid are confirmed with fluoroscopy. A second K-wire is placed for derotation, the screw length is measured, and the track is drilled. Based on the fracture location, a shorter than measured screw with threads crossing the nonunion site is placed. The palmar wrist capsule and radiocarpal ligaments are repaired. The skin is closed with subcuticular or nylon sutures. A thumb spica splint is placed postoperatively and switched to a removable splint at follow-up. If stable fixation is achieved, gentle wrist range of motion may be initiated at 2 weeks. Heavy manual labor or strenuous activity is not allowed till 12 weeks and confirmation of union.

Proximal Pole Nonunion with a Viable Proximal Fragment

Proximal pole nonunion with a viable proximal fragment is best managed with a nonvascularized bone graft through the dorsal approach. This approach provides the best exposure for the proximal pole and allows for stable fixation of the small proximal fragment minimizing the chance of displacement. It also ensures a better accuracy in central screw placement of the small proximal fragment. Often, the fracture line of a proximal nonunion occurs in a distal volar to proximal dorsal orientation. Therefore, screw placed from the volar side may not cross the nonunion and in fact may displace the proximal fragment [10]. A dorsal approach is relatively contraindicated in a scaphoid waist nonunion (especially with collapse).

Surgical Technique

A small longitudinal incision is made just radial to Lister's tubercle centering over the radiocarpal joint. The sheath of the extensor pollicis longus is released, and the scapholunate articulation is exposed by sharply incising the fourth extensor compartment and capsule from the dorsal lip of the radius. By flexing the wrist, the scapholunate ligament is visualized and the entry site for the screw is located adjacent to it. The nonunion site is identified with a needle and the nonunion plane is confirmed via fluoroscopy. The nonunion site is prepared with curettes and a burr to remove any sclerotic bone and fibrous tissue. Cancellous bone graft may be packed if needed. The guide wire for the cannulated screw is inserted up to the subchondral bone and its central position is confirmed fluoroscopically. After determining the screw length, the wire may be advanced into the trapezium so that it does not dislodge during drilling or tapping. A second K-wire can add rotational stability during screw placement. Some surgeons prefer placing a non-cannulated screw after drilling for the small proximal fragments so that it leaves a smaller footprint in the proximal pole cartilage.

Proximal Pole Nonunion with an Avascular Proximal Pole

Proximal pole nonunions of the scaphoid have the potential to heal with conventional bone grafting techniques and stable internal fixation with the rate of healing directly correlated with the vascularity of the proximal pole [10–12]. Although most studies with vascularized bone grafting have shown union rates from 80 to 100%, the majority of these patients in the studies did not have avascular necrosis [13, 14]. Other, more recent studies have shown union rates of only 60–70% with vascularized bone grafts in the presence of avascular necrosis [15]. However, a recent meta-analysis found union rates of 88% with vascularized bone graft compared to a 47% union rate with wedge bone graft and screw fixation in scaphoid nonunions with avascular necrosis [16]. Therefore, although the value of vascularized bone graft in the presence of avascular necrosis is questioned, the overall balance of data does suggest that a vascularized bone graft may improve healing in the presence of AVN. In the literature, vascularized bone grafts based on a pedicle from pronator quadratus, ulnar artery, volar carpal artery, periosteal distal radius flaps, and thumb or index metacarpal and even free vascularized grafts from iliac crest and medial femoral condylar region have been reported [17]. At present, grafts based on the dorsoradial aspect of distal radius, nourished by 1,2 intercompartmental supraretinacular artery (1,2 ICSRA) described by Zaidemberg, and the second metacarpal grafts are most frequently used [18, 19].

Vascular Anatomy

The blood supply to the distal radius and ulna is relatively constant and is comprised of the radial, ulnar, and anterior and posterior interosseous arteries. A series of longitudinal vessels which are best described by their spatial relationships with surrounding anatomic structures, i.e., the wrist extensor compartments and extensor retinaculum, form the basis for the pedicled vascularized grafts. These are considered intercompartmental if located between and compartmental if located within the wrist extensor compartment. Also, vessels that lie superficial to the extensor retinaculum are called supraretinacular.

The 1,2 and 2,3 intercompartmental supraretinacular vessels are fairly consistent and lie above the extensor retinaculum between the numbered extensor compartments. The retinaculum under these vessels separates the compartments and is adherent to the underlying bony tubercle. The 1,2 ICSRA originates from the radial artery 5 cm proximal to the radiocarpal joint, courses beneath the brachioradialis, and travels on the dorsal surface of the retinaculum. It enters the snuffbox distally to anastomose with the radial artery or the radiocarpal arch. It is the smallest of the four vessels and travels with a venae comitantes. It is this distal to proximal ascending irrigating branch as described by Zaidemberg which serves as an ideal graft for the scaphoid due to its close proximity and superficial location. One must be aware that it has a short arc of rotation and often is small in caliber [2].

The 2,3 ICSRA is a good alternative in some patients when the 1,2 ICSRA is small or absent. It originates proximally from the anterior interosseous artery and lies superficial to the retinaculum directly over Lister's tubercle, and it anastomoses distally with the dorsal radiocarpal arch, dorsal intercarpal arch, and fourth extensor compartment. Like the 1,2 ICSRA, its nutrient artery also penetrates deep into the cancellous bone, but it has a much larger arc of rotation and can serve as a graft for the entire proximal row.

Preoperative Considerations

A successful outcome following a vascularized bone graft depends on appropriate patient selection and meticulous surgical technique. Indications for the use of a vascularized bone graft are scaphoid waist or proximal pole fracture with avascular necrosis, whereas presence of a viable proximal pole demonstrated on an MRI and advanced arthrosis (SNAC stage II or more) are relative contraindications to vascularized bone grafting.

Surgical Technique (Fig. 9.1)

A dorsal or dorsoradial approach provides exposure for the graft as well as the nonunion site. The limb is elevated for exsanguination and an esmarch bandage should *not* be used prior to tourniquet inflation. A gentle curvilinear incision is

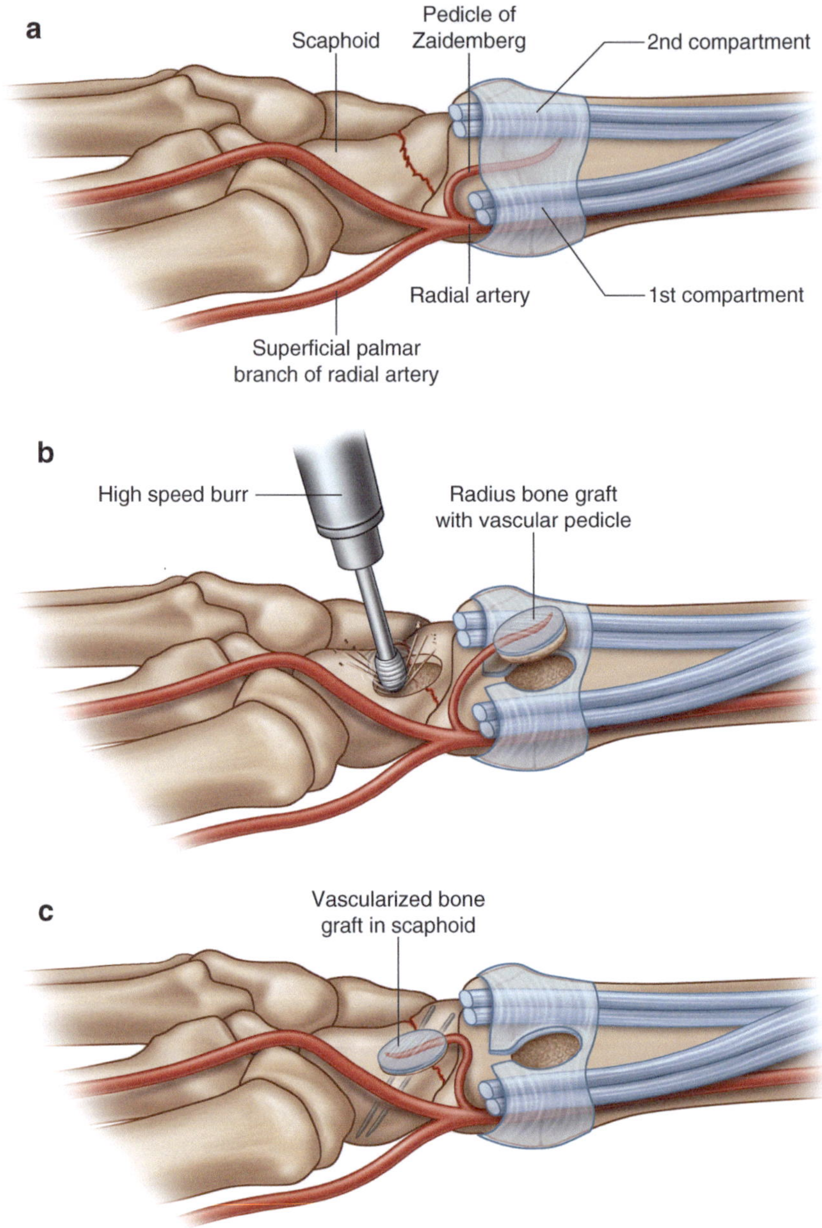

Fig. 9.1 1,2 intercompartmental supraretinacular artery (1,2 ICSRA) technique

made curving proximally between the first and second dorsal compartment and distally over the proximal scaphoid. The third dorsal compartment is exposed and the extensor pollicis longus is released to retract it radially. Branches of the superficial radial nerve are identified and gently protected. The extensor carpi radialis longus (ECRL) is retracted ulnarly. The 1,2 ICSRA and its venae comitantes are visible as a thin red line in a groove between the first and second dorsal compartment. The first dorsal compartment is released at its palmar surface (to prevent postoperative dorsal subluxation) and the tendons are retracted. Two parallel incisions are made in the periosteum between the two compartments, and the vessels are carefully dissected distally toward the anatomic snuffbox to their anastomosis with the radial artery. Prior to graft elevation, the scaphoid nonunion should be prepared by making a transverse radial capsulotomy to expose the scaphoid nonunion site. The nonunion site is prepared by removing the fibrous tissue: osteotomes or high speed burrs are utilized to prepare a graft recipient slot. With a proximal pole nonunion site, a dorsal inlay graft is appropriate. If the proximal pole fragment is too small, the graft is shaped to lie in the concavity of the proximal pole. The graft is centered 1.5 cm proximal to the radiocarpal joint in-line with the vessels. A 2–2.5-cm vascular pedicle is mobilized distal to the graft site from the radius and the underlying joint capsule, and subsequently, the periosteum around the donor site is incised as an elliptical or rectangle fashion. The proximal 1,2 ICSRA is ligated prior to graft elevation. Radial, ulnar, and proximal graft osteotomy is made using a fine oscillating saw with constant irrigation leaving the distal graft side as a hinge. Some surgeons prefer using osteotomes to cut the three sides of the graft to avoid thermal injury to the bone. The distal osteotomy is performed by gently levering with an osteotome to create a distally based pedicle. Once elevated, the tourniquet is deflated to observe bleeding from the bone graft. After satisfactory vascularity of the graft is determined, the graft is resized, passed beneath the wrist extensors, and gently rotated into the nonunion site; caution should be exercised to avoid any sharp turns or kinks in the pedicle. The construct can be provisionally stabilized with K-wires and definitively secured with screw fixation using the technique described in the dorsal approach. The capsule is loosely closed to avoid strangulating the pedicle and the extensor retinaculum is closed with nonabsorbable sutures.

Scaphoid Shortening and Humpback Deformity in the Setting of an Avascular Nonunion

In the setting of a scaphoid waist nonunion with an avascular proximal pole and a humpback deformity, it is essential to correct the deformity while addressing the nonunion. In this case, a vascularized wedge bone graft can be placed through the above-described dorsoradial approach [20]. The scaphoid should be prepared and the graft size needed should be determined prior to graft harvest. Any lunate extension should be corrected manually, and a radiolunate pin can correct the lunate extension deformity. Similar to the previous technique, a 1,2 ICSRA graft of sufficient size should be harvested in order to fill the dimensions of the defect as determined pre- and intraoperatively. This is achieved by trimming the graft to match the dimensions while protecting the vascular pedicle, which is technically demanding. When used as a wedge graft, it is placed with the vessels/pedicle facing palmarly, thus allowing the volar cortex of the graft to act as a strut for stability. Often, additional nonvascularized bone graft may be required to supplement the vascularized graft if the nonunion defect is large. The graft is secured with a screw in a similar fashion as described earlier in the chapter. In addition, removing the radial styloid can often aid in exposure or avoid later impingement if the scaphoid deformity is uncorrectable.

An Alternative Technique: Vascular Bundle Implantation and Bone Grafting in Proximal Pole Nonunions

Some authors have suggested alternative techniques for proximal pole vascularization with encouraging results. Hori et al. first demonstrated active proliferation of blood vessels

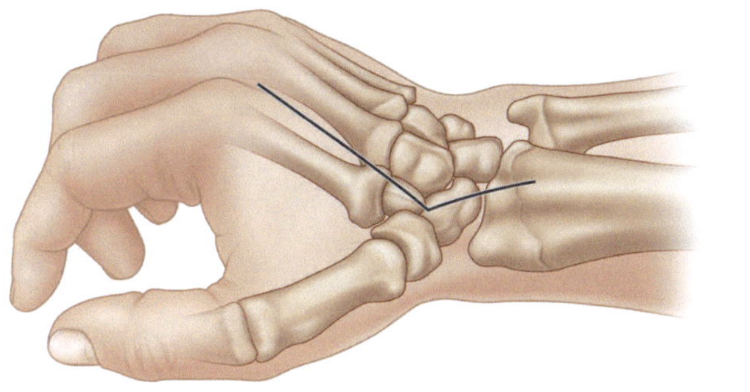

Fig. 9.2 Surgical incision for vascular pedicle graft from the second DMA

and new bone formation in an isolated or necrotic dog bone model when a vascular pedicle (an artery, vein, and perivascular tissue) was implanted [21]. This concept of vascular implantation has been reported in patients with Kienbock's disease with some success. Additionally, Fernandez et al. have reported excellent results with a combination technique of inlay corticocancellous strut grafting from iliac crest with a vascular pedicle implantation from the second dorsal metacarpal artery for proximal pole or scaphoid waist avascular nonunion. This technique may be used as an alternative or a potential rescue option in some select patients with proximal pole or waist avascular nonunions. Several other authors have reported excellent outcomes in revision scaphoid nonunions with this technique described by Fernandez and Eggli in 1995 [19, 20, 22, 23].

Surgical Technique (Fig. 9.2)

An extensive dorsoradial approach is utilized with the proximal incision starting at Lister's tubercle and extending distally approximately 4 cm parallel to the EPL tendon and terminating at the dorso-ulnar aspect at the base of the thumb metacarpal. Branches of the superficial radial nerve are identified and protected in the subcutaneous tissue. An interval between the ECRL and extensor carpi radialis brevis is developed. A wrist capsule is opened along the long axis of the scaphoid. The nutrient branches from the radial artery to the dorsal ridge of the scaphoid in the distal fragment are identified and protected throughout the procedure. The nonunion site is identified and prepared by removing the fibrous tissue and sclerotic bone. The proximal fragment is observed for punctuate bleeding, which should be evident even with the tourniquet inflated. If in doubt, the tourniquet may be released for confirmation. Once confirmation of an avascular segment is made, the proximal fragment is excavated with curettes and burrs (no more than 5 mm diameter) for an autogenous peg from the iliac crest. A rectangular trough is made in the dorsoradial aspect of the distal fragment with a small oscillating saw or chisel in an oblique fashion to accommodate the trapezoidal graft. After the trough in the

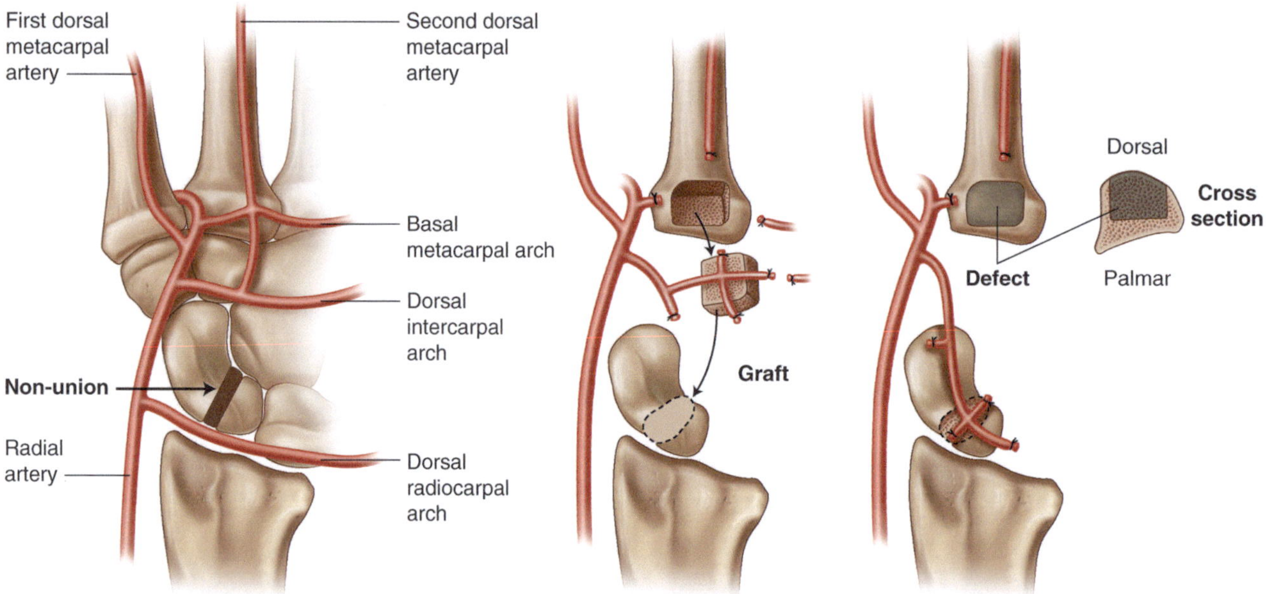

Fig. 9.3 Corticocancellous bone graft harvest from base of second metacarpal from FDMA

distal fragment and cavity in the proximal fragment are created, the scaphoid is reduced and the resultant defect spanning the segments is measured in all planes. A corticocancellous peg graft and some free cancellous bone chips are obtained per standard fashion from the iliac crest. Any cystic cavities and the nonunion site should be first packed with the free cancellous chips. Then the graft is trimmed to the measurements and inserted in the trough by gently spreading the nonunion site. One must take care and place the cortical surface dorsoradially and ensure that the graft is not oversized as it may distract the nonunion site. The construct is stabilized with a 1.0 or 1.2 K-wire on the most radial aspect of the scaphoid from the scaphotrapezial junction; if a second K-wire is required, it must be inserted on the most ulnar aspect of the scaphoid away from the vascular pedicle insertion site.

In order to raise a vascular pedicle, the incision is extended distally from the base of the thumb to the second dorsal web space, and the extensors to the index finger are retracted ulnarly. The second dorsal metacarpal vascular pedicle is identified between the first and second metacarpal. The vascular bundle travels under the thin fascia overlying the interosseous muscle. The fascia is incised longitudinally to the second web space, and the vascular pedicle with its perivascular areolar tissue is raised from a proximal to distal direction. Small collateral branches are coagulated and the pedicle is raised up to the web space. A long pedicle (5–6 cm) is raised by transecting and ligating the pedicle with a 5.0 monofilament suture. Subsequently, using a 2.7-mm drill bit, a hole is made just ulnarly to the iliac crest graft site, close to the scapholunate junction, in an oblique radio-volar direction. A fine resorbable suture is placed at the end of the pedicle, and the pedicle is passed from dorsal to palmar direction through the drill hole using a straight needle. At this point, the pedicle should be observed for any kinks or focal areas of constriction as it makes a turn toward its new bed. The suture is retrieved from the palmar side just radial to the FCR tendon. A small stab incision is made in the skin and the suture is tied over the palmar fascia. The tourniquet is deflated and the pedicle is observed for bleeding and any points of constriction. The capsule and skin are closed in standard fashion.

Postoperatively, a long-arm thumb spica cast for 4 weeks followed by another 4 weeks of short-arm thumb spica cast is utilized. The K-wires are removed at 8 weeks through small stab incisions under local anesthesia.

Correcting a DISI Deformity with a Vascularized Corticocancellous Bone Graft from the Second Metacarpal (Fig. 9.3)

Makino initially described a vascularized bone graft from the base of the second metacarpal as an option for treating scaphoid nonunions and Kienbock's disease [24]. Subsequently, Sawaizumi et al. in 2002 and 2004 reported on the use of this technique in scaphoid nonunions with a dorsal intercalated segment instability (DISI) deformity [19]. This technique can be applied to scaphoid nonunions with or without a DISI deformity with the addition of a small volar incision for graft placement in a DISI deformity. Advocated advantages of this procedure include ease of dissection and pedicle identification, smaller incision, and availability of adequate-strength corticocancellous bone from the base of the second metacarpal, sparing the iliac crest and preventing its potential complications.

A 4-cm curvilinear incision is made from the anatomical snuffbox to the shaft of the second metacarpal bone, and the branches of the superficial radial nerve are identified and protected. The radial artery is identified distal to the radial styloid, along with the dorsal intercarpal arch and the second dorsal metacarpal artery (originates from the radial artery at the snuffbox). The insertion of the ECRL is dissected and retracted exposing the second metacarpal base. These vessels are dissected to the level of the second metacarpal shaft, and identifying them on the periosteum at the ulnar margin of the ECRL aids in the dissection proximally and distally. The dorsal intercarpal and basal metacarpal arches travel under the wrist extensors, extensor pollicis longus, and superficial radial nerve. These structures are retracted and the branches of the dorsal intercarpal and metacarpal arch are identified and ligated, leaving the pedicle to the base intact. A square of periosteum is incised over the base of the second metacarpal and a hole is made at each corner with a 1.0 K-wire. Using an osteotome, the corticocancellous bone is carefully detached preserving its pedicle; the graft and its pedicle are carefully detached and elevated. The tourniquet is deflated to observe for graft viability. The scaphoid nonunion site is prepared as mentioned in previous techniques. The graft is trimmed as needed, inserted, and secured with a headless screw from the proximal pole.

In Scaphoid nonunions with a DISI deformity, an additional 3-cm curved incision is made over the scaphoid on the volar side. The scaphoid nonunion site is identified and prepared until cancellous bone is exposed. The deformity is then corrected by inserting a K-wire into the lunate from the dorsal incision and rotating the lunate and proximal scaphoid (via intact SL ligament) into neutral. Even though not mentioned in the original technique, one may consider placing a transient radiolunate pin for DISI deformity correction. Based on preoperative determination and intraoperative open wedge measurement, the graft is trimmed to the appropriate-sized wedge. The pedicled second metacarpal corticocancellous graft is then transferred to the nonunion site, which has been exposed through the volar incision. This is done by passing it beneath the abductor pollicis longus and extensor pollicis brevis tendons subcutaneously. The graft is stabilized with a headless screw.

Scaphoid Malunion (Table 9.2)

Scaphoid malunion may result from operative or nonoperative treatment of scaphoid fractures and can occur following a displaced fracture that heals after nonoperative management, a fracture that heals without any treatment, or a fracture that goes on to unite after surgical treatment without a reduction. Malunited scaphoid fractures have a higher incidence of osteoarthritis and poorer wrist function than those that have healed anatomically [4, 25]. It is well documented that a malunited scaphoid results in altered carpal kinematics and abnormal load distribution [26–28]. Several studies have shown that many patients with a malunited scaphoid continue to have disabling limitation in wrist motion, pain due to carpal overload, and grip strength weakness [29]. Often, unstable scaphoid fractures occur with some degree of perilunate ligamentous injury given the mechanism [30]. The proximal scaphoid fragment follows the lunate into hyperextension and the distal fragment follows the trapezium and the distal carpal row in flexion. If healed in this position, the scaphoid develops an apex dorsoradial angulation, also known as "humpback" deformity and DISI may be observed [31]. Therefore, wrist extension at both the radiocarpal and midcarpal joint is limited due to the flexion deformity of the scaphoid, and this loss of wrist extension accounts for the main clinical complaint of the patient. It has been shown that the degree of angular deformity is directly proportional to the loss of wrist extension, which occurs at 15° of angulation at the radiocarpal joint and 30° at the midcarpal joint [32]. The classic deformities of a malunited scaphoid are shortening (which may be a component of rotation), distal fragment flexion, ulnar deviation, and pronation, and the opposite being true for the proximal fragment (extension, radial deviation, and supination [29, 33]).

Table 9.2 Scaphoid malunion

Indications	Contraindications
Symptomatic malunion—pain, weakness, stiffness	Advanced periscaphoid arthritis
Early periscaphoid changes—halt progression	Avascular bony segment on MRI
Prophylactic	Marginal soft tissue envelope

The goal in malunion surgery therefore is to restore a normal anatomic relationship of the scaphoid in order to improve wrist function and delay or reduce the incidence of osteoarthritis. Ideally, a successfully managed scaphoid should unite without any deformity and maintain normal carpal alignment.

Scaphoid malunion has been recognized only in the past few decades as a potential problem in the literature. In the early 1970s, Segmuller identified scaphoid shortening as a detriment to carpal kinematics and proposed a technique of interposition or "sandwich" grafting using a rectangular corticocancellous iliac crest bone graft. He also stressed the importance of accurate screw placement for better union and shortened time for immobilization [34]. Later that decade, Fisk recognized the association of DISI pattern with a "humpback" deformity of the scaphoid. He recommended approaching the scaphoid through a radial incision, performing a radial styloidectomy, and fashioning a wedge graft from the resected styloid to correct the DISI deformity with a maneuver that palmarly translated the distal carpus. Fisk omitted internal fixation and relied on the soft tissue tension and 2–3 months of wrist immobilization to allow for healing [35]. Fernandez, in 1984, utilized the noninjured wrist radiographs to measure scaphoid length and deformity and measured the size of graft needed to fill the defect. He modified Fisk's technique and palmarly approached it using iliac crest bone graft and achieved stability using two or three Kirschner wires [36]. Few others since then have proposed variations of the technique maintaining the same principle. With the advent of CT scan and three-dimensional reconstruction, the need for a trapezoidal graft and complex deformity of the malunited scaphoid are well understood.

Indications and Contraindications

A thorough discussion explaining their current state, risks of benign neglect, and potential benefits of the intervention is paramount to any malunion surgery. The primary indication for scaphoid malunion surgery is pain and limitation of motion. Secondary indications include defined bony changes on radiographs which are amenable to correction and may halt or correct any progression of bony changes. Lastly, patient must have the desire to achieve a better function by understanding that a prophylactic surgery potentially halts degenerative changes and offers a long-term benefit with little short-term gain if one is minimally symptomatic. Patient's pain, weakness, and stiffness should be weighed against possible post-osteotomy risks which may be nonunion or avascular necrosis.

Contraindications are advanced periscaphoid arthritis, indications of a potential avascular segment, and marginal soft tissue integrity.

Preoperative Assessment

A detailed history of the patient's injury, previous treatments, and current symptoms should be elicited. Radiographs of both wrists should be obtained with the following views: PA view in neutral, radial, and ulnar deviation and lateral views in neutral, flexion, and extension. The additional views help assess the length of the scaphoid and assess limitation in intercarpal motion. A computed tomography (CAT) scan along the axis of the scaphoid with three-dimensional reconstruction provides abundant information on scaphoid shortening and deformity for preoperative assessment. Clinical parameters such as range of motion, grip and pinch strength, and assessment of pain status should also be recorded.

On plain lateral radiographs, carpal height ratio, intrascaphoid, radiolunate, capitolunate, and scapholunate angles should be measured. On the PA projection in ulnar deviation, scaphoid length and PA intrascaphoid angle should be determined. These parameters should be compared to the uninjured wrist. Intrascaphoid angle is measured by the angle between two lines drawn perpendicular to the proximal and distal articular surface. The lateral intrascaphoid angle varies between 15° and 34° and the AP intrascaphoid angle between 32° and 46°. Amadio et al. concluded that angulation of more than 45° on the lateral view poses an increased risk for functional wrist impairment. In addition, an MRI should be obtained in cases where avascular necrosis of the fragments is suspected.

Surgical Technique

Surgery is performed under general anesthesia as it is necessary to harvest an iliac crest bone graft. A nonsterile arm tourniquet is placed and an esmarch exsanguination is utilized. A palmar approach to the scaphoid is preferred. The incision is centered over the scaphoid tubercle which is easily palpable with the wrist in radial deviation. The proximal limb extends approximately 2 cm along the radial border of the FCR tendon, and the distal limb of the incision is gently curved toward the base of the thumb. Superficially, the palmar branch of the radial artery is ligated just proximal to the scaphoid tubercle as it crosses the palm. The FCR sheath is incised and the tendon is retracted ulnarly to expose the anterior capsule over the scaphoid. Distally, the origin of the thenar muscles is divided in-line with its fibers over the trapezium for deeper exposure.

The capsule is incised longitudinally from the tip of the radius to the distal scaphoid to expose the underlying scaphoid; care should be taken to avoid injury to the underlying articular surface. Proximally, the capsule and the radiolunate ligament appear as a thick labrum which should be carefully preserved for later repair. A small self retainer should be placed for a better visualization of the volar scaphoid surface. The malunion site is then identified via visual inspection and confirmed by fluoroscopy. Two 0.045 in. Kirschner wires are placed parallel to one another on each side of the planned osteotomy to use as joy sticks for fragment manipulation once the osteotomy is completed. These wires also serve to confirm, intraoperatively, the amount of intraoperative correction by determining their subtended angles (extension and derotation). The osteotomy is performed with an oscillating saw, and extra caution should be taken so as not to injure the dorsal ridge vessels. The wrist is then extended over a rolled towel which opens up the palmar gap and reveals the amount of palmar gap needed for the correction. The K-wires are manipulated to correct the flexion and pronation deformity of the distal fragment, which should restore full passive wrist extension, and the reduction is assessed intraoperatively by observing the new positions of the K-wires in both sagittal and horizontal planes as confirmed by fluoroscopy. Ulnar deviation is corrected by opening the osteotomy on the ulnar side with a small spreader clamp. Based on the preoperative graft measurements and intraoperative gap assessment, a corticocancellous wedge graft shaped to fit the defect is obtained from the iliac crest and inserted into the osteotomy site as the assistant holds the K-wires in the corrected position. The graft is provisionally held with a K-wire placed under fluoroscopy and should be placed such that it can serve as a derotational wire. Before definitive fixation, complete passive wrist extension should be tested. After fluoroscopic confirmation of adequate restoration of length and correction of the deformity, a headless screw of the surgeon's preference should be placed from the distal scaphoid. The redundant edges of the graft are smoothed off with a burr. The wrist capsule and radiocarpal ligaments are closed with interrupted absorbable sutures.

Postoperatively, a long opponens splint is applied and, after suture removal, a thumb spica cast is placed for 3 weeks followed by a removable thumb spica splint till the patient is comfortable. At 8 weeks postsurgery, scaphoid views and CAT scan are used to assess for union. Comparative radiographs from the contralateral wrist will allow for assessment of deformity correction and carpal alignment.

Alternative Technique: Correcting Scaphoid Malunion with a DISI Deformity Using 1,2 ICSRA [31]

The surgery is performed under axillary block with general anesthesia added later if necessary. A volar radial approach is preferred in this technique to allow for harvest of a vascularized bone graft. A curved or zigzag incision is made 5 cm proximal to the radial styloid and ending over the midportion of the thumb metacarpal; the dorsal superficial radial sensory branches are identified and protected. The deep fascia over the anatomic snuffbox is incised to expose the radial artery and its venae comitantes, and the ascending 1,2 intercompartmental suprarctinacular branch is identified on the radial styloid. The periosteum is incised 2 mm on either side of the identified vessel for approximately 2 cm and is further extended another 1–1.5 cm proximally, widening the periosteal incision to 5 mm; this ensures a wide exposure to the bone graft site. Several small drill holes are made at the periphery of the bone graft site with a 1-mm drill bit and completed with a fine osteotome. A corticocancellous graft approximately 5 mm deep is elevated, and the vessel is subperiosteally raised with the graft and dissected off the capsule to its origin from the radial artery. The graft and the pedicle are carefully protected with a damp saline sponge and brought out of the field distally. The palmar recurrent branch which penetrates the scaphoid tuberosity is identified from the radial artery and protected.

The capsule is then incised approximately 1.5 cm along the borders of the radial styloid. Using an osteotome, 1 cm of the radial styloid is removed transversely; this provides a better exposure to the radioscaphoid joint and removes any site of degenerative disease, as well as provides bone graft. Ulnarly distracting the wrist readily exposes the scaphoid, and the site of the old fracture is identified by looking for an articular cartilage defect or a ridge correlated with the radiographs and confirmed under fluoroscopy. After indentifying the plane of the old fracture, small drill holes are made and these holes are connected palmar to dorsal with a sharp osteotome. The dorsal soft tissues are preserved to protect the residual vascularity. The defect is wedged open like a book palmarly using an osteotome.

The lunate position is corrected by extending and ulnarly deviating the wrist and is held in its reduced position with an oblique percutaneous Kirschner wire from the radial styloid into the lunate body. The exposed bony surfaces of the osteotomized scaphoid are observed for signs of punctuate bleeding. A wedge graft is fashioned from the osteotomized radial styloid based on the preoperative plans and placed in the defect. The normal carpal relationship should be apparent in both planes and assessed under fluoroscopy.

After satisfactory alignment is obtained, a decision for bone grafting is made; options include a tricorticocancellous graft from iliac crest alone, pedicle graft alone, or pedicle graft augmented with iliac crest or radial styloid fragment bone. The authors of this technique prefer a composite approach by placing either the trimmed styloid fragment or iliac graft to hold the defect open palmarly and use the vascularized pedicle graft in the remaining defect. The pedicled graft is checked carefully for any torsion or kinking to the vessel. If the proximal fragment appears avascular, the dead trabecular bone is curetted and filled with trabecular bone and the pedicled graft. Subsequently, the construct is stabilized by two or more K-wires drilled percutaneously from the proximal pole before placing the graft and then advanced through the graft once the graft is inserted. The K-wires are drilled through the distal fragment and retracted until the wires are buried proximally within the scaphoid and cut distally above the skin. The authors of this technique state that a retrograde compression screw may be difficult from this exposure and potentially risks loosening the construct. After confirming the construct under fluoroscopy, the tourniquet is deflated and bleeding from the pedicled bone is checked before skin closure. A small suction drain is placed to prevent tamponade on the vascular pedicle. The skin is closed with subcuticular absorbable sutures.

Postoperatively, an above-elbow thumb spica splint is placed and the dressing is changed at 4–7 days. The K-wires are padded well and dressed with povidone-iodine dressing.

The cast is changed to a below-elbow cast at 6–8 weeks and subsequently removed at 12 weeks. The K-wires are left in place until 8–10 weeks if no adverse reaction is noted.

Complications

The primary complication of the techniques mentioned is failure to restore an anatomic relationship; therefore, one must be vigilant intraoperatively in obtaining adequate fluoroscopic images to assess intercarpal relationship. Often times, it is a result of difficultly in conceptualizing the three-dimensional deformity and its correction, lack of adequate exposure, placing a graft of inadequate size or configuration to maintain the correction, inadequate fixation such as loosening or infection from a K-wire, or over compression from a screw and potential graft slippage. Understanding the potential pitfalls allows one to avoid these complications.

Salvage Procedures for Failed Nonunion Surgery (Table 9.3)

Despite all our best efforts, oftentimes, the scaphoid fails to unite or progresses to a SNAC deformity. In other instances, patients present at a much later stage with arthritic changes and the available options for reliable symptomatic relief are limited. Watson and Ballet initially described the arthritic changes associated with the scaphoid in four stages. Stage I is a normal radioscaphoid articulation with radial styloid breaking and dorsal scaphoid osteophytes. In stage II, the process involves the radioscaphoid articulation but spares the proximal scaphoid-radius articulation in the early stages. In stage III, the capitolunate articulation is involved, and stage IV further involves all periscaphoid articulations sparing the lunate-radius articulation [37].

Every patient who presents with a scaphoid deformity, nonunion, or avascular necrosis should be carefully evaluated for the presence of arthritic changes. The goal of the surgery is relief of preoperative symptoms and if preoperative arthritic changes are ignored, even a successfully united scaphoid nonunion may have a poor outcome. In general, cystic changes in the scaphoid are noted 1 decade after fracture, radioscaphoid arthritis is expected after 2 decades, and panscaphoid arthritis is evident in the third decade in an untreated scaphoid [38]. Management of a SNAC wrist depends upon several variables: patient's age, activity level, functional needs, occupation, and SNAC stage. Nonoperative treatment with splints, anti-inflammatory medications, physical therapy modalities, and steroid injections should be exhausted before considering surgery. Stage I SNAC wrist is best managed with a radial styloidectomy with or without a scaphoid nonunion procedure. Options for a stage II SNAC wrist are motion preserving and include proximal row carpectomy (PRC), four-corner fusion with styloidectomy, and a four-corner fusion with scaphoid excision. Stage III can be treated with four-corner fusion with scaphoid excision and wrist arthrodesis. The best and most predictable option for stage IV is total wrist arthrodesis although a total wrist arthroplasty may be an option in stage IV. Malerich et al. have reported good results with distal scaphoid resection in patients with SNAC stages I and II [39].

Distal Scaphoid Resection Arthroplasty [39]

Distal scaphoid resection has been proposed as a minimally disruptive option to the traditional PRC and four-corner fusion for patients with early SNAC wrists (stages I and II). It is a relatively quick procedure, minimally disruptive to the intercarpal and radiocarpal ligaments, and does not require bone grafting or internal fixation. Its proponents initially

Table 9.3 Salvage procedures for failed nonunion surgery

Distal scaphoid resection arthroplasty	SNAC stages I and II wrists	Capitolunate arthritis
Proximal row carpectomy	SNAC stages I and II wrists	Loss of proximal capitate or lunate fossa cartilage (relative contraindication)
Adjuncts Interposition with capsular flap Proximal capitate excision	Failure of nonoperative management	Age less than 35 (relative contraindication)
Four-corner fusion	SNAC stage II or III wrists Younger patient Failure of nonoperative management	Radiolunate arthritis Ulnar carpal translation Active infection
Wrist arthrodesis	SNAC stage IV wrists Chronic wrist pain from variety of arthritic causes Failed partial arthrodesis Failed arthroplasty Failed wrist denervation procedure	Active infection

reported their results in 19 patients with all different stages of SNAC wrists. In their experience, patients with preoperative capitolunate arthritic changes faired the worse and went onto arthritic progression. Therefore, this procedure is contraindicated in patients with capitolunate arthritic changes. The authors reported an 85% improvement in the range of motion and 134% improvement in grip strength at an average follow-up period of 49 months.

Surgical Technique

A dorsal oblique incision approximately 5 cm long is made starting at Lister's tubercle along the EPL. The EPL is unroofed and retracted radially and the radiocarpal joint is entered at the floor of the EPL tendon. The first structure visualized is the dorsal scaphoid osteophyte from the distal scaphoid fragment. The nonunion site is identified with a needle and confirmed via fluoroscopy. The distal scaphoid is excised by placing a freer or key elevator at the scaphotrapezial-trapezoid articulation and delivering it dorsally. This will aid in excising all soft tissue attachments on that fragment and the distal scaphoid can be removed en bloc or piecemeal. Care must be taken as the radial artery is at risk during this dissection. If there is difficulty in detaching the volar soft tissues from the distal fragment, then a volar incision may be helpful. The surrounding articular surfaces are inspected if possible without any further dissection. No soft tissue interposition is required for this procedure. The wrist is examined for stability to ensure that important ligamentous constraints were not violated. The wrist should be immobilized for 2 weeks and then range of motion and strengthening should be initiated.

Proximal Row Carpectomy [40]

PRC is a useful procedure for degenerative arthritis of the wrist regardless of the cause and has been used to treat stages I and II SNAC wrists. Parameters such as functional disability, pain, and objective measures of motion and grip strength should be assessed preoperatively. Pathology of the proximal scaphoid, lunate, or triquetrum is not important as these bones are removed. One concern when considering PRC is proximal capitate involvement since the postoperative motion is achieved via the capitate-radius articulation. The main contraindication to PRC is cartilage loss at the head of the capitate and lunate fossa of the distal radius. However, in such cases, variations to the PRC such as resection with interposition or resection distraction can be adapted [41, 42]. Examining the distal radius and proximal capitates for pathology via arthroscopy before definitive surgery can help determine the need for any adjunctive procedures in conjunction with PRC. PRC in a young patient (<35 years) is considered a relative contraindication by some surgeons due to unfavorable results in some studies. Although others have found even in some young patients that PRC can be a durable option that lasts a lifetime.

Surgical Technique

A longitudinal, transverse, or oblique (proximal ulnar to distal radial) incision is made over the dorsum of the radius to expose the proximal and midcarpal rows. Subcutaneous dissection is carried down to the extensor retinaculum preserving all longitudinally oriented veins and nerves, and the proximal and distal ends of the extensor retinaculum are identified and incised longitudinally leaving a rim intact proximally. The EPL tendon is then identified and retracted radially by unroofing its retinaculum. The interval between the third and fourth dorsal compartments is developed and tendons are elevated in a subperiosteal fashion. The first, second, and third dorsal compartments are retracted radially and the fourth extensor compartment is retracted ulnarly. The posterior interosseous nerve is identified at the floor of the fourth compartment and transected proximally. Capsulotomy is performed in a transverse or T-shaped shaped fashion with the distal limb over the SL interval. If interposition of the dorsal capsule is expected, then the capsule should be incised as distal as possible off the carpal bones, and a flap for interposition could be created by making longitudinal incisions on the radial and ulnar aspects of the transverse incision. The capsulotomy will reveal the underlying diseased proximal row. Excision of the proximal carpal row is then performed. An osteotomy is used to divide the scaphoid at its waist. A Steinman pin may be placed in the proximal scaphoid dorsally and used as a joy stick to detach all capsular and soft tissue attachments using a combination of osteotomes, periosteal elevator, and beaver blades. In a similar fashion, the lunate and triquetrum are carefully excised from the surrounding soft tissues. It is acceptable to remove these bones in a piecemeal fashion and often may be a more expeditious alternative. An alternative approach is to place a 3.2-mm Steinman pin in the lunate and excise it first creating more space, then placing another Steinman pin along the long axis of the scaphoid will make its excision easier. At this point, both care and patience should be exercised to avoid injury to adjacent articular tissue and volar capsule-ligamentous envelope. Retaining the distal pole of scaphoid allows maintenance of the scaphotrapezial ligaments. However, some authors recommend complete excision of the scaphoid to avoid symptomatic distal scaphoid and radial styloid impingement. Once the proximal or entire scaphoid, lunate, and triquetrum are excised, the distal radius and capitate are inspected for pathology. The radioscaphocapitate ligament on the palmar capsule should be inspected for integrity as it is very important for radial support of the capitate once it rests in the lunate fossa and thus should therefore be preserved during proximal carpal row excision. If radial styloidectomy is performed, only 5–7 mm should be excised and the radioscaphocapitate should be preserved. Careful repair of the capsule should be performed to maintain capitate position. Temporary fixation across the new articulation with a pin is not required and, if placed, risks infection and pin migration. The wrist should be tested in flexion, extension, radial, and ulnar deviation for stability. The extensor retinaculum is repaired and the skin and subcutaneous tissue are closed in layers. A volar splint is placed for 2–4 weeks to allow for soft tissue healing. Early finger and wrist range of motion is encouraged.

For patients with capitate-radius pathology, several authors have suggested adjuncts to PRC with good success. The simplest method is to create a distally based capsular flap which could be sutured to the volar capsule and hence covers the head of the capitate. If a longitudinal capsular incision is made, then that split could be repaired with a nonabsorbable suture and still serve its role in interposition. Salomon and Eaton have reported favorable results resecting the proximal 2–4 mm of capitate in-line with the proximal articular surface of the hamate, creating a broader contact area of the proximal carpal row and better distribution of compressive forces. A distally based capsular flap then covers the broad capitohamate surface [41].

Four-Corner Fusion with Scaphoid Excision [43]

Four-corner fusion with scaphoid excision is another motion preserving option in SNAC stages I, II, and III. In this procedure, wrist motion is maintained through the preserved radiolunate and ulnocarpal joint. The principle is to remove the periscaphoid arthritis (scaphoid excision) and stabilize the midcarpal joint by either a capitolunate or a four-corner fusion. In this procedure, including the hamate and the triquetrum in the fusion mass has shown to increase the rate of fusion without losing any more motion; thus, a four-corner fusion is, by some, considered to be a better option. An ideal patient for a four-corner fusion would be one with a SNAC stage II or III wrist, with a painful wrist, and who has exhausted all nonoperative options. Contraindications to a four-corner fusion with scaphoid excision are radiolunate arthritis and ulnar carpal translation (long radiolunate ligament insufficiency) which results in incongruity at the radiolunate joint risking further degeneration.

Surgical Technique

Four-corner fusion can be approached through either two parallel dorsal transverse incisions as described by Watson [44] or a single longitudinal incision centered over the wrist. The distal transverse incision would overlie the radiocarpal joint and the proximal over the distal radius to obtain bone graft. In both approaches, the dissection is carried down to the extensor retinaculum while protecting the dorsal veins and nerve branches. The third dorsal compartment is incised along its course to gain access to the wrist capsule. The scaphoid is approached between the ECRL and ECRB. The wrist capsule is incised transversely and the underlying scaphoid is visualized. The scaphoid is carefully excised (piecemeal or en bloc) without injuring the adjacent radial and volar capsular structures. It is imperative to preserve the long radiolunate ligament to prevent ulnar carpal translation. Removing the scaphoid and longitudinal traction provides excellent visualization of the radiolunate articulation for confirmation that it is well preserved. Attention is then paid to the articulations between lunate, capitate, hamate, and triquetrum, and their cartilaginous articular surfaces are removed down to cancellous bone using a rongeur. Longitudinal traction may help create space between the intercarpal joints. Bone graft is obtained from the proximal aspect of the longitudinal incision or through a separate transverse incision proximally. The cancellous surfaces between the four bones are opposed and definitive fixation is achieved via either K-wires, staples, headless screws, or a plate-screw construct. The most important aspect of this procedure is correcting any DISI deformity at the time of the fusion as uncorrected carpal malalignment can lead to ultimate decrease in range of motion and persistent wrist pain from capitate impingement. DISI deformity is corrected by either placing a 0.062-in. K-wire in the lunate or placing a radiolunate pin. The capitate should be centered (displace it palmarly and ulnarly) in the lunate, and slight volar intercalated segmental instability is preferable as it improves wrist extension. Bone graft is packed between the fusion surfaces. Percutaneous K-wires (0.045 or 0.062) are placed from a distal to proximal direction as follows: one each in capitate, hamate, and triquetrum directed toward the lunate. One additional K-wire is placed between the triquetrum and capitate. The wrist capsule and extensor retinaculum are closed and skin is closed with subcuticular sutures.

Postoperatively, a long-arm splint with wrist in slight extension and elbow at 90° is placed. One week postoperatively, a long-arm thumb spica cast is placed including the metacarpophalangeal joints of the index and long finger flexed at 80°. At week 4 follow-up, the long-arm cast is switched to a short-arm thumb spica cast leaving the MP joints free for another 2 weeks. The pins are removed in the office at 6 weeks and range of motion is initiated at that time.

Plate Fixation: Spider Plate (KMI, San Diego, CA)

An alternative method of fixation is the conical spider plate which is seated below the dorsal surface of the carpus. The surgical approach is similar to the preceding technique. The capitate, hamate, lunate, and triquetrum are exposed; carpal malalignment corrected; and cartilaginous surfaces denuded. They are provisionally fixed with K-wires and a spider rasp is centered over the four-corner junction and rasped flush or below the dorsal surface of the carpus. Autogenous bone graft is packed in between and at the junction of the four-corner fusion site, and an 8-hole spider plate is placed at the junction such that two screws overlie each carpal bone. A 1.5-mm drill bit is used to place 2.4-mm self-tapping screws. Due to its conical shape, tightening each screw yields radial compression. Care should be taken to avoid entering the pisotriquetral joint when placing the triquetral screw. Provisional K-wires are then removed and proper hardware placement is confirmed via fluoroscopy.

Postoperatively, a short-arm splint is placed. A short-arm cast or removable splint is used for 3–4 weeks after surgery and early active range of motion of fingers and elbow is initiated. The senior author does not prefer this method of fixation. It is merely presented as an alternative.

Comparing Proximal Row Carpectomy and Four-Corner Fusion

PRC and four-corner fusion are both excellent options for early stages of SNAC wrist; however, controversy exists as to which procedure yields a better outcome. PRC is a reliable procedure with a long-term follow-up (>10 years). Even though postoperatively 60–70% of wrist motion and grip strength compared to the contralateral side can be expected, persistent wrist pain eventually necessitating wrist arthrodesis is seen in 5–20% of the patients. Four-corner fusion with scaphoid excision has shown similar results in long-term follow-up. Complications specific to four-corner fusion are nonunion, dorsal impingement, RSD, and superficial infection. According to a recent meta-analysis of 52 articles, range of motion was better with a PRC than a four-corner fusion and lacked the above mentioned complications. However, risk of subsequent osteoarthritis was significantly higher in the PRC group. No difference was found in grip strength, pain relief, and subjective outcomes between groups. The authors acknowledged the lack of unbiased trials which explains the existing controversy between the two procedures [45]. However, the authors prefer PRC in older patients and a four-corner fusion in the younger population.

Wrist Arthrodesis

Wrist fusion is a well-established procedure with reliable results in the literature. The goal is to provide a stable and painless wrist by eliminating motion in the arthritic segments. Relieving pain in the wrist allows one to concentrate on finger range of motion and strengthening. Results of wrist arthrodesis vary in the literature with reported pain relief in 70–100% of patients, with a mean time off work being 5–15 months and a high patient satisfaction rating [46, 47]. However, oftentimes, the pain is incompletely relieved, grip strength remains poor, and additional procedures are required in nearly half of the patients.

Indications for a wrist arthrodesis are chronic wrist pain that may result from a variety of inflammatory, metabolic, posttraumatic, and late stages of periscaphoid arthritis (SNAC stage IV). Commonly, it serves as salvage after failed partial wrist arthrodesis, arthroplasty, or denervation aiming to relieve pain. Contraindications to wrist arthrodesis are active infection if internal fixation is contemplated. Arthrodesis must be carefully selected in patients with bilateral disease and in patients with paralysis who may become less functional after surgery despite the wrist being in a better "functional" position. Immobilizing a patient preoperatively with a cast in a position of fusion for 1–2 weeks is extremely helpful for both the surgeon and the patient in determining if the pain relief or functional limitation is acceptable. The distal radioulnar joint (DRUJ) and length of ulna should be addressed with a partial resection, Sauve-Kapandji, or an implant to avoid postoperative impingement (due to shortened carpus) or DRUJ pain. The surgical technique of wrist arthrodesis is discussed elsewhere in this book.

Reoperative Issues Following Scaphocapitate Syndrome

Scaphocapitate syndrome consists of a fracture of the scaphoid waist and a concomitant fracture of the capitate neck such that the proximal capitate fracture fragment rotates 180° about its axis [48]. Scarcity of published literature regarding this injury attests to its rarity. It usually occurs from falls on a hyperextended wrist or in a pattern of a perilunate injury. This rare injury was first described by Nicholson in 1940 and subsequently coined "naviculocapitate fracture syndrome" by Fenton in 1956 in his case report of two patients with such an injury. He postulated that a hyperextended wrist in radial deviation causes the radial styloid to act as a "chisel" as it strikes the scaphoid waist which is supported by the capitate (anvil) medially. A moderately strong force causes the scaphoid to fracture; however, a strong violent force further leads to a capitate fracture and its malrotation [48]. Stein and Seigel in a cadaveric study challenged this theory and showed in a cadaveric experiment that in hyperextension, the dorsal lip of the radius strikes the capitate neck causing it to fracture and rotate 180° as the wrist returns to neutral [49]. Due to its rarity and difficulty in radiographic diagnosis, this injury is often missed. In this injury, persistent capitate malrotation can persist even after successful closed reduction and restoration of overall carpal alignment, which further leads to a delayed or missed diagnosis.

Complications are common to this injury despite adequate diagnosis and treatment. Nonunion, avascular necrosis, and functional limitations have been reported. The proximal capitate is completely covered by cartilage and the vascular foramina are located in the neck and waist. Hence, a completely malrotated proximal capitate fragment with minimal soft tissue attachment is vulnerable to nonunion and avascular necrosis. Several authors have reported on patients with a healed scaphoid and a persistently malrotated or nonunited capitate with a pain-free wrist and minimal functional loss [48, 50]. However, such an outcome with this injury is an exception rather than the rule; therefore, anatomical surgical reduction and internal fixation is recommended by most authors.

Reoperative options for avascular necrosis, nonunion, or delayed arthritic changes include bone grafting, midcarpal arthroplasty, midcarpal arthrodesis, and capitohamate arthrodesis [51–53]. Due to the sparse literature on this topic, treatment options and addressing their failures cannot be drawn. A few case reports of capitate pseudoarthrosis have shown favorable outcomes with cancellous bone grafting and internal fixation of capitate through a dorsal approach. Others have proposed excising the proximal capitate avascular fragment and performing an interposition arthroplasty. Intercarpal arthrodesis is a viable option eliminating the offending articular segment but at the expense of motion. Overall, little consensus exists given the low power in the studies and lack of long-term follow-up.

Reoperative Issues Following Hook of Hamate Surgery

Hook of the hamate fractures are rare (<2%) but should always be on the differential in volar- and ulnar-sided wrist pain. Current treatment of hook of hamate fractures includes immobilization, excision of the fragment, and open reduction internal fixation. Reoperative issues following hook of hamate surgery are persistent pain due to a nonunion, partial union, rupture of flexor tendons, and nerve injury [54, 55]. In order to understand the complications involving this bone, one must understand its anatomy. The hook projects 2 cm distal and radial to the pisiform in the hypothenar eminence. Its multiple attachments provide stability, and they include the transverse carpal ligament radially, pisohamate ligament ulnarly, and the muscles of flexor digiti minimi and opponens digiti minimi. The hamate forms the ulnar border of the carpal tunnel and the radial border of Guyon's canal. The base of the hamate serves as a pulley to the flexor tendons especially to the ring and small finger.

Treatment of painless hook of hamate nonunion is controversial. Advocates of surgery in these patients argue that removing the nonunion fragment averts potential for tendon fraying or neurologic injury. Options for painful hook nonunions include excision of the hook and revision ORIF with bone grafting. The hamate hook has a rich vascular supply; therefore, a nonunion is more likely due to the forces transmitted from its ligamentous and muscular attachments rather than vascular insufficiency. Excision of the hook of the hamate avoids potential attritional flexor tendon rupture or neurovascular injury. However, residual symptoms following excision, although uncommon, are mild weakness, painful grasp, altered sensibility, scar tenderness, and bone reformation [56]. Bishop et al. found residual symptoms in 10 of 17 (59%) after hook excision, with weakness of grasp being most frequent. Complications from excision (<3%) are injury to ulnar nerve and superficial palmar arch and median nerve paresthesias from traction. Careful dissection through the carpal tunnel and extraperiosteal excision can avoid these complications. Advocates of ORIF with bone graft argue that superior outcome in these patients is due to the restored pulley effect of the flexor profundus during power grip [57]. However, literature supporting this argument is scarce. Studies in literature comparing excision vs. ORIF have shown comparable outcomes [58, 59].

In our opinion, patients with hook of hamate nonunions that have failed previous excision or ORIF should be carefully evaluated for the following: location of pain, pain with flexor tendon excursion, flexor tendon integrity, ulnar nerve motor and sensory function, grip strength, patient age, occupation, and functional demands. An athlete requiring a power grip for racquet sports may potentially benefit from restoring the hook anatomy whereas someone with a sedentary lifestyle may not notice minor functional limitations. Therefore, treatment should be individualized for an optimal outcome.

Case 9.1: Malpositioned Screw

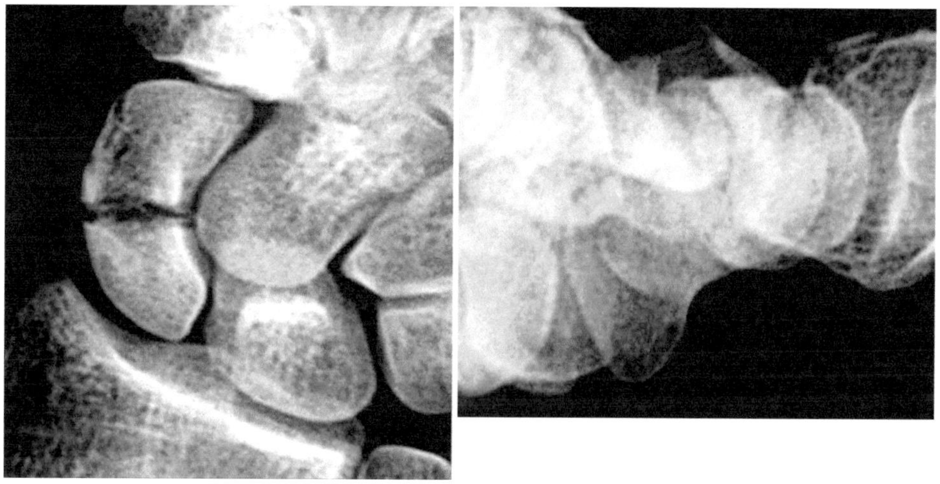

(a) Minimally displaced scaphoid waist fracture

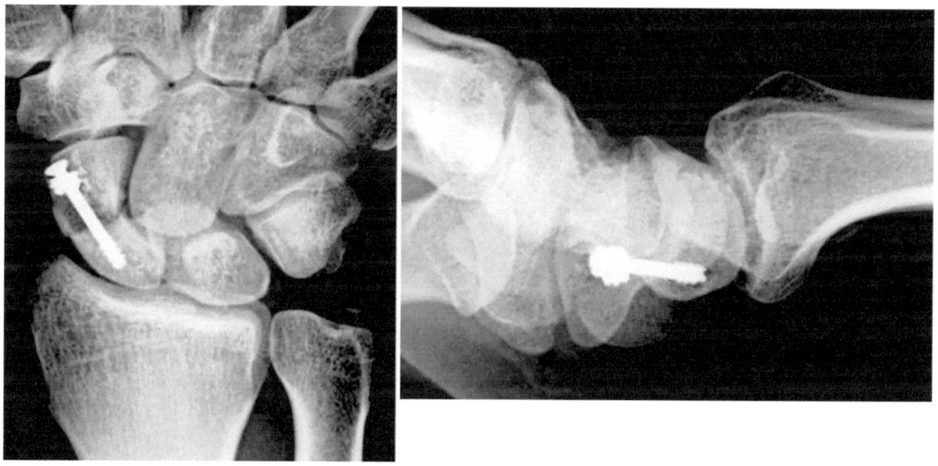

(b) Treated with a compression screw via percutaneous volar technique. Note that the malpositioned screw is too vertical, abutting the volar scaphoid cortex, and ideally should be center in both planes

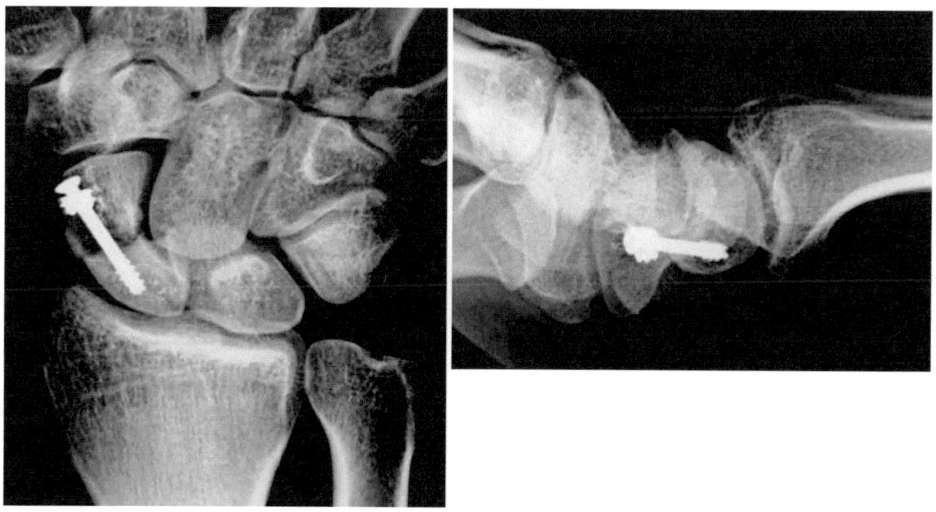

(c) A few months post-op: Hardware loosening and lucency around the screw due to poor proximal purchase

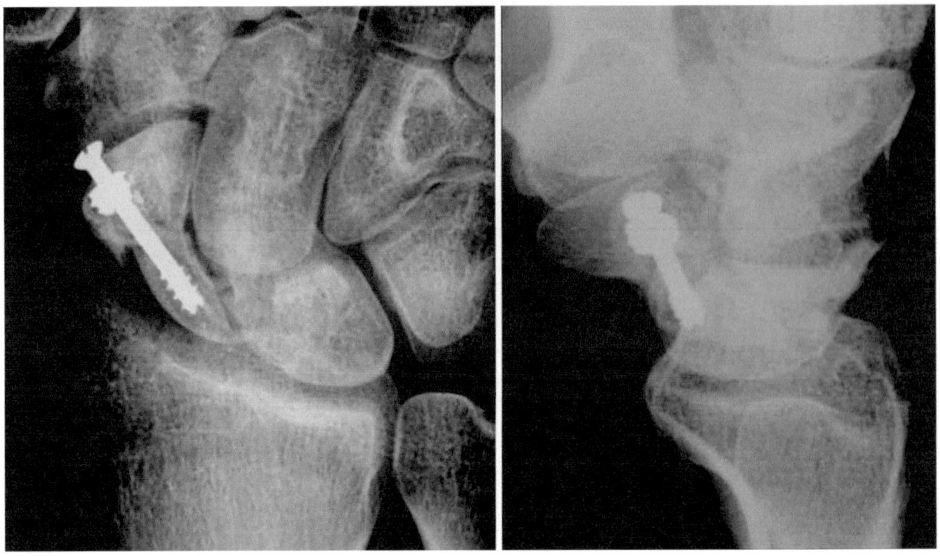

(d) Proximal migration of the hardware with a nonunion and proximal fragment trabecular collapse and minimal osteogenic activity at the fracture site

Case 9.2: Proximal Pole Nonunion After Failed Fixation. Healed After Intercalary Iliac Crest Graft and K-Wire Fixation

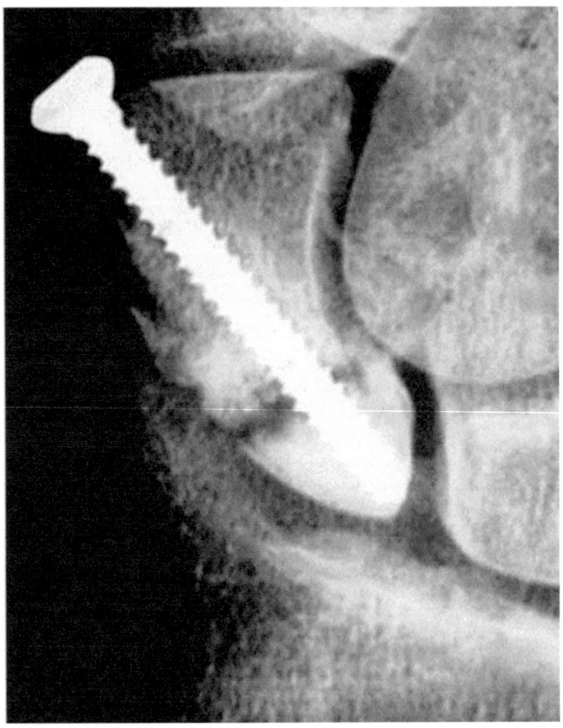

(a) Preoperative X-ray of patient who underwent percutaneous volar screw fixation of a proximal pole fracture that subsequently developed a nonunion

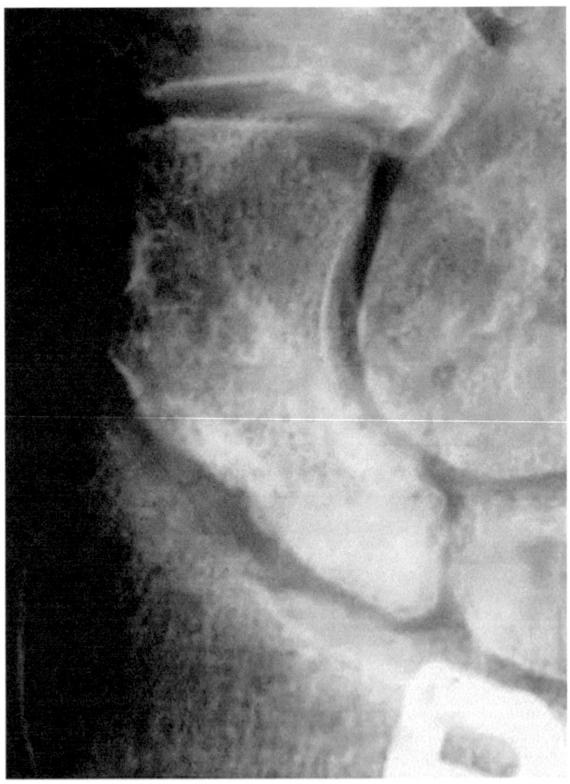

(b) One year post-op s/p hardware removal after undergoing intercalary bone graft and K-wire fixation of proximal pole nonunion

(c, d) 2.5 years post-op showing a viable proximal pole and some early degenerative process

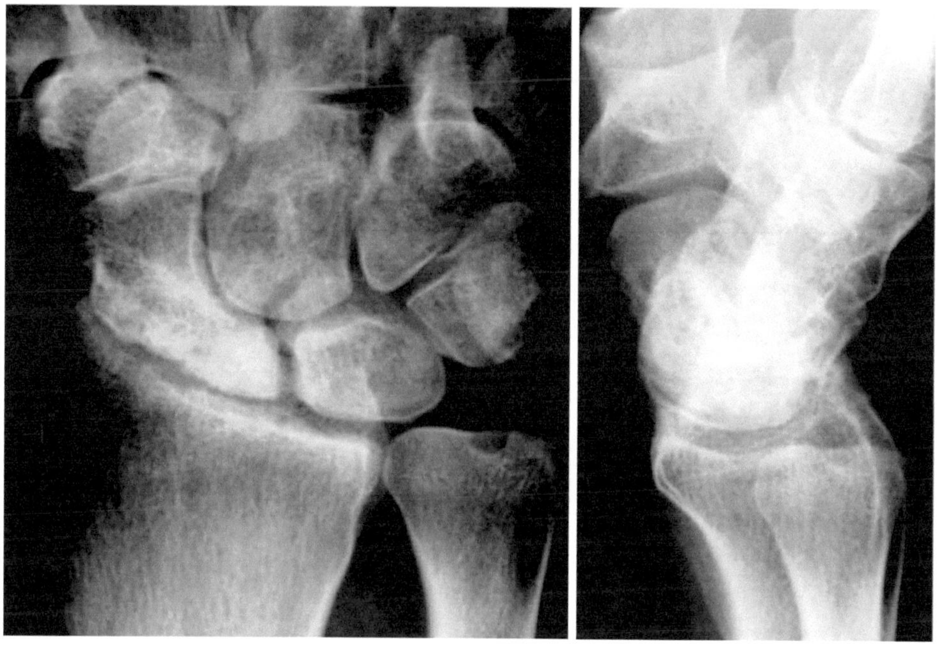

Case 9.3: Proximal Pole Nonunion Treated with 1,2 ICSRA

(a) Scaphoid nonunion after screw fixation with proximal pole collapse from impaired vascularity

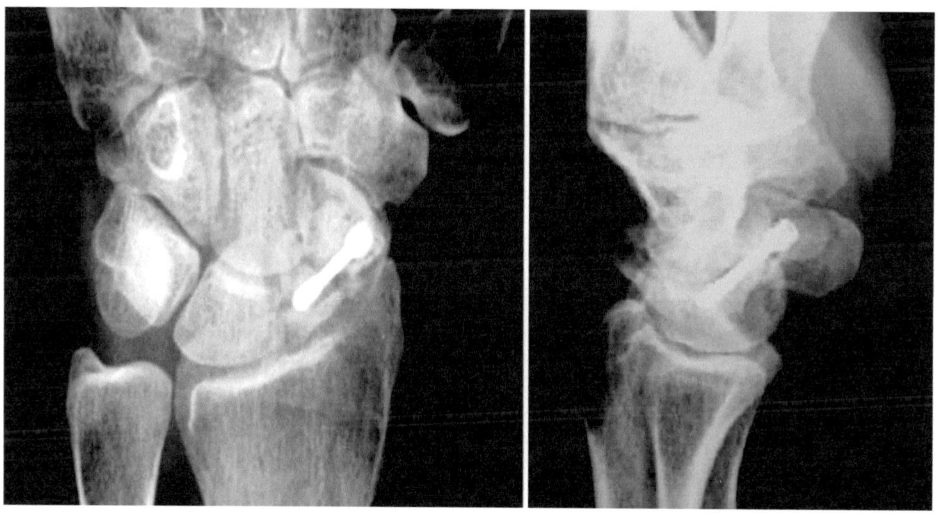

(b) CT scan confirming an established nonunion with sclerotic edges, a small proximal fragment, and bone loss

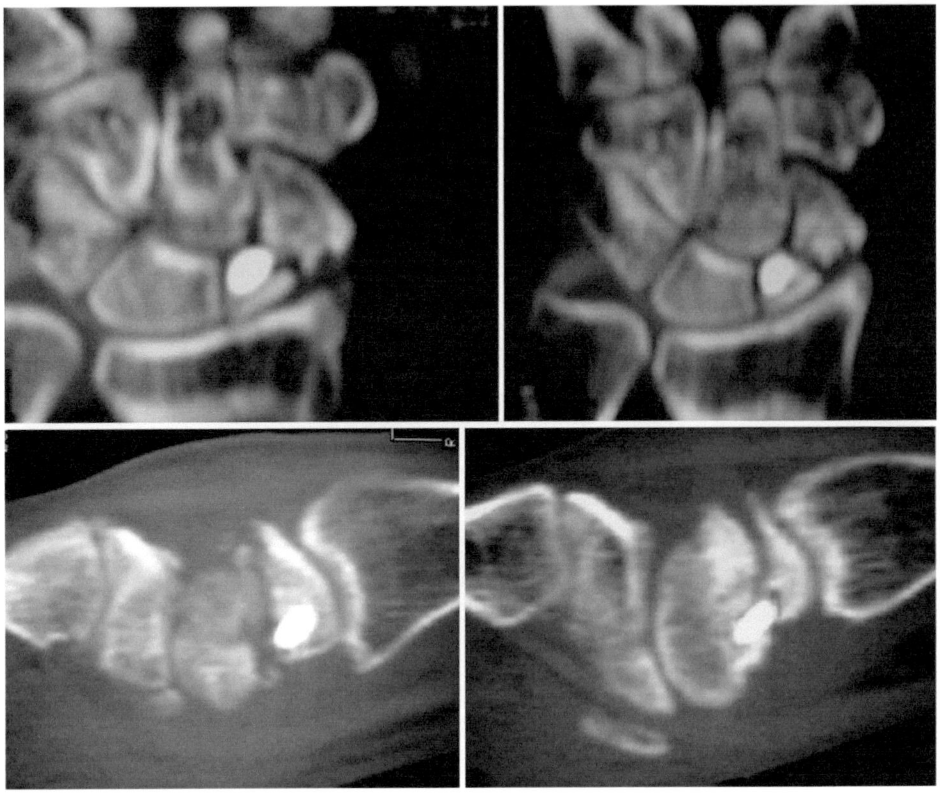

(c) MRI confirming proximal pole avascular necrosis. Determining the vascularity of the proximal pole preoperatively is important in determining if a vascularized bone graft is necessary

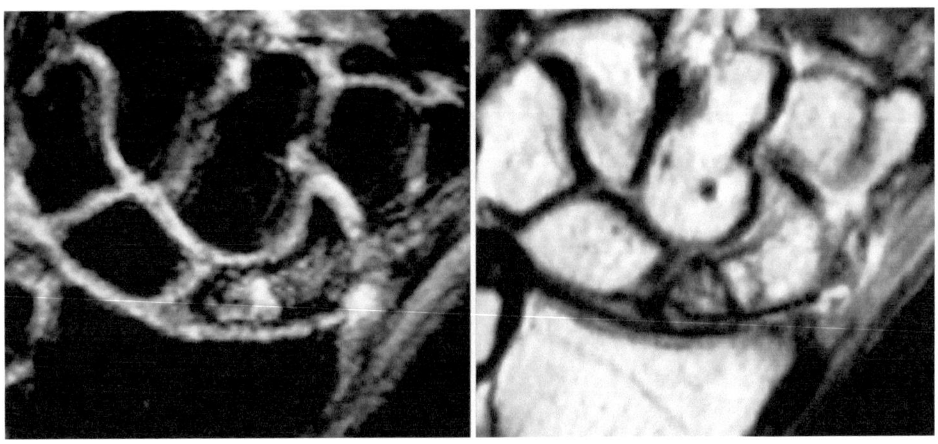

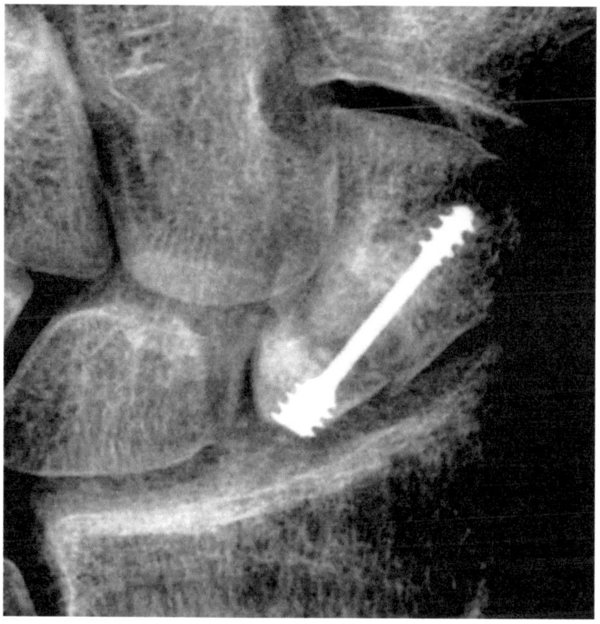

(d) Six weeks after revision fixation and 1,2 ICSRA

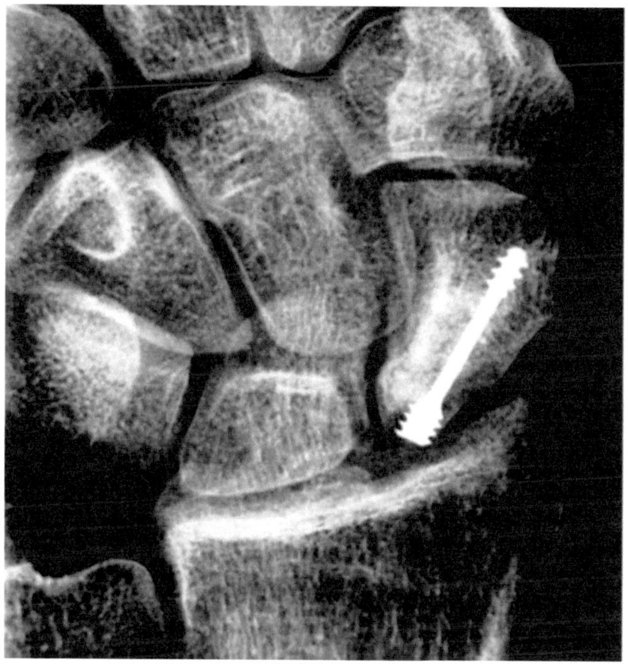

(f) Nine months post-op. Well-incorporated vascularized graft with a viable proximal pole

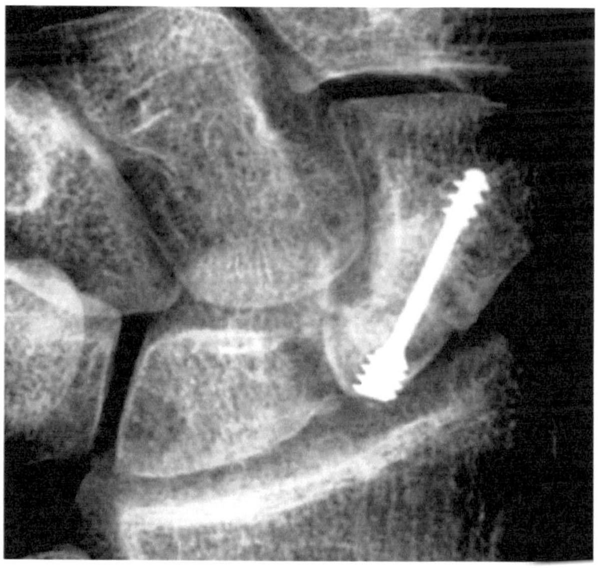

(e) Nine weeks after revision fixation and 1,2 ICSRA

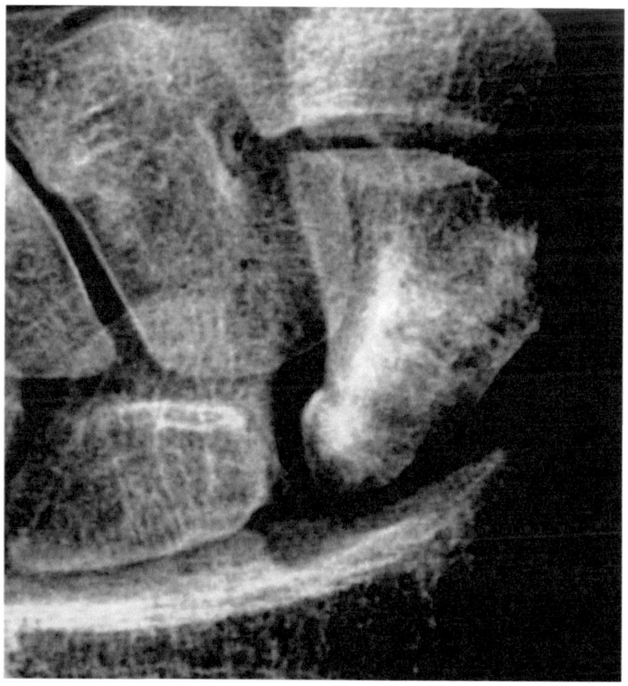

(g) 1.2 years post-op after hardware removal

References

1. Kawamura K, Chung KC. Treatment of scaphoid fractures and nonunions. J Hand Surg Am. 2008;33(6):988–97.
2. Jupiter JB, Shin AY, Trumble TE, Fernandez DL. Traumatic and reconstructive problems of the scaphoid. Instr Course Lect. 2001;50:105–22.
3. Gelberman RH, Menon J. The vascularity of the scaphoid bone. J Hand Surg Am. 1980;5(5):508–13.
4. Amadio PC, Berquist TH, Smith DK, Ilstrup DM, Cooney III WP, Linscheid RL. Scaphoid malunion. J Hand Surg Am. 1989;14(4):679–87.
5. Bain GI, Bennett JD, MacDermid JC, Slethaug GP, Richards RS, Roth JH. Measurement of the scaphoid humpback deformity using longitudinal computed tomography: intra- and interobserver variability using various measurement techniques. J Hand Surg Am. 1998;23(1):76–81.
6. Capo JT, Orillaza Jr NS, Slade III JF. Percutaneous management of scaphoid nonunions. Tech Hand Up Extrem Surg. 2009; 13(1):23–9.
7. Mazet R, Hohl M. Radial styloidectomy and styloidectomy plus bone graft in the treatment of old ununited carpal-scaphoid fractures. Ann Surg. 1960;152(2):296–302.
8. Russe O. Fracture of the carpal navicular. Diagnosis, non-operative treatment, and operative treatment. J Bone Joint Surg Am. 1960;42-A:759–68.
9. Tomaino MM, King J, Pizillo M. Correction of lunate malalignment when bone grafting scaphoid nonunion with humpback deformity: rationale and results of a technique revisited. J Hand Surg Am. 2000;25(2):322–9.
10. Robbins RR, Ridge O, Carter PR. Iliac crest bone grafting and Herbert screw fixation of nonunions of the scaphoid with avascular proximal poles. J Hand Surg Am. 1995;20(5):818–31.
11. Inoue G, Shionoya K. Herbert screw fixation by limited access for acute fractures of the scaphoid. J Bone Joint Surg Br. 1997;79(3):418–21.
12. Green DP. The effect of avascular necrosis on Russe bone grafting for scaphoid nonunion. J Hand Surg Am. 1985;10(5):597–605.
13. Merrell GA, Wolfe SW, Slade III JF. Treatment of scaphoid nonunions: quantitative meta-analysis of the literature. J Hand Surg Am. 2002;27(4):685–91.
14. Yuceturk A, Isiklar ZU, Tuncay C, Tandogan R. Treatment of scaphoid nonunions with a vascularized bone graft based on the first dorsal metacarpal artery. J Hand Surg Br. 1997;22(3):425–7.
15. Dailiana ZH, Malizos KN, Zachos V, Varitimidis SE, Hantes M, Karantanas A. Vascularized bone grafts from the palmar radius for the treatment of waist nonunions of the scaphoid. J Hand Surg Am. 2006;31(3):397–404.
16. Tsuyuguchi Y, Murase T, Hidaka N, Ohno H, Kawai H. Anterior wedge-shaped bone graft for old scaphoid fractures or non-unions. An analysis of relevant carpal alignment. J Hand Surg Br. 1995;20(2):194–200.
17. Trumble TE, Salas P, Barthel T, Robert III KQ. Management of scaphoid nonunions. J Am Acad Orthop Surg. 2003;11(6): 380–91.
18. Zaidemberg C, Siebert JW, Angrigiani C. A new vascularized bone graft for scaphoid nonunion. J Hand Surg Am. 1991;16(3): 474–8.
19. Sawaizumi T, Nanno M, Nanbu A, Ito H. Vascularised bone graft from the base of the second metacarpal for refractory nonunion of the scaphoid. J Bone Joint Surg Br. 2004;86(7):1007–12.
20. Henry M. Collapsed scaphoid non-union with dorsal intercalated segment instability and avascular necrosis treated by vascularised wedge-shaped bone graft and fixation. J Hand Surg Eur Vol. 2007;32(2):148–54.
21. Hori Y, Tamai S, Okuda H, Sakamoto H, Takita T, Masuhara K. Blood vessel transplantation to bone. J Hand Surg Am. 1979;4(1):23–33.
22. Fernandez DL, Eggli S. Non-union of the scaphoid. Revascularization of the proximal pole with implantation of a vascular bundle and bone-grafting. J Bone Joint Surg Am. 1995;77(6):883–93.
23. Bartelmann U, Kalb K. Treatment of difficult scaphoid pseudarthroses by bone transplantation and additional implantation of the second dorsal metacarpal artery using the Fernandez and Eggli technique—report of experiences. Handchir Mikrochir Plast Chir. 2001;33(6):379–86.
24. Makino M. Vascularized metacarpal bone graft for scaphoid nonunion and Kienbock's disease. J Reconstr Microsurg. 2000;16(4):261–6; discussion 6–8.
25. Shah J, Jones WA. Factors affecting the outcome in 50 cases of scaphoid nonunion treated with Herbert screw fixation. J Hand Surg Br. 1998;23(5):680–5.
26. Lynch NM, Linscheid RL. Corrective osteotomy for scaphoid malunion: technique and long-term follow-up evaluation. J Hand Surg Am. 1997;22(1):35–43.
27. Birchard D, Pichora D. Experimental corrective scaphoid osteotomy for scaphoid malunion with abnormal wrist mechanics. J Hand Surg Am. 1990;15(6):863–8.
28. Nakamura P, Imaeda T, Miura T. Scaphoid malunion. J Bone Joint Surg Br. 1991;73(1):134–7.
29. Fernandez DL, Martin CJ, Gonzalez del Pino J. Scaphoid malunion. The significance of rotational malalignment. J Hand Surg Br. 1998;23(6):771–5.
30. Mayfield JK. Mechanism of carpal injuries. Clin Orthop Relat Res. 1980;149:45–54.
31. Linscheid RL, Lynch NM. Scaphoid osteotomy for malunion. Tech Hand Up Extrem Surg. 1998;2(2):119–25.
32. Burgess RC. The effect of a simulated scaphoid malunion on wrist motion. J Hand Surg Am. 1987;12(5 Pt 1):774–6.
33. Barton NJ. Twenty questions about scaphoid fractures. J Hand Surg Br. 1992;17(3):289–310.
34. Fernandez DL, Eggli S. Scaphoid nonunion and malunion. How to correct deformity. Hand Clin. 2001;17(4):631–46, ix.
35. Fisk GR. Carpal instability and the fractured scaphoid. Ann R Coll Surg Engl. 1970;46(2):63–76.
36. Fernandez DL. A technique for anterior wedge-shaped grafts for scaphoid nonunions with carpal instability. J Hand Surg Am. 1984;9(5):733–7.
37. Watson HK, Ballet FL. The SLAC wrist: scapholunate advanced collapse pattern of degenerative arthritis. J Hand Surg Am. 1984;9(3):358–65.
38. Mack GR, Bosse MJ, Gelberman RH, Yu E. The natural history of scaphoid non-union. J Bone Joint Surg Am. 1984;66(4):504–9.
39. Malerich MM, Clifford J, Eaton B, Eaton R, Littler JW. Distal scaphoid resection arthroplasty for the treatment of degenerative arthritis secondary to scaphoid nonunion. J Hand Surg Am. 1999;24(6):1196–205.
40. Diao E, Andrews A, Beall M. Proximal row carpectomy. Hand Clin. 2005;21(4):553–9.
41. Salomon GD, Eaton RG. Proximal row carpectomy with partial capitate resection. J Hand Surg Am. 1996;21(1):2–8.
42. Fitzgerald JP, Peim CA, Smith RJ. Distraction resection arthroplasty of the wrist. J Hand Surg Am. 1989;14(5):774–81.
43. Enna M, Hoepfner P, Weiss AP. Scaphoid excision with four-corner fusion. Hand Clin. 2005;21(4):531–8.
44. Watson HK, Ryu J. Degenerative disorders of the carpus. Orthop Clin North Am. 1984;15(2):337–53.
45. Mulford JS, Ceulemans LJ, Nam D, Axelrod TS. Proximal row carpectomy vs four corner fusion for scapholunate (Slac) or scaphoid nonunion advanced collapse (SNAC) wrists: a systematic review of outcomes. J Hand Surg Eur Vol. 2009;34(2):256–63.

46. Rauhaniemi J, Tiusanen H, Sipola E. Total wrist fusion: a study of 115 patients. J Hand Surg Br. 2005;30(2):217–9.
47. Rayan GM. Wrist arthrodesis. J Hand Surg Am. 1986;11(3): 356–64.
48. Fenton RL. The naviculo-capitate fracture syndrome. J Bone Joint Surg Am. 1956;38(A(3)):681–4.
49. Stein F, Siegel MW. Naviculocapitate fracture syndrome. A case report: new thoughts on the mechanism of injury. J Bone Joint Surg Am. 1969;51(2):391–5.
50. Adler JB, Shaftan GW. Fractures of the capitate. J Bone Joint Surg Am. 1962;44-A:1537–47.
51. Rico AA, Holguin PH, Martin JG. Pseudarthrosis of the capitate. J Hand Surg Br. 1999;24(3):382–4.
52. Kimmel RB, O'Brien ET. Surgical treatment of avascular necrosis of the proximal pole of the capitate—case report. J Hand Surg Am. 1982;7(3):284–6.
53. Lowry Jr WE, Cord SA. Traumatic avascular necrosis of the capitate bone-case report. J Hand Surg Am. 1981;6(3):245–8.
54. David TS, Zemel NP, Mathews PV. Symptomatic, partial union of the hook of the hamate fracture in athletes. Am J Sports Med. 2003;31(1):106–11.
55. Fredericson M, Kim BJ, Date ES, McAdams TR. Injury to the deep motor branch of the ulnar nerve during hook of hamate excision. Orthopedics. 2006;29(5):456–8.
56. Bishop AT, Beckenbaugh RD. Fracture of the hamate hook. J Hand Surg Am. 1988;13(1):135–9.
57. Demirkan F, Calandruccio JH, Diangelo D. Biomechanical evaluation of flexor tendon function after hamate hook excision. J Hand Surg Am. 2003;28(1):138–43.
58. Scheufler O, Andresen R, Radmer S, Erdmann D, Exner K, Germann G. Hook of hamate fractures: critical evaluation of different therapeutic procedures. Plast Reconstr Surg. 2005;115(2):488–97.
59. Scheufler O, Radmer S, Erdmann D, Germann G, Pierer G, Andresen R. Therapeutic alternatives in nonunion of hamate hook fractures: personal experience in 8 patients and review of literature. Ann Plast Surg. 2005;55(2):149–54.

Secondary Procedures and Surgical Treatment of Distal Humerus Fractures

10

Rick F. Papandrea

Abstract

Every surgeon treating distal humeral fractures understands that perfection is usually an unobtainable goal. Sound surgical treatment with modern implants does usually render a functional and painless elbow, but complications do occur in properly treated distal humeral fractures. Fixation can fail, articular cartilage can be damaged beyond its ability to heal, and non-unions occur for mechanical and biological reasons. Understanding indications for revising distal humeral fracture treatment requires knowledge of extensile exposures to the elbow and current implant technology. Distal humeral articular surfaces that can not be reconstructed can now be partially or totally resurfaced, obviating the need for a salvage with a total elbow implant. Some distal humeral revisions are best treated with a linked total elbow implant. When considering revising a distal humeral fracture fixation, it is imperative to align patient and surgeon expectations and ensure both parties understand what potential complications can occur during any revision.

Keywords

Distal • Humerus • Fracture • Nonunion • Necrosis • Hemiarthroplasty

Key Points

- Early recognition of problems will allow for more options and optimize outcome.
- CT scanning early after the primary procedure will direct the need for and type of reoperation.
- Infection needs to be ruled out in nonunion and failed fixation.
- Monitor the ulnar nerve: tardy compression/neuropathy may cause atypical problems in the post-op period. Never make assumptions about the location of the ulnar nerve intraoperatively.
- Preserve native cartilage and joint whenever possible.
- Be prepared to make the definitive reconstruction decision intraoperatively.
- Off-label use of implants currently available may permit partial resurfacing of an irreparable portion of the joint, obviating the need for a total elbow replacement.
- If fixation is too tenuous to allow for some early motion, it probably is not rigid enough for success.
- Respect the soft tissue envelope, be prepared for potential wound breakdown.
- Align patient and surgeon expectations preoperatively.

R.F. Papandrea, MD (✉)
Partner, Orthopaedic Associates of WI,
1111 Delafield Street, Suite 120, Waukesha, WI 53188, USA
e-mail: rick@papandrea.net

S.F.M. Duncan (ed.), *Reoperative Hand Surgery*,
DOI 10.1007/978-1-4614-2373-7_10, © Springer Science+Business Media, LLC 2012

Introduction

Relatively few distal humerus fractures in adults are straightforward. Fortunately, by following current recommendations and using the appropriate implants, most of these injuries will not prevent return to function [1–4]. It is important for the patient and surgeon to be aligned in their goals and expectations after any injury. Even after a perfectly executed ORIF of a distal humerus, some loss of motion is typical and hardware complications are not unusual [2, 4].

Soft tissue problems early in the postoperative period may be from dehiscence or from necrosis, especially in the presence of the multiply operated elbow. Hematoma and seroma formation are common early problems that are usually readily managed by observation, occasionally aspiration, and rarely surgical debridement. If the wound edges are threatened due to poor vascularity in the presence of a pressure producing hematoma or seroma, surgical I&D should be considered to decompress the wound and allow for a tension-free closure. If a wound dehisces early, the cause needs to be identified. Too early or aggressive range of motion may cause problems, especially if the closure was not secure enough. Infection needs to be ruled out. At times, the pressure from a seroma or hematoma may be enough to dehisce a wound. Judicious use of tacking sutures from the skin flap to the fascia (the surgeon must be cautious to avoid cutaneous nerves with these sutures) can limit potential space for these fluid collections to occur. Postoperative drains can be useful to limit hematoma formation as well. Should necrosis of the surgical envelope ensue, care should include a surgeon skilled in multiple modalities of treatment including negative pressure/sponge dressings, local flaps, pedicle flaps, and even the rarely needed free flaps. Skin coverage procedures will not be covered further, as they are not specific to distal humerus fractures, but rather the principles apply to any elbow soft tissue problem.

Limitation of motion is expected, at least temporarily, with some potential for permanent limitations after distal humerus fracture fixation [2–5]. In spite of this, there should be the ability for some motion early, after the soft tissue equilibrates. Typically, rotation is least painful and restricted, but even flexion/extension should be comfortable in the middle of the available arc of motion. Lack of any comfortable motion, especially if combined with mechanical symptoms, may indicate a problem with an elbow after ORIF.

An insufficiently fixed fracture may completely fail, or there may be failure of individual fragments that were not adequately secured [6]. This is usually clear on radiographic examination. Early radiographic follow-up may also demonstrate that intra-articular fragments were not aligned in the optimum position. Clinical progression is usually delayed in this subset of patients. CT scans can be utilized in these situations to identify, confirm, or delineate the problem. Three-dimensional studies add another level of detail that may be indispensible, especially when planning the reconstruction.

When initial fixation is inadequate, revision may be considered. If the fragments are still displaced, but there is adequate bone for revision, maintaining the native cartilage and joint is preferred. If the articular surface is not reconstructible, it may be resurfaced. If only a portion is not reconstructable, partial resurfacing may be considered, depending on the location and the bone support in the area of question.

Intra-articular distal humerus fractures may heal the articular component, but go on to nonunion of the supracondylar region. In this situation, the joint is not in jeopardy. Revision or salvage is possible in this situation. If there is adequate bone, revision with bone grafting is the treatment of choice in the younger and/or more active patient. If the bone loss is significant, or the patient is frail, low demand, and of an advanced age, total elbow arthroplasty (TEA) can be considered [7].

When problems do occur after ORIF of a distal humerus, reoperation is often necessary to optimize outcome. The decision to revise a distal humerus fracture is one that should not be taken lightly. There are indeed times that the risks do not outweigh the possible benefits. The younger the patient, the more important articular alignment becomes, but there are some joints that cannot be made perfect. This is where the "art" of medicine and surgery must be combined with the science. No text can categorically state that a revision surgery will work, but there can be clear times where it makes sense to proceed with a revision.

When the decision to revise a distal humerus fracture is made, it should be planned with contingencies thought out. The preferred order of revision should be reconstruction, partial replacement, and lastly complete resurfacing. This revision ladder can be carried out intraoperatively. The revising surgeon should plan for a preferred method of reconstruction, but have contingencies planned such that the algorithm can be followed intraoperatively. This requires that the treating surgeon has the appropriate alternative equipment and implants available. If these modes of revision fail, or are not possible, salvage may need to be considered. Salvage may consist of total prosthetic replacement, interposition arthroplasty, total allograft replacement, or fusion. Total replacement for the posttraumatic elbow is carried out much like the osteoarthritic or rheumatoid elbow [8–10]. Interposition is usually reserved for patients deemed too young for a total elbow; its unpredictability has continued to limit any widespread acceptance for even salvage situations [11, 12]. Total allograft replacement has demonstrated a high complication rate and had limited success in few centers [13]. Fusion is the ultimate salvage and has been described as too debilitating to utilize. There is little literature to document outcomes, although a recent report in 14 patients demonstrates it does have utility [14, 15]. This chapter will only cover salvage of nonunion with a total elbow prosthetic replacement, as well as the entire reconstructive ladder.

Indications

- Failed fixation with impending nonunion
- Impending or established malunion (articular, extra-articular, or combined)
- Established nonunion

Contraindications

Absolute
- Infection

Relative
- Low demand patient with acceptable function
- Poor soft tissue envelope
- Bone loss
- Damage to proximal radius/ulna

Reconstruction is usually possible after a failed initial attempt at ORIF of the distal humerus. Short of the rare asymptomatic (usually low demand) patient, the failed distal humerus fracture should be reconstructed, unless it is infected. The first step is recognition of the problem as early as possible. It is imperative that frequent radiographic studies are obtained in the healing phase of the injury. Poor fixation will not get better with time, and unless healing has already stabilized the fracture fragments to some degree, hardware failure is a harbinger of trouble. If radiographs demonstrate loose hardware, or a significant shift in position of the fracture fragments, consideration for revision should be discussed between patient and surgeon. Likewise, if articular alignment is not ideal, arthrosis will ensue. Unfortunately, there is no solid science to guide one as the acceptable articular displacement. Clinical experience has shown that the younger the patient, the more critical articular alignment becomes.

The articular reconstruction should be scrutinized, and if more detailed assessment is necessary, a CT scan with 3D reconstructions should be obtained. Utilizing open source software, the treating physician can use a standard 2D CT in one plane to create a 3D reconstruction after the initial study [16]. When early follow-up reveals the congruity of the articular surface is suboptimal, revision of the alignment needs to be considered. Given the timing, the supracondylar portions of the elbow are typically not healed. Therefore, the reconstruction may involve revising all components of the fracture. Isolated intra-articular fractures (without supracondylar involvement) typically involve the capitellum, with the possibility of extension into the trochlea. Inadequate exposure combined with inadequate fixation often leads to incongruity of theses fractures. Distal humerus fractures in adults most often include intra-articular extension of varying degrees.

When internal fixation of the distal humerus fails, there are few indications to forgo revision. If radiographic follow-up demonstrates failure and yet the patient is functioning adequately and is comfortable, this would be one of the few times observation may be in order. When this is seen clinically, it is usually in a frail elderly patient receiving significant assistance for other medical reasons.

If the articular surface cannot be adequately reconstructed, a portion or the entire distal humerus may be resurfaced. These cases usually are those in which the fracture is a low supracondylar, shear capitellar/trochlea, or comminuted capitellar fracture. These injuries may not involve the supracondylar region, or if they do, it may heal by the time the patient needs to have the resurfacing. At times, initial fixation is adequate, but the damage to the subchondral surface and articular cartilage was so severe that incongruity or avascular necrosis results.

Supracondylar fractures of the elbow may go on to heal the intra-articular component, but fail to heal at the metaphyseal-diaphyseal junction. It is rare to develop a nonunion in this region, while the hardware remains stable. This unusual situation will not be covered in this chapter, but at times is amenable to bone grafting with or without other forms of bone stimulation.

When fixation fails only at the supracondylar region, then the choices for reconstruction are revision fixation or arthroplasty. In this case, the joint surface is adequate and therefore hemiarthroplasty does not offer much benefit, other than an additional mode of fixation of the much-needed columns and epicondyles. Linked TEA in this situation obviates the need for the epicondyles and the columns distal to the typical nonunion. A linked arthroplasty allows for the entire ununited fragment to be removed and discarded. The gap created allows for the implantation of the prosthesis with the triceps still attached [7, 17].

When planning to revise a distal humerus fracture, one needs to consider the contraindications to proceeding in a single stage to revision. The cause for failure should be determined and the possibility of infection needs to be ruled out. If infection is known or suspected, staged treatment should follow, with eradication of the infection taking precedence over reconstruction of the skeletal deformity.

A well-done revision will fail if covered in a troubled soft tissue envelope. The preoperative evaluation needs to consider the soft tissue envelope and whether it can sustain the trauma of another surgical intervention. If there were wound healing problems during the early postoperative period on the index surgery, or if at the time of the revision, the soft tissue has not healed, a surgeon comfortable in dealing with multiple forms of treatment needs to be involved. Soft tissue coverage is beyond the scope of this chapter, but the surgeon has to be capable of utilizing multiple modalities of soft tissue coverage techniques including negative pressure sponges, local and pedicled flaps, and even free flaps.

A relative contraindication is bone loss. Structural bone loss will prevent successful reconstruction regardless of which type is attempted. As long as the bone loss is recognized preoperatively, the patient and surgeon can agree on the solution chosen to accommodate for the loss. Support from autologous or allograft bone may be considered if the articular surface can be reconstructed. If implants are being utilized to resurface the distal humerus, support must be provided from native bone, or structural bone graft, to prevent loosening.

Preoperative History and Considerations

Details of the injury, with attention to ensure no concomitant injuries were missed, should be collected. Focus is on the elbow, but it is imperative to ensure the ipsilateral shoulder and wrist are not involved and that no other injuries were overlooked. The extent of the injury at the elbow needs to be appreciated. The primary injury will be obvious, but secondary injury at the radial head or neck, or the olecranon (especially the coronoid) cannot be neglected.

Operative notes from the previous surgery should be reviewed and a preoperative work-up should ensure there is no indolent infection.

Based on operative note and physical exam, the location of the ulnar nerve should be ascertained. Even when both the note and exam are corroborative, one should never completely assume the nerve is located as expected. Previous operative approaches should be considered and the details of any hardware utilized should be obtained. This will allow for the assurance that the proper equipment is available to remove the previously placed hardware. Preparations should always be made for the initial failure of hardware removal. There should be a preoperative plan to deal with stripped, broken, or stuck hardware, as well as retained cement. This should be communicated to the patient, so there is no surprise should some hardware be left in situ due to breakage or the inability to remove it without severe collateral damage.

Physical exam should not only attempt to identify the ulnar nerve, but the function of it should be documented by examination of both motor and sensory ability. While most ulnar nerve injuries are obvious and occur with the original injury or surgery, at times they are not well documented. An associated nerve deficit may not be significant enough even for the patient to specify as there may be a more significant problem dominating the clinical picture. For both medical-legal reasons and to align patient–physician expectations, preexisting nerve injuries need to be identified and explained to the patient. Although nerve deficit is often associated with the ulnar nerve, the radial and median nerve should be examined, ensuring that the median nerve exam includes the anterior interosseus nerve.

The arc of motion needs to be carefully examined and measured. While absolute range of motion in both flexion/extension and supination/pronation is important, attention needs to be paid to the quality of pain in motion. Crepitus and pain during mid-arc motion, especially with the joint loaded, may indicate intra-articular displacement or penetration of hardware. Pain at end arc of motion may indicate hardware or displaced bone in the olecranon or coronoid fossae.

The most critical preoperative step is to align expectations between physician and patient. There must be understanding of what the patient perceives as his or her disability and what the surgeon feels can be corrected. Often, there are multiple aspects of the problem, such as decreased range of motion, pain, weakness, instability, and cosmesis. Often, some of these may be improved with surgical intervention; but it is unlikely that the elbow will be returned to normal. Therefore, it is important that the patient and surgeon are clear in their expectations as to the surgery performed, the expected postoperative course, the possible complications, and the ultimate long-term outcome.

Operative Approach

Pearls for Operative Approach: Equipment

Consideration should be made to have access to the following:

- Structural bone graft
  - Autograft
  - Allograft
- Bone-stimulating substances
  - Demineralized bone matrix
  - Platelet gel
  - Osteoinductive proteins
- Appropriate fixations devices
  - Screw trajectory to fix fragments in question
  - Cerclage wires
    - Monofilament wires are less expensive
    - Multifilament wires may generate more debris if they break
  - Intraoperative imaging
    - Fluroscopic equipment that will allow adequate definition and access
  - Arthroplasty implants
    - Use is often off-label

- The patient should be notified of off-label use
- Industry representatives are often unable to give meaningful intraoperative advice on use for off-label indications
- The surgeon should be prepared to implant in a nonstandard fashion with little help from technique guides and industry representatives

Instruments for manipulating and stabilizing small articular fragments
- Dental picks
- Threaded k-wires
- Small gauge wire

Surgical Exposure

Once an operative plan is determined, the operative approach can be decided. The surgeon should consider previous exposures, but utilize additional ones as needed. A distinction can be made between the skin or superficial approach and the deep, or muscular approach.

The superficial approach, or skin incision, can be directly over the deep approach, which is usually posterior (for olecranon osteotomy), sometimes lateral (for isolated capitellar fractures), and rarely medial (for concomitant ulnar nerve decompression). Previous incisions may be incorporated into an extended incision for a universal deep posterior approach (Case 10.2). Unless there is a need to access the biceps tendon, there is typically never a reason to make an anterior skin incision or deep anterior incision. The coronoid, median nerve, and brachial artery usually don't need to be addressed, but if they do, a medial deep approach is most appropriate. Although the coronoid can be accessed from lateral if the radial head is removed, or posterior with olecranon osteotomy and joint subluxation.

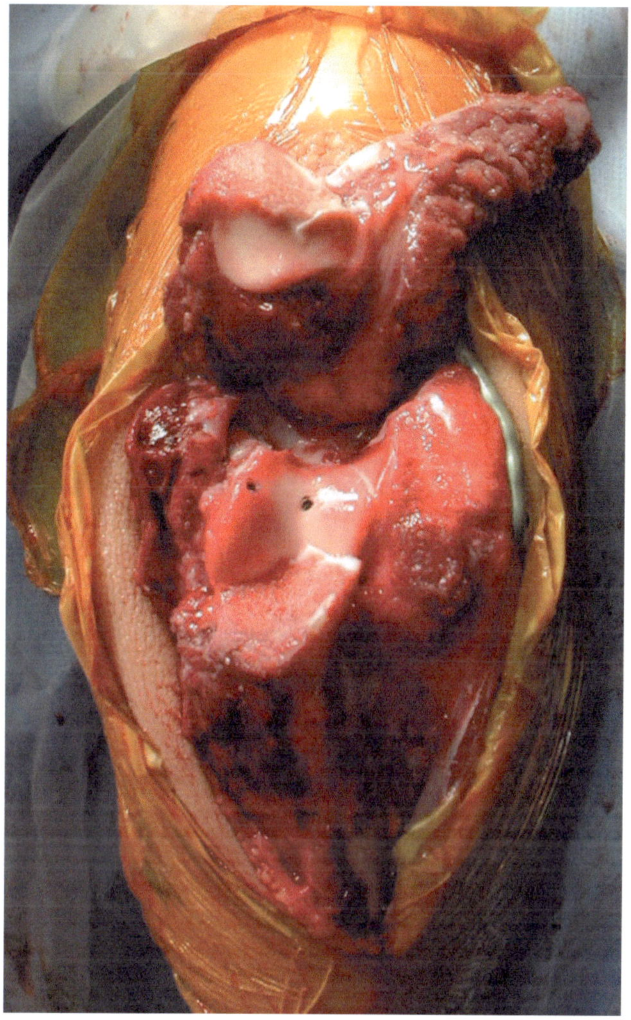

Fig. 10.1 The anconeus may be left attached to the olecranon tip when an osteotomy is done. Note the access to the distal humerus for fixation, and the lack of soft tissue obscuring visualization at the lateral joint due to the rotation of the anconeus proximal

Olecranon Osteotomy

Access to the entire distal humerus is usually gained by an intra-articular olecranon osteotomy. The TRAP approach has been described for treatment of intra-articular distal humerus fractures [18]. This involves a complete release of the soft tissue attachments of the triceps with the anconeus. While it can allow sufficient access for an experienced surgeon to repair a distal humerus fracture, this author does not find the visualization sufficient for revision situations.

If the anconeus is still intact, and an olecranon osteotomy is utilized, the anconeus can be dissected from distal to proximal, released off the posterior capitellum, and kept in continuity with the olecranon and the triceps (Fig. 10.1). Since the neurovascular pedicle to the anconeus goes through the triceps, it is kept intact. Steinmann has described this as the AFT approach [19]. The alternative to taking the aconeus with the olecranon is to transect it, which will devascularize it. If a previous olecranon osteotomy was done at the index surgery and the aconeus was transected, the tissue will have already undergone atrophy and there will be a loss of lateral soft tissue.

Extra-articular Nonunion

In some cases, the articular surface is anatomically aligned, but the extra-articular portion has developed a nonunion (Fig. 10.2). In this situation, if the patient is frail and low demand, and attempts at repeat ORIF are deemed high risk of failure, a TEA is a viable option. This is covered below.

If the need for revision is only due to a nonunion of the extra-articular portion of a distal humerus fracture, this is

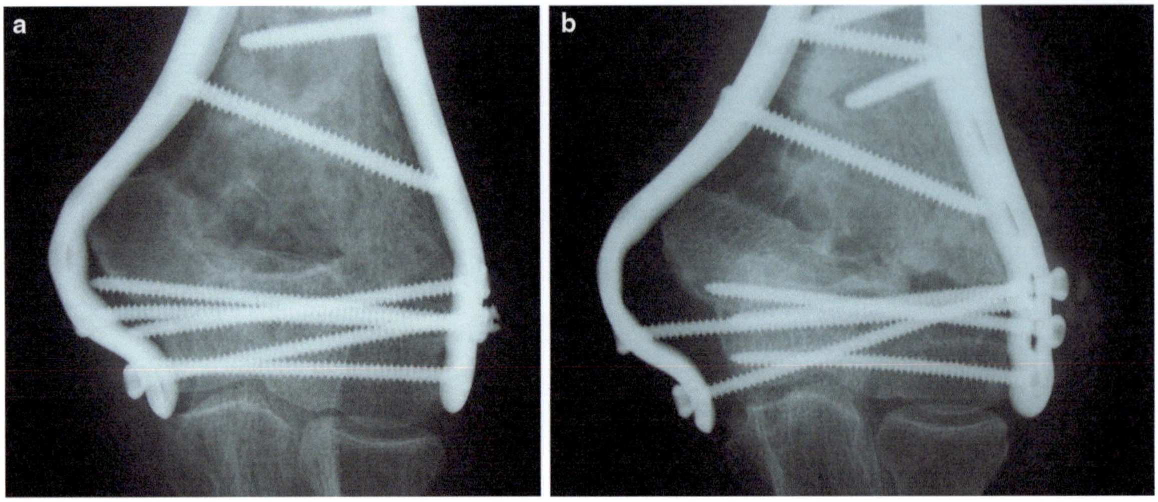

Fig. 10.2 (**a**) This extra-articular fracture was rigidly fixed in an elderly smoking patient (**b**) despite adequate appearing fixation, the fracture went on to an extra-articular nonunion

most commonly at the diaphyseal–metaphyseal junction. Depending on the timing of the revision, and the original approach, the previous olecranon osteotomy should be evaluated for healing.

If the osteotomy is not yet healed, yet access can be gained to the nonunion without repeating the olecranon osteotomy, the hardware for the olecranon can be left in place. Similarly, if the access of the osteotomy is not needed, and the olecranon has healed, the hardware may be removed if it is prominent. If there is any doubt about maturity of the union at the osteotomy, it should be left alone and the hardware should not be taken out an earlier than 6 months and only then if it is irritating the soft tissues. The decision to revise an extra-articular nonunion without an olecranon osteotomy is best left intraoperatively. Once the ulnar nerve is safely identified, access on either side of the triceps can be gained to the diaphyseal–metaphyseal juncture. If the initial fixation appears inadequate, and there is sufficient bone on the distal fragment, it is reasonable to revise with rigid fixation without repeating the olecranon osteotomy.

Repeating the olecranon osteotomy, regardless of whether or not it has healed, may be necessary. Reflecting the triceps proximal can allow better visualization. This can be especially important during a revision, since one may have to avoid previous screw placement tracts. If the nonunion is quite distal, and rigid fixation in the fracture fragment requires multiple long screws into the humeral trochlea, an osteotomy allows better visualization of the trochlea, to ensure that there is no penetration of the joint surface.

An attempt should be made to determine the reason for nonunion prior to revision. Infection needs to be considered; a negative laboratory evaluation or aspiration does not exclude infection. If it is felt that there is a nonunion due to inadequate fixation and the patient is otherwise healthy, then repeat fixation should be carried out. The need for bone grafting is a decision left to the surgeon. The cause for the nonunion should guide this decision. If there is adequate bone, but fixation was inadequate, rigid fixation with compression may be all that is necessary. This is especially true if the nonunion is hypertrophic. If there is poor biology, an atrophic nonunion, or the patient is a smoker, bone grafting should be utilized. While autologous bone is considered by many to be the "gold standard," the field of orthobiologics continues to advance at a rapid pace. Alternative bone grafting materials may be considered based on patient and surgeon preference or experience.

When there is structural bone loss at the diaphyseal-metaphyseal junction, a viable alternative to grafting the bone loss back to anatomic length is to shorten the humerus at the nonunion site. O'Driscoll et al. have described this method for acute treatment of highly comminuted fractures [1]. Because the shortening osteotomy goes through the olecranon and coronoid fossae, adjustments to the positioning of the distal humerus need to be made to allow flexion and extension of the elbow. The ununited fragment should be translated forward, to compensate for the lack of a coronoid and radial head fossa. In translating forward, flexion should be possible without bony impingement. In translating the distal humeral fragment anterior, the distal humeral shaft will now impinge on the olecranon tip with extension. Removal of posterior bone from the distal humeral shaft compensates for this and allows for improved extension (Fig. 10.3).

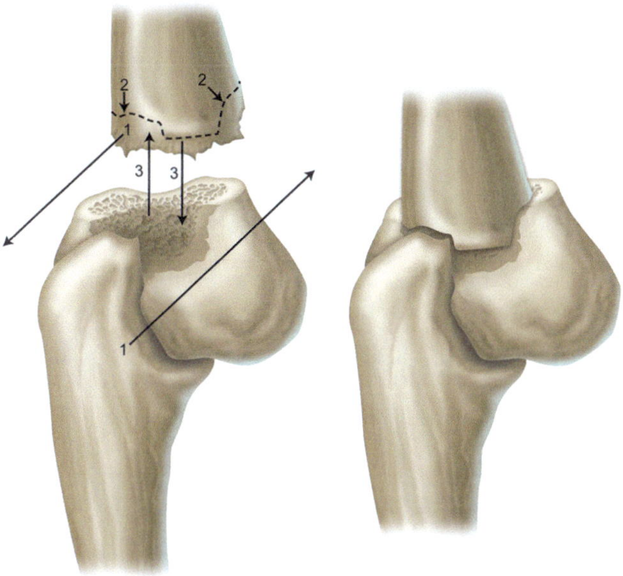

Fig. 10.3 Shortening osteotomy: (1) Anterior translation of the distal humerus relative to the shaft; (2) removal of a portion of the distal humerus to allow for shortening and for fit to the distal humerus in a translated position; (3) interfacing the two pieces together

Intra-articular Nonunion or Malunion (Case 10.1)

The decision to revise the distal humeral articular surface or partially resurface the joint or resurface the entire articular surface with a hemiarthroplasty is one that can be completed during the surgery if the patient and surgeon are prepared.

Adequate imaging preoperatively should give some idea of the joint derangement present (Case 10.1a–f). If the patient is young and active, every attempt should be made to reconstruct the distal humeral articular surface [20]. There are times that despite the desire of patient and surgeon, the damage is too severe to allow for successful reconstruction. If the surgeon and patient have considered this preoperatively, implants can be available for resurfacing of part or the whole distal humerus. At this time, this is accomplished with the off-label use (in the United States) of currently available implants.

Once exposure is adequate to examine the articular surface (Case 10.1g, h); the final decision can be made as to the reconstruction. If the articular surface is improperly aligned, it is quite possibly not healed. In these cases, the extra-articular component is often not healed as well.

The articular surface can be realigned only after the articular fragments are carefully released. This needs to be done with the remaining soft tissue attachments kept intact to maintain blood supply, and while protecting the articular cartilage. Dental picks and small curettes can be helpful to tease the fragments apart (Case 10.1i).

Once the articular surface has been disassembled, it can be repaired provisionally with smooth k-wires (Case 10.1j). At this time, any structurally significant bone loss needs to be assessed. If the bone loss is entirely extra-articular, the distal humerus may be shortened (see previous section on extra-articular nonunions and Fig. 10.3). If there is a focal area of bone loss, structural or nonstructural grafting can be considered. There is no literature to guide the surgeon as to the best decision, but if there is less than 50% native extra-articular bone present, consideration to shortening should be made; likewise, if there is more than 50% of the native structure present for support, grafting is a reasonable option. The best source of graft is not proven, although autograft is considered by many to be the "gold standard." If the distal articular fragments are deemed salvageable, yet there is little bone in them for fixation, consideration to supporting these fragments with structural graft should be made.

Once the articular surface has been provisionally reconstructed with bone graft, the selection of implants should be made. While it is critical for the surgeon to choose the necessary options preoperatively, the final decision is made at this time. The surgeon needs to understand the fixation options available prior to surgery. The length and location of the plates as well as the trajectory and locking ability of the screws are all important. The surgeon needs to choose a system that is familiar as well as flexible enough to deal with contingencies during fixation.

Fixation of the fracture fragment must be rigid. Failure is likely to recur if it is not and the risk of repeat operation will be for nothing if the articular reconstruction cannot be supported appropriately. While rigid fixation is imperative, healing depends on the viability of the fracture fragments. There must be a balance between enough implant to support the bone and adequate biologic viability to prevent avascular necrosis of the fragment.

If the articular fragments cannot be reconstructed, or are felt to be nonviable, replacement of the damaged articular surface should be considered. This can be either partial or complete resurfacing or replacement of the distal humerus.

Partial Resurfacing for Unreconstructable Articular Defects

If only a portion of the articular surface is damaged, there are commercially available implants that can resurface a portion or the entire capitellum, as well as a portion of the trochlea (see Table 10.1). These implants, if available in the United States, are off-label for the distal humerus as a hemiarthroplasty. All available implants require support from the distal humeral bone. If there is loss of a column or significant subchondral bone, it is unlikely that an implant used for partial resurfacing will be successful. If bone grafting is required to

Table 10.1 Implants available to resurface part of the distal humerus

Implant	Manufacturer	Available in US	FDA use as described in text	Surfaces applicable to	Fixation method
UNI-Elbow Radio Capitellum	Small Bone Innovations	Yes	Off-label	Entire capitellum	Press fit/cement
Lateral Elbow Replacement	Biomet	No	NA	Entire capitellum, proximal articulating surface of radial head	Press fit
Hemicap	Arthrosurface	Yes	Off-label	Partial capitellum, partial trochlea	Morse taper into titanium screw
Sorbie-Questor	Wright Medical	Yes	Off-label	Distal humerus	Cement
Latitude	Tornier	Yes (hemi option requires custom-ordered spool)	Off-label	Distal humerus (this device replaces, not resurfaces the distal humerus)	Cement

Note that none are available as FDA-approved devices in the United States. Their use is thus "off-label"

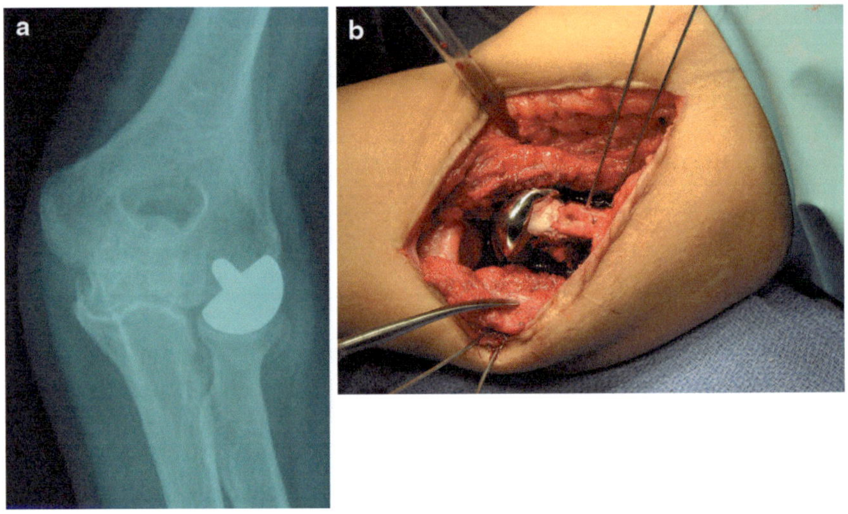

Fig. 10.4 (**a**) Lateral elbow replacement (LRE) capitellar component as a hemiarthroplasty (radiograph courtesy of Joe Pooley). (**b**) Capitellar component of the Small Bone Innovations (SBi) lateral elbow replacement implanted through a lateral approach and epicondylar osteotomy

support the entire partial resurfacing implant, its use should be abandoned. If there is a persistent fracture of the column, fixation can be carried out at the time of implantation. So long as the implant is stable in the native bone, and the fracture heals, the presence of the fracture should not change the outcome of the partial resurfacing.

If it is known prior to surgery that only the capitellum is going to be repaired or replaced, the alternative exposure described below may be utilized. If the decision is made intraoperatively, and an olecranon osteotomy has already been utilized, this exposure is often adequate.

Once it is deemed that a partial resurfacing of the distal humerus is appropriate, any column fractures should be rigidly fixed. If initial surgery was ORIF and the fracture has healed, but articular damage remains, the hardware may be removed.

At the current time, there are three different devices available that can be used to partially resurface the distal humerus. The Small Bone Innovations (SBi) lateral elbow replacement and Pooley device (Biomet—not available in the United States) are similar in that they both are designed to resurface the entire radiocapitellar articulation (Fig. 10.4). Both devices resurface the entire capitellum and are fixed by a central stem. Since the radial head is left in situ, access to the capitellum will most likely be limited and attention must be directed to gaining access for the implant to be utilized. Since use as a hemiarthroplasty is off-label, the technique may need to be modified from that of the manufacturers' recommendations. If access is limited with an olecranon osteotomy, a lateral epicondylar osteotomy can be combined to provide full access (see below—Alternative 1 and Fig. 10.10).

The HemiCap by Arthrosurface has some components that can be utilized for partial distal humerus replacement (Fig. 10.5). The particular implants are designed and approved for use in the foot (first metatarsal head) and knee. A threaded titanium modular central peg supports the device. The articular device designed for the distal first metacarpal head is convex with varying geometries. This can be utilized to resurface focal defects on the capitellum. Likewise, the femoral component of the patellar-femoral device may be

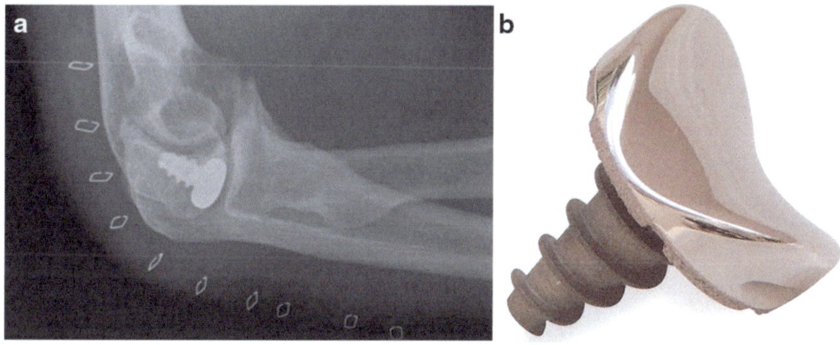

Fig. 10.5 (**a**) Hemicap first metatarsal implant implanted in a capitellar defect (radiograph courtesy of Todd Olsen, MD). (**b**) Arthrosurface Hemicap device for the femoral trochlea. Depending on geometry, this implant may reapproximate portions of the humeral trochlea

utilized to cover some isolated trochlear defects. These devices are not specifically designed to match distal humerus anatomy; the likelihood of a perfect match is unknown. Therefore, every effort should be made to preoperatively plan to determine proper match of the implant to the defect. If there is any uncertainty about the ability to fit the implant appropriately, a backup plan should be ready. The most appropriate backup plan is to have a hemiarthroplasty available (see below).

Hemiarthroplasty (Case 10.2)

If a distal humerus revision is deemed necessary, and the articular surface cannot be reconstructed, a distal humerus hemiarthroplasty may be indicated. Intact columns are not an absolute requirement for a hemiarthroplasty. If the columns are not intact, they must be reconstructable. Both columns must be able to support the hemiarthroplasty to prevent premature loosening.

While there are other options for exposure, this author's preferred technique is an olecranon osteotomy with the anconeus in continuity (the AFT approach—see Fig. 10.1). The triceps insertion on the olecranon is preserved. Postoperative stability is typically near normal, as the collateral ligaments are left intact. With experience, hemiarthroplasty can also be performed via an epicondylar osteotomy (medial or lateral), but it is not recommended that this be attempted until at least several cases are successfully completed with an olecranon osteotomy. Another alternative approach is to release the triceps, but this also requires release of the collaterals. Both these approaches require more extensive soft tissue releases than a simple olecranon osteotomy. Therefore, more restrictions during healing to prevent instability are required. The risk of triceps weakness or failure is introduced, whereas with an osteotomy, it is not a possibility. If an osteotomy is utilized, the collaterals can be kept intact, eliminating the need to protect the reconstructed elbow from varus or valgus stress.

An olecranon osteotomy is often already present in a failed distal humerus case. Repeat olecranon osteotomy or take down of healing osteotomy does not appear to impede healing after hemiarthroplasty.

As with the partial resurfacing, use of a device to resurface the distal humerus is off-label, as the devices available are FDA-approved for use as a total elbow replacement. Because of this, the technique described for placement of the hemiarthroplasty typically has to be varied for implantation via a transolecranon osteotomy.

There are currently two total elbow systems that can be utilized for distal humeral hemiarthroplasty. A requisite of any system for use as a hemiarthroplasty includes an anatomic articular design to allow appropriate congruency with the native proximal radius and ulna. The other design parameter that should be met for a distal humeral component is that there be an inherent restriction to posterior translation and rotation of the component. There are currently two designs available worldwide that this author is aware of that fit both of these categories. There have been other reports of different prosthetic elbows used as hemiarthroplasties, but neither is anatomic in its articular design [21, 22].

The Sorbie-Questor by Wright Medical is a stemmed, nonflanged component. It provides resistance to posterior forces and rotation by cupping the distal humerus (Fig. 10.6). Loss of this skeletal support (without repair or reconstruction) will cause increased stress on the implant, with probable early loosening. This device comes in three sizes each for left and right.

The Sorbie-Questor humeral instrumentation is designed for use with the elbow dislocated. As described above, there are advantages to implantation through an olecranon osteotomy. The options for implantation for reconstruction are to prepare the distal humerus "free hand" or modify the use of the instrumentation. The humeral cutting guide is positioned based on the center of rotation of the distal humerus. It uses an intramedullary guide as well. Depending on the anatomy, some of the landmarks for referencing the center of rotation may be missing or altered. Because of the intramedullary

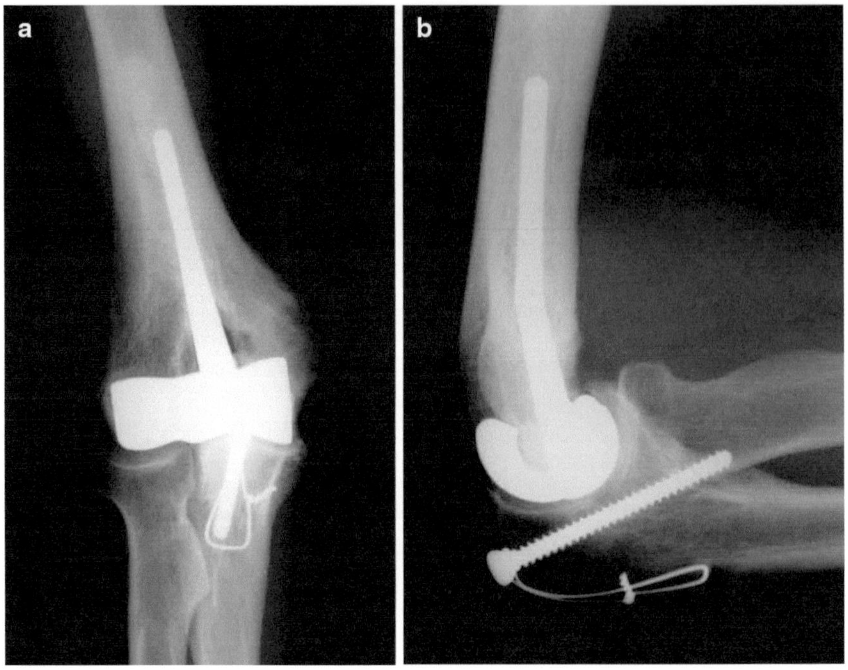

Fig. 10.6 The humeral component of the Sorbie-Questor Total Elbow System designed by Charles Sorbie and Marketed by Wright Medical. It is FDA-approved for use as a total elbow. Use as depicted is off-label in the United States. (**a**) AP radiograph: note the anatomic congruity with the native proximal ulna and radius. (**b**) Lateral radiograph: while there is no flange, rotational and translational forces are resisted by the distal portion of the device which "cups" the distal humeral bone from medial to lateral

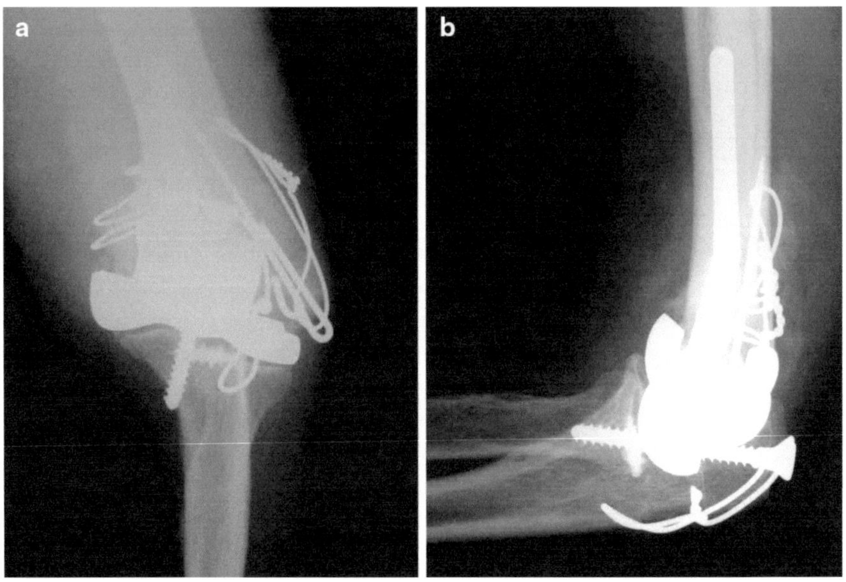

Fig. 10.7 Hemiarthroplasty with wire fixation of lateral column and medial epicondyle. The implant has gained support from the healed columns. Note: this is not the same patient as Case 10.2. This example is a hemiarthroplasty utilized for initial treatment of a distal humerus fracture (**a**) AP radiograph (**b**) lateral radiograph

guide, only one point of the center of rotation is necessary to align the guide, so long as the intramedullary portion of the guide is used (Case 10.2f, g).

If a chevron osteotomy is used, the proximal portion of the ulnar shaft may impinge on the guide. Because of this, a transverse osteotomy is recommended to allow the cutting guide to align properly with the collaterals still intact (Case 10.2g).

If the columns are fractured, they need to be stabilized. Since the intramedullary portion of the implant will provide some support, the fixation need not be as rigid as a plate and screws. While a plate may be used, one must be careful to avoid crossing the IM canal with hardware that will preclude placement of the hemiarthroplasty device. A simple technique is to utilize k-wires and tension bands (Fig. 10.7). Suture or wire may be used for the tension band. The author prefers wire, as it can be further tightened after initial fixation and does not tend to stretch or loosen as suture may. Regardless of the fixation method, the preliminary fixation should be done with the trial implant in place, to ensure that alignment is proper and hardware will not prevent the final implant from insertion.

If the columns are damaged or missing, one has to be prepared to bone graft to provide support for the implant (Case 10.2c, h). The graft may be held with plates and screws or wires. Wires are lower profile, highly variable in placement, and more cost-effective than plates and screws (Case 10.2i–l).

Once the distal humerus bone has been prepared and repaired or replaced as needed, the trial device can be utilized to ensure the mechanics to the elbow have been restored. With the device in place, the elbow should be able to go through a near normal range of motion. If there was significant stiffness preoperative, the anterior capsule may be removed from the humeral shaft without need for additional exposure. The centralized stem of the Sorbie-Questor device may limit flexion due to coronoid impingement. This occurs at approximately 125°. While some coronoid may be removed to allow for increased flexion, stability should not be sacrificed and a functional arc of motion will be obtained even if this impingement occurs.

The other device amenable for use as a hemiarthroplasty is the Tornier Latitude total elbow system. The humeral component has a nonanatomic "spool" that mounts on the humeral stem and articulates with the ulnar and radial components [23]. While this off the shelf set-up is not appropriate for use as a hemiarthroplasty, a custom spool may be ordered. This custom spool is anatomic in shape and articulates appropriately with the native ulna and radius (Fig. 10.8). This device gains posterior and rotational support with a flange. This must be bone-grafted during insertion. The body is wider (there are two columns for distal support) creating a fenestration. This prevents problems with the coronoid or olecranon impinging with motion. Reconstruction of the columns may be more difficult because the design places the supports at the medial and lateral columns. The major potential advantage of the Latitude design is the ability to convert to a total elbow without removing the cemented humeral stem. The custom spool may be removed, as it is modular, and a standard spool applied at a later time, if and when wear at the proximal radius and ulna necessitates revision to a total elbow.

Once trial implantation demonstrates proper alignment and length, the canal should be prepared for cementing and final device implantation. Reconstruction of the distal humerus with a hemiarthroplasty is typically done in active patients. The goal is to restore motion and eliminate or decrease pain. The length of time that a hemiarthroplasty will last is currently unknown, although there is a case report of a custom implant with good function at 20 years [24]. Implantation should be performed to allow for the easiest revision possible, while using the most durable techniques available. The intramedullary canal should be irrigated, cleaned, and dried. A cement restrictor should be used to prevent excess cement from going proximal and to allow for pressurization of the cement.

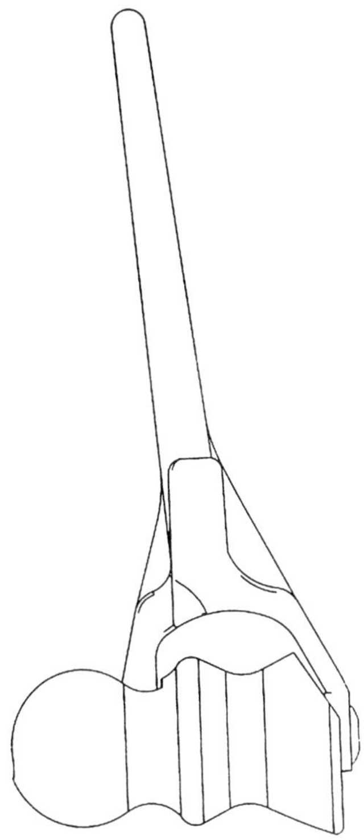

Fig. 10.8 Custom anatomic spool on a standard humeral stem with the Tornier Latitude system

Commercially available cement restrictors may be used, but are not necessary, and are often not sufficient. The humeral medullary canal usually tapers distally. In some instances, even an expanding cement restrictor will not obtain sufficient fit to prevent migration during cement pressurization. While bone from the excised distal humerus may be fashioned into restrictors, it may be difficult to get the bone plug to stay in the desired location. Additionally, should a revision be necessary later, a well-healed bone plug may obliterate the canal. An alternative cement restrictor, which is readily available, is oxidized cellulose (Surgicel, Johnson & Johnson). This is available in most operating rooms and can be cut into square sheets two to three times larger than the diameter of the canal in question. A smooth instrument (Frasier suction tip, DeBakey forceps, etc.) can be utilized to push the "wadding" down to the appropriate level. This is done until sufficient resistance is felt such that the conglomerate of cellulose will not move without significant force. Besides working in any size canal, the other advantage of this technique is the eventual resorption.

Before starting the operation, the surgeon should ensure that the cement system utilized has small-sized nozzles to allow cementation to the appropriate depth in the humerus. Using colored cement aides removal in the event of a revision. Utilizing commercially available PMMA that is already colored or adding methylene blue during mixing can accomplish this.

Two steps may help to decrease the risk of infection. The first is to instill 1 g of cefazolin mixed in 50 cc of normal saline in a peripheral vein after exsanguination and inflation of the tourniquet [25]. Many surgeons routinely also utilize PMMA with antibiotics mixed in during preparation.

Once the device is implanted, repair of the olecranon osteotomy utilizing the surgeon's preferred technique will allow for early range of motion. If the collaterals were not injured previously, and the columns are intact or rigidly fixed, stability should be normal in the immediate postoperative period. Restrictions should be based on allowing the osteotomy to heal as well as any concerns with the columns or collaterals if repaired. Typically, full range of motion with limitations of resisted or forceful extension is all that are necessary.

Alternative 1: Lateral Ostetomy for Capitellar Access

Most often, if an initial distal humerus fracture fixation has failed, a wide exposure will be necessary. There may be times though that the repeat operation needs a more focused approach. This would include the situation where the fracture is limited to the capitellum, or the remaining problem is located only in the capitellum. If access is needed only laterally, an olecranon osteotomy may be more surgical insult than is necessary, and at times may not provide the extent of exposure needed to the lateral aspect of the elbow joint. A lateral approach may provide more exposure.

If a limited, lateral approach is being considered, there should be a well-defined plan as to what will be accomplished from that approach. Preoperative imaging, especially CT scans, will help identify the extent of the damage to determine if access from the lateral side alone will be sufficient. If there is concern about the adequacy of a lateral only approach, a universal posterior incision can be made, with the lateral approach performed deeply. In this way, if there is need to also perform a more extensive approach, an olecranon osteotomy may be combined through this single skin incision.

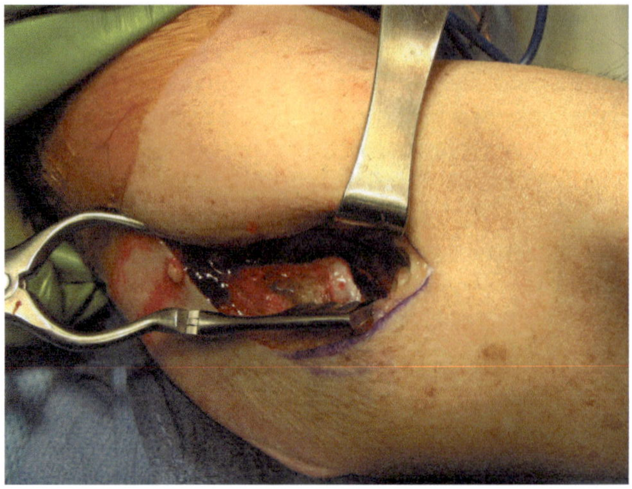

Fig. 10.9 Straight lateral exposure to the capitellum. Proximal extension should include common extensors, capsule, and may include part of the brachioradialis. The distal one-half of the lateral epicondyle is left undisturbed, maintaining integrity of the lateral collateral ligament

A straight lateral muscle splitting approach allows for better access to the capitellum, while preserving the lateral collateral ligament (Fig. 10.9). The exact interval between the mobile wad muscles and digital extensors need not be found. Rather, a split of the extensor musculature in line with the lateral epicondyle to Lister's tubercle for about 4–5 cm will provide sufficient exposure. The supinator should be identified, and the posterior interosseus nerve palpated and/or exposed for safety. If the supinator cannot be delineated from the undersurface of the extensor muscles, dissection distal to the radial neck should only be performed after identifying the radial nerve proximally. By leaving the distal 50% of the soft tissue attached to the lateral epicondyle, the lateral collateral ligament is protected and stability of the joint is maintained. Dissecting proximally along the lateral column, releasing the remaining common extensor origin, and proceeding to the brachioradialis, including the capsule, can increase the exposure to the capitellum. Dissection must proceed proximally with the radial nerve in mind. Various measurements can be utilized to identify the safe proximal extent. Measuring the distance between the epicondyles (the transepicondylar distance) provides a patient-specific reference. The radial nerve has been demonstrated to always be greater than 70% of the transepicondylar distance, as measured from the lateral epicondyle [26].

When a capitellar fracture has extension into the trochlea, a simple lateral approach, even with proximal extension, as described above, may not be sufficient. When this occurs, more extensile exposure of the distal humerus is necessary.

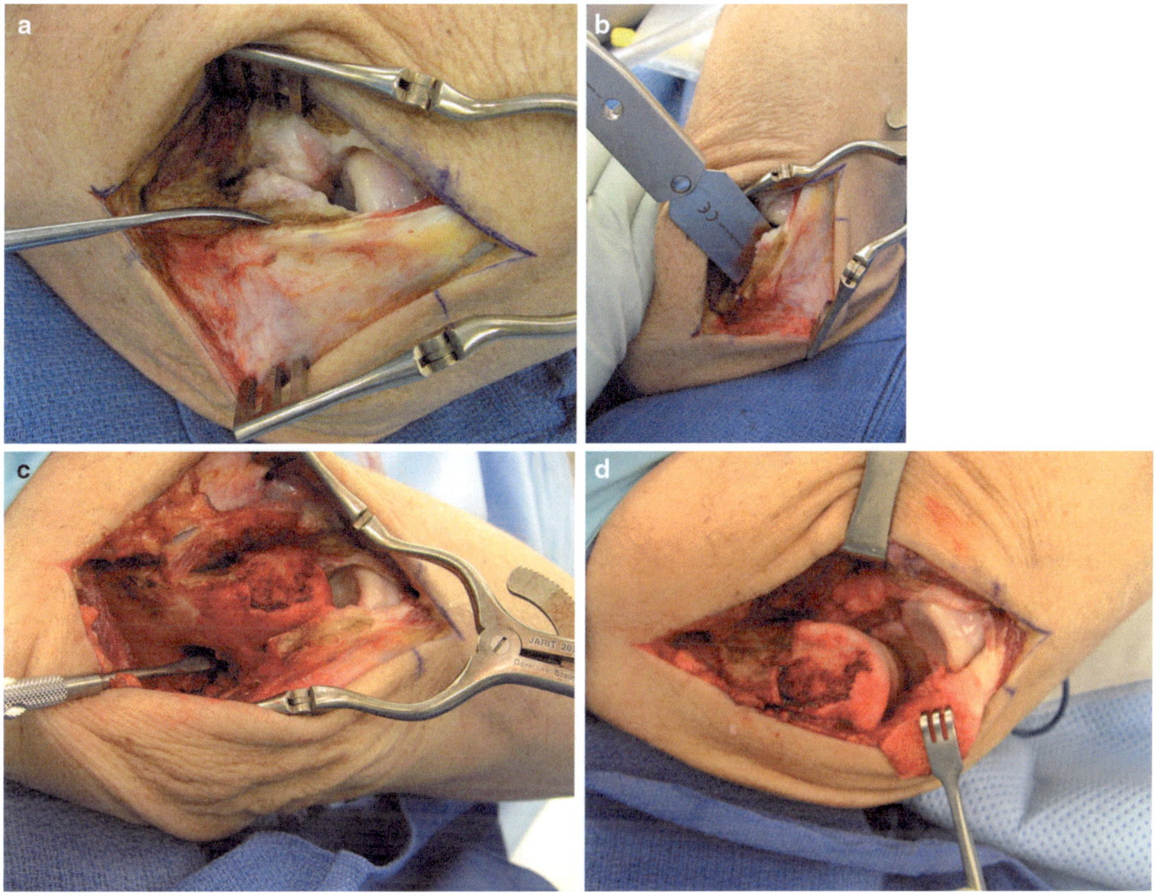

Fig. 10.10 (**a**) Lateral soft tissue exposure. The soft tissue attachments to the posterior one-half of the epicondyle are left intact. (**b**) A transverse counter cut has already been made at the proximal extent of the osteotomy. A sharp, thin osteotome is utilized to cut into the lateral epicondyle just at the edge of the capitellar articular surface. Care is taken to prevent the osteotome from taking articular capitellum, especially posteriorly. (**c**, **d**) Access after osteotomy. Note the view all the way to the coronoid. The elbow may also be subluxed with this release

This can be accomplished by an lateral epicondylar osteostomy or by taking down the lateral collateral ligament. A lateral epicondylar osteotomy allows for the isometry of the lateral soft tissues to be restored with little to no error, and fixation is usually rigid, so that rehabilitation is not hindered postoperatively. Combining the lateral soft tissue exposure with the lateral epicondyle osteotomy will allow complete exposure of the capitellum. The joint may be subluxed which allows access to the entire trochlea. If there is extensive comminution of the medial trochlea, this approach may not be sufficient for reduction or instrumentation, and an olecranon osteotomy may allow better access for implant placement (Fig. 10.10).

If lateral access is sufficient with only soft tissue dissection and preservation of the LCL, this exposure can be closed with #1 or #2 nonabsorbable suture. The lateral soft tissues should not be stressed in varus, but specific protection is not necessary as long as stability was intact during the procedure.

If the lateral epicondyle was osteotomized, this can be repaired with lag screws, headless compression screws, or cerclage wires. The fixation should be rigid enough to allow immediate motion. While varus stresses should be avoided, bracing is usually not needed and full range of motion may start once the soft tissue healing is adequate.

Alternative 2: Total Elbow Arthroplasty

If the distal humerus has been deemed to be unreconstructable, a linked TEA can be considered. The concept of replacing only the distal humerus (hemiarthroplasty) is relatively new and the determination of whether the elbow is best treated by hemiarthroplasty or TEA is, at this time, made on experience, opinion, and implant availability.

A definite advantage of a linked TEA for a failed internal fixation of the distal humerus is the lack of need of the

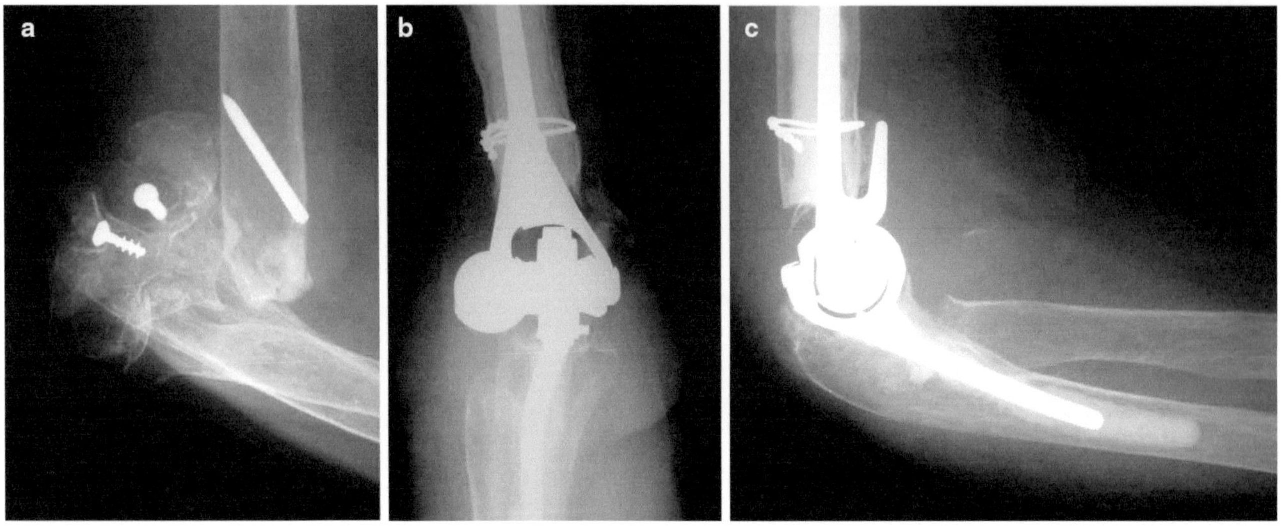

Fig. 10.11 This patient represents an ideal candidate for a total elbow arthroplasty (TEA) for distal humeral nonunion. Her original treatment was more than 10 years from the decision to revise, making union of this osteopenic bone unlikely. She was in excess of 70 years of age and had been living with a flail limb. The improvement in function after TEA was dramatic, and she was easily able to comply with the recommended restrictions (**a**) Preoperation radiograph. Note the sclerosis at the distal humer, (**b**) AP radiograph after total elbow arthroplasty (**c**) Lateral radiograph

epicondyles and collateral ligaments [27]. Because of this, there is no need to obtain union of the ununited segments [7, 28]. This consideration makes TEA for nonunion a consideration in those patients whose comorbidities make union after revision unlikely. A secondary advantage is that the procedure may be performed through the gap left by excising the distal humeral fragments from the epicondyles distal. This allows the triceps to be left undisturbed. With the linkage preventing dissociation of the implant and an intact triceps which does not need postoperative protection, recovery can proceed immediately to the permanent restrictions of TEA.

The typical patient appropriate for a TEA for nonunion of the distal humerus is one who can comply with the restriction of a TEA, who is unlikely to heal a revision ORIF with bone grafting and will be unlikely to need a revision in the future (Fig. 10.11). This option should be considered the last resort, and reconstruction or revision of a nonunion is recommended for the younger, more active patient. This includes any patient who will not comply with the lifting or activity restrictions of the TEA, as well as younger patients. There is no absolute age cut-off for a TEA, and the clinical situation should determine the proper course for the surgeon, but most patients of normal health less than 65 are appropriate for an attempt at revision of a nonunion before placing a TEA. This age is, of course, arbitrary and should be moved up for the active patient who wants to play tennis, golf, or perform other stressful activities. Likewise, the age can be moved down for the patient who is sedentary, especially if they have comorbidities likely to shorten their life span.

The surgical approach to remove the failed implants and place a TEA is typically the same as that which was used during the index operation. Once the ulnar nerve is located and protected, dissection can proceed to the failed implants. Care should be directed to the radial nerve at the proximal hardware. Prominent or painful hardware should be removed. Knowledge of the TEA implants is important if all the hardware cannot be removed. Any hardware impeding placement of the implants needs to be dealt with. Attention should be paid to the screw holes, as cement can extrude from them during TEA implantation. This is especially critical in the region of the radial nerve. The heat generated by the curing methylmethacrylate may damage a nerve if in direct contact.

Once the pertinent hardware is removed, the ununited distal humerus fragment(s) can be removed. If the nerves are protected as noted above, electrocautery allows for efficient removal of the bone (Fig. 10.12). The excision of bone creates a large gap between the humeral shaft and the proximal ulna. The humeral shaft can be exposed through the radial or ulnar side of the triceps. The ulnar nerve may dictate the direction. Preparation of the humerus differs by manufacturer, but most, if not all, initial implant specific steps (such as trochlear cutting and distal humeral shaping) are not necessary. Typically, the only necessary step is to utilize the final broaches to size and shape the humeral shaft and intramedullary canal. At this time, a trial humeral component can be placed. While there are several implants commercially available for TEA, utilizing a TEA for distal humerus nonunion requires some requisites. Removal of the epicondyles

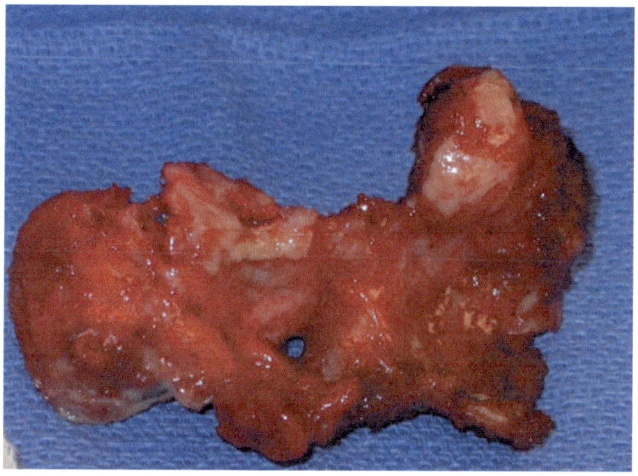

Fig. 10.12 The entire distal humeral fragment from the case in Fig. 10.11 was removed in one piece

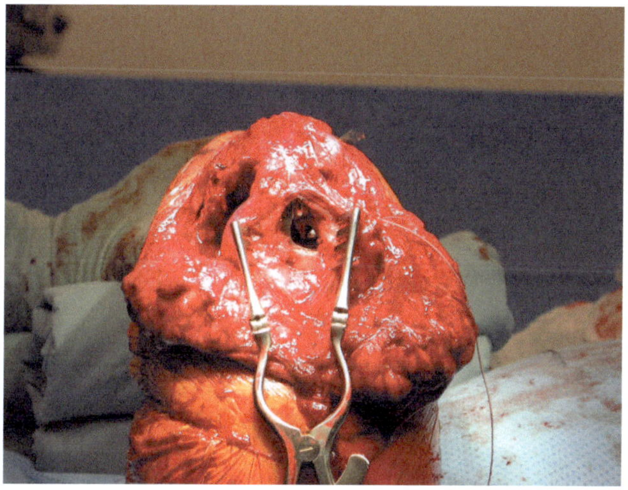

Fig. 10.13 A triceps split allows for access to the intramedullary canal of the ulna, if it is difficult to obtain from either side. It may also allow for placement of locking caps in convertible prosthetic designs

necessitates a linked component. The other required design feature is an anterior flange. This supports the posterior vector of force on the distal humerus to decrease chances of failure. The flange also provides resistance to torsional forces on the distal humerus implant. Standard TEAs obtain some torsional support from the lateral and medial columns supporting the implant. With these removed for a nonunion case, only the shape of the implant/humeral canal and the flange provided resistance to rotation. Failure to use an implant with an anterior flange will lead to early failure of the humeral component.

Access to the ulna is obtained through the defect left from excising the distal humeral bone. The triceps should be left attached; its presence will not prevent insertion of an ulnar component, although there are some simple steps to simplify unhampered access.

The proximal most attachment of the triceps can be released for a few millimeters; this will allow for the proximal 3–4 mm of bone to be removed as well. Depending on the implant system used, the ulnar component can often be placed from the lateral or medial interval. If there is any uncertainty because the soft tissue inhibits the bony anatomy, fluoroscopic guidance should be utilized. Alternatively, a split in the distal most triceps can add collinear access to the intramedullary canal of the ulna (Fig. 10.13). Many of the TEA systems were developed for use in the patient with softer bone due to inflammatory arthritis. When these systems are utilized in the patients discussed herein, the bone quality in the proximal ulna is usually such that additional attention needs to be paid to preparation for the ulna. Often, a burr is helpful to widen the intramedullary opening prior to broaching.

Depending on the TEA system utilized, the native radial head may or may not articulate with the humeral implant. If an implant is utilized which has a capitellar component, and the native radial head is normal, it may be left to articulate when the ulnar component is linked. Since the components are linked, the radial head will not increase stability, but it will share some load distally, thereby reducing load on the ulnar component. If the native radial head is damaged or articulates improperly, it should not be left to articulate with the distal humerus and should be excised.

If an implant is utilized which does not have a capitellar articular surface, the surgeon needs to know if the native radial head will articulate with the distal humeral component. If it does not, and the proximal radio-ulnar joint is normal, the native radial head should be left in situ, to prevent the possibility of proximal radial shaft instability after resection. Radial head excision should be carried out if the native head would articulate with a noncapitellar distal humeral component.

Commercially available cement restrictors may be used, but are not necessary, and are often not sufficient. The humeral medullary canal usually tapers distally. In some instances, even an expanding cement restrictor will not obtain sufficient fit to prevent migration during cement pressurization. The ulnar medullary canal is often too small for the smallest commercially available restrictors. While bone from the excised distal humerus may be fashioned into restrictors, the problem with adequate fixation in the humerus as well as premature incarceration in the ulnar canal exist. An alternative cement restrictor, which is readily available, is oxidized cellulose (Surgicel, Johnson & Johnson). This is available in most operating rooms and can be cut into square sheets two to three times larger than the diameter of the canal in question. A smooth instrument (Frasier suction tip, DeBakey forceps, etc.) can be utilized to push the "wadding" down to the appropriate level. This is done until sufficient resistance is felt such that the conglomerate of cellulose will not move without significant force. Besides working in any size canal, the other advantage of this technique is the eventual reabsorption.

Before starting a TEA operation, the surgeon should ensure that the cement system utilized has small-sized nozzles to allow cementation to the appropriate depth in the humerus and especially the ulna. Cementing the ulnar and humeral components in their own stage, while more time-consuming, may prevent problems properly seating the components due to premature curing of the PMMA.

Even though a TEA for this indication is utilized in those patients where revision is unlikely, using colored cement aides removal in the event of a revision. Utilizing commercially available PMMA that is already colored or adding methylene blue during mixing can do this. There is a higher risk of infection after TEA; the risk will increase in the multiply operated TEA. Two steps may help to decrease the risk of infection. The first is to instill 1 g of cefazolin mixed in 50 cc of normal saline in a peripheral vein after exsanguination and inflation of the tourniquet [25]. Many surgeons routinely also utilize PMMA with antibiotics mixed in during preparation.

Once the final implants are properly cemented in place, they can be linked. The soft tissue intervals medial and lateral may be closed, attaching the flexor and extensor origins to the triceps. Since the medial intermuscular septum was excised or released with the distal humeral resection and there is no longer a medial epicondyle, the ulnar nerve's position is one of inherent decompression such that a formal transposition is superfluous.

Because of the nature of revision surgery, the tourniquet should be let down and hemostasis obtained. Use of a drain is up to the discretion of the surgeon, but should be considered, since seroma and hematoma formation is a common postoperative complication (see below).

Twenty-four to forty-eight hours of compression and elevation may help to prevent seroma or hematoma; once motion is started it may commence as tolerated as long as the soft tissues allow. Since the TEA is linked, and the triceps attached, "routine" activities limited only by the TEA may start. Most surgeons follow the recommendations of allowing only 10 lb maximum lift push or pull as a single event, with 1–2 lb repetitive use allowed. Additionally, activities such as golf, tennis, or swinging a hammer heavier than a finishing hammer should be avoided to prevent catastrophic failure of the TEA.

Pearls for Revision Section (Technique)

Be prepared to bone graft
  Structural vs. cancellous vs. synthetic
Gain control of ulnar nerve
  Transpose if not already done
Understand the capabilities and limitations of implants
Resurface if not repairable
Use intraoperative imaging

Pearls for Partial Resurfacing Section

Preoperatively discuss with patient the implications of "off-label" use if practicing in the United States
Prepare for alternative implantation techniques
- Manufacturer recommendations will be for other uses
- Retaining the native radial head may make "standard" implantation difficult
- Trial implantation in the planned method in a cadaver or "saw bones"

Have a contingency plan if partial resurfacing is not technically possible, or if the geometry of the implant does not match the distal humerus
- Complete distal humerus resurfacing (distal humeral hemiarthroplasty) may be necessary

Pearls for Lateral Exposure only Section

Increase exposure with osteotomy of the lateral epicondyle
- Utilize a sharp, thin osteotome for the LE osteotomy

Release up the column to allow the joint to sublux
Add olecranon osteotomy if exposure is inadequate
Use intraoperative imaging

Pearls for TEA Section

Understand implant selection
  Radiocapitellar articulation
Keep triceps attached
Have cement applicator tubes that fit up the canals
Utilize oxidized cellulose for cement restrictor
Utilize antibiotics and dyed cement
Cement in two stages
"Regular" activity level can commence once the soft tissue envelope allows
  Make sure patient understands permanent TEA limitation

Optimizing Outcomes

- Align expectations between patient and surgeon
- Allow for early ROM
  - If the elbow has to be completely immobilized, fixation is not optimized
- Respect the ulnar nerve
  - Document function pre-op
  - Decompress
  - Transpose
- Prepare for contingencies
  - Bone graft as needed
    Structural bone graft when needed
    Consent for bone grafting
- Have proper instruments
  - Dental picks
  - Cerclage wires (monofilament)
- Have a variety of implants
  - Understand capabilities
    Locking
    Screw trajectory
    TEA
      Linkage
      Capitellar component
  - Understand limitations
    Size
    Location
    Fixation
- Obtain adequate exposure
  - Utilize previous incisions/approaches only when appropriate
  - Perform osteotomies when necessary
    Olecranon
    Lateral epicondyle
- Shorten extra-articular nonunions

Complication and Side Effects

Fortunately, in careful hands, common complications are manageable and less serious, while serious complications should be uncommon. When preparing a patient for revision surgery after distal humerus fracture, the surgeon should describe to the patient the common complications and their treatment. Recovery is much less traumatic to the patient when he or she has heard of the issues that may arise during their recovery.

The most common complication after a revision surgery for a distal humerus fracture is seroma or hematoma formation. Full thickness skin flaps often need to be raised for these surgeries and it is not uncommon for fluid to collect postoperatively. Although there are no evidence-based reports to support personal experience, it appears that some simple perioperative steps can decrease the incidence of hematoma or seroma. At times, during revision surgery, there is a well-defined bursal like lining on both the skin flap and the deeper fascial layers. At revision surgery, this should be roughened with a rasp or carefully scraped or scored with a scalpel to encourage healing of the skin to the deeper tissues. The dermis or fat (if there is excessive subcutaneous fat) on the flap should be sutured down to the fascia. This will decrease the potential space for fluid to collect postoperatively. Care must be used when doing this to prevent suturing a cutaneous nerve. The tourniquet should be released after the procedure is completed, or when felt to be necessary to decrease the risk of ischemic complications. Any brisk venous bleeding and any arterial bleeding should be controlled. Depending on the type of surgery done, slow venous bleeding may be too diffuse to stop completely.

A drain placed intraoperatively should also decrease the amount of fluid collection, whether from bleeding or serous collection. The drain is best placed both deep and superficial with its exit through muscle. The triceps is usually the safest and most accessible muscle with sufficient mass to allow placement of the drain. By having the drain exit the muscle, the tract closes to the deep tissues upon removing it, limiting drainage after removal. Clinical experience has also shown that uniformly compressive postoperative bandages can help with not only swelling, but also accumulation of seroma or hematoma. Twenty-four hours of elevation appears to help swelling and fluid accumulation as well.

Various degrees of wound breakdown are not uncommon after revision surgery for the distal humerus. This can be precipitated by a fluid collection. The pressure in a hematoma or seroma will increase with elbow flexion, which can often precipitate a wound dehiscence. Secondary surgical insult may also disrupt blood flow to already thin flaps, allowing for some necrosis at the wound edges.

With initial wound problems, the possibility of infection needs to be considered. This could be the cause or a by-product of the wound breakdown. Besides treating any infection, the wound should be given a chance to settle down and declare itself. Unless there is gross contamination and full thickness skin loss, judicious use of immobilization and uniformly compressive bandages should be utilized. Although motion is critical to a functional elbow, wound healing will trump mobilization. It is better to save the soft tissue envelope and gain motion later with operative or nonoperative means, rather than sacrifice the skin for early motion. Once the wound declares itself, a decision can be made to proceed with motion or not. The wound may be debrided and allowed to heal, left with eshar as a "biologic bandage" (Fig. 10.14), treated with topical bandages for serial debridements, or treated with more advanced therapies. Wound breakdown may involve exposure of some underlying hardware. In the

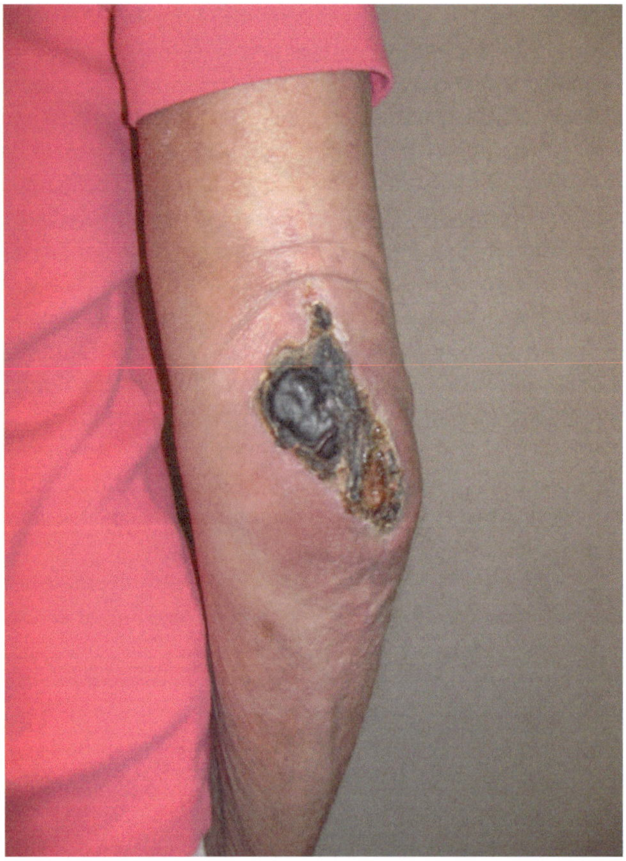

Fig. 10.14 Two months after an ORIF (primary), this elbow has a contracting wound with a thick eschar. Since there was full ROM and no signs of infection, observation was chosen for treatment

multiply operated elbow, this may be unavoidable, and at times is best treated with dressing changes until the offending hardware may be removed. As difficult as it may be for patient and surgeon to be looking at exposed hardware, it is important to understand that its presence does not preclude a successful outcome (Fig. 10.15). When a decision has been made to leave the hardware exposed, this author's preferred treatment is twice daily wet-to-dry dressings with 50% Dakin's solution.

The scope of this chapter does not include the more intensive treatments for wound breakdown. Options such as negative pressure vacuum bandages, local flaps, and even free flaps are sometimes necessary. When simple measures do not solve the wound issues, a surgeon well-versed in all the options should be involved.

Stiffness after revision surgery should be expected after surgery. The only variable is its duration. While some may not consider it a true complication, it is definitely an untoward event after surgery and is therefore considered in the context of complications for this chapter. The patient should be notified that their elbow would definitely be stiff after surgery (i.e., it will not have full range of motion). Depending on the preoperative condition and range of motion, as well as the procedure performed, the total arc of motion may be the same, better, or worse than the preoperative measurements. The patient should be educated as the expected course, as well as the main goals of surgery. A major reconstruction to realign the articular cartilage may cause a transient decrease in range of motion, but preserve the longevity of the joint. The patient needs to understand the expectations, and that motion will come with proper therapies. There are also times where motion will need to be gained at yet another time, such as when wound breakdown requires immobilization for soft tissue stabilization.

While not as ubiquitous as stiffness, hardware complications are common after revision elbow surgery. The subcutaneous prominences of the elbow, which often serve as anchor points to fixation, make for common sources of irritation when hardware is placed over them. During a revision situation, hardware may need to be placed in a less than ideal location to maximize the chance of successful healing. Rigid fixation will supersede idealized implant location in the revision setting. The patient should be informed preoperatively that hardware placed may be irritating, and that another procedure to remove it may be necessary once healing is confirmed by radiologic studies. Depending on the nature of the revision, removal of hardware should be delayed typically 6 months, preferably a year, or more.

Depending on exposure, neuropraxia can be another postoperative complication. If the exposure requires dissection of a nerve or nerves, it should be described to the patient as a possibility. If the dissection is a revision neurolysis, or if there is significant scarring or heterotopic bone around the nerve, the patient should be notified that a neuropraxia is likely. Meticulous dissection should preserve the continuity of the nerves, but may not prevent neuropraxia. In severely scared areas, or in regions with extensive heterotopic bone, transection to the nerve may occur by avulsion, or even laceration. Although this severe complication should be rare, the patient should be notified that it is possible if the dissection proceeds in areas as noted above. If sharp transection occurs during reconstruction, repair should be completed. If the ulnar nerve is involved, transposition may allow for removal of any scared or damaged portion of the nerve and primary repair. Motor recovery in an adult after transection of a nerve at the elbow will be variable to the hand, but sensory recovery should occur to some degree. Recovery will take over 1 year.

When exposure is in the proximity of the nerves, exposure of the nerve will allow for its protection, as well as guide treatment and expectations should dysfunction follow surgery. If a careful neurolysis and/or transposition are followed by nerve dysfunction, and one knows the nerve is intact, then treatment consists of supportive care for the defect with the expectation that nerve recovery should ensue. Splints should be used for support, while range of motion should be performed to prevent stiffness or contractures in the hand. If

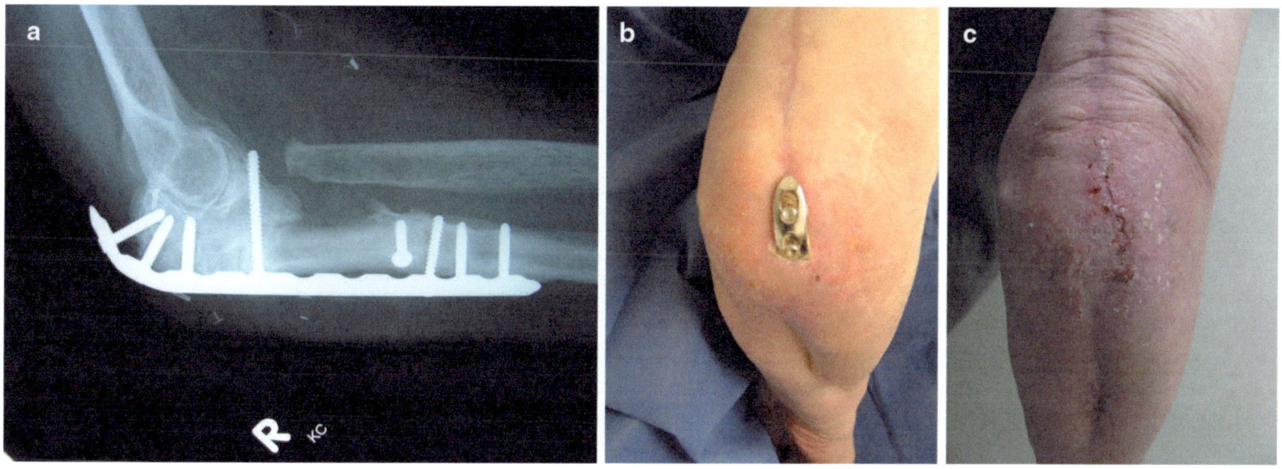

Fig. 10.15 This multiply operated ulnar fracture was eventually successfully treated with a vascularized fibula. (**a**) A locking plate was applied during surgery and primary skin coverage was obtained. (**b**) At 6 months postoperatively, the wound broke down, exposing the proximal portion of the plate. Healing was incomplete and there were no signs of infection. The plate was left exposed, treated as described in the text, and removed uneventfully at 1 year postoperatively, once the graft had healed completely. (**c**) The wound was closed primarily at hardware removal and healed uneventfully

no function returns by 3 months, baseline nerve conduction and electromyographic studies can be performed. Repeat studies can follow improvement 6–8 weeks later.

Should a permanent deficit follow a neuropraxic or other injury, reconstruction can often be done to allow for improvement in function. This may consist of tendon transfers, nerve transfers, or selected distal fusions or tenodeses. The delayed reconstruction of permanent nerve injuries about the elbow is beyond the scope of this chapter. The most successful recoveries from these severe injuries will occur when a patient has a preoperative understanding that there was this possibility, and when the patient's postnerve injury course is guided by a physician trained in this type of reconstruction.

Infection may represent the most vexing problem after a revision to a failed distal humerus. This complication is a very real possibility that is potentially caused by an indolent infection not detected prior to or at revision, poor soft tissue coverage, or avascular bone. Many patients who fail initial fixation of a distal humerus fracture are at high risk with comorbidities such as diabetes, osteopenia, poor nutritional status, obesity, or poor soft tissue coverage of the elbow.

As with all complications, prevention is paramount. The routine work-up of a patient prior to revision surgery should include a thorough history of any questionable signs of infection with the primary procedure. Preoperative imaging and lab work should rule out infection when needed. Aspiration can be done in questionable cases, and when in doubt, tissue specimens prior to antibiotic administration should be obtained. The use of frozen specimen evaluation intraoperative to rule out infection is somewhat dependent on surgeon and pathologist experience. If there is any question, it is better to stage the procedure and perform a thorough debridement, saving the reconstruction for a later time, when infection has been ruled out or treated.

Prevention should include the proper preoperative prophylaxis with a preoperative scrub prior to the patient coming to the hospital, the proper and complete scrub in the operating room, and prophylactic antibiotics. Regional administration of antibiotics (akin to a Bier block, but with Cephazolin instead of local anesthetic) has been demonstrated to give a high local concentration of antibiotics [25]. This unique administration should be considered in revision situations.

When infection occurs after a revision distal humerus fracture, it should be treated aggressively. Serial debridements with removal of devitalized tissue should be carried out with the appropriate antibiotic treatment. Salvage of a postoperative infection may ultimately require a prosthetic arthroplasty, even further necessitating the eradication of any postoperative infection. The clinical situation needs to be assessed with a salvage plan in mind during the treatment of a deep infection. Retention of hardware and articulating or supporting bone will need to be balanced with the likelihood of success and need for possible joint replacement. When doubt or uncertainty exists, it is best mitigated with serial debridements and the understanding from the patient that the treatment plan will evolve given the response to the treatment of the infection.

Postoperative Care

While the specific postoperative care may vary given the exact treatment rendered, or the patient's condition or comorbidities, there are certain general statements about the care.

Immediate

Swelling is common after any surgery for a distal humerus fracture, but more so in the revision situation. Lymphatic flow often has not returned to normal after the initial injury and surgery, and another surgical insult often exacerbates this. As noted above in the discussion on seromas and hematomas, a well-padded compressive bandage, elevation for at least 24 h, and immobilization with elevation will limit postsurgical swelling.

Mobilization should commence at 24–48 h after surgery. Clear communication must exist between the surgeon and any treating therapist in relation to the allowed range, weight bearing status, as well as any concerns about undue stress. If there is any concern about the lateral elbow's structural support, the patient must be educated on avoiding the obligatory varus stress that occurs with shoulder abduction.

Efforts should be made to reconstruct the elbow such that support is not needed from braces or splints. Individual preference as well as knowledge of the actual construct may lead to the use of resting splints or hinged braces. While hinged braces can be helpful in limiting range of motion when needed, and supporting against varus and valgus forces, they may be counterproductive. If a hinged brace slips distal, or twists, the center of rotation of the brace does not align with the center of rotation of the elbow. This may incur increased forces on fixation. Difficulty with the center of rotation is more common in arms with abundant soft tissue envelopes.

There are instances where revision surgery is felt to be adequate if tissues are allowed to heal, but inadequate for range of motion. If this presents, it is reasonable to immobilize the elbow until the tissues heal, then obtain motion if possible. In these situations, a planned additional surgical release may be needed. Prior to commencing with a revision of the distal humerus fixation, this possibility should be discussed if felt to be a possibility.

The soft tissue envelope should be monitored for healing. Especially in a revision situation, infection is always a concern. If an old incision was utilized for surgical exposure, the sutures or staples should be left in beyond "normal" wound healing time. This author usually waits between 2 and 3 weeks. Epidermal healing may occur such that a wound is sealed, but deeper healing is not sufficient to withstand the stress of elbow motion (especially if there is a residual fluid collection). Dehiscence should be treated aggressively, usually with a trip to the operating room for irrigation, deep culture acquisition, debridement, and closure (over a drain if necessary).

Long-Term Postoperative Care

If a revision of the elbow is successful and native tissue (with or without bone graft) has healed in an anatomic fashion, there should be no long-term restrictions. Certainly, limitations in motion may persist, and posttraumatic degenerative changes may occur in the elbow. These may cause limitations for the patient and the physician should guide the patient as to how any limitation may impact their future. If posttraumatic changes are significant, longevity of the elbow may be impacted by stressful activities such that avocation or occupational changes may need to be considered.

The use of partial or hemiarthroplasty resurfacing of the distal humerus is recent enough that the longevity of these implants is unknown. Case reports and intermediate individual results indicate that these implants may last beyond 10 and towards 20 years or longer [24, 29]. This author does not impose limitations after partial resurfacing or distal humeral hemiarthroplasty, although it is recommended to avoid highly stressful or impact activities or sports. Tennis and golf are allowed, but heavy weight training and using a jack or sledgehammer are discouraged.

When a linked elbow arthroplasty is utilized as a salvage, an advantage is the immediate function it provides. The linkage prevents dislocation and obviates the need to limit shoulder abduction. Triceps function is intact and need not be protected because the implant is inserted with the triceps attachment left intact. The only limitations are the arbitrary, yet near universally accepted, restrictions on lifting no more than 1–2 lb repetitively, or 10 lb as a single event [28].

Conclusion

Distal humeral fractures are rarely simple, and complications are not uncommon. Stiffness, at least temporarily, is universal. Highly comminuted fractures may be difficult or impossible to reconstruct anatomically. The possibility of nonunion, malunion, and loss of fixation should be discussed with a patient when undertaking the index procedure for a distal humerus fracture.

Given the complexity of these injuries, and the inherent difficulty with fixing them, there should be an understanding that revision may become necessary, should the index procedure not result in the outcome expected.

Revision consisting of revising the fixation, shortening the extra-articular portion of the fracture, resurfacing part or the entire distal humerus, or even replacing the entire elbow may allow for recovery of a dysfunctional elbow.

The physician treating distal humerus fractures ideally should be aware of these options. When necessary, they can turn a hopeless situation into a functional outcome.

Case 10.1

A woman in her 30s sustained a ground level fall resulting in a knee fracture and trochlear fracture with proximal lateral column extension. Persistent mechanical symptoms and limitations in motion at 3 months prompted a referral.

Plain radiographs (**a**, **b**) demonstrate an incongruity of the trochlea notable between the radial and ulnar facets of the trochlea. A CT scan (**c**) demonstrates the proximal column portion has healed, but the trochlea is ununited and impacted along the articular aspect.

Three-dimensional renderings of the CT scan (**d–f**) more clearly delineate the deformity.

Intraoperative photographs (**g**, **h**) prior to mobilizing the fragment demonstrate the displacement. The fragment was mobilized (**i**) taking care to keep its soft tissue attachments at the lateral epicondyle intact. Provisional fixation was held with k-wires out of the position of planned hardware (**j**). Note the anatomic alignment of the trochlea. Additionally, one can appreciate some early wear between the trochlea and capitellum that was caused from the malposition of the fragment. Final alignment with plate fixation in place (**k**, **l**).

Postoperative radiographs demonstrating multiple points of fixation in the fracture fragment and anatomic alignment of the trochlear joint surface (**m–o**).

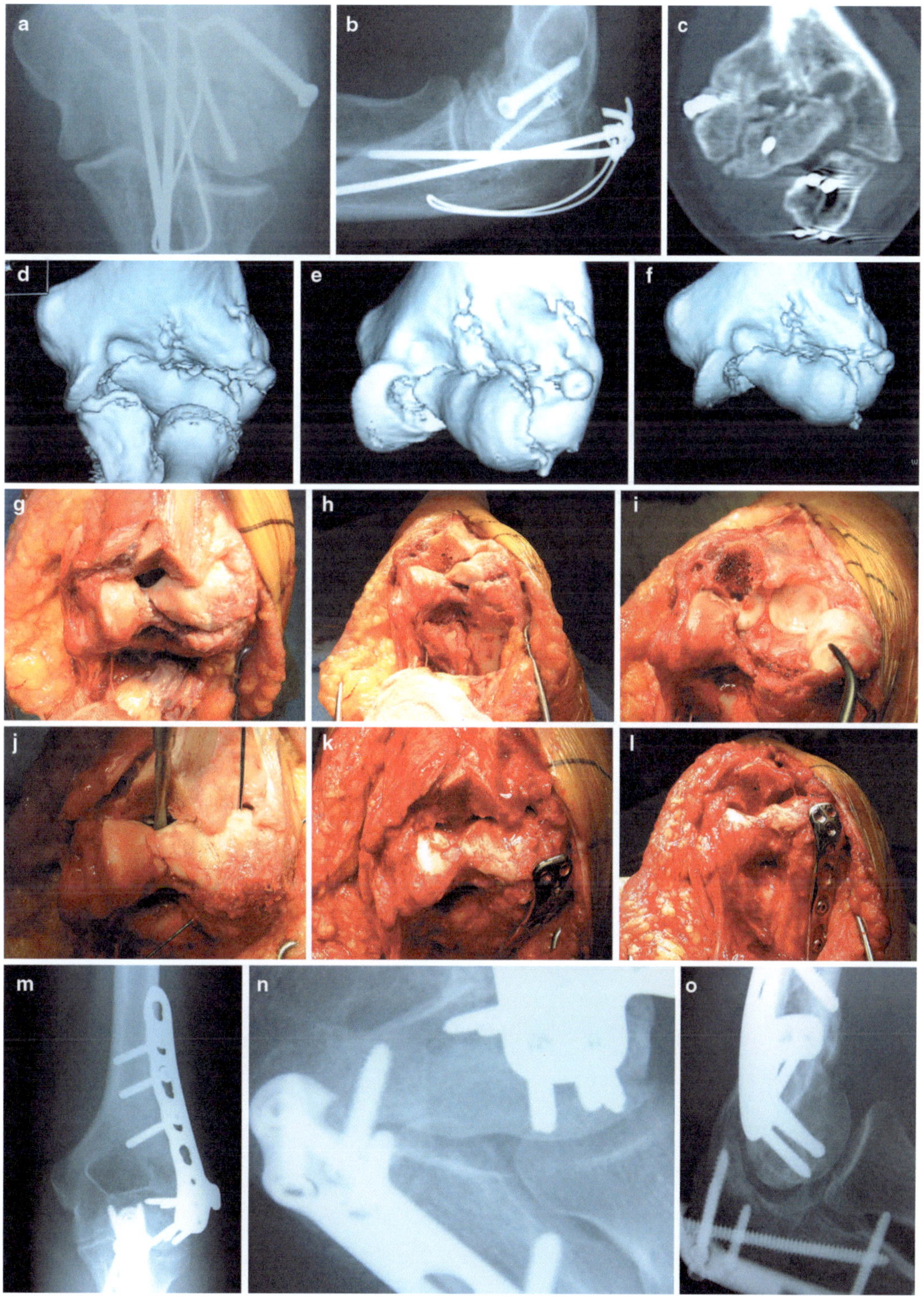

Case 10.2

A right-handed male in his 50s sustained an isolated right distal humerus fracture. (**a**) AP radiograph after initial attempt at fixation from a lateral approach. Note the incongruity of both the capitellum and trochlea. (**b**) A second attempt at fixation included repeating the lateral approach and adding an anterior approach. Articular congruity was not improved. (**c**) After AFT osteotomy and removal of the hardware, significant loss of the capitellum and trochlea is noted. (**d**, **e**) Trial stems are used to size the component. The center of the capitellum should be in the center of the radial head, while the trochlear notch aligns. If the elbow is between sizes, clinical experience has suggested choosing the smaller implant. (**f**) Intramedullary guide is in place. Utilizing the intact medial column and epicondyle aligns cutting jig. Both rotation and length are correctly accounted for by referencing off this one point. The bone loss laterally does not preclude use of the cutting guide. (**g**) The soft tissue is left intact on the medial epicondyle, therefore the guide pin for the medial center of rotation must be placed around or through the soft tissue. (**h**) Trial implant. Note the loss of support for the lateral aspect. Failure to provide support to this part of the implant would allow for excessive rotational and posterior forces. (**i**) Final implant. Prior to cementing the device, an allograft cancellous block was sculpted to interlock into the remaining lateral column and support the device. Smooth k-wires were utilized to secure it. (**j**) The bone graft gains additional support from the implant, while providing resistance to rotation and posterior forces. (**k**) AP radiograph: Note the congruency of the implant to the radius and ulna. (**l**) Lateral radiograph (**m**–**q**). Postoperative motion at 4 months, the patient has no pain. Note the initial lateral incision was incorporated into an extended incision for a deep posterior approach.

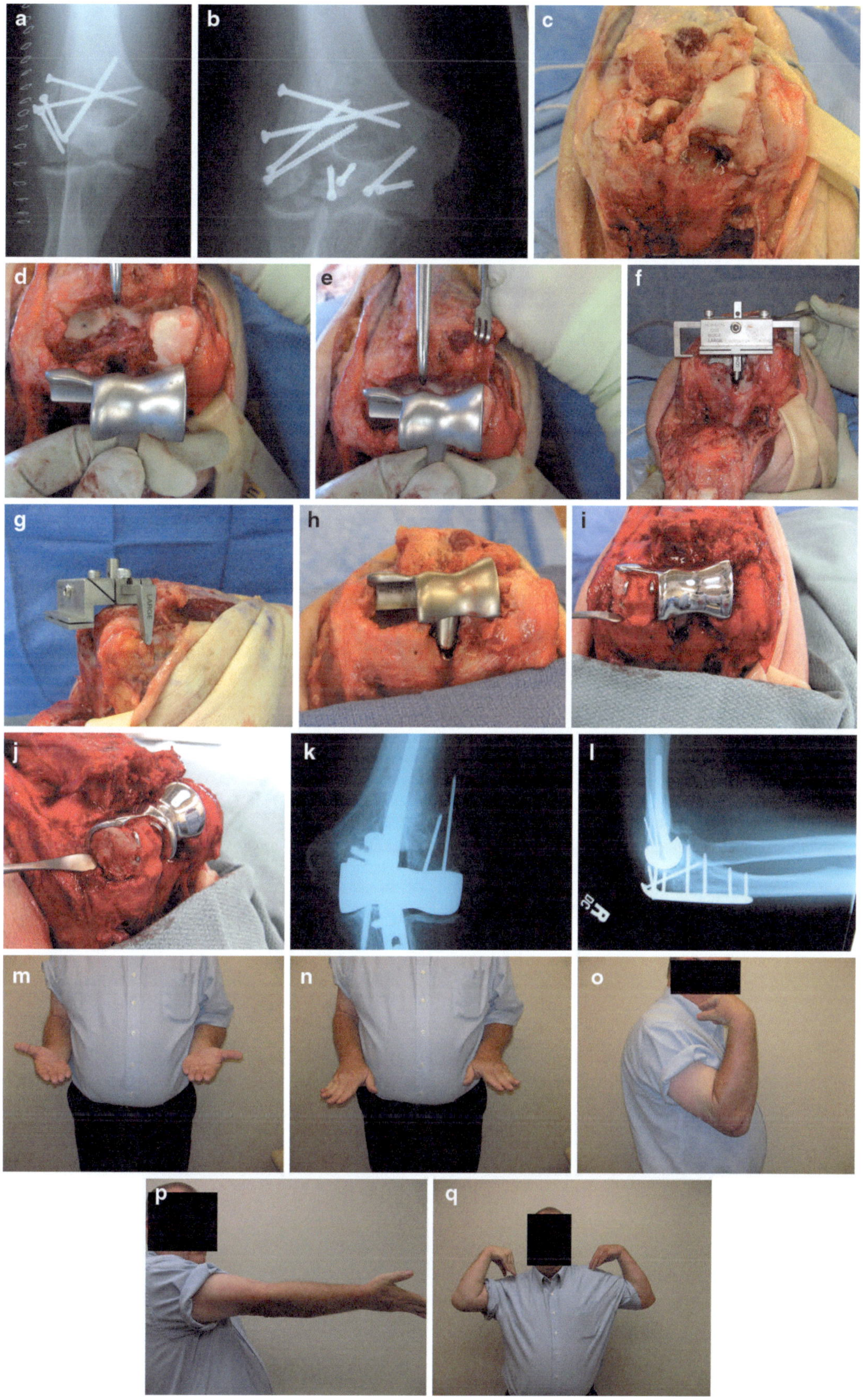
a
b
c
d
e
f
g
h
i
j
k
l
m
n
o
p
q

References

1. O'Driscoll SW, Sanchez-Sotelo J, Torchia ME. Management of the smashed distal humerus. Orthop Clin North Am. 2002;33(1):19–33, vii.
2. Sanchez-Sotelo J, Torchia ME, O'Driscoll SW. Complex distal humeral fractures: internal fixation with a principle-based parallel-plate technique. J Bone Joint Surg Am. 2007;89(5):961–9.
3. Doornberg JN, van Duijn PJ, Linzel D, Ring DC, Zurakowski D, Marti RK, et al. Surgical treatment of intra-articular fractures of the distal part of the humerus. Functional outcome after twelve to thirty years. J Bone Joint Surg Am. 2007;89(7):1524–32.
4. Gofton WT, Macdermid JC, Patterson SD, Faber KJ, King GJ. Functional outcome of AO type C distal humeral fractures. J Hand Surg Am. 2003;28(2):294–308.
5. McKee MD, Veillette CJ, Hall JA, Schemitsch EH, Wild LM, McCormack R, et al. A multicenter, prospective, randomized, controlled trial of open reduction—internal fixation versus total elbow arthroplasty for displaced intra-articular distal humeral fractures in elderly patients. J Shoulder Elbow Surg. 2009;18(1):3–12.
6. Ali A, Douglas H, Stanley D. Revision surgery for nonunion after early failure of fixation of fractures of the distal humerus. J Bone Joint Surg Br. 2005;87(8):1107–10.
7. Cil A, Veillette CJ, Sanchez-Sotelo J, Morrey BF. Linked elbow replacement: a salvage procedure for distal humeral nonunion. J Bone Joint Surg Am. 2008;90(9):1939–50.
8. Aldridge III JM, Lightdale NR, Mallon WJ, Coonrad RW. Total elbow arthroplasty with the Coonrad/Coonrad-Morrey prosthesis. A 10- to 31-year survival analysis. J Bone Joint Surg Br. 2006; 88(4):509–14.
9. Little CP, Graham AJ, Karatzas G, Woods DA, Carr AJ. Outcomes of total elbow arthroplasty for rheumatoid arthritis: comparative study of three implants. J Bone Joint Surg Am. 2005;87(11):2439–48.
10. Moro JK, King GJ. Total elbow arthroplasty in the treatment of posttraumatic conditions of the elbow. Clin Orthop. 2000; 370:102–14.
11. Nolla J, Ring D, Lozano-Calderon S, Jupiter JB. Interposition arthroplasty of the elbow with hinged external fixation for post-traumatic arthritis. J Shoulder Elbow Surg. 2008;17(3):459–64.
12. Larson AN, Morrey BF. Interposition arthroplasty with an Achilles tendon allograft as a salvage procedure for the elbow. J Bone Joint Surg Am. 2008;90(12):2714–23.
13. Dean GS, Holliger EH, Urbaniak JR. Elbow allograft for reconstruction of the elbow with massive bone loss. Long term results. Clin Orthop. 1997;341:12–22.
14. Koller H, Kolb K, Assuncao A, Kolb W, Holz U. The fate of elbow arthrodesis: indications, techniques, and outcome in fourteen patients. J Shoulder Elbow Surg. 2008;17(2):293–306.
15. Rashkoff E, Burkhalter WE. Arthrodesis of the salvage elbow. Orthopedics. 1986;9(5):733–8.
16. Rosset A, Spadola L, Ratib O. OsiriX: an open-source software for navigating in multidimensional DICOM images. J Digit Imaging. 2004;17(3):205–16.
17. Morrey BF, Adams RA. Semiconstrained elbow replacement for distal humeral nonunion. J Bone Joint Surg Br. 1995;77(1):67–72.
18. O'Driscoll SW. The triceps-reflecting anconeus pedicle (TRAP) approach for distal humeral fractures and nonunions. Orthop Clin North Am. 2000;31(1):91–101.
19. Athwal GS, Rispoli DM, Steinmann SP. The anconeus flap transolecranon approach to the distal humerus. J Orthop Trauma. 2006;20(4):282–5.
20. Ring D, Jupiter JB. Operative treatment of osteochondral nonunion of the distal humerus. J Orthop Trauma. 2006;20(1):56–9.
21. Adolfsson L, Hammer R. Elbow hemiarthroplasty for acute reconstruction of intraarticular distal humerus fractures: a preliminary report involving 4 patients. Acta Orthop. 2006;77(5):785–7.
22. Swoboda B, Scott RD. Humeral hemiarthroplasty of the elbow joint in young patients with rheumatoid arthritis: a report on 7 arthroplasties. J Arthroplasty. 1999;14(5):553–9.
23. Gramstad GD, King GJ, O'Driscoll SW, Yamaguchi K. Elbow arthroplasty using a convertible implant. Tech Hand Up Extrem Surg. 2005;9(3):153–63.
24. Shifrin PG, Johnson DP. Elbow hemiarthroplasty with 20-year follow-up study. A case report and literature review. Clin Orthop. 1990;254:128–33.
25. Miller BS, Harper WP, Hughes JS, Sonnabend DH, Walsh WR. Regional antibiotic prophylaxis in elbow surgery. J Shoulder Elbow Surg. 2004;13(1):57–9.
26. Kamineni S, Ankem H, Patten DK. Anatomic relationship of the radial nerve to the elbow joint: clinical implications of safe pin placement. Clin Anat. 2009;22(6):684–8.
27. McKee MD, Pugh DM, Richards RR, Pedersen E, Jones C, Schemitsch EH. Effect of humeral condylar resection on strength and functional outcome after semiconstrained total elbow arthroplasty. J Bone Joint Surg Am. 2003;85-A(5):802–7.
28. Sanchez-Sotelo J, Morrey BF. Linked elbow replacement: a salvage procedure for distal humeral nonunion. Surgical technique. J Bone Joint Surg Am. 2009;91 Suppl 2:200–12.
29. Parsons M, O'Brien RJ, Hughes JS. Elbow hemiarthroplasty for acute and salvage reconstruction of intra-articular distal humerus fractures. Tech Shoulder Elbow Surg. 2005;6(2):87–97.

Reoperative Concerns in Fractures of the Radial Head and Proximal Ulna

11

Scott G. Edwards

Abstract

Traditionally, proximal ulna and radius fractures have been underestimated as to their importance in providing stability and contributing to the long-term outcome of elbow fractures. Most of the research and clinical discussions have revolved around supracondylar injuries; however, the tight tolerances of elbow anatomy make it such that the olecranon, coronoid, and radial head also have important roles in reestablishing elbow function after injury. Most elbow surgeons now agree that the medial coronoid facet is very important to restore after trauma. Furthermore, the importance of the radial ulnar joint as well as the ulnohumeral joint cannot be underestimated to the long-term prognosis of elbow reconstruction after fracture. There are now a multitude of implant types, including the standard plating varieties with locked and unlocked screw options, as well as intramedullary devices. In recent years, there has been a development of several systems that can reestablish radial head anatomy as well as radial head replacements. The elbow surgeon now has more options than ever to help in the reconstruction of the patient's elbow. However, despite all of these new tools, issues such as nonunion, malunion, posttraumatic arthritis, and continued instability may result. This chapter looks into those treatment options and identifies pearls that may be useful in both the primary and revision settings.

Keywords

Olecranon • Fracture • Coronoid • Facet • Ulnohumeral • Radioulnar

Key Points

- The distal portion of the elbow joint traditionally has been underappreciated and consequently harbors many problems that remain unresolved.
- Although early motion is desirable in any elbow surgery, it may need to be sacrificed in order to maintain a concentric reduction and achieve successful union.
- Implants currently on the market are not optimal in terms of hardware prominence, soft tissue adherence, and fixation failure with loss of reduction.
- Fixed-angled intramedullary devices for olecranon fractures offer potential solutions to some historic problems.
- The proximal ulna, especially the coronoid, cannot be considered a 2D structure. Often 3D imaging, such as CT scan, is required fully to appreciate the challenges posed by the fracture.

(continued)

S.G. Edwards, MD (✉)
Center for Hand and Elbow Specialists,
Georgetown University Hospital, 1-Main West,
3800 Reservoir Road, NW, Washington, DC 20007, USA
e-mail: sgel@gunet.georgetown.edu

S.F.M. Duncan (ed.), *Reoperative Hand Surgery*,
DOI 10.1007/978-1-4614-2373-7_11,

- Careful consideration must be given to the reduction and fixation of the coronoid process, the medial coronoid facet, and medial wall of the coronoid.
- Allograft and autograft reconstructions of coronoid and radial head should be avoided.
- Protect soft tissue repairs and tenuous bony fixation with hinged external fixation.
- Complications are far more easily prevented than treated.
- Outcomes in treating posttraumatic contracture and heterotopic ossification are more predictable than nonunion, malunion, and instability.

Introduction

Traditionally, the discussion pertaining to elbow fractures tends to focus on supracondylar humerus fractures. Receiving less attention is the very important, and arguably more complex, distal portion of the joint. It is comprised of three separate articulations, the ulnohumeral, radiohumeral, and radioulnar joints, each with their own goals for function and series of complications following trauma. Further, any pathology present in the elbow inevitably influences the function at the adjacent wrist either directly or indirectly. The elbow remains an unforgiving joint, and the room for error is very small when addressing traumatic injuries to the proximal ulna and radius. Consequently, complications with elbow trauma are inevitable. Elbow revision surgery is one of the most difficult orthopedic surgeries in the anatomy, both conceptually and technically. This chapter is intended to assist surgeons in avoiding problems before they happen and managing these problems when they happen.

Indications and Contraindications

- Traumatic elbow surgery should be performed definitively within 24 h from the initial injury.
- Olecranon fractures must be identified as stable or unstable injuries in order to allocate appropriate treatment.
- The metaphyseal-diaphyseal junction is an area of high risk for nonunion and malunion and should be scrutinized carefully. Patients should be counseled appropriately.
- Clinical presentations, rather than radiographs, determine the operative indications for radial head and neck fractures.

In order to prevent certain complications, surgical intervention to a traumatic elbow should be performed within 24 h from the initial injury [1–4]. If the patient is medically unstable, delayed intervention may be elected until the patient is more stable. It is also preferable for the initial surgical intervention to be definitive and resist the temptation to return to the operating room for a staged procedure, particularly in the acute phases of the injury. Therefore, if an injury is outside the limits of the surgeon's comfort level, it is our belief that the patient's outcome would be better if the surgeon delayed the surgery until more expertise may be consulted. In other words, if given the choice of provisionally fixing the elbow or delaying surgery until definitive fixation may be obtained, the surgeon should choose the latter.

The indications for operative treatment vary depending on the particular injury. The following paragraphs summarize the indications for operative intervention for each part of the anatomy.

Proximal Ulna

Olecranon

Only completely nondisplaced olecranon fractures may be treated nonoperatively. Even with nondisplaced cases, patients may opt for operative management in order to avoid prolonged immobilization in a cast. Any displacement of the olecranon cannot be reduced and stabilized by closed means and requires open reduction and internal fixation.

Ulna Metaphysis-Diaphysis Junction

Comminuted fractures and all displaced fractures distal to the midpoint of the semilunar notch are considered unstable and require operative intervention. Although simple nondisplaced fractures of the metaphyseal-diaphyseal junction may be treated nonoperatively, vigilance is required as these fractures tend to drift into displacement with time even with proper immobilization and compliant activity modification. The degree of fracture displacement in the metaphyseal-diaphyseal junction is often difficult to assess with common radiographs. Despite this challenge, it is imperative that the alignment of the proximal ulna be anatomic or the effects at the proximal radioulnar joint will be detrimental.

Radial Head and Neck

The radial head and neck heal very well nonoperatively, making operative intervention only indicated in three situations: (1) open fracture, (2) bone fragments blocking supination or pronation, or (3) the buttress of the radial head is required to stabilize the elbow that otherwise has been compromised by associated ligamentous or other bony injuries. Certainly, there are parameters reported in the literature to predict joint blocking or instability, but the most reliable method to definitively determine the need for operative intervention is to take the joints through an arc of motion under local, regional, or general anesthesia. For example, local anesthesia may be easily administered in the office setting to evaluate for bony blockage during the pronosupination arc. General anesthesia should be reserved for cases that are highly suspicious for instability or blockage so that the surgeon is prepared to surgically intervene in the same sitting.

Combination Injuries

Combined injuries often impart complex instability patterns to the elbow and usually require operative intervention. If fracture patterns do not necessarily suggest a need for fixation by themselves but the joint stability remains uncertain, examination under anesthesia tends to be the best way to determine the need for operative management. In these cases, general anesthesia should be used so that the surgeon is prepared to surgically intervene in the same sitting.

Preoperative History and Considerations

When managing isolated injuries to the proximal ulna and radius, preoperative management is similar to other orthopedic injuries. A history of the injury itself is important to determine if the energy is appropriate to cause such an injury or whether the bone is osteopenic or pathologic. Careful examination is necessary to exclude other less obvious injuries. Equally important as trauma clearance is the patient's medical clearance. Proper consultations may be required to determine the patient's operative and anesthetic risks.

Proper preoperative planning is necessary for every operative candidate. Isolated fractures of the proximal ulna or radius require little more diagnostic studies than common radiographs. An oblique view of the proximal radioulnar joint may be helpful in some cases. CT scans, particularly with 3D reconstructions, are reserved for more complex or combined injuries, especially injuries involving the coronoid and radial head. An assessment of associated ligamentous stability, either by physical exam or indirectly from imaging studies, should be attempted, but discussions of these techniques are beyond the scope of this chapter.

Once the magnitude of the injury has been established and the areas of anatomy have been identified requiring operative intervention, the surgeon must determine the best approach to the problem or problems. Ideally, the incision or incisions chosen should expose the necessary anatomy to achieve all operative goals without inflicting needless dissection.

Certain injuries are at particular high risk of developing heterotopic ossification. Patients with fracture-dislocations involving the radial head should be considered candidates for some sort of prophylaxis, as should patients who undergo delayed, repeat, or revision surgery.

Surgical Treatment

Proximal Ulna

Olecranon

Operative Approach

A longitudinal posterior incision is traditionally required for adequate exposure of the olecranon. The length of incision begins at the most proximal point of the olecranon, curves laterally around the olecranon prominence, and continues distally along the subcutaneous border of the ulna enough to expose the fracture and place the necessary hardware. The subcutaneous flaps are retracted with the deep fascia and periosteum in a full-thickness manner.

Stable

Transverse, displaced fractures proximal to the midpoint of the semilunar notch may be treated with several options. Traditionally, tension banding techniques have been reserved for this fracture pattern. The technique was described to theoretically convert the bending forces of the olecranon fragment to compressive ones. It is important to realize that this conversion of bending to compression forces has not been proven either clinically or in a biomechanics laboratory [5] Despite this, the technique has been popular for many years. Recently, there has been a trend away from this technique for more rigid constructs, such as plating. Most would agree that plating provides a more rigid construct over tension banding [6, 7]. While it has been well accepted that tension banding has a lower profile than plating and theoretically will have less need for hardware removal, this has not been demonstrated in the literature. Removal rates of 20–100% have been reported for tension banding [7–10], nearly equal to that of plating [11–13]. The recent application of intramedullary nailing to olecranon fractures has been proposed as a method that combines the strength of plating with the relative imperceptibility of nailing [14]. These claims have not yet been validated, but the concept has merit and appears promising.

Fractures are usually reduced with a tenaculum under direct visualization. It is important to expose the fracture medially and laterally to assess the adequacy of reduction and remove any interposed tissue. Extending the elbow and reducing tension of the triceps tendon may facilitate reduction until provisional fixation may be placed. Once reduced, either two parallel 0.062-in. Kirschner pins or a 7.3-mm partially

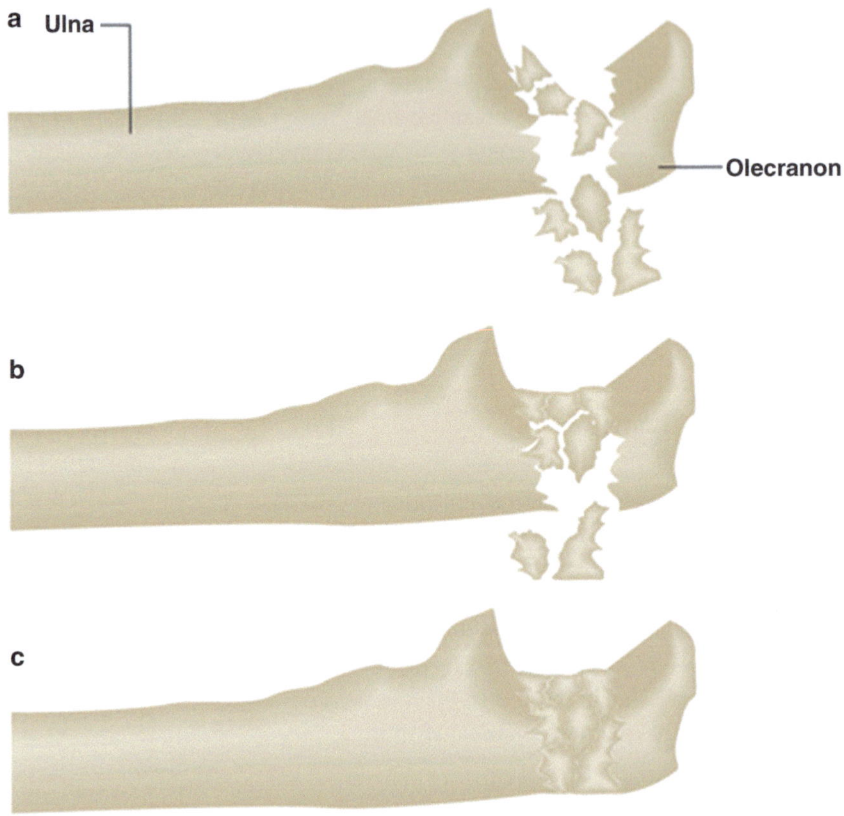

Fig. 11.1 Layer technique for comminuted olecranon fractures. Reduction begins with the fragments of the articular surface. Sequentially reduce fragments working toward the posterior cortex. Note the progressive reduction depicted in images (a), (b), and (c)

threaded cancellous screw may be placed antegrade across the fracture site. Traditionally, 18-gauge stainless steel wire is used to tension the construct in a figure eight fashion. Some surgeons have advocated using #5 braided suture for the same purpose, with the intention of avoiding the soft tissue irritability of the metal wire. Whether this is successful is entirely anecdotal.

Unstable

Comminuted fractures or fractures extending distal from the semilunar notch are considered unstable and are not amendable by any form of tension banding. Plating has been the standard fixation for these fractures [15, 16]. While these implants are strong and reliable, they have high rates of soft tissue irritation and often require hardware removal [11–13]. Recently, intramedullary nails have been developed to overcome the shortcomings of traditional olecranon fixations in terms of soft tissue irritation and the subsequent need for removal. Of the three intramedullary nails currently on the market, only one (OlecraNail™, Mylad Orthopedic Solutions) is indicated for unstable comminuted fractures. Similar to a locking plate, this particular nail has a fixed-angled design and rigidly stabilizes bone fragments in all planes. A recent biomechanical study compared nailing to locked plating for unstable olecranon fracture fixation in a cadaveric model [14]. Both implants controlled fragments equally well and survived an equal number of cycles. The nail, however, held fragments stable under statistically significantly greater maximal loads, suggesting that nailing may be of benefit to patients that must weight-bear with their upper extremities in the immediate postoperative period. At the very least, nailing appears biomechanically comparable to locked plating for unstable fractures and may have an advantage clinically of less soft tissue irritation.

Regardless of the fixation method chosen, the majority of complications arising from unstable olecranon fracture management arise from improper reduction. The sigmoid notch must be scrutinized. Anything short of a perfectly anatomic reduction will result in loss of motion in the short term and posttraumatic degeneration in the long term. One common method utilized by surgeons is to reduce the easily visible posterior cortex and assume that the anterior surface followed. While this technique may work well for simple fracture patterns, one must realize that in comminuted fracture patterns, the articular portion of the olecranon is often detached from the posterior cortex. With these fractures, the joint surface may be completely malreduced despite an anatomic reduction of the posterior cortex. A more appropriate technique is to reduce the bone in layers beginning with the articular surface (Fig. 11.1). Once the joint is anatomically reduced, the next layer of fragmented bone just posterior to the joint is reduced before moving on the next layer. Some fragments may be

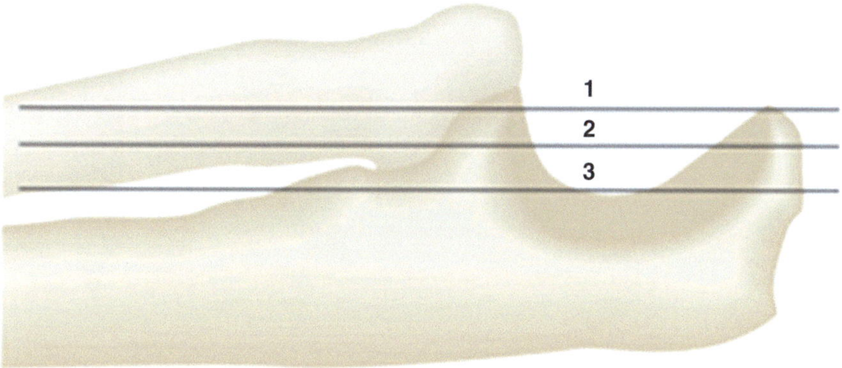

Fig. 11.2 Classification of coronoid fractures based on fracture size according to Regan and Morrey [17]: type I, avulsion of the tip of the coronoid process; type II, a fracture involving less than 50% of the coronoid process; type III, a fracture involving more than 50% of the coronoid process

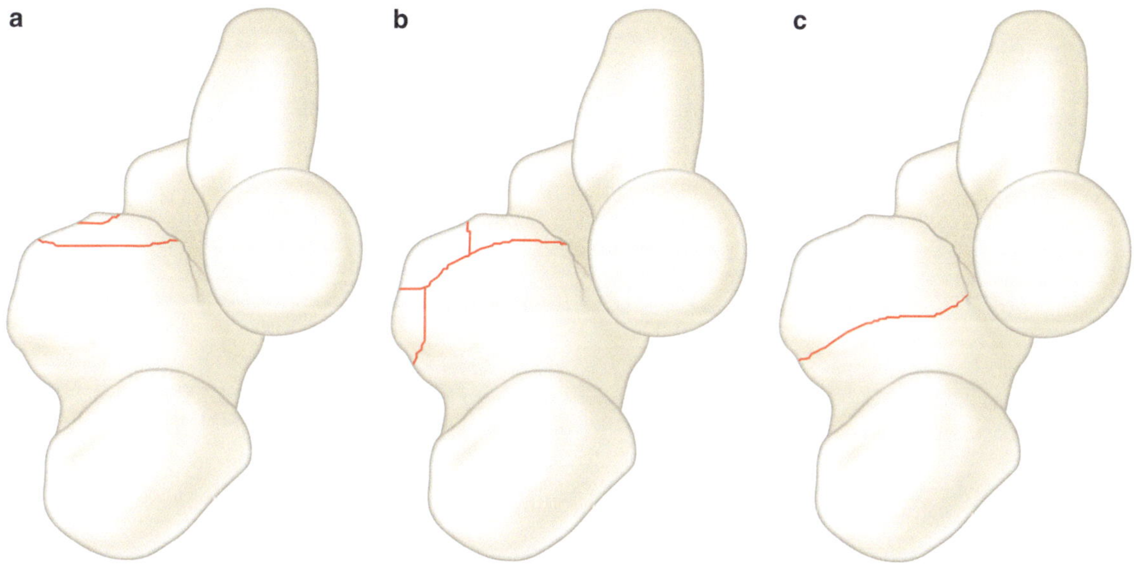

Fig. 11.3 O'Driscoll et al. classification of coronoid fractures based on the fragmentation pattern: type I, a transverse fracture of the tip of the coronoid process; type II, a fracture of the anteromedial facet of the coronoid process; type III, a fracture of the base of the coronoid process

trapped between two other fragments, while others may need provisional fixation such as 0.045-in. Kirschner wire. With this technique, the posterior cortex is the last layer, not the first, to be reduced. After all layers have been reduced and provisional fixed, definitive fixation is placed, usually one or more plates and screws, or a fixed-angled intramedullary device.

Coronoid

Management of coronoid fractures has been evolving in recent years. Only recently has the importance of its three-dimensionality been appreciated, but still not fully understood. Morrey proposed a classification system based on the 2D lateral view of the elbow radiograph (Fig. 11.2) [17]. According to this familiar classification, type I (tip) fractures rarely require surgical treatment, type II (midportion) fractures may require surgical treatment, and type III (base) fractures usually require surgical treatment. The coronoid can no longer be thought of as a 2D image viewed on the lateral elbow radiograph. While fractures may appear to fragment in this fashion on plain radiographs, in actuality, coronoid fracture patterns are far more complex and often cannot be fully realized without 3D imagery (Fig. 11.3) [18]. Specific indications for coronoid fixation based on radiographic evaluation, even sophisticated 3D analysis, are still evolving and, at this time, are best determined by intraoperative evaluation for stability.

The coronoid may be thought of as three separate regions: (1) the coronoid process, (2) the medial facet, and (3) the medial wall. Each region, if compromised, may impart instability to the elbow and consequently must be individually addressed. Deforming forces generally tend to displace fragments anteriorly and distally (Fig. 11.4). Fixation must resist these substantial forces, ideally, in order to allow early postoperative motion. Unfortunately, early motion may not be

Fig. 11.4 Deforming forces on coronoid fractures. Once the coronoid is fractured (**a**), the triceps pulls the ulna posteriorly as the elbow moved into extension (**b**)

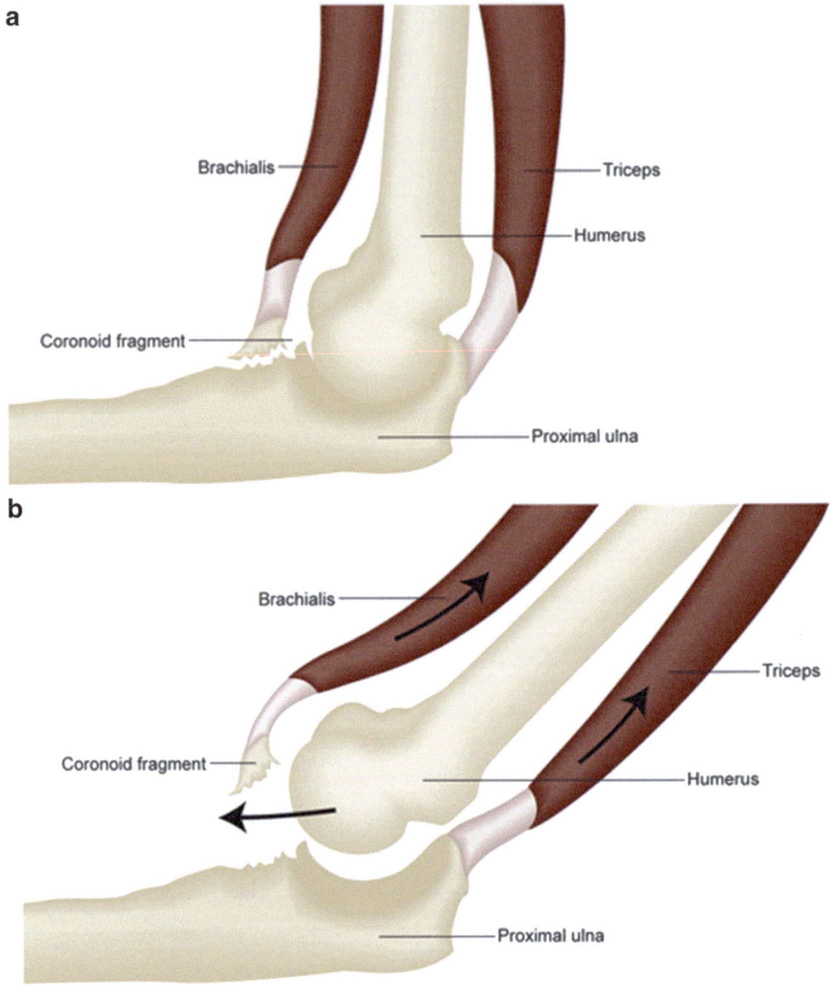

possible when dealing with these fractures. Many fixation options are tenuous and may require protection with joint immobilization. Alternatively, hinged external fixation may neutralize the deforming forces during joint motion and should be considered in select cases.

Operative Approach

Challenges of managing coronoid fractures reside in three categories: (1) identification of fracture pattern, (2) surgical approach and reduction, and (3) rigid fixation. Each category builds on the one before. As previously stated, identification of the fracture pattern and operative planning can be greatly assisted with 3D imagery techniques. Once it is determined which fragments need to be addressed, surgeons must plan their approach. This may take other associated injuries into consideration. Skin incisions tend to be relatively irrelevant since subcutaneous tunnels may be developed readily and circumferentially around the elbow. The decision to approach the joint through facial planes seems to be more of an important issue.

We rarely use an anterior approach, though others have used it very well. We prefer to either address the coronoid from either a posteromedial or anteromedial approach. A posteromedial approach is well suited for the reduction of smaller coronoid fragments or anchoring the anterior capsule back to bone (Fig. 11.5). After exposing the posterior ulna, the medial portion of the ulna adjacent to the coronoid is dissected in a subperiosteal fashion. At the level of the coronoid, the ulnar nerve typically will lie in the flexor carpi ulnaris (FCU) and should be safe from a dissection remaining on the bone, but care must be exercised. Also at risk is the medical collateral ligament (MCL) which is attached to the medial facet. Detachment of the ligament should be avoided as it will compromise the vascularity of the fragment and sacrifice the stability of the joint. If reduction proves impossible without detachment of the ligament, then it should be detached at its origin on the humerus and reattached with bone tunnels or suture anchors. This proximal repair is far more predictable than reattaching distally.

Reduction of the coronoid may be facilitated if there is an associated olecranon fracture. Access to the coronoid may be achieved through the window provided by a displaced olecranon fracture. After the coronoid is reduced and fixed, the olecranon may be repaired. While this technique makes conceptual sense, its practical execution can be problematic since it is often difficult to reconfigure the semilunar notch without an intact or anatomically reduced olecranon to guide the reduction of the coronoid.

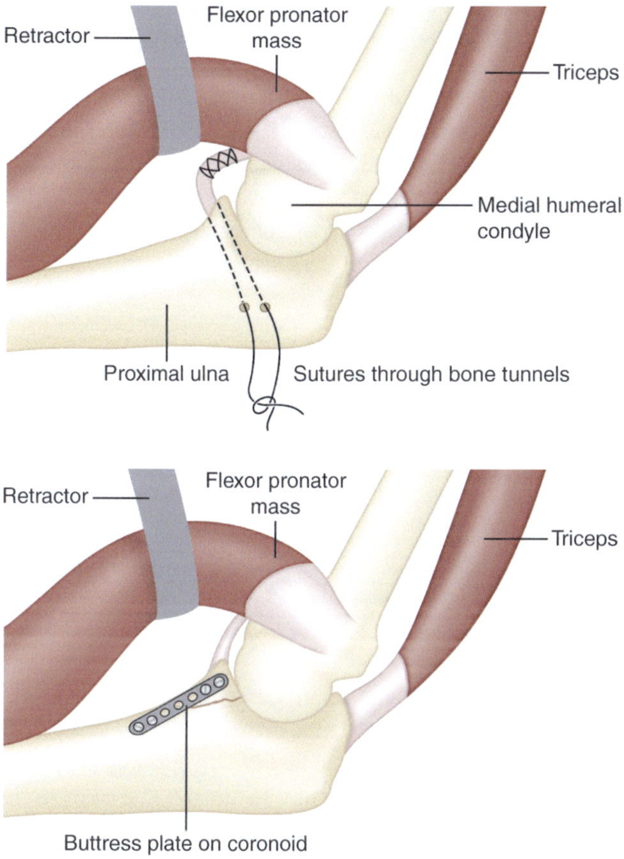

Fig. 11.5 Posteromedial approach to the coronoid and anterior capsule. (**a**) Anterior capsule is repaired to ulna with suture through bone tunnels; (**b**) buttress plate repairs coronoid to ulna

If the coronoid involvement is extensive, more exposure may be necessary. In these cases, we prefer an anteromedial approach through the FCU (Fig. 11.6) [19]. It is preferable for postoperative rehabilitation to leave the posterior aspect of the FCU attached to the medial epicondyles. Once the anterior FCU is detached from the medial epicondyles and reflected distally, the exposed brachialis is retracted anteriorly for a complete view of all portions of the coronoid. We routinely decompress the ulna nerve, but do not transpose. The same considerations are given to the MCL as with this approach and as with the posteromedial approach previously described.

Once the fragments are reduced, the surgeon has an assortment of fixation techniques from which to choose. Larger fragments may be secured with screws directed either posterior to anterior, or anterior to posterior depending on the particular approach. It is important to understand the limitation of screw fixation. They simply grasp the fragment rather than buttress it. Consequently, in many cases, this fixation must be protected with either temporary immobilization or neutralization with a hinged external fixator for 3 weeks. Plates may be used to buttress the deforming forces, but the amount of hardware necessary to capture all aspects of the coronoid can be substantial if multiple fragments are involved. Small fragments may be excised, and the anterior capsule may be repaired to the remaining coronoid using bone tunnels or suture anchors. While this soft tissue repair can impart stability to the joint, it should be protected by a hinged external fixator for 3 weeks, especially if a relatively large portion of the coronoid is excised.

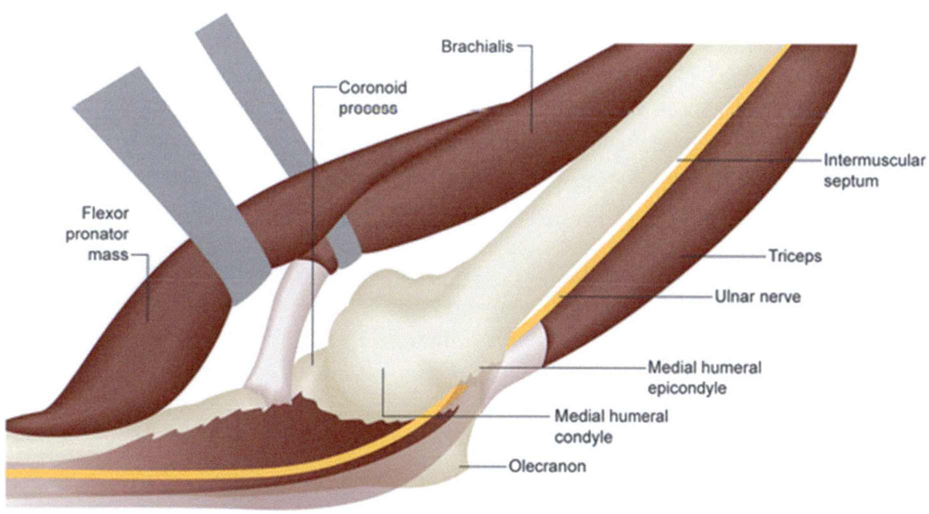

Fig. 11.6 Anteromedial approach to the coronoid and anterior capsule

Optimizing Outcomes

- Tension banding is not appropriate for unstable olecranon fractures.
- If tension banding or plate fixation is used, counsel patients that hardware removal may be necessary at a future date.
- Fixed-angled intramedullary nailing seems promising as it offers rigid fixation without the need for hardware removal.
- Repair the comminuted olecranon in layers beginning with the articular surface and progressing posteriorly.
- With comminuted olecranon fractures, use the humeral trochlea as a template to confirm anatomic reduction rather than the posterior cortex.
- Involvement of the proximal to middle third of the ulna has a high incidence of malunion and nonunion.
- Coronoid fractures must be visualized in 3Ds. All three aspects must be stabilized: coronoid process, medial facet, and medial wall.
- Rigid fixation is recommended for coronoid stabilization. If rigid fixation cannot be achieved, consider a hinged external fixator to allow early motion or resort to prolonged immobilization until adequate healing.

Complications

Nonunion

The most common site for nonunion is at the junction of metaphysis and diaphysis of the ulna [20]. This may be due in part by relative paucity of vascularity and in part by surgeon error. As in many other high-risk areas for nonunion, a relative vascular "watershed" phenomenon occurs at this part of the ulna [21]. As a result, technical errors are less tolerated, such as poor apposition of bony fragments, improper fixation methods, or poor alignment.

> *Pearls and Pitfalls*: Fractures at the metaphyseal-diaphyseal junction need special attention as it is a common area for nonunion. Good bony apposition, anatomic alignment, minimal soft tissue stripping, and rigid fixation are imperative.

A fracture in this area should alert the surgeon to scrutinize the reduction carefully but, at the same time, minimize soft tissue stripping. This poses a challenge since this area is difficult to visualize without significant stripping.

Once a nonunion has occurred, it has been our experience that changing the biologic milieu to encourage healing can be extremely challenging. Bone quality quickly deteriorates, so fixation may be compromised and hardware may loosen or pull out of soft bone. Segmental defects and gaps of missing bone are commonplace. In other areas, these gaps would normally be closed and the bone shortened in order to achieve acceptable bony apposition. Closing periarticular gaps, however, such as this in the olecranon, will shorten the radius of the semilunar notch and likely will result in joint incongruity. Therefore, significant compression in these intra-articular nonunions should be avoided. Consequently, in addition to rigid fixation, aggressive use of autograft and even off-label use of bone morphogenic protein (BMP) have been routine in our practice. In our series evaluating BMP use for upper extremity nonunions, we observed that fracture defects of less than 4 cm and the presence of vascularized soft tissue are good prognostic indicators for success using BMP techniques.

> *Pearls and Pitfalls*: If BMP is being used, be sure the carrier is in contact with vascularized tissue, as opposed to dense fibrous tissue. This will allow the BMP to bring the necessary viable cells into the area. In the setting of nonunion, localizing healthy vascularize tissue may be difficult. If no vascular periosteum is available, approximate the BMP carrier against exposed muscle tissue.

Should nonunion repairs be unsuccessful, alternative measures must be considered. If the proximal fragment is small, the olecranon may be excised and the triceps attached to the distal ulna stump. It is important to attach the triceps to the posterior portion of the ulna to maximize the leverage allowing for strong elbow extension. In our experience, we tend to use bone tunnels, though some have successfully reported on suture anchors. With either method, the repair needs to be protected. We typically immobilize the elbow in 45° of extension for 4 weeks and progressively allow 10° of additional flexion each week.

When the size of the proximal olecranon fragment exceeds 50% and joint stability is compromised, linked total elbow arthroplasty (TEA) can be effective in that it bypasses the nonunion and stabilizes the joint. In these nonunion cases, greater portions of olecranon must be excised, and reattachment of the triceps becomes challenging.

> *Pearls and Pitfalls*: Avoid attempting to attach the triceps tendon directly to the prosthetic implant. Achieving a direct repair is far more predictable. Fractional lengthening of the triceps or an anconeus tendon transfer may add the necessary length. While extending the triceps with tendon graft is less predictable, it is preferable to attaching the triceps to metal.

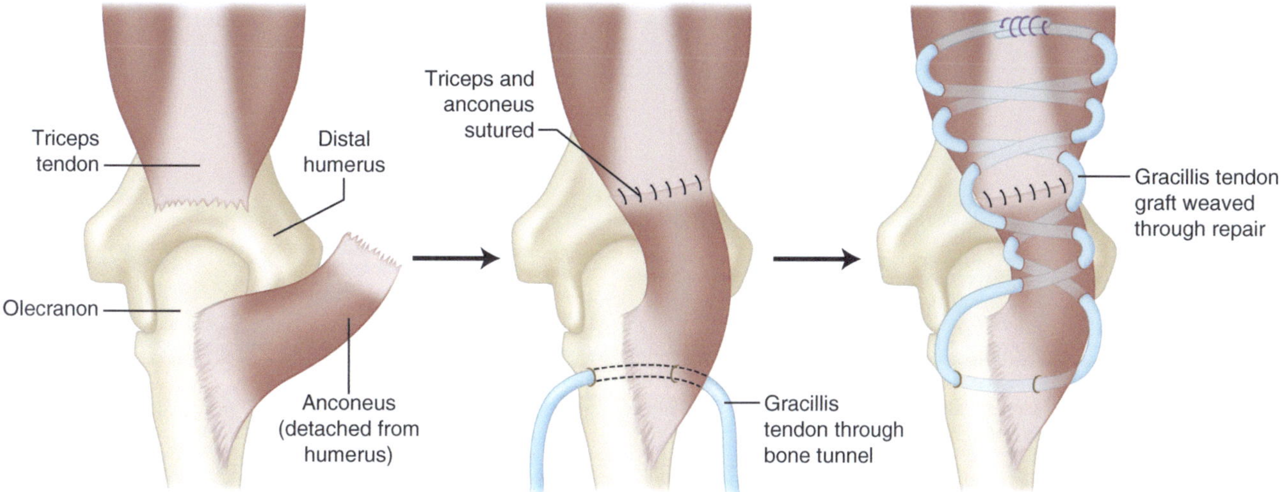

Fig. 11.7 Triceps tendon reconstruction. (**a**, **b**) Anconeus is detached from humerus and is sutured to triceps tendon stump; (**c**) repair is augmented by weaving gracilis tendon graft

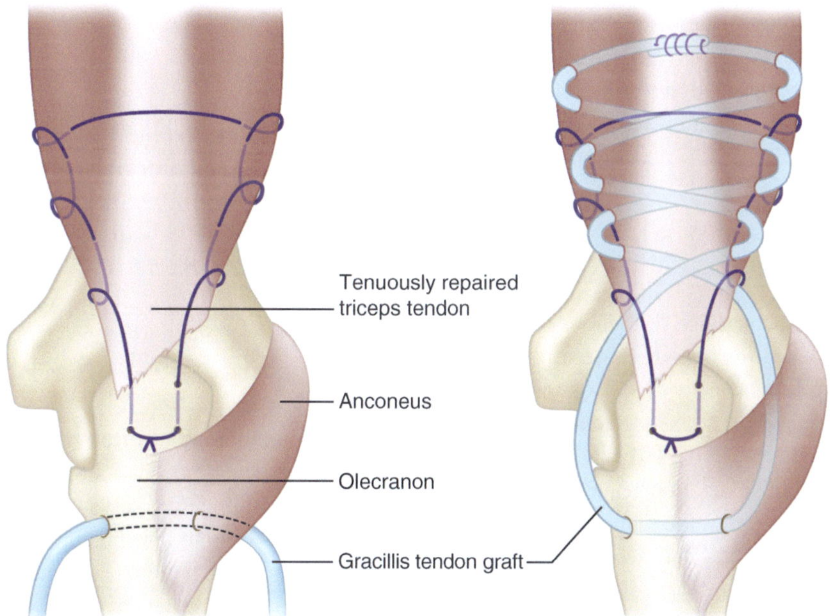

Fig. 11.8 Triceps tendon augmentation. (**a**, **b**) A tenuous repair of the triceps tendon to the olecranon may be augmented by weaving gracilis tendon graft through tendon and anchoring the graft through bone tunnels in the ulna

In our experience, attaching tendon to the metal of the prosthesis usually always results in triceps avulsion within a year. Fractional lengthening of the triceps has been used successfully in our practice to gain up to 6 cm of length which decreases the tension of the repair. If more length is desired, the anconeus may be detached from its proximal attachment on the humerus and used as an extension bridge for triceps attachment or as augmentation for tenuous repairs (Fig. 11.7). In most repeat surgeries, however, the anconeus is fibrotic and not a good option for transfer or augmentation. Extension graft using autograft or allograft gracilis tendons may serve as a bridge graft for attachment or augmentation of a tenuous repair (Fig. 11.8). In our experience, these graft reconstructions are unpredictable and often result in failure.

Traditionally, allograft reconstructions following excision of large portions of the proximal ulna have been disappointing, resulting in resorption or infection. We have used allograft reconstruction successfully in one instance and attributed this success to the fact that the portion of the ulna replaced by allograft was flanked on either side by viable bone with its own vascular supply (Fig. 11.9). This attempt

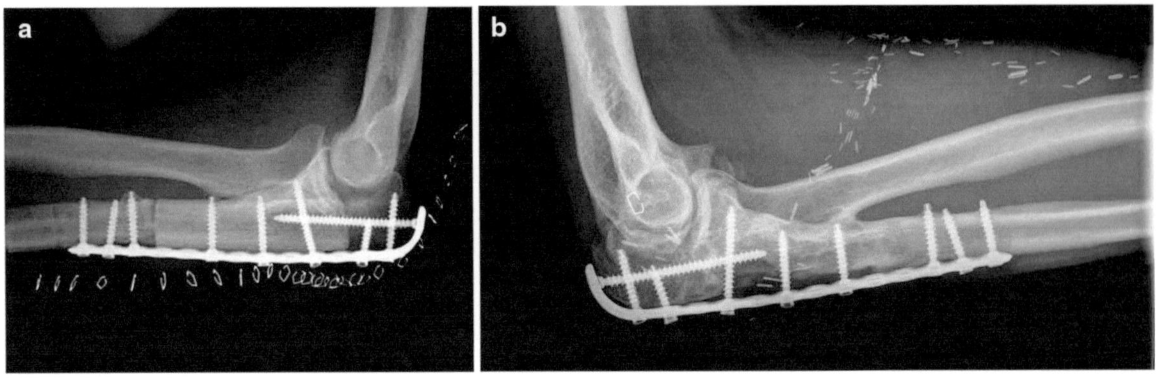

Fig. 11.9 Proximal ulna reconstruction using allograft. (**a**) Segmental bone was used to reconstruct an unsalvageable proximal ulna fracture; (**b**) 5 years after surgery, the allograft remains viable

differed from previous failed attempts in that previous grafts tended to be terminal portions of olecranon which relies entirely on the vascularity from the distal stump which, we believe, is inadequate to revascularize the graft. While in our particular situation, the reconstruction resulted in a successful outcome, we still advocate that en bloc allograft reconstruction is an unpredictable surgery and should be avoided if possible.

Malunion

Malunions at the olecranon can result in loss of motion and degeneration due to joint incongruity. Malunions occur more commonly with comminuted fractures because of the greater risk of inadequate fragment management or improper application of fixation. The previously described technique of "layer" reduction as well as implementation of rigid fixation will reduce the chances of malunion. Should fixation be judged to be inadequate to allow for early motion of the joint, it is far better to immobilize the elbow until union and accept a stiff elbow. Should it be necessary, it is much more predictable to surgically release a stiff elbow than to correct a malunited elbow joint.

Pearls and Pitfalls: Despite the goal of early motion for all elbow injuries, tenuous fixation must be protected even if it means prolonged immobilization. Joint contracture is more predictable to manage than joint incongruity.

Overly aggressive compression of olecranon fragments may change the radius of the semilunar notch and result in malunion. For this reason, compression of intra-articular portions of the proximal ulna should be monitored closely intraoperatively and probably avoided in most unstable fracture patterns. In these situations, locking screw technology lends itself well (Fig. 11.10).

Pearls and Pitfalls: Compression of nonunion bony defect involving the intra-articular portion of the joint is contraindicated. Locking nails and plates provide a fixed-angled construct that will allow for optimal fragment control without relying on compression and friction to augment the stabilization. Patients will be able to rehabilitate the elbow joint safely without fear of losing reduction and fixation.

Intra-articular malunions often result in rapid joint degeneration so that by the time a patient presents with pain, malunion correction is futile and a salvage procedure must be considered, such as facial interpositional arthroplasty or TEA, depending on the patient's goals and activity demands. Facial interpositional arthroplasty is reserved for younger patients but often will require revision to a TEA in subsequent years. TEA is reserved for low-demand patients, and patient expectation must be adjusted appropriately. In cases of malunion leading to symptomatic degeneration, unlinked TEA may perform well. In our experience, however, linked TEA has been more predictable with fewer complications.

Extra-articular malunions typically occur at the junction of the metaphysis and diaphysis. Patients with these malunions typically present with either reduced motion or subluxation. Often these patients are misdiagnosed as having residual posterolateral instability or an incompetent annular ligament. This is a bony problem, not a soft tissue one. Correction involves surgical osteotomy. Since nonunions commonly occur in this area of the metaphyseal-diaphyseal junction due to a potential relative vascular insufficiency, osteotomy

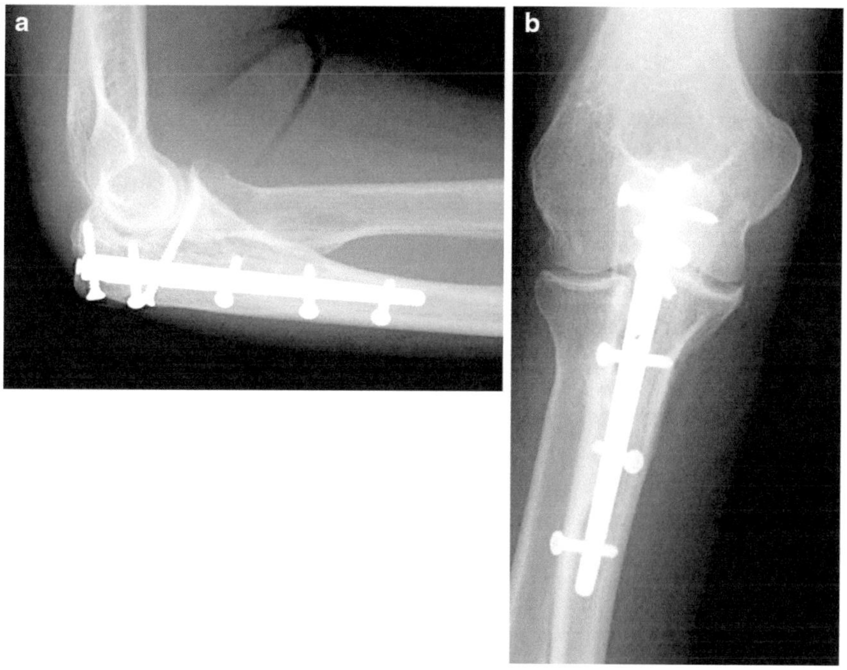

Fig. 11.10 Fixed-angle intramedullary nail addressing a comminuted fracture-dislocation on anteroposterior (**a**) and lateral (**b**) views, now healed (Courtesy of OlecraNail®, Mylad Orthopedic Solutions, McLean, VA)

should be undertaken very carefully. In addition to scrutinizing the realignment of the ulna, careful attention must be given toward appropriate bony apposition, rigid fixation, and consideration of bone grafting and even BMP use.

Subluxation

The two most common instances when subluxation of the elbow occurs following proximal ulna fracture are in cases of a malreduced Monteggia fracture or when the proximal portion of the olecranon has been excised. Even experienced surgeons may believe that the proximal ulna has been reduced anatomically, only to be surprised that the radial head has dislocated by the time of the first postoperative visit. Liberal use of intraoperative fluoroscopy and clinical assessment for subluxation can help to reduce this problem. It is important to acknowledge that the radial head subluxation probably is not the result of an incompetent lateral ligament complex. The only solution is a corrective osteotomy of the ulna, not a lateral collateral or annular ligament repair or reconstruction.

Regarding olecranon excision, while it has been reported that up to 60% of the olecranon may be excised without biomechanical detriment to the elbow [22–24], we believe that all but the smallest excision in the acute traumatic setting has untoward consequences and should be avoided if possible. Only the most comminuted proximal fragment with the poorest bone quality in the lowest-demand patient should be considered for excision. The chances of subluxation rise with associated bony or ligamentous injuries.

Loss of fixation of the coronoid can result in subluxation and dislocation. Without the bony buttress of the coronoid neutralizing the forces across the elbow during normal motion, the humerus will translate anteriorly and distally relative to the ulna. Because coronoid fragments tend to be small and of relatively poor quality, rigid fixation can be very difficult to achieve.

Infection

The elbow lacks an ample soft tissue envelope compared to other joints. As a result, the risk of infection and wound problems should be taken seriously. If a postoperative wound becomes erythematous or dehisces, aggressive measures should be taken. It is not acceptable to place the patient on oral antibiotics for outpatient follow-up. Because of the paucity of soft tissue, it can be assumed that any superficial infection is already, or will soon develop into, a deep infection. Admission with intravenous antibiotics and close monitoring is recommended. If improvement is not measurable within 24 h of initiating treatment, the surgeon should have a low threshold for surgical debridement. In cases of severe infection involving the joint and bone, frequent debridements that may sacrifice the joint architecture may be necessary to eradicate the infection. Using a static external fixator and antibiotic beads or spacers may help in these cases. After at least 6–12 weeks on antibiotics, we recommend waiting an additional 12 weeks to obtain appropriate blood tests to clinically validate that the infection has been eradicated before considering reconstructive efforts.

> *Pearls and Pitfalls*: Observe a patient for several weeks after all antibiotics have been discontinued before embarking on definitive reconstruction.

Some might feel that this protocol is overly conservative; however, the author believes that there is only one good chance for reconstructive efforts to be successful and is not willing to jeopardize that chance because of impetuousness.

Optimizing Outcomes

- The junction of the metaphysis and diaphysis is particularly at risk for nonunion for a variety of reasons and should be treated aggressively.
- Intra-articular nonunions of the proximal ulna should not be compressed, but spanned with locking nails or plates and augmented with autograft.
- In cases of olecranon excision, make every attempt to repair the triceps tendon to native ulna rather than resorting to graft reconstructions or repairing to metal prostheses.
- In general, outcomes for linked TEA have been more predictable than unlinked TEA.
- Residual instability should call attention to either a malreduced ulna or insufficiency of the olecranon or coronoid.
- Aggressive treatment of infections should be followed by patience to resist the temptation to proceed with definitive reconstruction prematurely.

Proximal Radius

Operative Approach

Radial head and neck fractures may be approached through a Kocher incision. This incision may be extended proximally by detaching the extensor wad from the lateral epicondyles, but the dissection must remain anterior to the lateral collateral ligament in order to preserve its integrity. Should detachment be necessary, it is removed at its proximal origin on the humerus to be later reattached with suture anchors or bone tunnels. Distal extension of the Kocher incision may be made by pronating the forearm, which pulls the posterior interosseous nerve out of the operating field.

> *Pearls and Pitfalls*: It is preferable to preserve the annular ligament. Sacrificing the annular ligament does not lead to the instability as previous teachings have stated [25, 26], but its incision and repair will likely cause more fibrosis that may limit supination and pronation.

Simple radial head fractures may be treated with headless compression screws. A commonly displaced fragment from the anteromedial portion of the radial head, however, is not directly accessed through a lateral approach. Extreme manipulation in supination and pronation may help to gain access to this problematic fragment. In some cases, screws may need to be advanced through intact bone as the displaced fragment is lagged into proper position. Overcompression of osteopenic or comminuted radial head fragments can cause the articular surface to deform and result in loss of reduction (Fig. 11.11). Bone grafting used in conjunction with adjustable compression screws currently on the market offers a good solution to this problem.

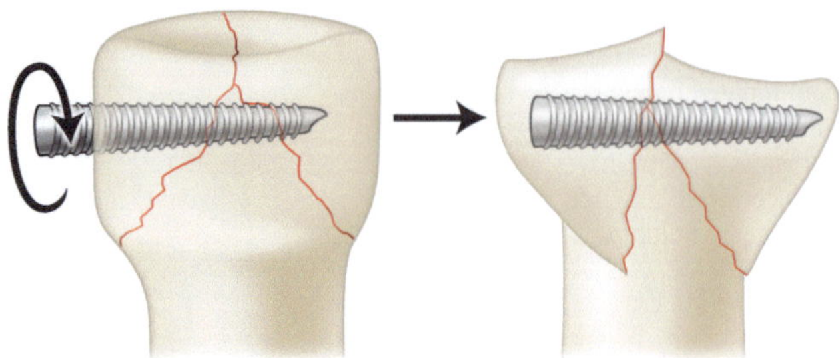

Fig. 11.11 Overcompression of radial head by a headless compression screw

Plastic deformation of the radial head fragments during the time of injury may compromise reduction and overall outcome. If the radial head does not reduce easily or if it does not appear concentric with the capitellum following reduction attempts, the surgeon must suspect that some degree of plastic deformation has occurred. To remedy this problem, the articular surface must be reduced using the adjacent capitellum as a template.

> *Pearls and Pitfalls*: In cases of severe radial head deformation, use the capitellum as a template to reconstruct the normal architecture of the radial head articular surface.

This will inevitably leave gaps at the base of the fragment which should be grafted with autologous corticocancellous bone from the olecranon or bone substitute. We prefer corticocancellous grafts primarily for the adjuvant stability they provide to the fixation of the construct. Once the reduction is anatomic and the bone graft is in place, definitive fixation is implanted.

In comminuted articular fractures that involve the radial head and neck, it is helpful to assemble the radial head on the back table. Once the articular surface has been repaired, the head can be secured to the shaft with a plate (Fig. 11.12). Alternatively, screws can be used, but we have found this to be less stable. In especially comminuted cases, rigid fixation is important since union may be delayed. The drawback to this rigid plate fixation is that this requires a significant amount of hardware to remain on the surface of the bone and soft tissue adhesions could pose a problem. Traditionally, we favor stainless steel, low-profile locking plates, given their strong screw tensile strength for providing a fixed-angled

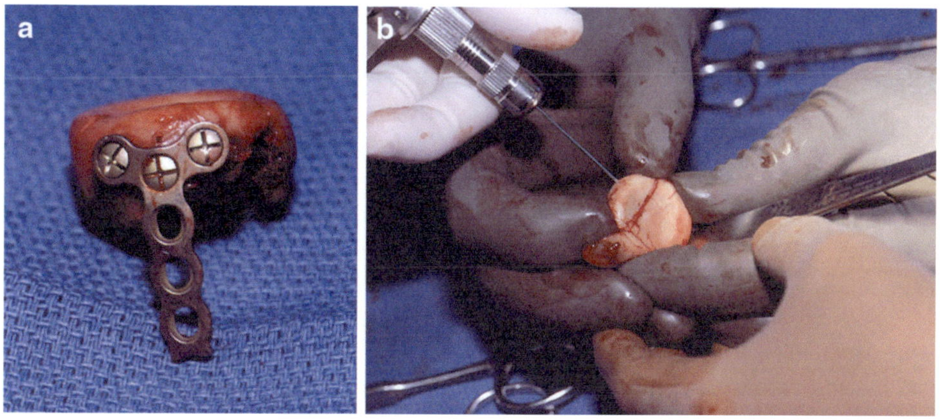

Fig. 11.12 (**a, b**): Radial head repair on the back table in preparation for reimplantation

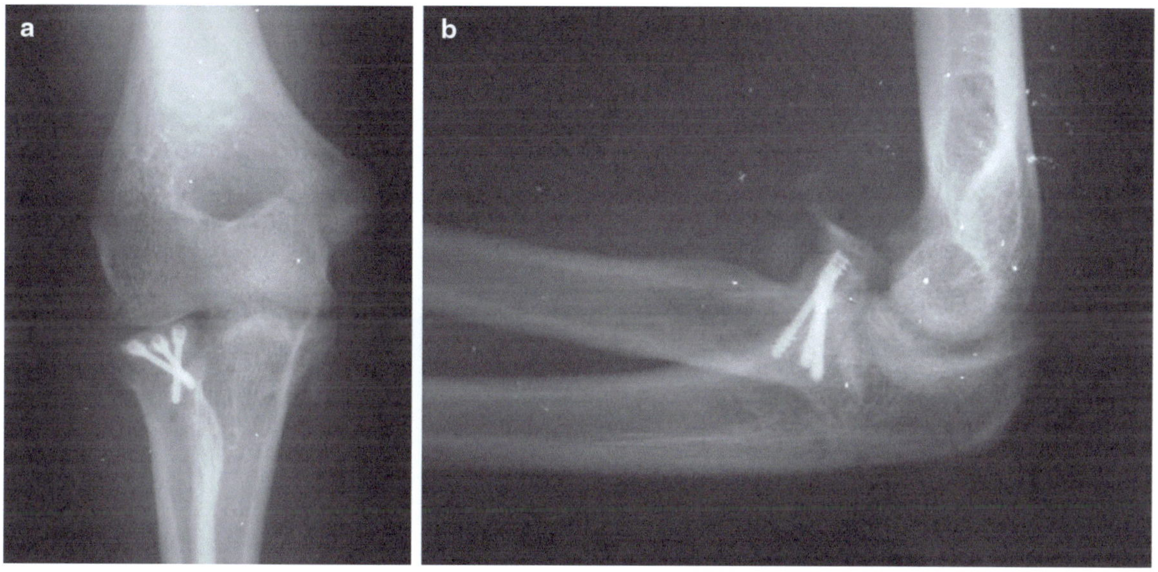

Fig. 11.13 Radial head reconstruction using autograft iliac crest graft. Three years following surgery, the graft remains viable (**a, b**)

buttress and low propensity for adhesions. Recent titanium implants have improved their polishing processes, which have lessened their adhesion potential, but the tensile strength concerns still remain a question in our minds.

Another commonly debated topic is radial head replacement. There has been a recent trend to replace, rather than repair or excise, radial heads [27]. This has led to many reports of complications ranging from chronic pain and capitellar degeneration to rotary instability [28, 29]. Improvements in design and techniques have addressed some of these complications, but surgeons should counsel patients that once a prosthetic radial is implanted, it is likely to require removal in the future. While we prefer to repair the radial head when possible, including up to four-part fractures, we acknowledge the short-term benefits of replacement. Radial head integrity, either comprised of bone or metal, plays an essential role in traumatic complex elbow instability. While experts disagree on whether replacement is preferred to excision in cases of chronic radiocapitellar degeneration, most would agree that excision has no place in the acute setting, particularly if the medial collateral ligament has been compromised [30, 31].

> *Pearls and Pitfalls*: Excision of the radial head in the acute traumatic setting should be avoided.

For these cases where the radial head is irreparable, replacement greatly helps to stabilize the lateral column of the elbow and allows for early postoperative motion.

Our experience with partial or complete allografts has been disappointing as resorption is common within months, which is consistent with previous reports [32]. Alternatively, we have attempted fashioning autograft iliac crest to resemble partial or complete radial heads (Fig. 11.13). Anecdotally, incorporation of these autografts tends to be slightly more reliable, with partial grafts fairing much better than complete grafts. We believe that these autografts should only be considered when other options, such as prosthetic head or hinged external fixator, are not available.

Optimizing Outcomes

- Begin with establishing the articular surface of the radial head before repairing it to the radial shaft.
- Repair with rigid fixation, rather than prosthetic replacement, whenever possible.
- Consider the rigidity, strength, and soft tissue adhesion potential of every implant.
- Be aware of plastic deformation of radial head fragments.
- Reconstitute the articular surface using the capitellum as a template, and fill in the void with bone graft.
- Corticocancellous graft strengthens the overall fixation construct.
- Counsel patients that radial head replacement will probably need to be removed in the future.
- Avoid partial or complete radial head allografts or autografts.

Complications

Malunion

It has been our experience that malunions are particularly challenging to repair satisfactorily for two reasons: First, the bone often is quite compromised, and even the most diligent bone grafting fails to restore its integrity. Second, a malunion at the radiocapitellar joint frequently is subject to significant aberrant forces that accelerate degeneration at the joint. Patients with malunions most commonly present with pain which is more likely than not caused by joint degeneration. At this point, a salvage procedure must be considered since correcting the biomechanics of the malunion will not alleviate the pain.

Placing a radial head prosthesis in areas of degeneration can be problematic since capitellar wear will not be remedied. We reserve radial head replacement (1) for cases in which we suspect medial collateral ligament incompetence, such as a significant previous trauma or autoimmune arthropathy, or (2) in patients who will place significant repetitive stress across the elbow, or (3) if we are fortunate to diagnose the malunion prior to degeneration. Otherwise, we prefer excision.

In cases where radiocapitellar wear is present and excision is contraindicated, radiocapitellar arthroplasty is possible (Fig. 11.14). While this technique has limited indications, it has been a unique solution to an uncommon but devastating problem. The implant lacks long-term data, but the short-term data seems promising.

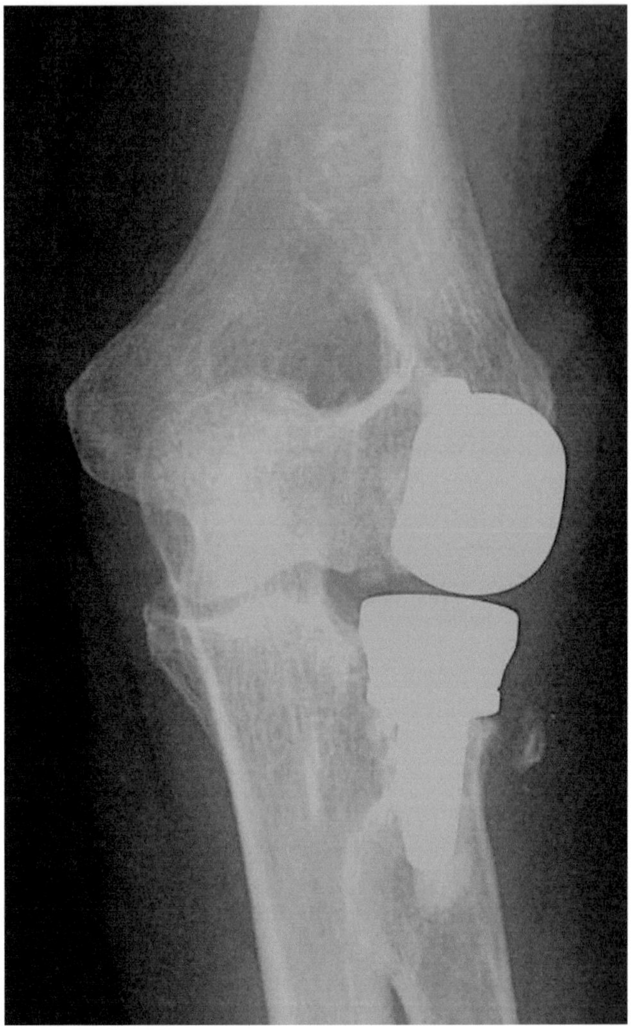

Fig. 11.14 Radiocapitellar arthroplasty (Courtesy of Small Bone Innovations, Morrisville, PA)

Nonunions

It has been our experience that once a radial head or neck has established a nonunion, it becomes very difficult to change the biologic milieu to achieve union. Should repair be attempted, we would recommend considering rigid fixation, liberal use of autologous bone graft, and even BMP. Use of BMP for this nonunion is considered "off-label" and even somewhat debatable, but we have used it successfully on several occasions. Some surgeons are reluctant to use BMP about the elbow, particularly in such close proximity as the radial head for fear of iatrogenic heterotopic ossification (HO), but in our series of BMP for upper extremity nonunion,

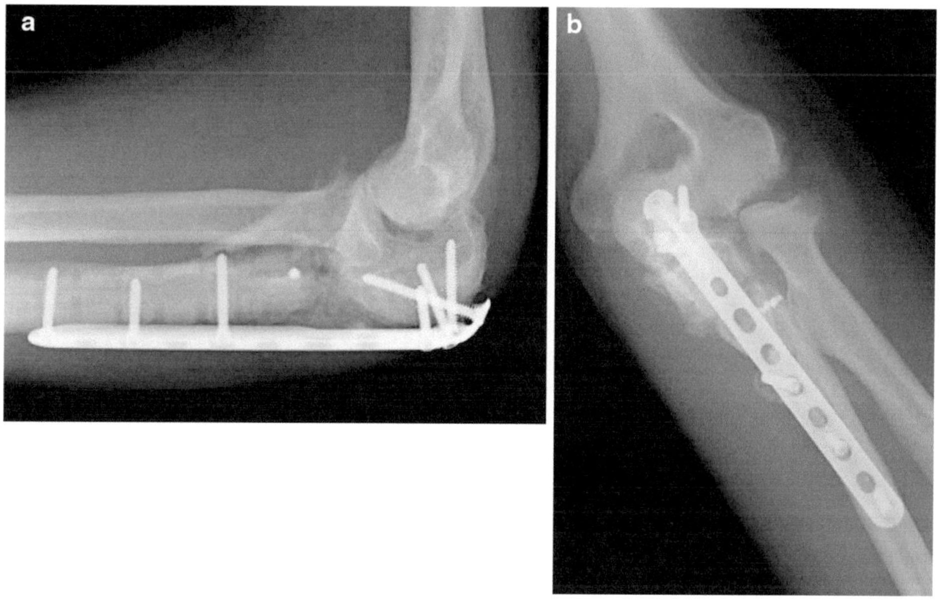

Fig. 11.15 (**a, b**): Proximal ulnar malunion causing subluxation of the radial head. This patient underwent two failed soft tissue procedures, as evidenced by the suture anchor, in a misguided attempt to correct the subluxation. Note the degeneration of the radiocapitellar joint

we could not demonstrate an increased incidence of HO over the normal population.

Generally, we treat radial head nonunions with the same algorithm as we treat radial head malunions. The quality of the bone, the status of the joint, and presence of associated injuries must be evaluated prior to determining which definitive surgical treatment should be recommended.

> *Pearls and Pitfalls*: In cases of radial head malunion and nonunion, it is advisable to have a very low threshold to replace or excise the radial head, rather than attempt repair.

Instability

Residual radial head subluxation is most commonly the result of a malreduced associated proximal ulna fracture. If the subluxation is not associated with a proximal ulna fracture, assess for posterolateral instability and reconstruct if indicated. We prefer to reconstruct with autograft gracilis tendon given its low donor morbidity, adequate length for reconstruction, and comparable strength of tissue to the native LCL. Occasionally, residual rotational instability following a dislocation may occur despite adequate reduction and no or minimal presence of bony injury on plain radiographs. These patients typically present after undergoing one or two needless soft tissue reconstructions only to be still unstable (Fig. 11.15). In perplexing cases like these, CT scans are often helpful in identifying missed bony injuries, especially to the radial head or coronoid, not easily visualized on plain radiographs.

Heterotopic Bone Formation (HO)

Concern for the development of HO begins at the time of elbow injury, as this is the most effective time to start prophylactic treatment. The time between injury and the onset of heterotopic bone formation is generally about 2 weeks, at which point osteoid formation has begun and there is radiographic evidence of soft tissue ossification. Unfortunately, by the time HO is visualized on plain radiographs, the window of opportunity for effective preventative intervention has closed. Therefore, prudent clinicians must identify patients who are at risk for developing HO before it occurs.

While repeat or revision surgery on the elbow has been identified as a major risk factor for HO, surgical technique has been scrutinized as a possible cause as well. McLaughlin recommended that a surgeon should focus on complete excision of loose fragments, avoid formation of bone dust from burring, utilize careful hemostasis, and prevent hematoma formation. Although not based on any scientific data, these sensible recommendations initially proposed over 50 years ago have largely been accepted as dogma.

In severe traumatic injury or revision surgery, especially involving the radial head, we routinely implement prophylactic treatment. The literature continues to debate the merits of preventive measures such as perioperative radiation or

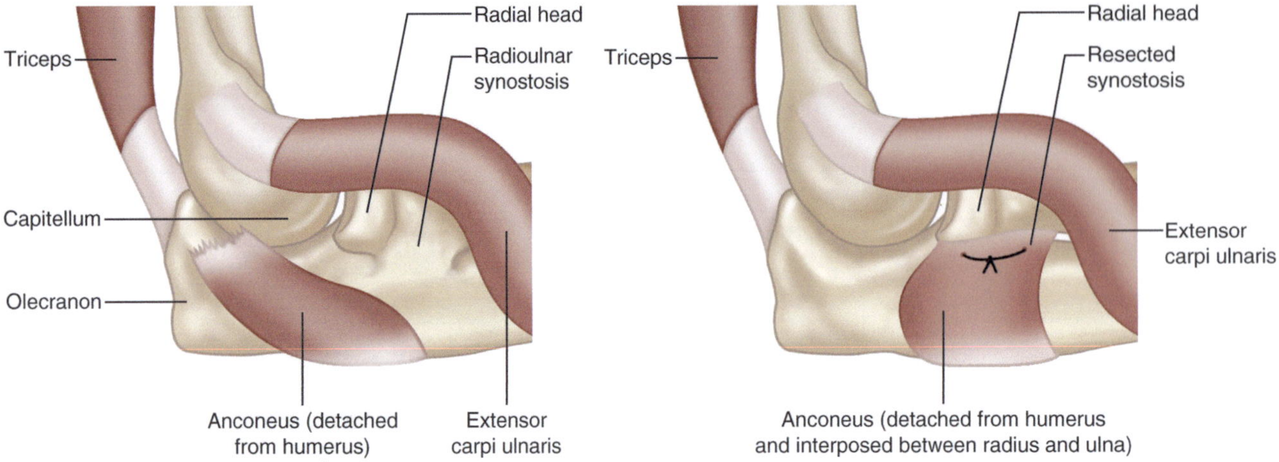

Fig. 11.16 Radioulnar synostosis resection with anconeus flap interposition

nonsteroidal anti-inflammatory use. It seems clear, however, that in order to reap the benefits of any preventative therapy, it must be initiated within the first 24–48 h for the initial insult, be it trauma or surgery. A minority of investigators would argue that current preventive therapy is not efficacious for HO in the elbow. This is debated, but most clinicians would opt for any reasonable measure, however questionable, to reduce the changes of HO formation.

Pearls and Pitfalls: Once HO develops, treatment options become more invasive and less predictable, so early attempts at prevention tend to lead to better patient outcomes.

Radiographic assessment is essential to determine the most appropriate treatment. Plain radiographs can be misleading, and CT scans are recommended to visualize not only the extent and involvement of HO but, more importantly, the status of the joint. A malunion, nonunion, or significant degeneration of the joint will have to be addressed, often in staged procedures, regardless of the HO present.

Because of the variable involvement of posttraumatic HO and individual patient goals, treatments should be customized for each patient. The majority of cases are asymptomatic, and these patients are simply treated with the therapy required for their elbow injury. However, when motion becomes limited and unresponsive to nonoperative modalities, the decision for treatment becomes more difficult. Surgical resection is indicated in those patients with significant functional limitations who have exhausted all nonoperative means and are capable of completing the necessary rehabilitation protocols. While some cases of elbow contracture with minor involvement of HO may be treated arthroscopically, we recommend that more involved cases of HO should be managed by open means.

HO resection is a technically challenging procedure of which the goal is to remove ectopic bone and contracted capsule until range of motion is restored. This needs to be performed in a manner that will allow for stable and immediate range of motion postoperatively. The important steps were well described by Viola and Hastings: use of adequate incision(s) allowing for complete resection, decompression of compromised nerves, resection of HO, excision of contracted capsule while sparing the collateral ligaments, if possible, clearing the coronoid fossa, debriding the coronoid process, clearing the olecranon fossa, excising the terminal olecranon, correcting post-op elbow instability if needed, and possible transposition of the ulnar nerve. Fortunately, not all patients require every step. Along with a thorough clinical and radiographic evaluation of the elbow, a comprehensive discussion of the patient's goals will largely determine which of these steps are necessary to perform.

Synostosis

This rare complication represents a variation of heterotopic ossification between the ulna and radius. It is difficult to excise the synostosis without sacrificing the LCL. While some advocate reconstruction of the LCL in these instances, others shun the reconstruction because of the theoretical risk of recurrence given the necessity of creating bone tunnels and an invasive "pathway" between the radius and ulna on which heterotopic bone may form. In actuality, neither stance is supported in the literature because of the paucity of reports. In our experience, we try to avoid reconstruction unless elbow instability is severe. We also recommend interposing viable tissue between the radius and ulna, usually the anconeus (Fig. 11.16). Following resection of heterotopic bone, the anconeus is detached from its proximal origin on the humerus and reflected into the posterior defect between the radius and ulna. The flap must remain attached to the ulna in order to remain viable. Mattress sutures can be placed deep to help pull the anconeus flap into the defect. The posterior interosseous nerve is at risk, particularly during bone resection and securing the anconeus flap deep in the defect. A long-standing synostosis may require a contracture release at the distal radioulnar joint (DRUJ) as well in order to achieve a good outcome. Postoperatively, patients begin gentle motion the following postoperative day with emphasis on supination and pronation. Postoperative radiation or oral anti-inflammatory drugs should be used for recurrence prophylaxis.

Posttraumatic Contracture

Even minor trauma to the elbow can result in contracture in flexion-extension and/or supination-pronation. Elbow rehabilitation tends to plateau around 4–6 months. Once this plateau is reached, it is unlikely that the patient will regain more motion through nonoperative means and surgery may be considered. For as long as the patient's motion improves, however, surgical release should be avoided.

> *Pearls and Pitfalls*: Regarding the timing of a contracture release, listen to the patient. If there has been any improvement, even small, resist the temptation to proceed with release. Conversely, if improvement has plateaued for several weeks, it would be reasonable to consider surgical intervention.

In considering surgery, patients must decide whether the burden of their functional deficit outweighs the risks surgery and the inconvenience of a prolonged recovery.

Surgical management historically has been indicated to restore the functional arc of 30–130° of flexion-extension and 50–50° of supination-pronation when nonoperative modalities have failed to do so. Recently, however, the goals in achieving supination and pronation tend to be individualized, as each patient has different functional priorities. One patient, for example, may want to maximize supination to facilitate feeding and grooming, while another patient may want to maximize pronation to maintain productivity as a keyboardist. Further, individuals with particular personal or vocational needs may often require a larger arc of motion than previously recommended, which has broadened the indications for surgery.

Currently, there is no consensus on indications for either arthroscopic or open release. It is generally accepted that contractures involving altered anatomy, including previous ulnar nerve transpositions, presence of heterotopic ossification, and contractures requiring hardware removal, are best addressed by open means. Recently, arthroscopic indications have been broadening to include these conditions, as techniques continue to evolve. Surgeons should rely on their comfort and skill level to guide their surgical strategy in treating elbow contractures. Regardless of preferred technique, surgery should only be contemplated for patients that are clearly motivated and have relatively high thresholds to overcome the challenges of postoperative pain.

Any combination of anterior, medial, lateral, and posterior approaches can be performed for open release depending on the focus of pathology. The approach chosen must be able to provide access to the pathologic structures as well as the ulnar nerve, if decompression or transposition is required. After contracture release, if even mild preoperative ulnar nerve symptoms are present, these symptoms will often progress. The sudden gain in elbow motion will pull the ulnar nerve through a fibrosed area with many intrinsic adhesions, causing traction ischemia to the nerve. For this reason, even patients without ulnar nerve symptoms prior to release have a high likelihood of developing symptoms postoperatively.

> *Pearls and Pitfalls*: Regardless of whether a contracture is released by open or arthroscopic means, the ulnar nerve needs to be at least decompressed and incisions need to be planned to accomplish this. If it is not, the nerve likely will tether and inhibit rehabilitation.

We recommend at least simple decompression, and transposition if preferred, provided that access to the ulnar nerve is at all convenient. This does not add a significant amount of dissection or operative time and decreases the need for additional surgery at a later time. Each approach will be discussed briefly.

Through the anterior approach, only the anterior capsule is accessible. Consequently, this approach is best indicated for isolated flexion contractures in elbows that allow full flexion. Improvement of 25–48° in the flexion-extension arc has been demonstrated in retrospective studies. However, isolated flexion contractures rarely occur without associated posterior pathology, such as olecranon osteophytes or debris within the olecranon fossa blocking extension, especially in long-standing contractures. As a result, we do not recommend the anterior approach unless combined with other approaches.

The medial approach is the workhorse approach for most contractures and provides the best access to the ulnar nerve if decompression is indicated. To expose the anterior capsule, the origin of the flexor-pronator mass is taken down from the medial supracondylar ridge to the epicondyle and continued longitudinally, leaving the most posterior fascia of the FCU attached to the medial epicondyle. Sparing this attachment facilitates rehabilitation without compromising exposure to the brachialis and anterior capsule. The dissection continues deep to the brachialis to expose the anterior compartment.

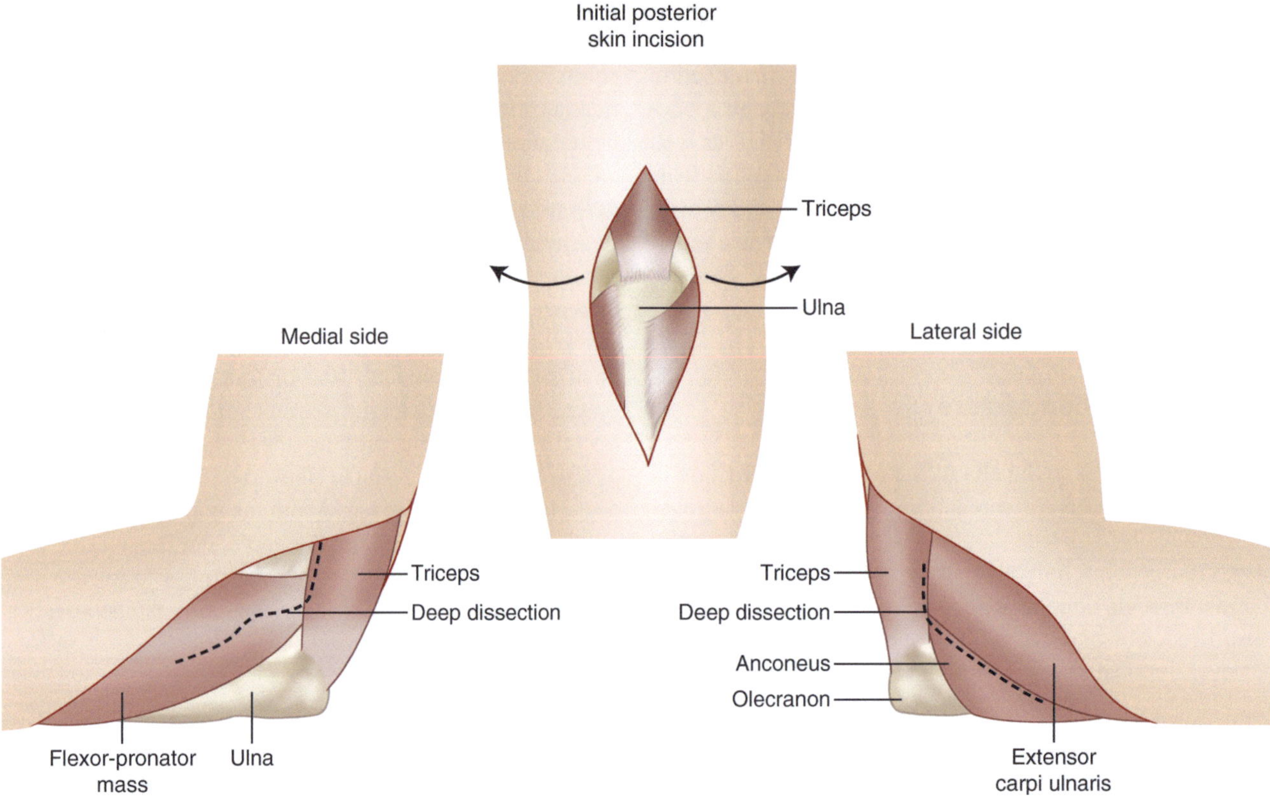

Fig. 11.17 Posterior approach. (**a**) A posterior skin incision allows for full-thickness subcutaneous flaps to be created medially and laterally; (**b**) reflecting the medial flap, the dissection continues between the triceps and brachialis and through the flexor carpi ulnaris; (**c**) reflecting the lateral flap, the dissection continues between the triceps and brachialis and between the anconeus and extensor carpi radialis ulnaris

From the same medial incision, the posterior compartment is exposed by elevating the medial portion of the triceps off of the humerus. Every attempt is made to spare the collateral ligaments as they impart stability to the joint.

The lateral approach, also known as the column procedure, allows release of the anterior and posterior capsules. However, this does not conveniently allow for decompression of the ulnar nerve. Often, a second incision is needed if the ulnar nerve is to be treated. To expose the posterior capsule, the anconeus and triceps are reflected posteriorly. Anteriorly, the origin of the extensor carpi radialis longus and distal fibers of the brachioradialis are released off of the humerus. Distally, the dissection continues between the extensor carpi radialis longus and brevis. This provides exposure of the capsule without injuring the collateral ligaments. One can expect 45–55° of improvement in the arc of motion with this approach.

With most severe or chronic contractures, or contractures involving extensive heterotopic bone or hardware, all aspects of the elbow must be addressed and frequently require multiple incisions. Alternatively, a single posterior skin incision will allow access posteriorly, anteriorly, medially, and laterally through the elevation of subcutaneous flaps (Fig. 11.17). Certainly, this approach offers more appealing cosmetic results, but it is unclear at this time whether functional outcomes are superior. Given its versatility, the posterior approach is our most commonly used open approach for severe contractures.

The intraoperative algorithm is far more important than the type of technique or approach utilized for contracture release. As stated previously, there are intrinsic and extrinsic causes for contracture releases, and all must be appropriately addressed. To address too few will result in incomplete release; to address too many will result in needless surgical dissection and consequent chronic instability or increased fibrosis and risk of motion loss.

> *Pearls and Pitfalls*: The general concept to following a sensible algorithm for elbow contracture release is to first release the tethering soft tissue, then progress from simple to more complicated bony procedures to address residual mechanical blocking.

When planning for surgical release of a flexion contracture, we prefer to excise the anterior capsule and lyse the intra-articular adhesions anteriorly, posteriorly, medially, and

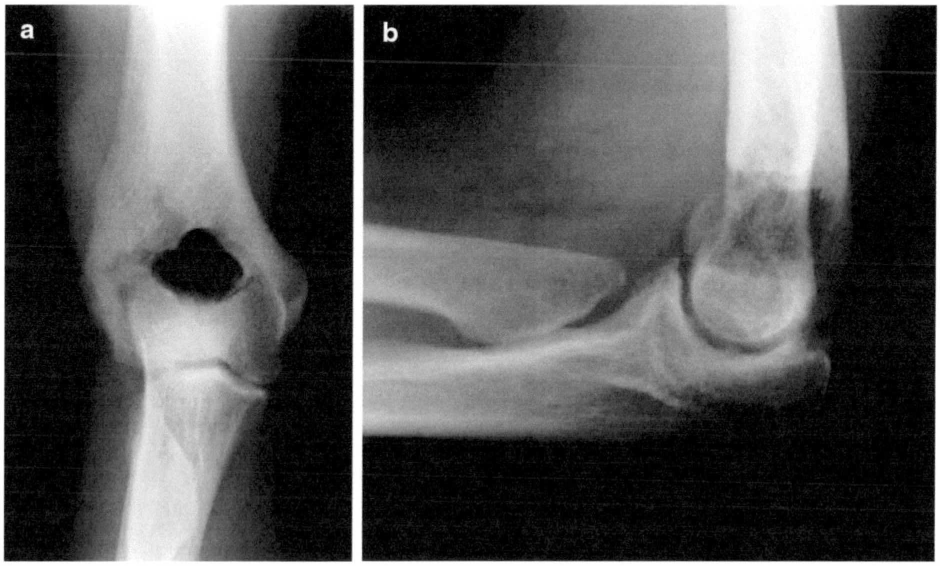

Fig. 11.18 (**a**, **b**): Outerbridge-Kashiwagi technique. Fenestration through the distal humerus removes the bony blockade against the coronoid and olecranon

laterally. A generous capsulectomy is performed, keeping the brachialis as a protective barrier between the dissection and all neurovascular structures located anteriorly. As the capsulectomy proceeds laterally, however, care should be taken to protect the radial nerve from injury as the brachialis does not extend to that extent laterally. Gentle manipulation will reveal the effectiveness of this simple soft tissue release. If the goals of the patient have not been met by removing the tethering to extension, then the next step is to remove the posterior obstruction to extension. This can involve debris removal from the olecranon fossa, osteophyte excision, or partial olecranon excision, usually in that sequential order to achieve the desired effect. A similar algorithm can be applied to extension contractures or mixed contractures. It is rarely necessary to incise the collateral ligaments; all other potential limitations of motion should be evaluated prior to disrupting these structures. Occasionally, the ligaments are too contracted and must be sacrificed, which may cause the joint to become grossly unstable through its arc of motion. If the collateral ligaments are sacrificed, it is important to have a hinged external fixator available should the ulnohumeral joint demonstrate subluxation when positioned within 40° of full extension.

One elegant method of addressing a mixed flexion and extension contracture that has failed soft tissue releases is the Outerbridge-Kashiwagi technique, known as the "O.K. procedure" (Fig. 11.18). This allows for simultaneous removal of anterior and posterior blocking by creating a transhumeral osteotomy which allows the coronoid and olecranon to pass without limitation. While the "O.K. procedure" was originally described as an open technique, we find that it lends itself quite nicely to arthroscopic applications.

The technique for arthroscopic contracture release follows the same algorithm as open techniques. Alternating through an anteromedial portal and an anterolateral portal, at least 1–2 cm of anterior capsule is excised from the humerus with a 4.0-mm full-radius shaver in a proximal to distal fashion. Particular care must be taken both medially and laterally to avoid injury to the ulnar and radial nerves, respectively. Keeping the shaver as proximally as possible on the lateral side and remaining anterior to the intermuscular septum on the medial side will allow a relatively safe dissection. Once the anterior soft tissue tether has been removed, a minor manipulation to gently rupture the last remaining adhesions should allow for improved extension. If not, then the mechanical block in the posterior aspect of the elbow must be addressed, as in open procedures. Likewise, in patients with limited flexion, the posterior soft tissue tether must be released first. Again, caution must be exercised as an excision of the posteromedial capsule will often expose the ulnar nerve and make it particularly susceptible to injury. Once the posterior tether has been removed, attention must be turned to the anterior mechanical block if flexion is still limited. Although a 2.7-mm arthroscope and similarly sized instruments have been recommended for the tight constraints of the posterior compartment, we have found the 2.7-mm shaver to be not aggressive enough in dealing with this tough tissue, and maneuvering a 4.0-mm shaver has not been difficult. Radiofrequency ablation should be used sparingly, especially in the vicinity of nerves medially and laterally.

Pearls and Pitfalls: A helpful technique during arthroscopy to decrease the chance of nerve injury is to use retractors to aid in visualization and retraction of the nerves from cutting instruments. In addition, care should be taken during portal development, nerves should be carefully explored if their position is in question, the capsule should be dissected away bluntly from the humerus to increase capsular volume, suction should not be used, and cutting equipment should always be directed away from nerves.

Contractures of supination or pronation occur less commonly than contractures of flexion or extension and are much more difficult to treat. Typically, they respond less predictably to nonoperative and operative treatment, so prevention is the best course. Release for supination and pronation is possible but should be staged apart from any other contracture releases. We have observed that patients become easily overwhelmed with the rehabilitation required for all directions of motion and usually perform better when allowed to focus on one or two motions.

Pearls and Pitfalls: It may be unreasonable to expect that patients can effectively rehabilitate both flexion-extension and supination-pronation contracture releases simultaneously. We prefer to stage these procedures.

Should heterotopic bone be involved, we also believe that the extent of surgery required to release all directions of motion may increase the risk of heterotopic bone recurrence more than if separated into two relatively smaller procedures. Lastly, if a patient is unable to rehabilitate a simpler release for whatever reason, then any further releases will surely be doomed for failure and should not be attempted.

Release of supination or pronation contractures begins at the proximal radioulnar joint with a Kocher incision laterally over the radiocapitellar area. If present, bony or hardware mechanical blocking must be removed, which may involve radial head resection with or without radial head replacement. If the radial head remains, careful lyses of the intra-articular adhesions should be performed with preservation of the annular ligament (Fig. 11.19). If the annular ligament has been disrupted previously or incompetent, it must be reconstructed, and contracture release must be deferred until after complete healing. Usually, surgical release of the proximal radioulnar joint is not sufficient by itself to regain satisfactory supination or pronation, especially more severe and chronic ones. Often, the DRUJ must be released concomitantly. The integrity of the triangular fibrocartilage complex (TFCC) must be confirmed clinically or arthroscopically before proceeding with a capsular release in order to avoid creating an unstable DRUJ.

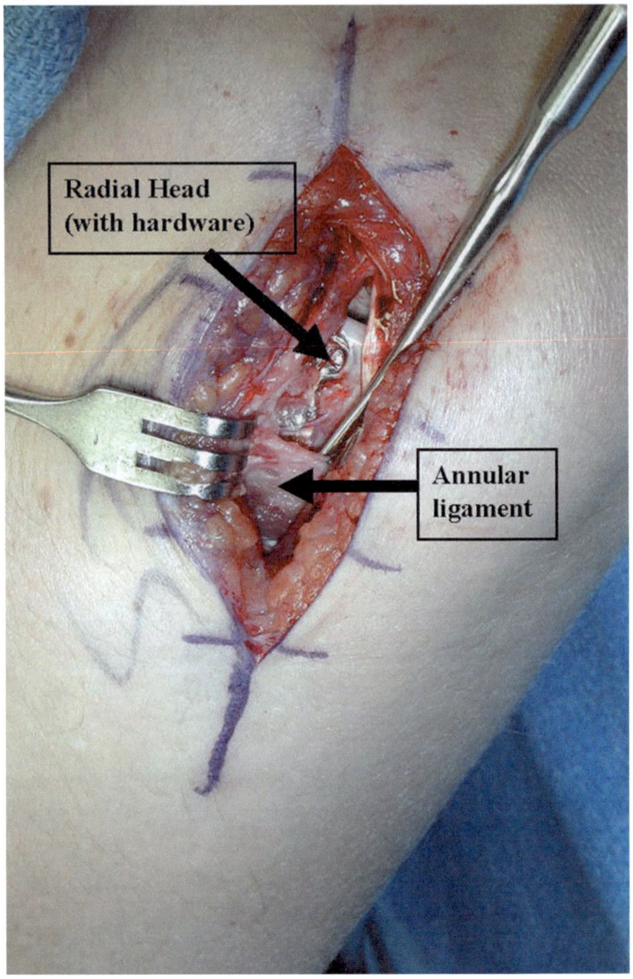

Fig. 11.19 Lysis of the intra-articular adhesions (around radial head hardware) performed with preservation of the annular ligament

Pearls and Pitfalls: As the primary stabilizer of the DRUJ, the TFCC must be competent prior to releasing the majority of the secondary stabilizers, the ulnar extrinsic ligaments.

Contractures of supination require a dorsal incision, while contractures of pronation require a volar incision (Fig. 11.20). Usually, patients present with contractures of both and consequently require either two skin incisions or access to the anterior and posterior capsules through a single volar skin incision. Alternatively, the DRUJ may be released arthroscopically, but we have no experience with this.

It is imperative to start motion early after contracture release in order to maintain the motion achieved at surgery.

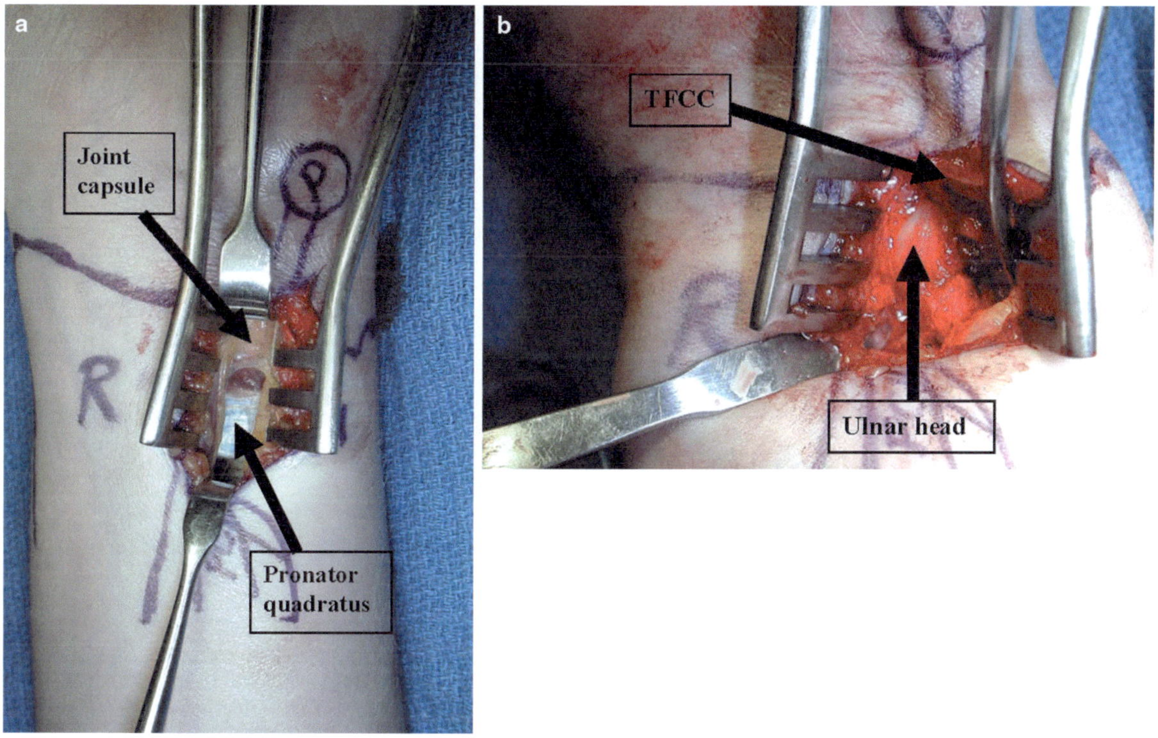

Fig. 11.20 Distal radioulnar joint contracture release. (**a**) Exposed capsule, (**b**) resected capsule, sparring the TFCC

Continuous passive motion (CPM) devices have been utilized for other joints postoperatively and have even met with some success in the elbow, but our experience has been somewhat disappointing. CPM is time-consuming and cumbersome, leading to compliance issues, and it has frustrating insurance reimbursement issues. We have also observed that patients inappropriately tend to consider the CPM machine as the primary component of their postoperative rehabilitation, rather than an adjuvant to a more comprehensive program. Instead of CPM, we routinely administer long-acting axillary blocks for postoperative pain and discharge patients to qualified physical therapists to be seen on the day of surgery.

Pearls and Pitfalls: Long-acting perioperative axillary blocks have been invaluable in our practice. Not only do patients benefit from immediate motion, the anesthesia provides a powerful psychological tool as patients are able to witness their elbows moving unhampered by postoperative pain. Consequently, patients begin to believe that they can overcome their limitations and greatly improve their chances for success.

Optimizing Outcomes

- Because malunions and nonunions of the radial head and neck are problematic for several reasons, excision or prosthetic replacement is preferred to repair.
- Residual instability should call for scrutinization of bony injury and malalignment before soft tissue reconstruction is contemplated.
- During HO excision, sparing of the collateral ligaments is preferred but may not be possible. Should collateral ligaments be sacrificed, a hinged external fixator should be applied if instability ensues.
- An anconeus interposition flap following synostosis resection may help to reduce the chances of recurrence.
- The DRUJ often may need to be released with the proximal radioulnar joint in order to achieve the desired result.
- Follow a systematic approach for each contracture release. Begin with soft tissue restraints and move toward bony blocks. Not every patient needs to follow the algorithm to its end.
- Flexion-extension contractures should be released separately from supination-pronation contractures.
- Immediately following contracture release, consider physical therapy under long-acting axillary nerve blocks to help patients build confidence in battling the challenges of rehabilitation.

Conclusion

The only thing more challenging than repairing a traumatized elbow is to revise what had failed. A large portion of this chapter focuses on aspects of the management of acute trauma because prevention of potential complications cannot be overemphasized. Despite adhering to the dogma presented in this chapter, outcomes can be unpredictable in the elbow, and complications occur even in the best of hands. Revision elbow surgery is almost the norm rather than the exception. Unfortunately, the literature has very little guidance for revision surgery. It describes very well that problems of the proximal ulna and radius exist but fails to clearly indicate what to do when these problems occur. This chapter attempts to supplement what is known in the literature with the author's anecdotal experience. While some of the recommendations lack scientific support, they are based on several years of trial and observation. With this chapter, it is the author's hope that the reader may learn from his successes and his failures without having to discover them firsthand. There is good reason for a wave of angst to overcome surgeons first gazing at radiographs depicting a traumatized proximal ulna and/or radius. Surgeons know that there will be a very good chance they will be seeing these patients for a very long time, and the journey will not be easy for either.

References

1. O'Driscoll SW. Optimizing stability in distal humeral fracture fixation. J Shoulder Elbow Surg. 2005;14(1 Suppl S):186S–94S.
2. Sanchez-Sotelo J, Torchia ME, O'Driscoll SW. Complex distal humeral fractures: internal fixation with a principle-based parallel-plate technique. Surgical technique. J Bone Joint Surg Am. 2008;90(Suppl 2 Pt 1):31–46.
3. Plancher KD, Lucas TS. Fracture dislocations of the elbow in athletes. Clin Sports Med. 2001;20(1):59–76.
4. Constant CR. Injuries to the elbow. J R Coll Surg Edinb. 1990;35(6 Suppl):S31–2.
5. Hutcinson DT, Horwitz DS, Ha G, Thomas CW, Bachus KN. Cyclic loading of olecranon fracture fixation constructs. J Bone Joint Surg. 2003;85-A(5):831–37.
6. Newman SD, Mauffrey C, Krikler S. Olecranon fractures. Injury. 2009;40(6):575–81.
7. Hume MC, Wiss DA. Olecranon fractures. A clinical and radiographic comparison of tension band wiring and plate fixation. Clin Orthop Relat Res. 1992;285:229–35.
8. Lindenhovius AL, Brouwer KM, Doornberg JN, Ring DC, Kloen P. Long-term outcome of operatively treated fracture-dislocations of the olecranon. J Orthop Trauma. 2008;22(5):325–31.
9. Rommens PM, Küchle R, Schneider RU, Reuter M. Olecranon fractures in adults: factors influencing outcome. Injury. 2004; 35(11):1149–57.
10. Macko D, Szabo RM. Complications of tension-band wiring of olecranon fractures. J Bone Joint Surg Am. 1985;67(9): 1396–401.
11. Bailey CS, et al. Outcomes of plate fixation of olecranon fractures. J Orthop Trauma. 2001;15(8):542–8.
12. Lindenhovius AL, Brouwer KM, Doornbers JN, Ring DC, Kloen P. Long-term outcome of operatively treated fracture-dislocations of the olecranon. J Orthop Trauma. 2008;22(5):325–31.
13. Rommens PM, et al. Olecranon fractures in adults: factors influencing outcome. Injury. 2004;35(11):1149–57.
14. Klimkiewicz JJ, Argintar E, Martin BD, Hsieh A. Nail vs plate: biomechanical comparison in unstable olecranon fractures. Poster presentation. Annual Meeting, American Society for Surgery of the Hand, San Francisco, CA, 3–5 Oct 2009.
15. Buijze G, Kloen P. Clinical evaluation of locking compression plate fixation for comminuted olecranon fractures. J Bone Joint Surg Am. 2009;91(10):2416–20.
16. Sahajpal D, Wright TW. Proximal ulna fractures. J Hand Surg Am. 2009;34(2):357–62.
17. Regan W, Morrey BF. Classification and treatment of coronoid process fractures. Orthopedics. 1992;15(7):845–8.
18. O'Driscoll SW, Jupiter JB, Cohen MS, Ring D, McKee MD. Difficult elbow fractures: pearls and pitfalls. Instr Course Lect. 2003;52:113–34.
19. Kasparyan NG, Hotchkiss RN. Dynamic skeletal fixation in the upper extremity. Hand Clin. 1997;13:643–63.
20. Rotini R, Antonioli D, Marinelli A, Katusi D. Surgical treatment of proximal ulna nonunion. Chir Organi Mov. 2008;91(2):65–70. Epub 2008 Mar 3.
21. Wright TW, Glowczewski F. Vascular anatomy of the ulna. J Hand Surg Am. 1998;23(5):800–4.
22. Iannuzzi N, Dahners L. Excision and advancement in the treatment of comminuted olecranon fractures. J Orthop Trauma. 2009; 23(3):226–8.
23. Moed BR, Ede DE, Brown TD. Fractures of the olecranon: an in vitro study of elbow joint stresses after tension-band wire fixation versus proximal fracture fragment excision. J Trauma. 2002; 53(6):1088–93.
24. Veillette CJ, Steinmann SP. Olecranon fractures. Orthop Clin North Am. 2008;39(2):229–36, vii.
25. Bhaskar A. Missed Monteggia fracture in children: is annular ligament reconstruction always required? Indian J Orthop. 2009; 43(4):389–95.
26. Cohen MS, Hastings H. Rotatory instability of the elbow. The anatomy and role of the lateral stabilizers. J Bone Joint Surg Am. 1997;79(2):225–33.
27. Ring D, Quintero J, Jupiter JB. Open reduction and internal fixation of fractures of the radial head. J Bone Joint Surg Am. 2002;84 (A(10)):1811–5.
28. Calfee R, Madom I, Weiss AP. Radial head arthroplasty. J Hand Surg Am. 2006;31(2):314–21.
29. Birkedal JP, Deal DN, Ruch DS. Loss of flexion after radial head replacement. J Shoulder Elbow Surg. 2004;13(2):208–13.
30. Pike JM, Athwal GS, Faber KJ, King GJ. Radial head fractures—an update. J Hand Surg Am. 2009;34(3):557–65.
31. Rosenblatt Y, Athwal GS, Faber KJ. Current recommendations for the treatment of radial head fractures. Orthop Clin North Am. 2008;39(2):173–85, vi.
32. Karlstad R, Morrey BF, Cooney WP. Failure of fresh-frozen radial head allografts in the treatment of Essex-Lopresti injury. A report of four cases. J Bone Joint Surg Am. 2005;87(8):1828–33.

12 Reoperative Concerns for the Unstable Elbow

Paul Maloof and Virak Tan

Abstract

The unstable elbow can be caused by not only problems with the bony anatomy but of course the soft tissue envelope as well. The unstable elbow may require correction of any bony deficits as well as reconstruction of ligaments in order to obtain an elbow that the patient feels confident in from a stability standpoint. The dissection after previous surgeries in these areas can be difficult because of bone loss as well as significant scar tissue about neurovascular structures. Frequently these surgeries may require more than one procedure in order to rectify anatomical deficiencies in a step-by-step fashion. Ultimately, if reconstructive efforts fail, the patient may be looking at elbow arthroplasty or fusion in order to find usage and stability from the arm.

Keywords

Elbow • Instability • Collateral • Ligament • Reconstruction

Key Points

- Realistic patient expectations.
- More than one surgery may be required.
- Plan for extensile surgical approach.
- Respect surgical planes.
- Recreate normal anatomic planes, if possible.
- Repair or reconstruction of bony architecture, if possible.
- Reconstruction of lateral ulnar collateral ligament (LUCL), if needed.
- Hinged external fixation, if needed.
- Elbow arthroplasty in acceptable patients.
- Fusion as last option.

P. Maloof, MD • V. Tan, MD (✉)
Department of Orthopedics, University of Medicine and Dentistry of New Jersey and University Hospital, 90 Bergen Street, Newark, NJ 07103, USA
e-mail: tanvi@umdnj.edu

Overview

The elbow is a complex trochoginglymoid joint with motion in multiple planes, allowing for flexion/extension as well as pronation/supination. These motions are afforded by the bony articulations at the distal humerus with the proximal radius and ulna. The ulnohumeral, radiocapitellar, and proximal radioulnar joint (PRUJ) are the three articulations of the elbow joint.

Stability of the elbow is provided through a combination of the bony articulations as well as the capsuloligamentous structures surrounding the joint. Conventional thought is that 50% of elbow stability is due to the highly congruent ulnohumeral joint. The olecranon and coronoid process are the greatest contributors to the bony stability. With loss of 50% of the coronoid process, the elbow joint becomes highly unstable [1]. The radial head acts as a secondary stabilizer of the elbow. Valgus stress is initially resisted by the medial collateral ligaments, and when the MCL is intact, absence of the radial head does not lead to instability [2]. If the MCL complex is compromised, the radial head then becomes essential to elbow stability and becomes a major stabilizer as it acts to buttress the joint.

S.F.M. Duncan (ed.), *Reoperative Hand Surgery*,
DOI 10.1007/978-1-4614-2373-7_12, © Springer Science+Business Media, LLC 2012

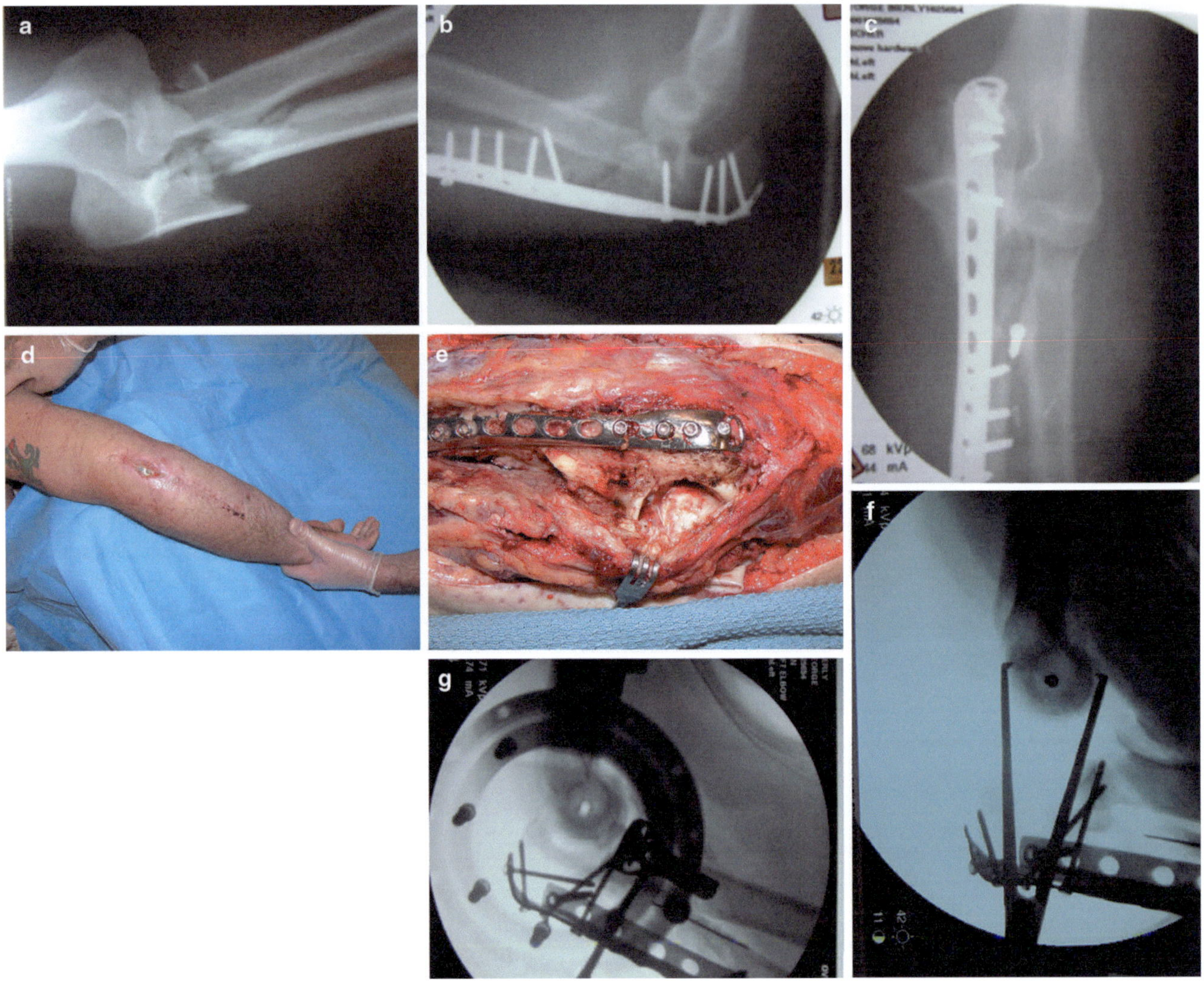

Fig. 12.1 (**a**) Traumatic injury to the elbow joint showing signs of a complex fracture dislocation. (**b**, **c**) Patient underwent ORIF at an outside institution and presented to our clinic with X-rays showing a complete elbow dislocation. (**d**) Clinical photograph showing exposed hardware. (**e**) Intraoperative photograph showing that the proximal ulna had been fixed in 90° of malrotation relative to the ulnar shaft. (**f**, **g**) This patient required revision ORIF of the ulna and radial head and placement of external fixation to obtain stability

The capsuloligamentous structures provide the other 50% of elbow stability. The medial collateral ligament consists of anterior, posterior, and transverse segments. The anterior bundle is considered the primary stabilizer of the ulnohumeral joint and is the only discrete bundle that can be easily seen. Its proximal attachment is from the large anteroinferior surface of the medial epicondyle of the humerus, and it inserts on the sublime tubercle of the coronoid process of the ulna. The posterior and transverse bundles have not been shown to be significant contributors to stability of the elbow [3] (Fig. 12.2).

The lateral collateral ligament complex of the elbow joint consists of the annular ligament, the radial collateral ligament, and the lateral ulnar collateral ligament (LUCL). The LUCL originates from the lateral epicondyle of the humerus with its fibers blending with the radial collateral ligament. It inserts distally on the tubercle of the supinator crest of the ulna and has been shown to be significant in preventing posterolateral rotatory instability (PLRI) of the elbow [4].

Instability of the elbow joint is usually the result of a traumatic injury. Simple elbow instability has been defined as the unstable elbow in the absence of any fractures, and most can be successfully managed without surgery. Complex instability involves disruption of soft tissues as well as bony architecture of the joint [5]. The bony injury may include a fracture of the coronoid process, radial head, and/or olecranon.

Definitive treatment for complex elbow instability usually involves surgery because these injuries are highly unstable and are prone to complications when inadequately treated [6]. With operative treatment, one should attempt to restore elbow stability by reestablishing periarticular bony anatomy and/or competent collateral ligaments.

When the primary surgical procedure to restore elbow stability fails or when new occurrence of instability presents

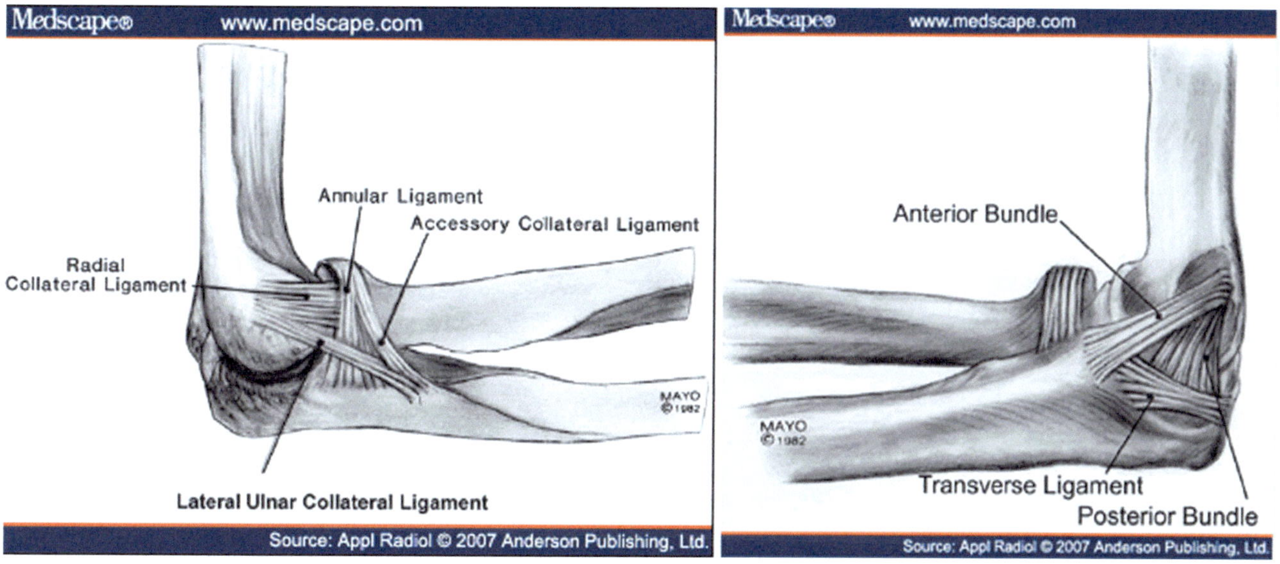

Fig. 12.2 Lateral view of the elbow demonstrating the lateral ulnar collateral ligament (LUCL) and annular ligaments (*right*). Medial view demonstrates medial collateral ligaments (*left*)

postoperatively, these situations can often be quite challenging to manage due to several factors. First, diagnosis of recurrent instability may be difficult because physical examination may be limited by postoperative pain, swelling, and restriction of motion. Second, any retained hardware may obscure visualization of the joint on radiographic images. Finally, when the revision surgery is undertaken, scarring, altered anatomy, and distorted surgical planes will make the procedure more technically difficult. The focus of this chapter is on revision elbow surgery and what to do when the primary procedure fails to achieve stability.

General Considerations

There are a few general principles to consider when performing revision elbow surgery for instability. First, patients need to be counseled to have realistic expectations, including postoperative rehabilitation, decreased range of motion and strength, and possible further elbow surgery. Second, preoperative planning is essential to determine hardware/implant and instrumentation required during the case.

In considering the technical aspect of the revision surgery, plan a skin incision that will allow for an extensile approach. If possible, incorporate the previous incision but do not compromise the exposure because of the location of the prior skin incision. In most cases, a posterior approach, raising medial and lateral skin flaps, will allow access to all structures. With the deeper dissection, even though the anatomy is distorted by scarring, it is important to try to follow the normal interstructure planes as much as possible. Doing so will minimize further tissue disruption by the approach and allow for anatomic repair of the structures at closure. Once the elbow is exposed, the bony architecture needs to be established. For example, if the proximal ulna is malaligned, the radial head will continue to be unstable. Likewise, if the radial head had been excised and there is valgus instability, then a prosthetic radial head replacement is necessary. After the bony anatomy is reestablished, attention is turned to reassessing stability, and repair or reconstruction of the ligament(s) are undertaken as needed. In the majority of cases, the elbow will be stable at this point and no further procedure is required. In the few cases where stability is not established, then a dynamic articulating external fixator is used to hold concentric reduction and control elbow motion.

Management of the Unstable Elbow

The Unstable Elbow After Tennis Elbow Surgery

Elbow instability may uncommonly occur after open treatment of lateral epicondylitis. Iatrogenic injury to the LUCL during debridement of the origin of the ECRB can lead to PLRI. The instability encountered in these cases may be extremely subtle. Diagnosis requires a high index of suspicion. Examination should include the pivot shift test [4]. Because this test can be difficult to perform in an awake patient, another simple maneuver that can be done is to ask the patient to perform a push-up from the floor or from the seated position. These movements put the elbow joint in a similar position to the pivot shift and will produce apprehension in PLRI. Examination under anesthesia may be needed to confirm the diagnosis. Once this diagnosis has been made, surgical treatment is preferred.

A lateral skin incision should suffice in this scenario. The deep exposure is through a modified Kocher approach exposing

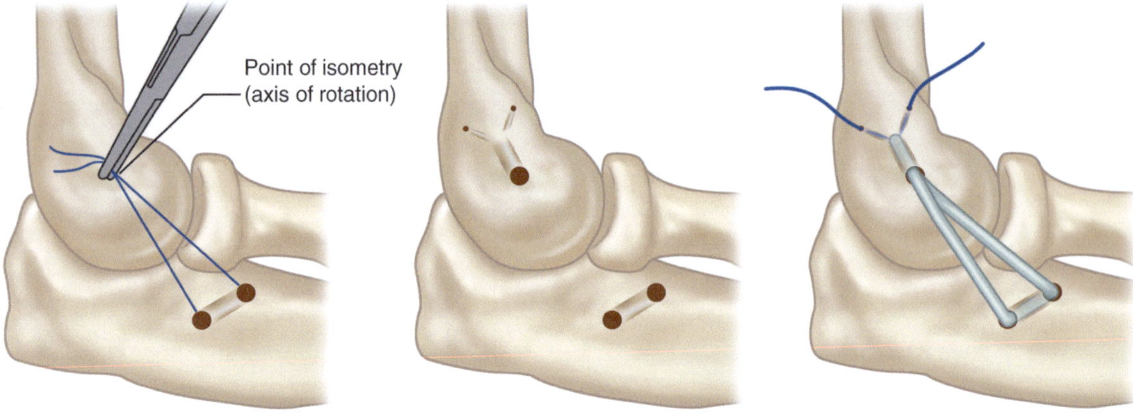

Fig. 12.3 Reconstruction of the LUCL. The position of ulnar bone tunnels at the supinator crest and the humeral isometric point (*top left*). Humeral and ulnar tunnels (*top right*). A tendon graft is passed through the ulnar tunnel and the two ends are docked into the humeral tunnel (*bottom*)

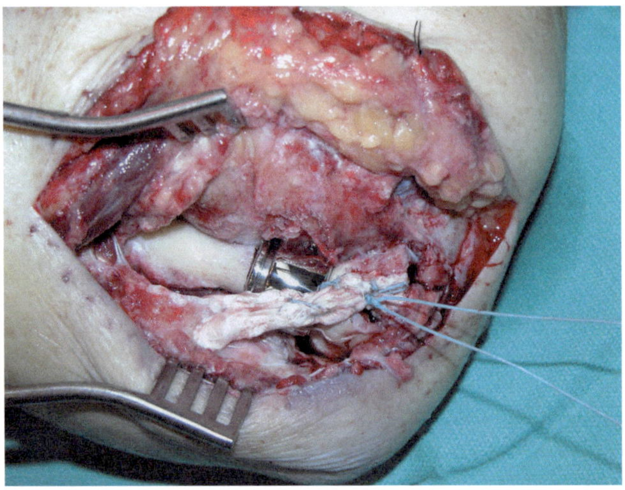

Fig. 12.4 Intraoperative photo of LUCL reconstruction with a tendon graft. Note the radial head replacement

the lateral epicondyle to the supinator crest of the ulna. The extensor carpi ulnaris (ECU) is reflected anteriorly with the common extensor tendon origin by sharp dissection off the capsuloligamentous complex. The anconeus is reflected posteriorly.

At times, a remnant of LUCL may be present. If enough competent tissue is available, then a primary repair can be done by reattaching the ligament to the lateral epicondyle with sutures through drill holes or suture anchors. The ligament is tensioned with the elbow flexed to 90° and the forearm in full pronation.

If adequate ligament is unavailable, reconstruction is performed using tendon autograft or allograft [7]. The ipsilateral palmaris longus or a strip of triceps tendon is the preferred autograft. Semitendinosis or plantaris can also be used. A bone tunnel is then created in the ulna from the tubercle of the supinator crest to a point proximal and posterior along the olecranon. The bone bridge should be 1–1.5 cm to avoid fracture. The humeral tunnel is created at the isometric point on the lateral epicondyle. This point can be found intraoperatively by passing a suture through the ulnar tunnel and holding it over the capitellum while taking the elbow through the flexion/extension arc. The isometric point is the point of rotation at which the suture strands remain taut throughout a range of motion of the joint. A bone tunnel is created at the humeral isometric point with two drill holes exiting proximally [8] (Fig. 12.3).

Nonabsorbable sutures are passed through the free ends of the tendon graft. The graft is looped through the ulnar tunnel and the free ends are docked into the humeral one. The sutures are delivered through the drill holes and tied over the bone bridge (Fig. 12.4). Tensioning is performed by placing the elbow in 90° of flexion and full pronation. The elbow is then taken through a range of motion. Provocative testing with progressive elbow extension and supination is performed to assess stability. If the radial head is found to be stable, the interval between the ECU and anconeus is closed. Postoperatively, the elbow can be ranged from 30° to full flexion. Full supination and pronation should only be done at 90° of flexion initially. Range of motion should be advanced accordingly.

The Unstable Elbow After Complex Dislocation Without Adequately Addressing the Bony and/or Ligamentous Injuries

Monteggia Malunion or Nonunion

Monteggia fracture of the proximal ulna and dislocation of the radial head require anatomic reduction of the ulna to achieve congruent reduction of the radiocapitellar articulation. Any malalignment of the ulna (sometimes a little as 5–10°) will lead to persistent radial head subluxation or dislocation (Fig. 12.5). Reoperative options in these cases include corrective osteotomy of the ulna (for malunion), repair of nonunion, or radial head excision [9, 10].

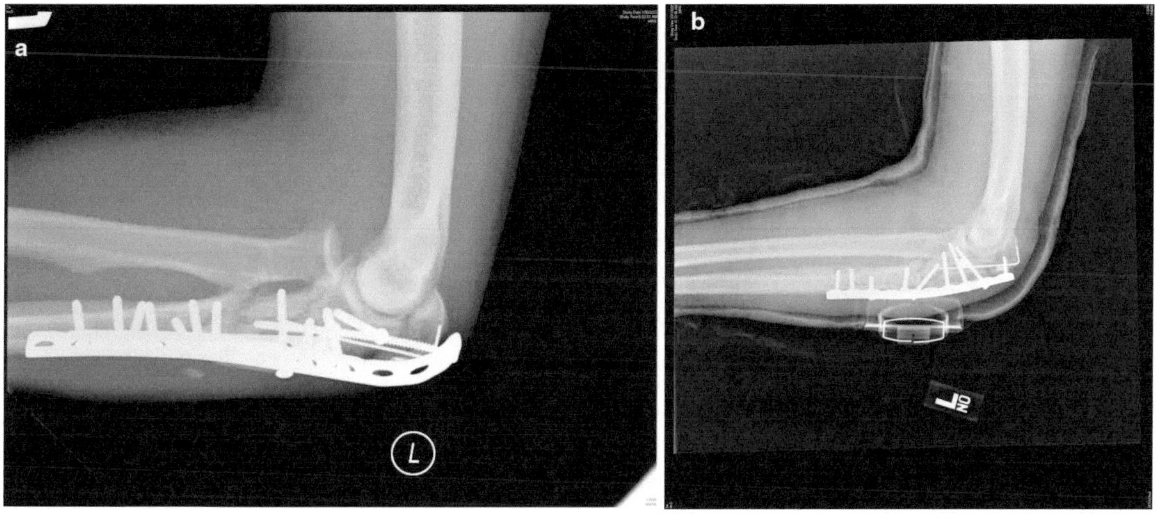

Fig. 12.5 (**a**) Malreduction (extension) of a proximal ulna fracture (in the sagittal plane) leading to persistent radial head subluxation. (**b**) Revision ORIF in more flexion at the fracture resulted in a stable radiocapitellar articulation

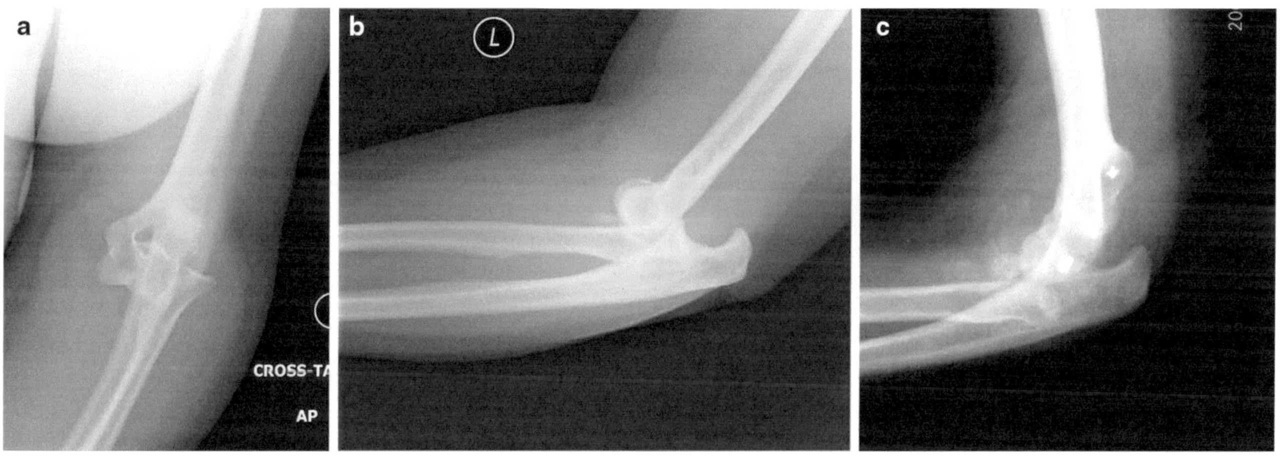

Fig. 12.6 (**a**, **b**) AP and lateral views of the elbow revealing a dislocation in the presence of a radial head and coronoid fracture, the so-called terrible triad. (**c**) X-ray showing redislocation after surgical intervention failed to adequately address the bony injury. Note the suture anchors used to repair the ligamentous structures only

Our preferred technique is to surgically address the alignment of the ulna and retain the native radial head. After exposure of the posterior aspect of the ulna, any retained hardware is removed. The radiocapitellar joint is opened and scar tissue within the joint and PRUJ is excised. The proximal ulna osteotomy or nonunion is provisionally stabilized in the anatomic alignment. This maneuver will allow for the radial head to reduce onto the capitellum. After confirming radiocapitellar joint reduction, definitive plate fixation of the ulna is done, using structural bone grafting as needed. Repair of the LCL complex is usually not necessary in adult patients.

Postoperatively, the elbow is immobilized for approximately 4 weeks to allow for the lateral soft tissues to heal. For posterior radial head dislocation, the forearm is immobilized in pronation, while anterior dislocation is immobilized in supination.

Terrible Triad

The terrible triad is the well-described constellation of radial head and coronoid fractures with dislocation of the ulnohumeral joint (Fig. 12.6a, b). The goals of surgical intervention are to restore bony as well as ligamentous stability [6]. Acute failure of the primary procedure in this scenario is usually due to inadequate attention to the bony anatomy [11] (Fig. 12.6c). Unfortunately, the instability pattern is not always fully appreciated and the radial head is excised at the index procedure. At times, even when fixation of the radial head is done, failure and collapse can occur (Fig. 12.7). In both cases, instability persists and radial head implant with repair or reconstruction of the lateral collateral ligament is indicated. Additionally, displaced coronoid fragment may need fixation to achieve stability.

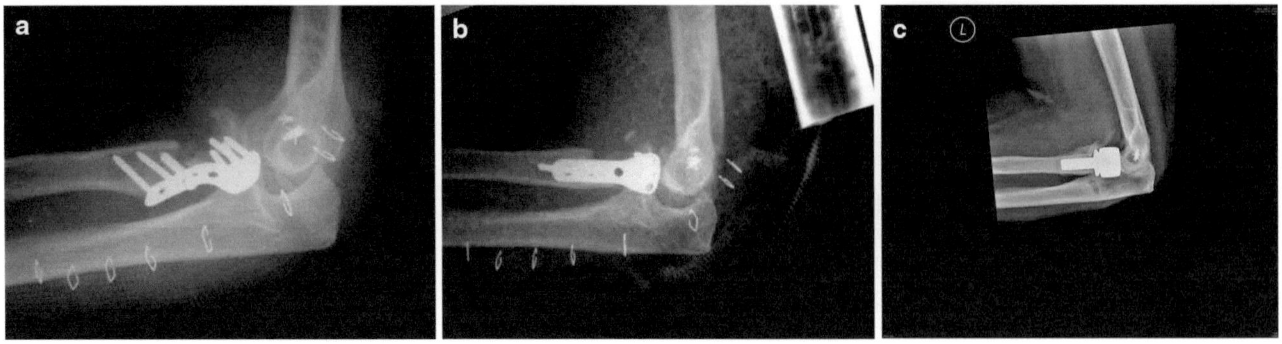

Fig. 12.7 (**a**, **b**) Films show attempted ORIF of a radial head fracture resulting in a nonunion. (**c**) Patient subsequently had a reoperation with radial head replacement and LUCL reconstruction

Surgical incision should follow the previous scar. If a lateral approach was used prior, it may be difficult to access the medial structures. One must consider using a posterior approach in order to work medially, if necessary. Otherwise a two incision approach may be needed [12].

For the radial head replacement, standard techniques are employed [13] and a modular implant is preferred. The use of a monoblock implant is not recommended as the proximal radius must be overdistracted for insertion, a maneuver best avoided in the unstable elbow. Attention to detail is necessary as to avoid overstuffing the joint. If available, the excised radial head as well as contralateral X-rays should be used for sizing the implant. The proximal aspect of the prosthesis should lie approximately 1 mm distal to the tip of the coronoid in order to sit in the appropriate location in the radial notch of the ulna.

With the trial radial head implant in place, provocative testing of the elbow must be done to assess ligamentous stability as well. If the LUCL is found to also be incompetent, then it needs to be addressed later in the case.

Any coronoid reconstruction should be done prior to definitive radial head implant and LCL repair/reconstruction to take advantage of the unstable elbow. In the revision case, primary osteosynthesis of the coronoid is rarely possible and reconstruction should be planned. Access to the coronoid may be possible through the lateral arthrotomy by mobilizing the common extensor muscles anteriorly, off the supinator. The underlying supinator muscle is then released from the radius from a posterior to anterior direction. The forearm is held in full pronation during this part of the dissection to protect the posterior interosseous nerve. Alternatively, the coronoid can be exposed through an anteromedial approach. After mobilization and protection of the ulnar nerve, the ulnar origin of the flexopronator mass is elevated off the medial proximal ulna to expose the coronoid.

Deficient Coronoid/Coronoid Reconstruction

Many techniques to address a deficient coronoid have been described including bone grafting from the tip of the olecranon, a piece of the discarded radial head, or iliac crest [3]. The bone graft is contoured to be flush with the remaining coronoid and with the articular surface (of olecranon or radial head) oriented toward the trochlea. Fixation is with screws alone or a precontoured coronoid plate. Oftentimes, this will be a nonanatomic reconstruction but should achieve the goal of restoring an anterior buttress.

After reconstructing the coronoid process, implantation of the actual prosthetic radial head is done, followed by definitive repair or reconstruction of the LCL as previously described. The medial collateral ligament complex does not usually require reconstruction because (1) it will likely heal, and (2) for most patients, valgus stress at the elbow is not commonly seen for activities of daily living.

The authors prefer to place the elbow in a static posterior elbow splint with the forearm in neutral position postoperatively. Rehabilitation is initiated within a couple of days with the supine overhead protocol (Fig. 12.8).

The Unstable Elbow Requiring a Hinge External Fixator

The situation will arise in which fixation and/or reconstruction of bony and ligamentous structures (including both collateral ligaments) of the elbow will fail to produce a stable ulnohumeral joint. Whenever revision surgery for a suspected or obvious unstable elbow is undertaken, the surgeon should consider having a hinged external fixator available. The hinged external fixator is rarely done as a stand-alone procedure for elbow instability [14]. The application of a fixator will function to add structural support to the repaired or reconstructed structures, as well as to help maintain a concentric reduction of the joint. With a fixator in place, early postoperative motion can begin soon after the procedure. In addition, the range where the elbow is stable can be determined intraoperatively, and the external fixator can be used to limit movement beyond those positions during the rehabilitation process.

Two types of fixators are available: multiplanar and unilateral. The purported advantages of unilateral frames are a

NEW JERSEY MEDICAL SCHOOL · DEPARTMENT OF ORTHOPAEDICS
NORTH JERSEY ORTHOPAEDIC INSTITUTE

Overhead Elbow Exercises

(These exercises are done lying flat on your back.)

Bending and Straightening the Elbow

1) Start by lying down flat on your back.

2) Put your arm over your chest, then remove the splint but keep the elbow bent.

3) Begin by placing your bent elbow so that it is directly above your shoulder (in other words, keep the upper arm perpendicular to the floor). Do not let the arm sag to the side (sagging will tend to push the elbow out of joint).

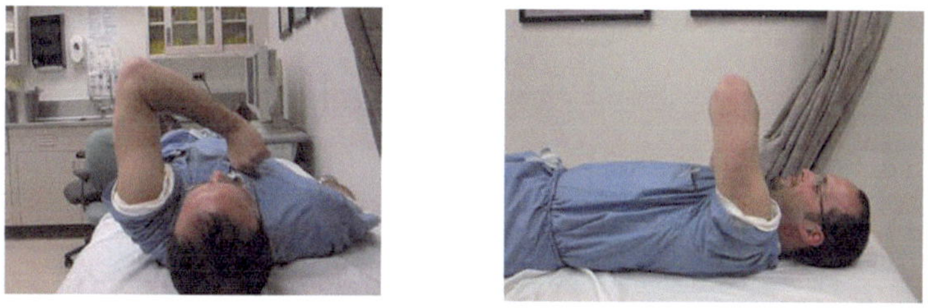

4) With the arm perpendicular to the floor, straighten the elbow. You may use the other (in this case the right) hand to help support and straighten the injured arm.

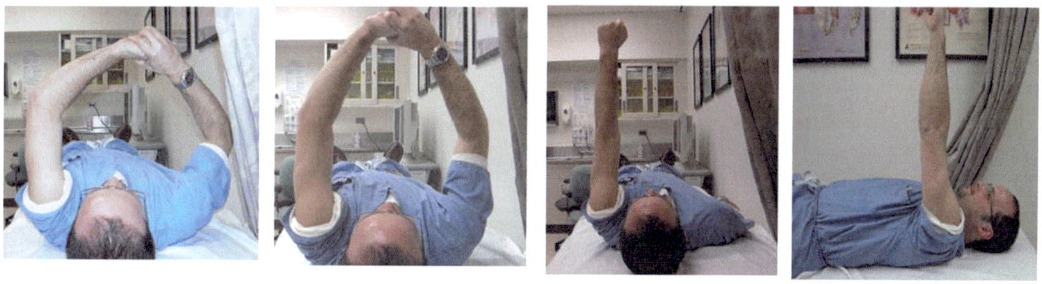

5) Then bend the elbow back down toward your chest.

6) Repeat steps 3 to 5, for 10 repetitions.

Virak Tan, M.D.; Professor; Hand, Upper Extremity & Microvascular Surgery
http://orthodoc.aaos.org/VirakTanMD/

Fig. 12.8 Supine overhead protocol for elbow rehabilitation. (**a**) Elbow flexion and extension ranging. (**b**) Forearm rotation at 90° of elbow flexion

b

NEW JERSEY MEDICAL SCHOOL • DEPARTMENT OF ORTHOPAEDICS
NORTH JERSEY ORTHOPAEDIC INSTITUTE

Overhead Elbow Exercises
(continue)

Rotating the Forearm

1) With the elbow bent at 90°, turn your forearm so that your palm is facing away from you (ie facing the ceiling). Hold it for 10 seconds.

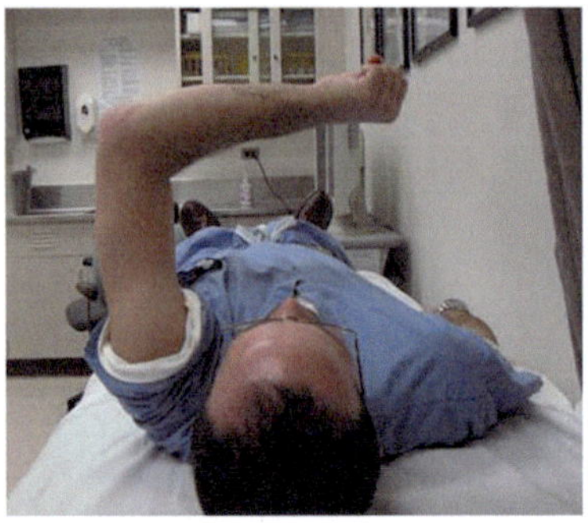

2) Now rotate your forearm in the opposite direction, so that your palm is facing down. Hold it for 10 seconds.

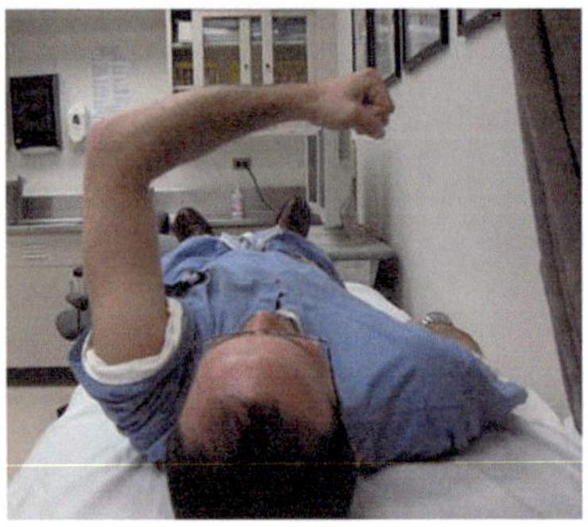

3) You may use the other (in this case, the right) arm to help with the forearm rotation.

4) Repeat steps 1 & 2, for 10 repetitions.

5) At the end of the exercises, put your elbow splint back on.

Virak Tan, M.D.; Professor; Hand, Upper Extremity & Microvascular Surgery
http://orthodoc.aaos.org/VirakTanMD/

Fig. 12.8 (continued)

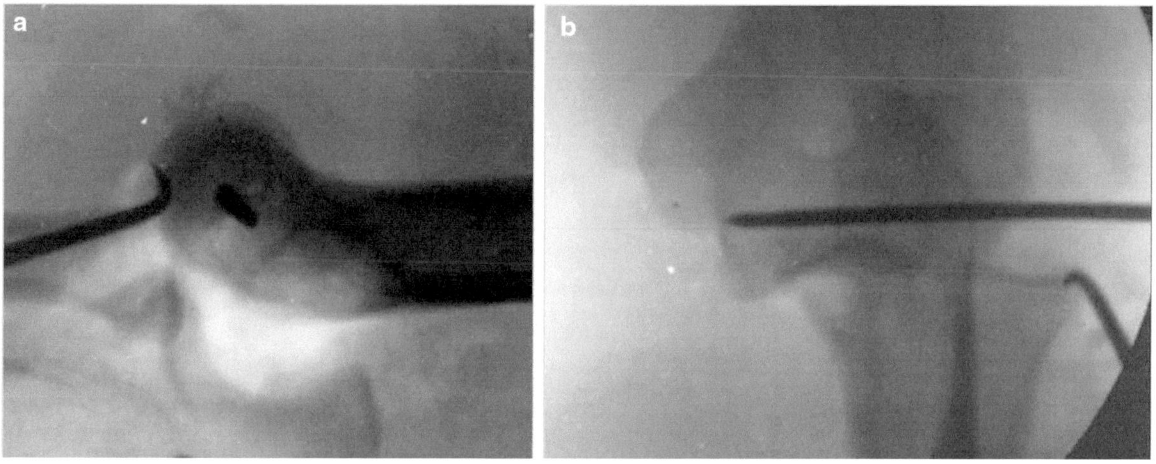

Fig. 12.9 (**a**) Fluoroscopy showing the point of entry for external fixation axis pin on the lateral view. (**b**) AP view with pin traveling parallel to the joint line

less ulnar nerve irritation, lower profile, and ease of application. The multiplanar design offers more rigidity and better control of coronal plane movement and joint distraction, but with the trade-off of being more cumbersome and more challenging to apply. Meticulous surgical technique is important and the most critical step is placement of the axis pin into the center of rotation of the elbow joint. This axis lies at the center of the capitellum and trochlea, and anatomic landmarks are used to define the entry point. Medially, it lies at a point distal and anterior to the medial epicondyle, while laterally, it is just distal to the lateral epicondyle. Fluoroscopic guidance is used to target the starting point before pin placement. Care must be taken to avoid disruption of the humeral anchor points for the collateral ligament reconstruction during insertion of the axis pin. After slowly advancing the guide pin, AP and lateral views should confirm placement parallel to the joint and as a dot within the center of the trochlea, respectively (Fig. 12.9). The AP view should show the pin traversing the distal humerus parallel to the joint line with the normal valgus angulation of the elbow joint maintained. With a unilateral frame, the axis pin does not need to completely traverse the bone; only adequate purchase must be obtained while ensuring proper alignment. When applying a multiplanar style fixator, one pin may be driven across from lateral to medial, or the distal humerus can be approached with two pins, one medial and one lateral meeting in the middle. With either technique, great care must be taken to avoid iatrogenic ulnar nerve damage.

The external fixator frame is next assembled around the axis pin using multiple half pins, which should be carefully placed to avoid impaling any muscle-tendon units or threatening the neurovascular structures. Humeral pins are usually easiest to place first due to patient positioning. Lateral placement should avoid the radial nerve while medially based pins should be done through an open approach to avoid the ulnar nerve. Bicortical purchase is required on all pins.

Once a concentric reduction is obtained, the ulnar pins may be inserted. Positioning the limb in the overhead position, with the elbow flexed, makes pin insertion easier while the weight of the forearm will aid in holding reduction. Pins can be inserted in a dorsal to volar or a lateral to medial direction. Once the pins are inserted, the frame is secured to the ulna. If a highly unstable elbow is encountered, a large Kirschner wire can be inserted across the joint to temporarily hold reduction before the ulnar pins are inserted.

Once all connections are secure, the axis pin is removed and the elbow is taken through a range of motion under fluoroscopy to ensure that a concentric stable reduction is maintained. Skin clearance by the half pins should be checked and the ulnar nerve should be felt during flexion and extension of the elbow. Fine-tuning of the frame to ensure proper varus/valgus alignment, as well as adequate distraction, should be done as the last step.

The Unstable Elbow Requiring Total Elbow Arthroplasty

In the event that all other options to stabilize the elbow joint have failed, a semiconstrained prosthetic arthroplasty can be considered [15]. Patient selection is of utmost importance when considering a total elbow replacement. These patients usually will have had multiple surgeries on the elbow and there is commonly severe joint surface incongruity and/or bone loss. The ideal candidate is an elderly patient with low functional demands. Consideration in the young patient with incapacitating instability can also be made with knowledge that revision elbow arthroplasty is expected in the future.

Contraindications for the standard total elbow arthroplasty include those with active infection, massive bone loss, soft tissue compromise, and poor healing potential, as well as paralysis. In the face of infection, surgical debridement with deep cultures must be performed, and staged prosthetic reconstruction

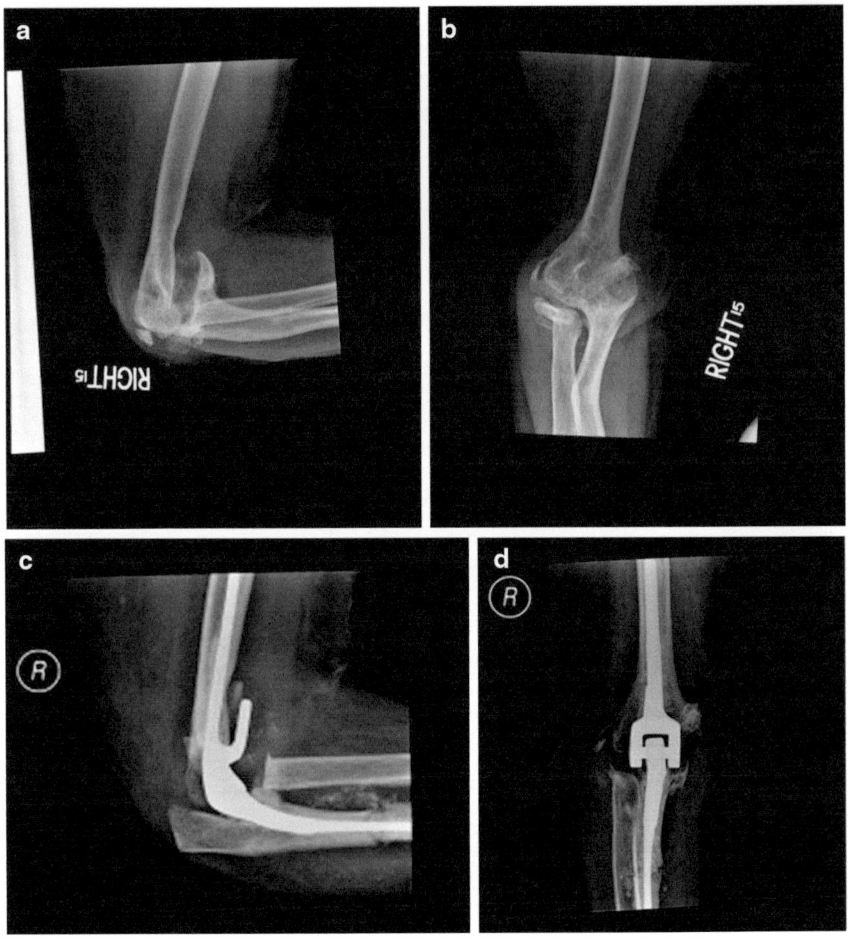

Fig. 12.10 (**a**, **b**) Radiographs demonstrating elbow arthropathy and instability after a failed distraction interpositional arthroplasty. The malalignment of the proximal ulna required osteotomy for insertion of the ulnar stem. (**c**, **d**) Postsurgical films show successful conversion to a total elbow arthroplasty

can be done. Any soft tissue defects should be addressed to ensure adequate coverage either prior to or at the same sitting as the prosthetic replacement. Noncompliance is a concern and patients need to be counseled on the limits of the procedure. A lifting restriction of 5–10 lb must be fully comprehended by the patient. Complications of elbow arthroplasty in the young patient have been reported due to dominant side involvement, activity level, and a traumatic etiology [16].

Previous surgeries to correct elbow instability or a chronically unstable elbow may pose specific difficulties not encountered in a primary elbow arthroplasty. Distorted anatomy may create special considerations when converting prior attempts at stabilization to an arthroplasty (Fig. 12.10). Attention to location of the ulnar nerve is important and history of prior ulnar nerve transposition should be obtained if possible [17]. Often, the chronically unstable elbow will be malaligned and careful soft tissue releases must be performed medially and/or laterally to ensure proper soft tissue balance which will help to avoid eccentric polyethylene wear [3]. Because of the instability, often times the joint can be "booked open" without having to take down the triceps insertion.

Adequate bone stock must be present to accept the prosthesis. Preparation of the canals may be more difficult due to intramedullary callous or bony malalignment. The surgeon should avoid use of aggressive reaming or broaching into the canal to minimize perforation of the cortex. Dedicating the appropriate time and judicious use of a burr to enlarge the canal or corrective osteotomy at site of deformity and fluoroscopy will be helpful during this step.

Humeral bone loss may lead to significant shortening with displacement of the forearm in any plane and may necessitate a long-stem humeral component. Ulnar bone loss may require the use of strut grafts to reconstruct the olecranon and provide an insertion for the extensor mechanism.

The Unstable Elbow Requiring Arthrodesis

In the event that all prior attempts, including prosthetic arthroplasty, have failed to provide a stable elbow joint, the salvage procedure is elbow arthrodesis [18]. The scenario in which this procedure is typically indicated involves a multiply operated elbow suffering from infection, bone loss with debilitating instability, and/or severe soft tissue compromise. Fusion of the elbow joint can relieve pain and leave the patient with a relatively functional upper extremity and avoid the morbidity associated with a flailed extremity. Elbow arthrodesis should be strongly considered in the young laborer.

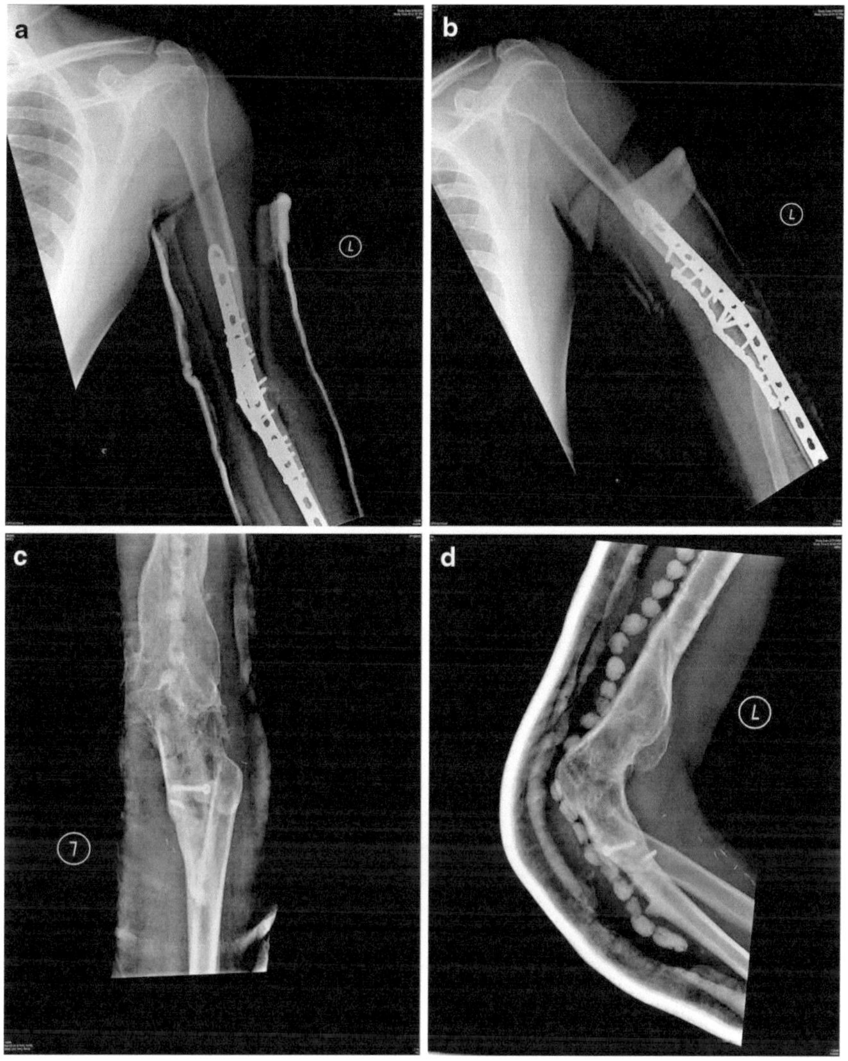

Fig. 12.11 (**a**, **b**) This patient chose to have his elbow fused in a position of relative extension. His goals were to be able to continue swinging a golf club. (**c**, **d**) Another patient requiring arthrodesis requested a position of more flexion in order to continue his job as a laborer. This allowed him to carry heavy objects while at work

The main obstacle to a successful outcome lies in the fact that an ideal position for fusion of the elbow joint does not exist. The most important activities are feeding and self-care and no angle of fusion is easily amenable to both. One must consider the individual demands of the patient (Fig. 12.11). Prior to the fusion, it is advisable to cast the elbow in a number of possible positions in an effort to determine the angle of most functionality for that particular patient.

Another obstacle in this procedure is the difficulty in obtaining a solid fusion. By the time that the patient needs a fusion, there is relatively little bone available. Each patient requires individual consideration when determining the technique to be used. Ideally, internal fixation with a 4.5-mm dynamic compression plate contoured to the appropriate angle should be utilized. If posterior soft tissues are tenuous, then a posterior approach should be avoided. The radial head should be resected except in the rare circumstance when its joint surface is pristine.

Maximal bony contact is the basic principle applied to achieve solid fusion. Autologous bone graft should be utilized and fibular strut grafts can be used if large defects are noted to provide the greatest chance at obtaining a solid fusion mass. Shortening of the humerus is not contraindicated as it brings the hand closer to the mouth as well as relieving soft tissue tension at the elbow. Postoperatively, cast application to protect the construct is recommended. In the case of severe soft tissue compromise, external fixation should be considered.

Summary

Elbow instability is a potentially debilitating condition unlikely to be corrected without surgical intervention. Meticulous attention to a proper history and physical exam utilizing the appropriate provocative maneuvers must be employed in addition to critical evaluation of appropriate radiologic studies. Patient goals must be combined with surgical goals; both parties must be willing to compromise and be realistic with regard to possible outcomes. Focus must be directed toward restoring bony anatomy before attempting to reconstruct soft tissue stabilizers. Previous surgical procedures as well as skin incisions must be considered when performing reoperative surgery of the elbow.

Restoration of bony anatomy should be followed by ligamentous reconstruction. Once deemed stable, a strict protocol of postoperative range of motion must be followed. If attempts at stabilization fail to yield adequate results, an external fixator should be applied and stability reassessed. If stability still cannot be achieved, then conversion to a total elbow arthroplasty should be considered. Only in the most severe cases of end-stage instability should a fusion be performed. Careful planning as well as patient education should not be underestimated as critical steps toward a successful outcome.

References

1. Regan W, Morrey B. Fractures of the coronoid process of the ulna. J Bone Joint Surg Am. 1989;71(9):1348–54.
2. Morrey B, Tanaka S, Kai-Nan A. Valgus stability of the elbow. Clin Orthop Relat Res. 1991;265:187–95.
3. Morrey BF. The elbow and its disorders. 4th ed. Toronto: Saunders; 2008. p. 839–41.
4. O'Driscoll SW, Bell DF, Morrey BF. Posterolateral rotatory instability of the elbow. J Bone Joint Surg Am. 1991;73:440–6.
5. Mathew P, Athwal G, King G. Terrible triad of the elbow: current concepts. J Am Acad Orthop Surg. 2009;17:137–51.
6. McKee M, Pugh D, Wild L, Schemitsch E, King G. Standard protocol to treat elbow dislocations with radial head and coronoid fractures. J Bone Joint Surg Am. 2005;87:22–32.
7. Nestor B, O'Driscoll S, Morrey B. Ligamentous reconstruction for posterolateral rotatory instability of the elbow. J Bone Joint Surg Am. 1992;74:1235–41.
8. Sanchez-Sotelo J, Morrey B, O'Driscoll S. Ligamentous repair and reconstruction for posterolateral rotatory instability of the elbow. J Bone Joint Surg Br. 2005;87-B:54–61.
9. Jepegnanam TS. Salvage of the radial head in adult Monteggia fractures. J Bone Joint Surg Br. 2006;88-B:645–8.
10. Ring D, Jupiter J, Simpson S. Monteggia fractures in adults. J Bone Joint Surg Am. 1998;80:1733–44.
11. Ring D, Jupiter J, Zilberfarb J. Posterior dislocation of the elbow with fractures of the radial head and coronoid. J Bone Joint Surg Am. 2002;84:547–51.
12. Ring D, Jupiter J. Reconstruction of posttraumatic elbow instability. Clin Orthop Relat Res. 2000;370:44–56.
13. King G, Patterson S. Metallic radial head arthroplasty. Tech Hand Up Extrem Surg. 2001;5(4):196–203.
14. Tan V, Daluiski A, Capo J, Hotchkiss R. Hinged elbow external fixators: indications and uses. J Am Acad Orthop Surg. 2005; 13(8):503–14.
15. Bennett J, Mehlhoff T. Total elbow arthroplasty: surgical technique. J Hand Surg Am. 2009;34A:933–9.
16. Celli A, Morrey B. Total elbow arthroplasty in patients forty years of age or less. J Bone Joint Surg Am. 2009;91:1414–8.
17. Ramsey M, Adams R, Morrey B. Instability of the elbow treated with semiconstrained total elbow arthroplasty. J Bone Joint Surg Am. 1999;81:38–47.
18. Koller H, Kolb K, Assuncao A, Kolb W, Holz U. The fate of elbow arthrodesis: indications, techniques, and outcome in fourteen patients. J Shoulder Elbow Surg. 2008;2(17):293–306.

Reoperative Conditions Following Total Elbow Arthroplasty

13

Jeffrey C. King

Abstract

Revision elbow arthroplasty is a very technically challenging and demanding procedure. The nerves and vessels about the elbow may be scarred and may no longer be in their usual anatomic locations. The bone stock can also be quite minimal leading to difficulties with further implant fixation. Moreover, the soft tissue envelope is easily compromised about the elbow, and this can lead to problems with wound breakdown and infection. Structural allografts can be helpful in trying to reinforce thinned-out bone. However, in some cases the patient may be better served by resection arthroplasty, especially in many cases of infection.

Keywords

Elbow • Arthroplasty • Revision • Complication • Reconstruction

Key Points

- Prevention is always better than revision. Patient selection is paramount to minimizing complications and failures in total elbow arthroplasty "TEA."
- Survival of a revised TEA is generally inferior to the index procedure, and the complication rate is higher; this should be a consideration in the recommendation of TEA in younger, more active patients.
- Infection of TEA is more common than with total knee arthroplasty "TKA" and total hip arthroplasty "THA," antibiotic impregnated cement, and meticulous tissue handling appear to have lowered this disastrous complication.
- Previous incisions should be used whenever possible to minimize stress to the skin flaps. If the soft tissue envelope is poor, consider a staged procedure to improve the soft tissue envelope prior to joint revision. Meticulous attention to the position and vascular supply of the nerves is required to minimize injury and dysfunction.
- Bushing wear and aseptic loosing occur with all types of implants and is load and cycle dependent. Different implant designs have been developed to minimize this problem, but the ideal design has not been achieved. Activity modification is still required for patients with TEA to preserve implant longevity.
- Implant and cement removal is frequently required during reoperations for elbow replacement failure. This process is difficult and time-consuming and requires careful protection of the nerves and bone

(continued)

J.C. King, MD (✉)
Division of Hand and Elbow Surgery, Michigan State University College of Human Medicine and Kalamazoo Center for Medical Studies, HealthCare Midwest, 601 John Street, Suite M-230, Kalamazoo, MI 49007, USA
e-mail: jking@hcmw.org

S.F.M. Duncan (ed.), *Reoperative Hand Surgery*,
DOI 10.1007/978-1-4614-2373-7_13,

preservation. Creation of bone windows to remove residual cement is preferable to unexpected fracture.

- Periprosthetic fractures frequently accompany osteolysis and implant loosening. Structural and nonstructural allografts are useful to restore bone stock and assist in the stabilization of fractures. Commercially available implants are usually sufficient for these revisions, and custom-made implants are rarely necessary.
- Triceps insufficiency is common, and likely underreported. This complication is related to the approach used to expose the joint during replacement. Techniques that preserve the attachment of Sharpey's fibers to the olecranon appear superior. Reconstruction techniques using local tissue and allograft, if required, can restore extension force against gravity and limit functional impairment.
- Nonreimplantation options for the salvage of failed TEA exist, including resection arthroplasty, elbow fusion, and above-elbow amputation, but are less frequently employed with the improvement of revision techniques. The most common of these is resection arthroplasty, which may be indicated in specific cases of TEA infection.

Introduction

The burden of revision surgery following TEA is increasing (Fig. 13.1). The cause of this increase is multifactorial. The absolute number of primary TEAs performed, although significantly less than "TKA" and "THA" is increasing [1] (Table 13.1). Reasons for this include an increased interest in, and understanding of surgical reconstruction of the elbow by orthopedic surgeons, more orthopedic implant companies designing and promoting implants, and a growing demand for improved elbow function by our patients. Unfortunately the "all cause" rate of revision surgery for TEA is higher than for other joint arthroplasties [2]. Although the total number of TEAs performed is smaller than TKA and THA, the proportion of revision surgery is higher. Second, although there seems to be a decrease in the number of TEAs done for the traditional indication of rheumatoid arthritis (RA), in part due to better medical management, there are an increasing number of elbow replacements performed for posttraumatic arthritis (PTA), acute fractures (AF) (Fig. 13.2a, b) [58], and distal humerus nonunions (NU) (Fig. 13.3). The survival of TEA performed for PTA, AF, and NU is worse than for RA and other inflammatory arthritic conditions [2], increasing the ratio of elbow implants requiring revision surgery.

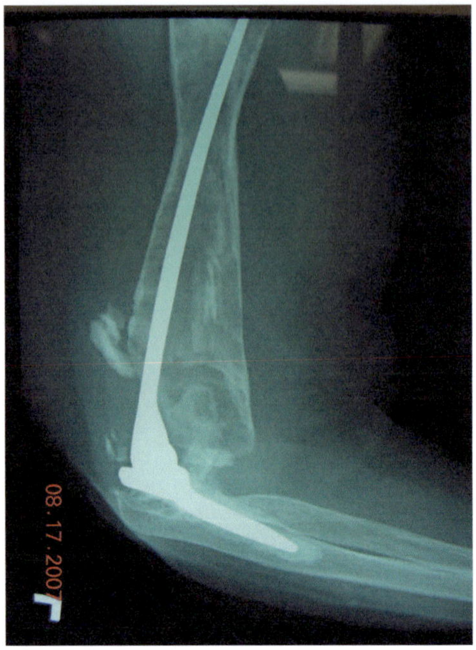

Fig. 13.1 Failed linked total elbow arthroplasty (TEA) with implant loosening, osteolysis, and pathologic fracture. Note the reactive bony deformity of the proximal anterior humeral cortex; this occurs more frequently with implant designs which lack an anterior flange

Additionally, survival of the revision TEA procedure is worse than for the index procedure [3]. The most common indications for reoperation following failed TEA are infection [4–6], periprosthetic fracture [7], aseptic loosening/bushing wear [8–10], instability [11], and triceps insufficiency [12]. This chapter will address current reconstructive surgical techniques utilized to manage these difficult problems.

Bushing Exchange

Introduction

Bushing wear and the subsequent osteolysis, which may result from the particulate debris generated, is a major concern [13]. The frequency with which it occurs is related to the implant used [14], the age and activity level of the patient [15], and the degree of preoperative deformity [10]. Rates of bushing wear are highest in the Pritchard II and GSB implants with rates of 12% [16] and 5%, respectively. The Coonrad–Morrey device has a reported 1.3% reoperation rate for bushing wear [8]. The true incidence of problematic bushing wear is probably under reported as early identification is difficult, and the underlying problem of bushing wear may be masked by its manifestations of osteolysis, implant loosening (Fig. 13.4) and periprosthetic fractures [10] (Fig. 13.5). Diagnosis may be difficult in the early stages but becomes

Table 13.1 Total elbow replacement procedures 1998–2006

Procedure name	1998	1999	2000	2001	2002	2003	2004	2005	2006
Total elbow replacement	1,254	1,553	1,441	1,904	1,780	2,400	2,568	2,473	2,762

Source: HCUP Nationwide Inpatient Sample (NIS) [1]

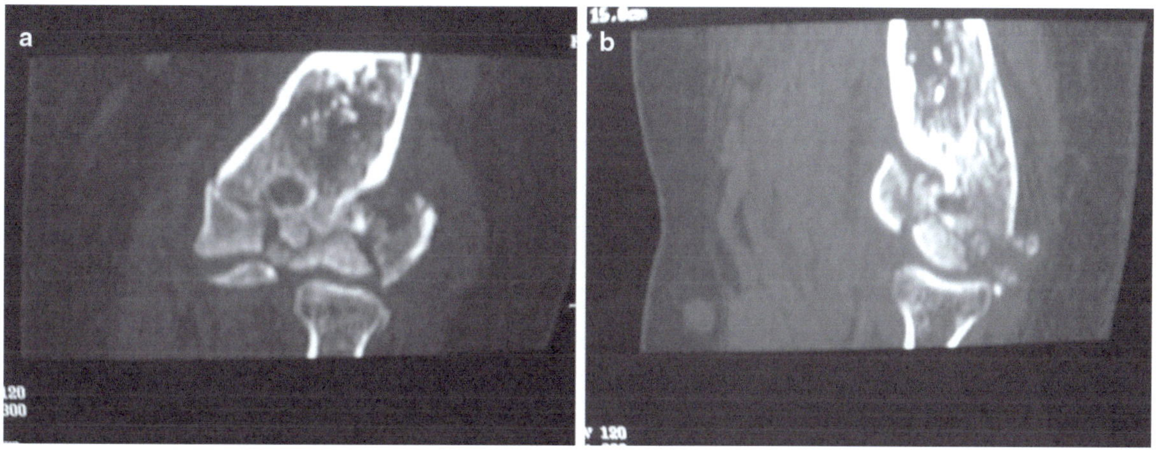

Fig. 13.2 (**a**, **b**) Coronal and sagittal CT images demonstrating significant intracapsular and intra-articular comminution

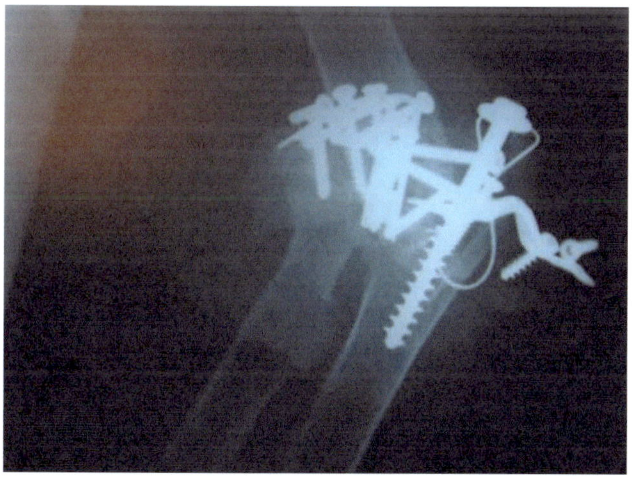

Fig. 13.3 Failed fixation of a complex distal humerus fracture/nonunion

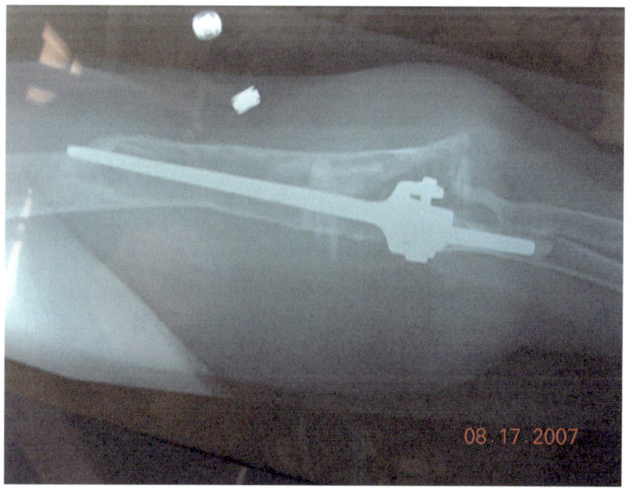

Fig. 13.4 Osteolysis and implant loosening likely secondary to excessive bushing wear

evident once bushing failure occurs. Clinical signs of squeaking or grinding may be present, especially with varus load. Patients may or may not experience a sense of elbow laxity. Radiographic evaluation with stress views in the true AP plane shows an increased angle of intersection between the longitudinal axis of the humeral implant and medial or lateral surface of the articular portion of the ulnar implant (Fig. 13.6). The normal laxity of the Coonrad–Morrey implant is 7–10°, greater than this indicates excessive wear of the poly bushing [17]. Extreme angulation is often an indicator of metal-on-metal articulation (Fig. 13.7).

This procedure has been described as simple and straightforward [9]; however, great care should be taken to avoid additional complications. The procedure should be approached as any TEA procedure with respect to the risk of infection, including the use of a laminar flow environment,

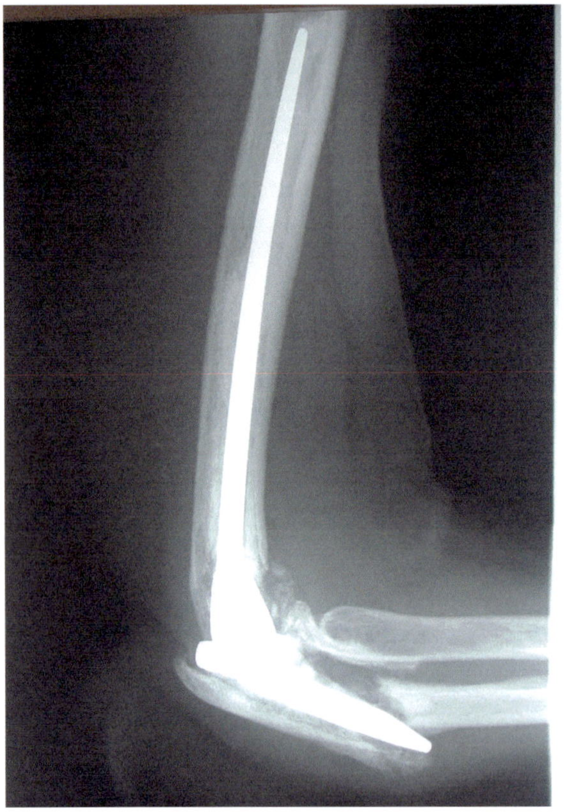

Fig. 13.5 Periprosthetic fracture of the ulna

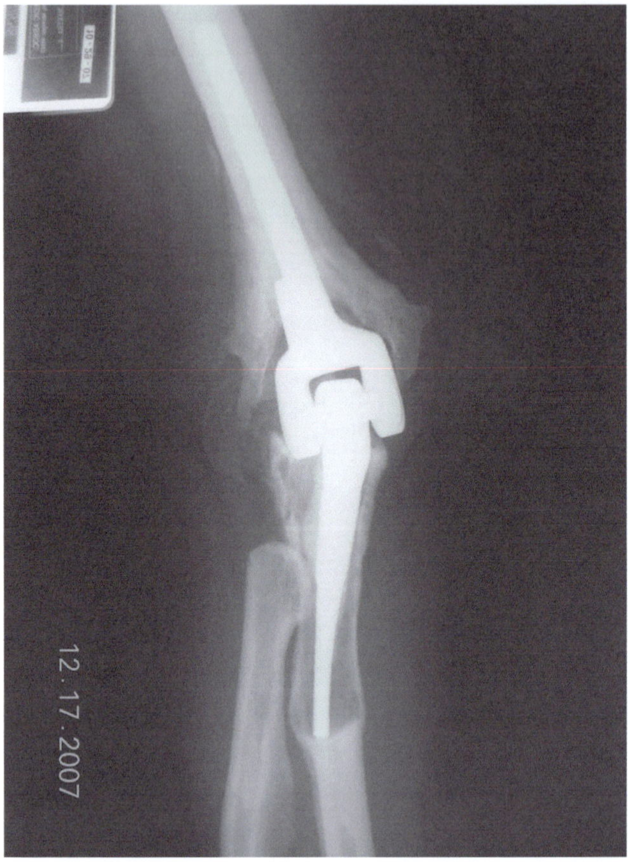

Fig. 13.6 Increased angulation of the ulnar implant relative to the humeral yoke indicates increased bushing wear

space suits, etc. Care is required while disarticulating the implant if the triceps is preserved to avoid fracturing the olecranon, especially in patients with RA or significant osteopenia. One should resist the urge to try to perform this procedure through a "keyhole" incision because it is "just a bushing exchange." The surgeon should be prepared to address any issue, including soft tissue rebalancing, supplementing the cement mantle, even replacing the implants if they are found to be loose or malpositioned. Proper preparation and careful attention to detail will minimize the chance of further complications.

Indications

- Symptomatic bushing wear, i.e., squeaking, grinding, pain etc.
- Asymptomatic patient with angulation >10° on stress radiographs
- In conjunction with other associated TEA procedures, i.e., triceps repair or reconstruction, washout for acute infection, etc.
- All implant revision surgery cases

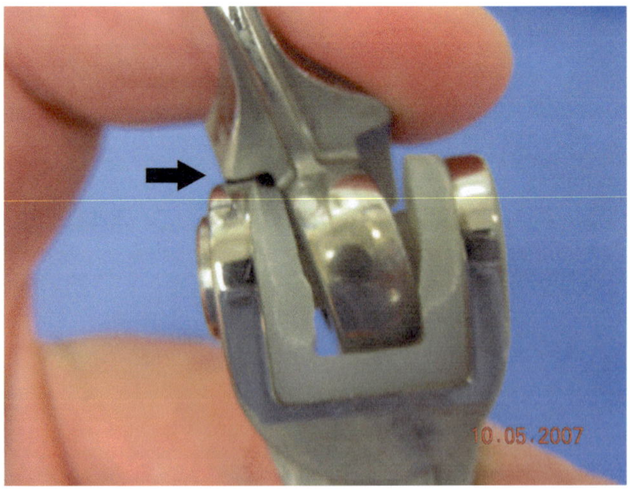

Fig. 13.7 Metal-on-metal articulation (*arrow*) is easily seen in this worn and explanted implant

Contraindications

- Asymptomatic low demand patient with medical contraindications to surgery

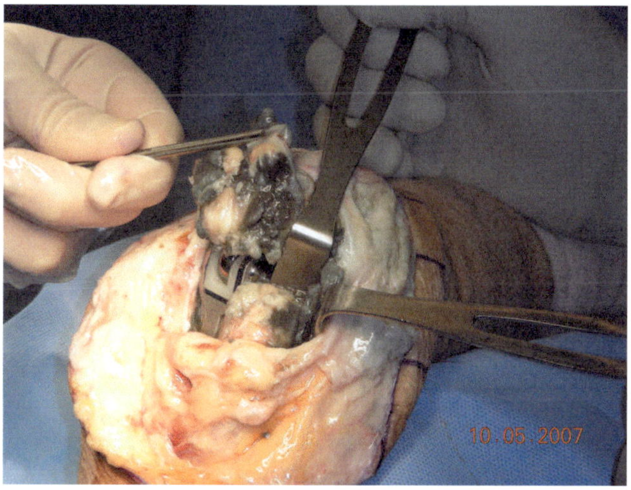

Fig. 13.8 Significant metallosis present due to excessive bushing wear allowing metal-on-metal contact (same case as Fig. 13.7)

Procedure

The patient is positioned supine with the arm across the body. The arm is exsanguinated and the tourniquet inflated. The previous skin incision is utilized, and full thickness flaps are carefully raised. The ulnar nerve is identified and protected. Medial and lateral approaches to the implant are performed. The triceps is left attached to the olecranon if possible. If the condyles are intact, sufficient anterior bone is removed to allow clear access to the locking mechanism. Some implant designs allow access to the bushing from the rear and can be accessed through a triceps split without removing bone. The linkage is uncoupled and the joint disarticulated. Complete muscle paralysis is often helpful during this stage. Removal of the polyethylene bushing should be accomplished without scratching the metal surface of the implants. The implants are inspected for metal-on-metal wear, and depressions in the surface, which could accelerate wear of the replacement bushing. Theoretically, if the implant shows sufficient surface wear to compromise support of the replacement bushing, the implant should be removed and replaced, although I have not had to do this.

Thorough synovectomy is performed, especially if metallic debris is present (Fig. 13.8) [18]. The bone–implant interfaces are examined for resorption. If present, the soft tissue is carefully removed and the gaps filled with polymethyl methacrylate bone cement [9]. Use of a 10-cc syringe with a large bore angiocatheter (12 or 14 g) is helpful for this process. The new bushings are inserted, and the joint is coupled. Range of motion of the joint should demonstrate the ulna tracking though the middle of the available varus/valgus play in the articulation. If the ulnar implant is tracking along one edge of the humeral articulation, this indicates soft tissue imbalance, which will accelerate wear of the new bushing. In this situation, soft tissue releases to balance the joint are required. The flexor pronator mass is released for varus imbalance, and the extensors released for excessive valgus stress. The triceps, if reflected or released, is reattached at this time. The released tendinous origins are repaired to the respective edge of the triceps during closure.

Pearls and Pitfalls

- Increased bushing wear is associated with some implant designs, males, young age, activity level, PTA, and especially preoperative deformity.
- Approach "simple" bushing exchange with all of the care you would a TEA.
- It is probably better to consider bushing exchange a bit too early, than too late. Delay in bushing exchange may lead to metallosis which is more damaging to the soft tissues, bone and the joint, and should be avoided if possible.
- If leaving the triceps intact, be very careful to avoid fracturing the olecranon during disarticulation, especially in RA patients.
  - If the olecranon fractures, it can be repaired with a tension band wire, or plate with unicortical screws, or cables, although persistent nonunion is common [19].
- Identify and fill osteolytic voids with polymethylmethacrylate (PMMA) during bushing exchange.
- Soft tissue balancing is important to minimize stress on the bushing and implant.

Postoperative Care

The patient is placed in a splint in full extension for 36–72 h and discharged home. If the triceps was not released, early active range of motion is started at that time. If triceps repair was performed, further immobilization and/or restrictions may be appropriate depending on the technique used and the surgeon's preference.

Implant and Cement Removal

Introduction

Despite advances in surgical techniques and instrumentation, the removal of well-fixed humeral and ulnar implants continues to be difficult and fraught with complications [7, 20]. Newer implant designs with increased modularity allow for easier replacement of worn surfaces, and even conversion of the implant from an unlinked to linked configuration, without removing the cemented stems [21]. There will always be, however, instances that require the removal of the implants and cement mantle [6].

Indications

- Infection
- Aseptic loosening/osteolysis
- Malposition of the implants
- Conversion of implant
  - Nonlinked to linked
  - Hemi to TEA
  - Obsolete to current designs

Contraindications

- Medically unstable
- Antibiotic suppression vs. implant removal

Removal of the implant and all of the cement is required in the setting of infection. If infection is not present, the option exists to reimplant into a prepared existent cement mantle. This minimizes the risk and simplifies the revision procedure considerably. There are several steps that can be performed at the time of the index procedure to minimize the difficulty and complexity of cement removal. First, the use of cement restrictors limits the extrusion of cement beyond the desired area for implant fixation. Cement restrictors are commercially available, and may contain radiopaque beads to aid in localization. Bioabsorbable cellulose or bone graft may be used as well and does not require specific removal during revision (Hughes, personal communication 2002). The restrictor should be placed approximately 1 cm beyond the tip of the implant. The opening of the humerus is often smaller than the internal diameter of the humeral canal, so care must be taken to prevent the placement of the restrictor more proximal than anticipated. The addition of a few drops of methylene blue or other dye during cement preparation allows easier identification of the cement bone interface at the time of removal, and does not affect the strength of the cement. Finally, the addition of antibiotic powder to the cement during preparation has become widely accepted in joint arthroplasty literature [22, 23] and may lower joint infection rates. The use of i.v. regional antibiotics during total joint arthroplasty has been reported as well [24] and has been utilized with excellent results in one center (Hughes, personal communication 2001).

The ulnar [25] and radial [26] nerves must be identified initially. The radial nerve is at specific risk at the level of the spiral groove if it is not identified and protected. Iatrogenic cortical fracture or cortical perforation from cement removal techniques place the nerve at risk for direct mechanical injury from the instruments, contact from cement extrusion during reimplantation [27], or thermal injury from ultrasonic cement removal devices [28]. The position of the nerves must be respected during cable fixation of osteotomies or strut grafts as well.

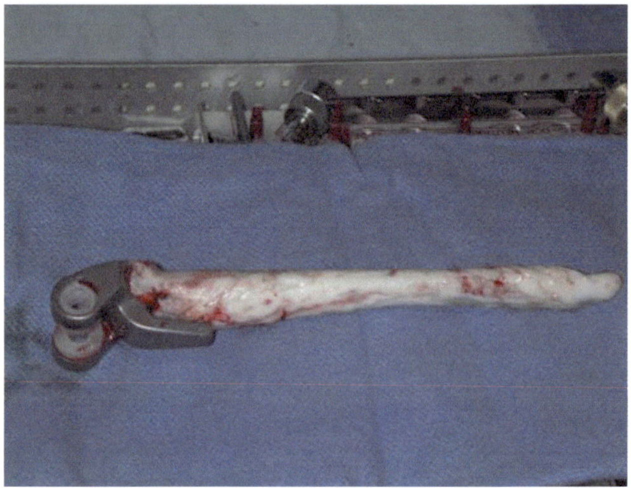

Fig. 13.9 Humeral implant extracted by hand with an intact cement mantle

Surgical Technique

The patient is positioned supine with the arm across the chest. A sterile tourniquet is used to allow proximal access to the humerus. The previous incision is typically utilized and may be extended proximally or distally as the situation dictates. The ulnar and radial nerves are identified and protected. The triceps is released or reflected as appropriate and the implant exposed. Following the manufacturer's recommendations, the implant is uncoupled or separated. In cases of advanced infection or osteolysis, the implant may be sufficiently loose that it can be removed by hand. The cement mantle may or may not be attached (Fig. 13.9). In all other cases, significantly more work is involved. An extraction tool may be attached to the implant and a longitudinal traction force applied. Often, a slap hammer can provide the appropriately directed force to break the connection between the implant and the cement. Commercially available vice grip pliers with an attached slap hammer are available as well. If the implant does not release at this point, the cement mantle must be removed from around the implant, specifically around any roughened or bead coated portion of the implant. This can be accomplished with the use of small osteotomes and great patience. Small burrs can be used, but great care should be used to prevent damage to the bone or showering the wound with metal debris. If the implant is not extractable by removing the distal cuff of cement, an osteotomy may be required to facilitate extraction. Performing a controlled osteotomy is clearly preferable to an uncontrolled fracture of the humerus or ulna during attempted implant removal.

Humerus: A trapezoidal osteotomy is created on the posterior aspect of the humerus with the wide part distal (Fig. 13.10). The bone window should extend beyond the textured surface of the implant, but allow for at least two

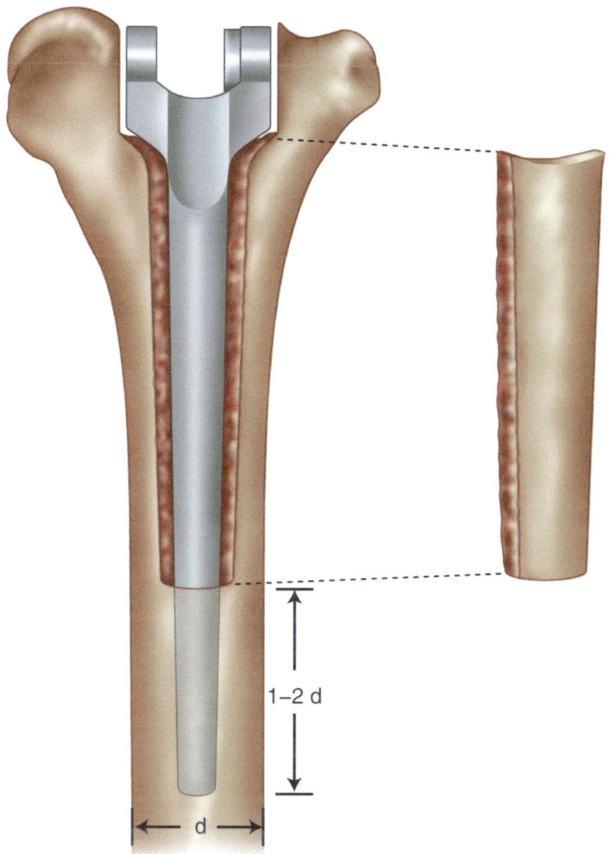

Fig. 13.10 Removal of a trapezoidal portion of the humerus improves exposure and facilitates cement removal

diameters of circumferentially intact cortex beyond the tip of the window. The osteotomy can extend all the way to the tip of the implant if needed, however, the next longer sized implant is required for reimplantation. A pencil tip burr is used to remove the cement from around the sides of the implant and the slap hammer used to extract the implant. Once the implant is removed, the exposed cement may be carefully removed with osteotomes and specific cement removal instruments. The core of cement beyond the tip of the implant is removed by drilling through the cement core (Fig. 13.11a) and placing a guide wire through the drilled hole. Flexible cannulated reamers can be used to remove the remaining cement (Fig. 13.11b). Use of fluoroscopy is helpful to minimize the chance of cortical perforation by the drill or reamers (Fig. 13.11c). A headlight may be helpful at this stage as well to improve visualization. Reilly et al. [29] reported the use of a 30° arthroscope and a 3-mm burr to aid in the removal of cement from inside the medullary canal. The use of an Ultradrive to remove cement can be helpful; however, it must not be used near the spiral groove as the elevated temperatures can injure the radial nerve [28]. Once all of the cement is removed, the inner walls of the canal are scraped with a ring curette to remove any residual infected material. Pulsatile irrigation is used at this stage as well.

Ulna: The ulnar osteotomy is created on the medial aspect of the proximal ulna. The trapezoidal window, if needed, extends from the sigmoid notch to just past the textured portion of the implant. A second rectangular window may be required, and is created as proximally as possible, but still allows access to the tip of the implant and distal cement (Fig. 13.12). Again, a pencil burr is used to remove cement from around the implant to allow a slap hammer to remove the implant. When drilling distally, or using the flexible reamers, be sure there is sufficient clearance in the sigmoid notch to allow for colinear passage of the drill down the canal. Failure to do so increases the risk of penetration of the ulnar cortex dorsally and laterally.

If the elbow joint is not infected, a well-fixed cement mantle can be retained and a new implant cemented into it [7]. All loose cement should be removed and then the canal prepared with a drill and flexible reamers. Standard rasps are typically ineffective at broaching intact cement. Unpublished data from the Mayo Clinic indicates that the failure rate of this procedure is higher if the underlying bone quality is poor [30].

Fixation

The osteotomized bone plates are reapproximated and held with cerclage wires or cables. The osteotomy site can be reinforced with strut allografts as well if the quality of the bone is poor.

Complications

- Iatrogenic fracture, including cortical perforation
- Injury to ulnar or radial nerves
- Failure to remove all cement in cases of infection

Pearls

- Removal of a well-fixed implant and cement is a tedious and complex exercise. The risks of injury to the radial nerve and iatrogenic fractures should be anticipated and avoided.
- The use of controlled osteotomies, fluoroscopy, a headlight and arthroscopy facilitate implant and cement removal.
- High-speed burrs and ultrasonic cement removal devices should be used with caution to avoid injury to the remaining bone and neurologic structures.
- Removal of all of the cement is not required for revision of noninfected implants. The new implant may be cemented into a well-fixed cement column.
- Attention to detail in the index procedure can limit the need for, and complexity of, cement and implant removal.

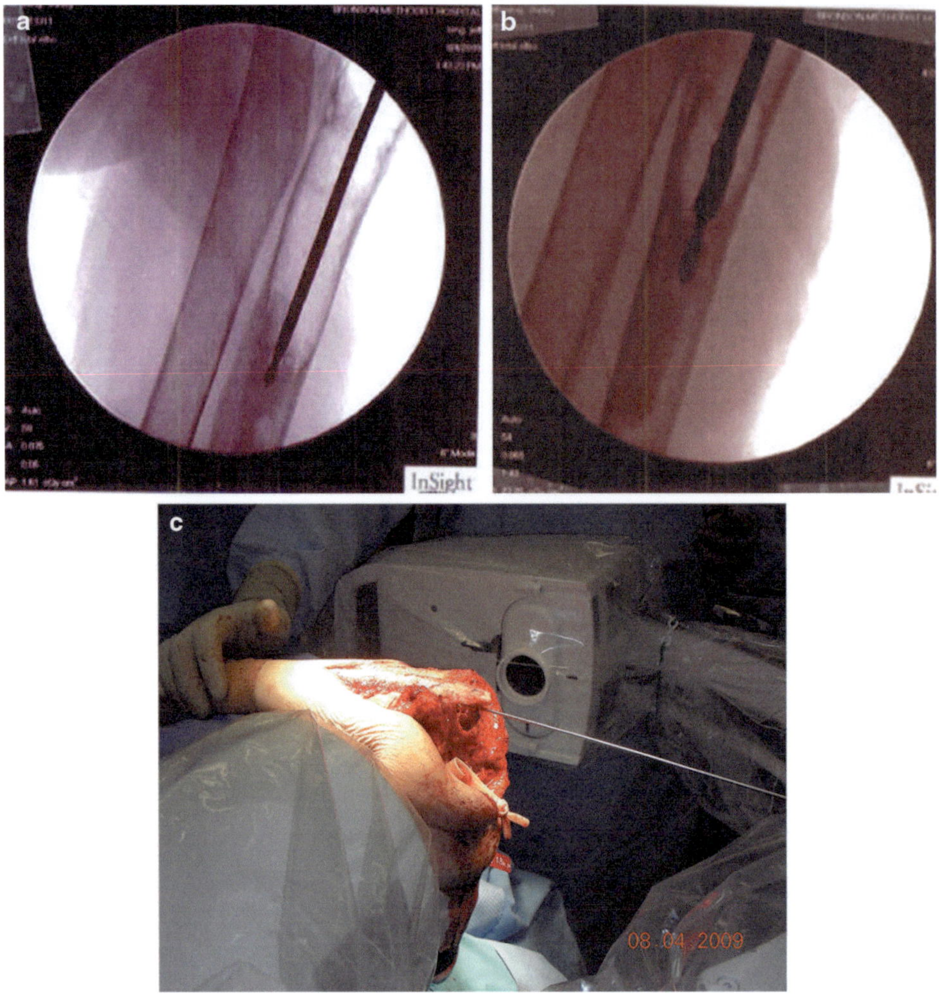

Fig. 13.11 (**a**) Fluoroscopic image of a drill tip guide wire being placed through the well-fixed distal cement mantle of an ulna. (**b**) Fluoroscopic image of a cannulated reamer placed over the previously placed guide wire. (**c**) Mini fluoroscopy unit in place during guide wire placement. Standard sized fluoroscopy may be used as well

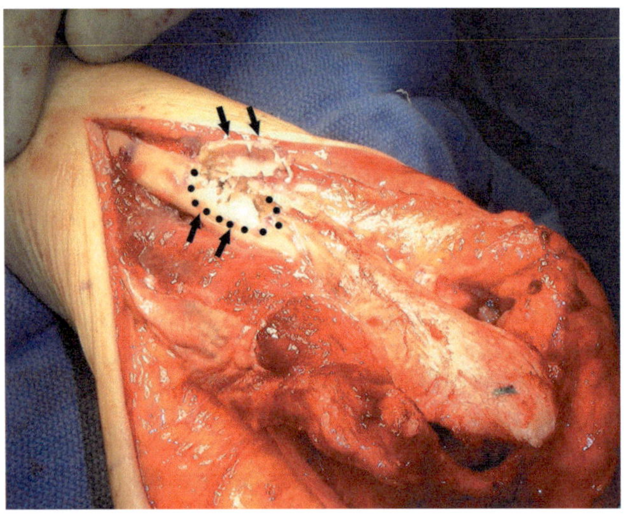

Fig. 13.12 Clinical photo of distal osteotomy of the ulna (*arrows*) to remove the distal cement plug

Managing Bone Loss and Periprosthetic Fractures

Introduction

Loss of the osseous support for TEA implants can be a significant element of TEA failure. The loss of support can occur gradually as osteolysis due to infection, reaction to wear debris, unbalanced mechanical forces (Fig. 13.4), or acutely via periprosthetic fractures (Fig. 13.5). Bone deficiency can be categorized as a loss of length (i.e., deficient humerus or ulna), loss of structural integrity (i.e., fracture) or compromise of bone quality (i.e., thinned patulous canals secondary to osteolysis and implant loosening). Restoration of the integrity of the humerus and ulna to support their respective implants is critical to the success of revision surgery. The Mayo classification of periprosthetic fractures divides these fractures

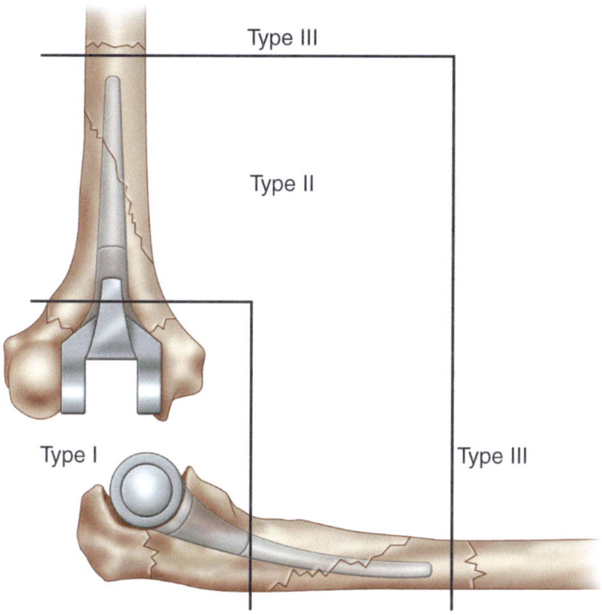

Fig. 13.13 Mayo classification of periprosthetic fractures about the elbow. The types II and III are typically managed with strut grafting

into (I) proximal (metaphyseal), (II) with stem involvement, or (III) proximal or distal to the implant tip (Fig. 13.13). Sanchez-Sotelo et al. [25] reported the utility of strut grafts for the reconstruction of type II and type III fractures.

There are several techniques that can be used alone or in combination to restore the osseous stability for the TEA implants. These techniques include impaction grafting, mechanical strut grafts, anatomic allografts (APC: allograft-prosthetic composite), and rarely vascularized autografts (such as a vascularized free fibula). Additionally, implant selection is critical to the success of these complex revisions. Although the use of custom implants has been described [31], commercially available linked implants in a variety of interchangeable sizes have been successfully utilized in almost all revision situations [3, 6, 25].

Indications

- TEA revision for
  - Periprosthetic fractures
  - Aseptic loosening
  - Infection (treated and controlled)
- Impaction grafting
  - Patulous canal, cortical shell intact
- Allograft struts
  - Restore length
  - Support diaphyseal fracture site
  - Support window osteotomy site
  - Reinforcement of thinned intact cortex
  - Restore triceps moment arm (ulna)
- APC
  - Significant loss of length
  - Reinforcement of thinned intact cortex
  - Restore triceps moment arm (ulna)
- Vascularized bone graft
  - Chronic nonunion of periprosthetic fracture

Contraindications

- Uncontrolled infection
- Unsatisfactory soft tissue envelope
- Medically unstable patient

Impaction Grafting Procedure

The patient is positioned supine with the arm across the chest. A sterile tourniquet is used to allow proximal access to the humerus. The previous incision is typically utilized and may be extended proximally or distally as the situation dictates. The ulnar and radial nerves are identified and protected. The triceps is released or reflected as appropriate and the implant unlinked. Take care not to fracture the thinned cortex during this process. Typically, the implant is loose in this clinical situation and is easily removed. Occasionally, there is deformity of the humeral or ulnar shaft, which can make extraction difficult (see section "Implant and Cement Removal"). Following implant and cement removal, the cortex is inspected for perforations or fractures. If defects are identified, strut grafts are utilized to span the defective cortex. Anterior and posterior strut grafts can also be utilized to reinforce the thinned and fragile cortex (see strut graft application). There is usually a membranous lining within the canal that must be removed. The intramedullary canal is then cleaned and dried, and the non-affected portion of the canal identified if possible, beyond the affected area. A long guide wire can be helpful for this step, and if there is any question, fluoroscopic imaging in orthogonal planes confirms appropriate positioning. There are commercially available devices (Zimmer, Inc.) to simplify the impaction bone grafting process, although they are not required to satisfactorily perform the process. If these are used (Fig. 13.14), the inner tube is place over the guide wire to a depth of approximately two diameters into normal bone. An outer (larger) tube is placed over the first tube to the depth of the compromised bone. Morselized allograft or autograft cancellous bone chips measuring 2–4 mm are then impacted circumferentially around the outer tube, filling the space between the outer tube and the cortex. A tamp is utilized to compact the bone graft tightly. The space is completely filled and compacted. Bone cement

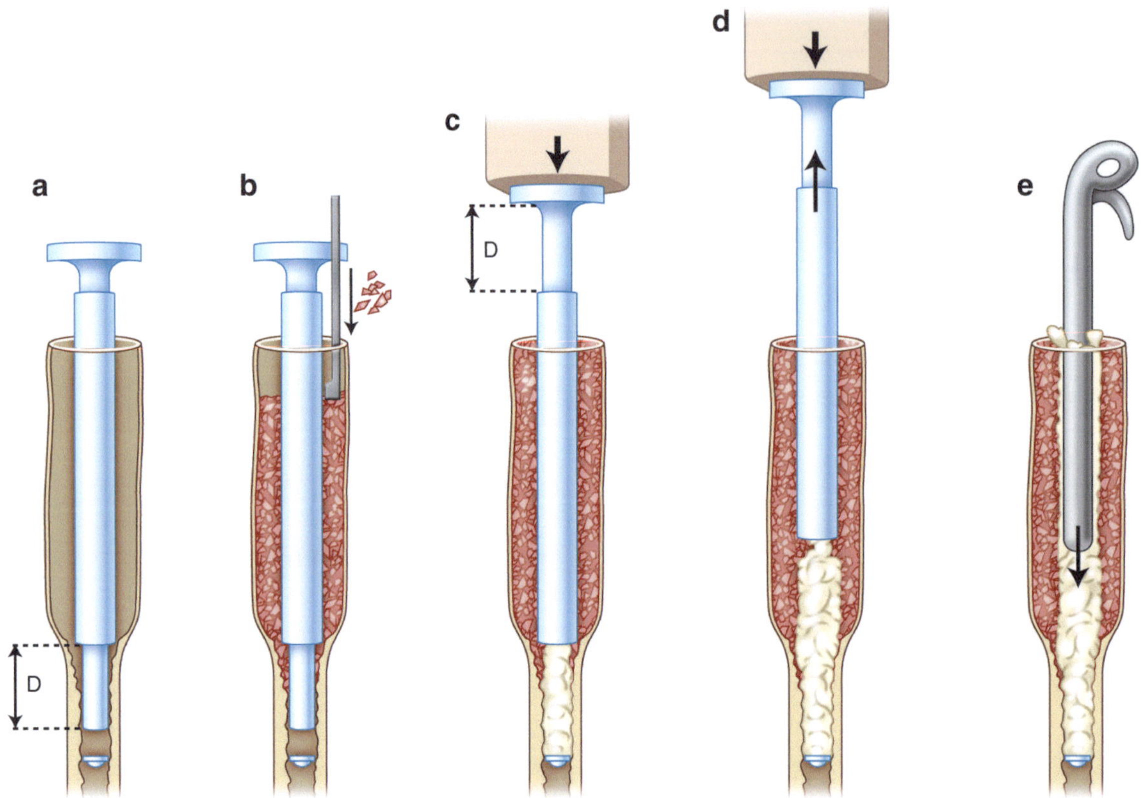

Fig. 13.14 The technique of impact grafting. (**a**) A smaller diameter tube is inserted through a larger diameter tube and extends past the larger diameter tube for a distance (*D*) by approximately two cortical diameters into the normal host bone. The outer diameter tube is inserted to the depth of the osteolytic segment. (**b**) Small chips on cancellous bone are tightly impacted around the outer diameter tube. (**c**) The cement cartridge is attached to the inner diameter tube, which is withdrawn to the level of the larger outer tube while cement is being injected. (**d**) At this point, both tubes are withdrawn together while cement continues to be delivered through the inner tube. (**e**) The implant is inserted through the cement and impacted graft composite and into normal host bone

is injected through the inner tube into the native canal, and the inner tube is withdrawn to the level of the outer tube. The outer and inner tubes are carefully withdrawn as the cement is injected into the neo-canal. The implant is then inserted into the cement-filled neo-canal with either a small bone "cookie" under the anterior flange, if applicable, or with the preplaced strut graft under the flange. The length of the implant may be long enough to enter the intact canal, or left short of the junction, but should not end at the junction of the normal and abnormal cortex. If a shorter implant is utilized, it is wise to supplement the reconstruction with strut grafts.

The impaction grafting technique without the use of the "tube in a tube" technique is similar in concept, with the following modifications. After preparation of the canal and addition of struts if necessary, the largest size trial implant is placed in the canal, being sure the tip enters the normal canal. While maintaining the implant in the center of the dilated canal, the cancellous chips are impacted tightly around the implant until the canal is filled. The trial implant is then carefully removed from the canal and a narrow cement nozzle is introduced down the "neo-canal." The cement is then injected and the next smaller size actual implant inserted. The issue of implant length and anterior flange support are unchanged from above. This technique is slightly more difficult as the walls of the "neo-cortex" may dislodge during trial extraction or nozzle introduction, which could block implant insertion. Special care in compacting the graft can minimize this problem.

Pearls

- Autograft is more compressible than allograft but has not been shown to have superior results.
- Allograft femoral head can be prepared for this procedure with a bone mill.
- The radial nerve must be protected when working around the spiral groove.
- Strut grafts are often used in conjunction with impaction grafting to reinforce the thin or violated cortex.

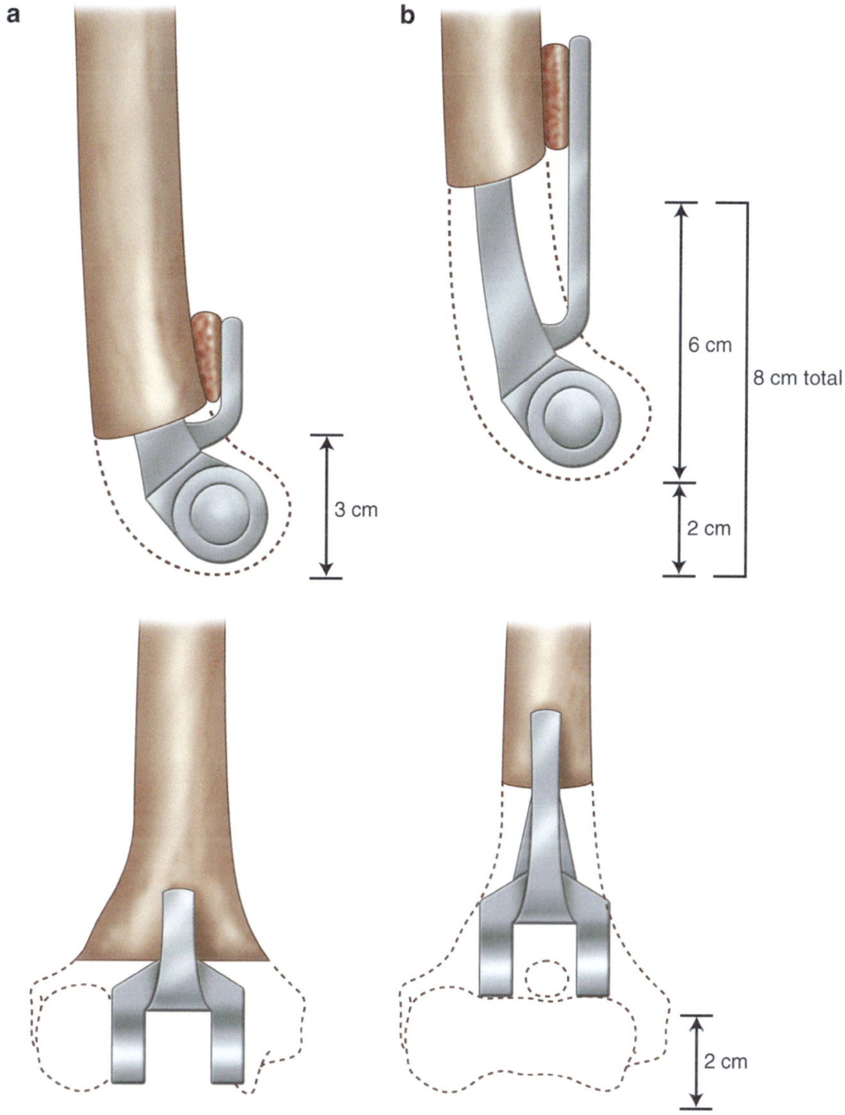

Fig. 13.15 (**a**) The distal 3 cm of the humerus is not required for proper position and flexion. (**b**) Deficiencies up to 8 cm in length can be addressed by a 4-cm extension of graft to span the anterior defect and by accepting a 2-cm shortening of the extremity

Placement of Bone Strut Grafts

Patient positioning and preparation are similar to impaction grafting. A sterile tourniquet is recommended if revision of the humerus is planned. The joint is exposed and the triceps is mobilized medially and laterally. The ulnar nerve is identified and protected. If revision of the humerus is planned, the radial nerve is localized at the spiral groove and protected. The implants and cement are removed as described previously. Humeral and/or ulnar osteotomies are utilized as needed.

Humerus

The triceps is released posteriorly and the brachialis anteriorly from the humerus. The radial nerve is identified and mobilized if the strut graft is expected to pass proximal to the spiral groove. If there is a loss of length of the humerus, the amount of bone loss is estimated. Up to 2 cm of shortening of the humerus is tolerated without significant functional alteration [32] and does not need to be restored. Beyond 2 cm of loss, anterior strut grafts are used to restore functional length. Up to 8 cm of bone loss can be reconstructed by using an anterior strut and an extended flange humeral component. There must be some overlap of the proximal end of the flange and the host bone, which defines the amount of bone loss corrected by this technique (Fig. 13.15). The "shuck" test [30] is helpful in determining the depth of insertion for the humeral component when the distal humerus is deficient (Fig. 13.16). Deficiencies beyond 8 cm may be addressed by an APC along with strut grafts.

Common sources of allograft struts include the femur and tibia; of the two, femoral grafts are preferable as they contour more easily. If available, humeral strut allograft is ideal, as the dimensions are more comparable. Tapering the ends with a burr or saw eases insertion of the graft and dissipates the stress riser associated with the end of the graft. The strut graft should extend beyond the tip on the implant if possible, and where

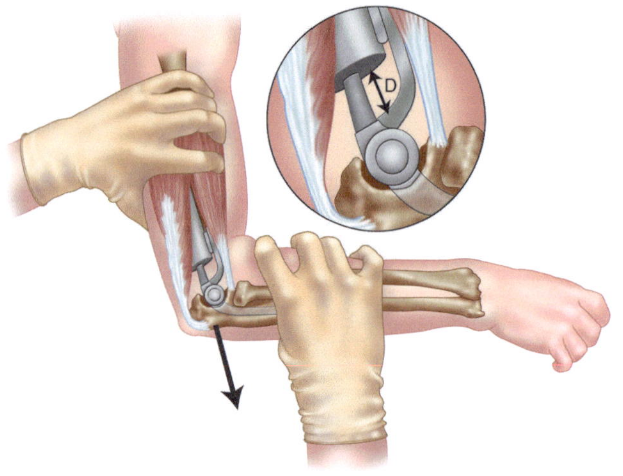

Fig. 13.16 The so-called Shuck test assists in determining the proper depth of the insertion of the humeral component in the absence of the distal humerus. The humeral implant is inserted down the canal and is articulated with the ulnar trial. At 90° flexion, the forearm is then displaced distally. The position of the humeral component defines the optimum position for implant insertion

multiple struts are used, they should be of different lengths. The strut graft should not end at the level of the tip of the implant. Struts used to span periprosthetic fractures and cortical defects should extend two to three diameters beyond the lesion. Use caution when sliding a strut proximally on the dorsum of the humerus to confirm passage under the radial nerve at the level of the spiral groove. A second strut on the opposite side will prevent the cables or wires from cutting into osteoporotic bone. Heavy gauge (18–20 gauge) wire (Fig. 13.17) or commercially available cable systems (Fig. 13.18) are used to hold the struts in place. While the wire is cheaper, the cables have the advantage of being able to loosen and tighten as necessary; two to three cables or wires are used above and below a fracture site, less are needed if supporting intact but thinned cortex. Avoid the radial nerve along the lateral intermuscular septum distal to the spiral groove. Wire twists or crimp blocks should be placed posterior or posterior lateral to minimize risk to the ulnar nerve medially and subcutaneous placement should be avoided. Strut grafts should be placed prior to impaction grafting. Provisional placement of anterior and posterior struts and wires is performed with the trial implant in place. The wires are not definitively tightened until after the actual implant has been placed. Premature tightening may make the trial implant difficult to remove, or worse, make the actual implant difficult or impossible to insert. When dealing with a fracture or cortical perforation, the use of fluoroscopy during actual implant insertion can prevent unexpected malposition of the implant (Fig. 13.19). Autogenous cancellous bone graft can be placed around the fracture site but is usually not necessary.

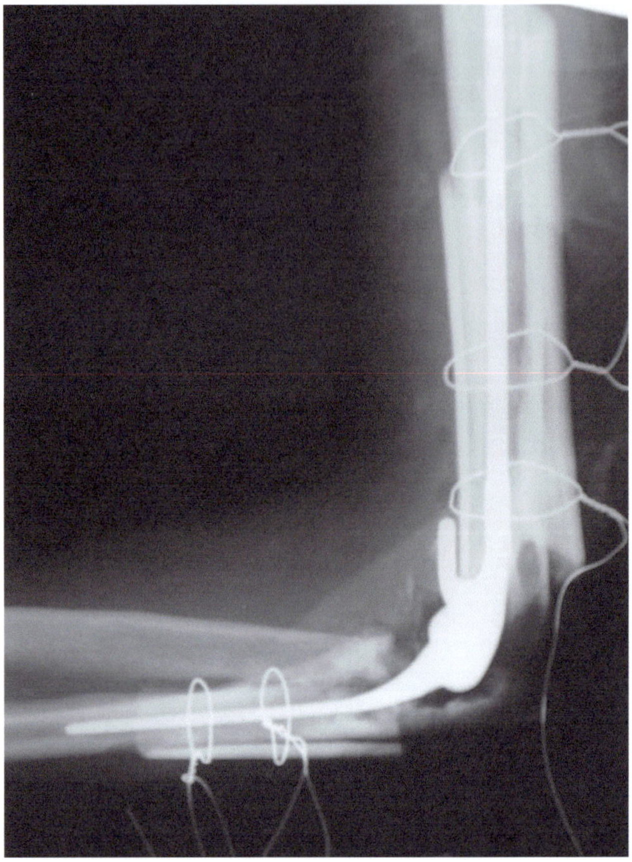

Fig. 13.17 Twisted 20-gauge wire fixation of strut allografts of the ulna and humerus

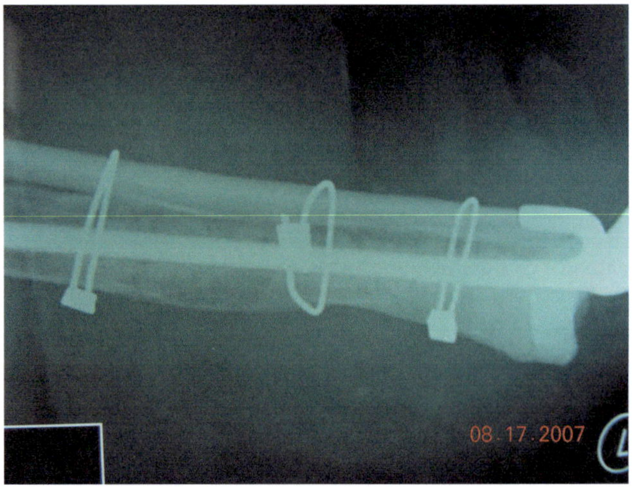

Fig. 13.18 Cable fixation of humeral allograft strut

Ulna

Basic considerations for graft application for the ulna are similar. The subcutaneous position of the ulna makes visualization easier but soft tissue coverage more problematic. Kamineni and Morrey [33] described four main applications

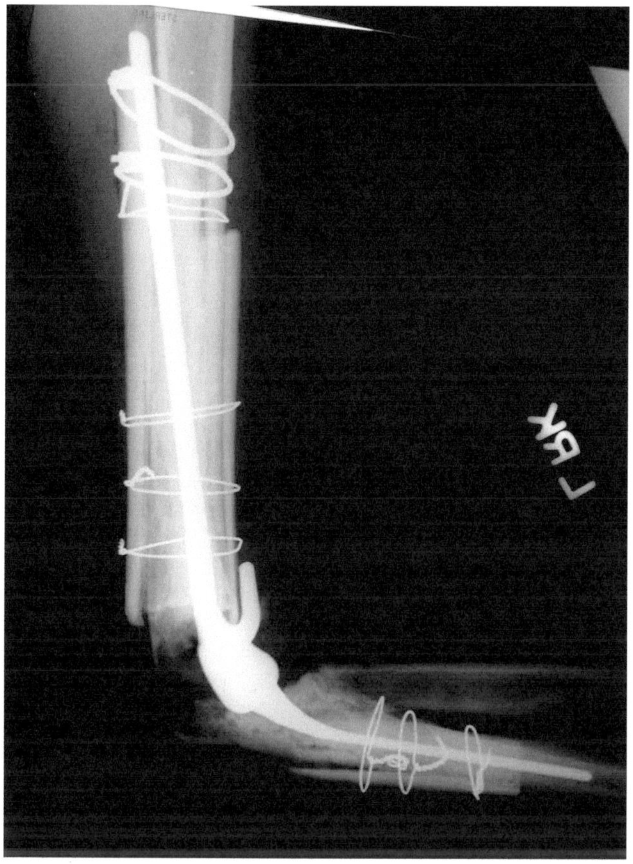

Fig. 13.19 The humeral component is malpositioned. The tip passed out of a cortical defect, under the strut allograft during cementing. Use of fluoroscopy during implant placement may have prevented this complication. The decision was made to leave the well-cemented implant in place and add a supplemental cable around the tip. The patient is asymptomatic at 10 years postsurgery

of strut grafts around the ulna. They are as follows: containment struts for focal defects in the cortex (three sides intact), splinting struts to span fractures, augmentation struts used in conjunction with impaction grafting, and posterior strut grafts to improve or reconstruct the moment arm of the triceps. The proximal end of a fibula allograft, split and hollowed out, applied posteriorly fits well for support and augmentation of the proximal ulna. Additionally, iliac crest autograft [34] and calcaneus allograft attached to an Achilles tendon graft have been used for reconstruction of the triceps moment arm as well. Where possible, avoid placement of containment, splinting, and augmentation strut grafts on the lateral border of the ulna to avoid interference with forearm rotation. The grafts should be contoured with a burr to maximize contact with the host bone to promote healing.

The radial head, if present, is a useful landmark to determine the depth of insertion of the ulnar component [35], if not, the residual coronoid may be referenced. In cases of severe bone destruction or deformity, few landmarks may be available. In this instance the desire to maintain accurate ulnar length is balanced by the need to support the proximal aspect of the ulnar implant to prevent implant fracture. Reabsorption of extended posterior strut grafts, without underlying bony support has been reported [33]. Of course, accurate rotational positioning of the ulnar implant is critical and can be referenced from the flat dorsal aspect of the proximal ulna or, if not present, from the tip of the ulnar styloid.

Pearls

- Strut grafts should extend two to three diameters beyond the fracture site.
- Use a second strut on the opposite side of the bone to prevent the cables/wires from cutting into osteoporotic bone.
- Accurately reduce and compress across the fracture site to prevent cement extrusion into the fracture site.
- Provisionally place the cables or wires around the struts with the trial implant in place. Do not perform final tightening until the final implant is cemented in place and its position is confirmed.
- Use fluoroscopy to monitor placement of the implant to prevent the implant from passing out of the canal through the fracture site.

Allograft-Prosthetic Composite Procedure

The use of proximal ulna or distal humerus allografts may be indicated in the event of significant bone loss. This includes a greater than 8 cm deficit of distal humerus, or deficiency of the ulna which extends distal to the coronoid. The use of APCs for the ulna is more common than for the humerus. Although, with the change in the precoat of the Zimmer ulnar implant in 2000, the incidence of massive osteolysis of the proximal ulna seems to have decreased. The traditional method of mating the APC to host bone involved a step cut osteotomy, fixed with metallic plates, uni- and bicortical screws and wires. This required precise cuts and resulted in a small area for healing. Complication rates were high with deep infection and nonunion most common [36]. Several additional techniques for the improved fixation of the ulnar APC have recently been described by Morrey and Sanchez-Sotelo [30] (Fig. 13.20). The key to improved bone integration appears to be maximizing linear contact at the host graft junction.

Surgical Technique, Ulna

Following removal of the ulnar implant, cement and bony fragmentation, the degree of bone deficiency is determined. Strut grafting, as described above, is utilized if possible to support the implant and restore bone stock. If this is not possible, then an APC is considered. A size-matched proximal ulna or proximal fibular allograft is most commonly used. The distal aspect of the graft is cut to length and prepared depending on the technique chosen, as described below. The medullary canal of the graft is opened and prepared with a burr and rasps, and an appropriately sized implant may be cemented in on the back

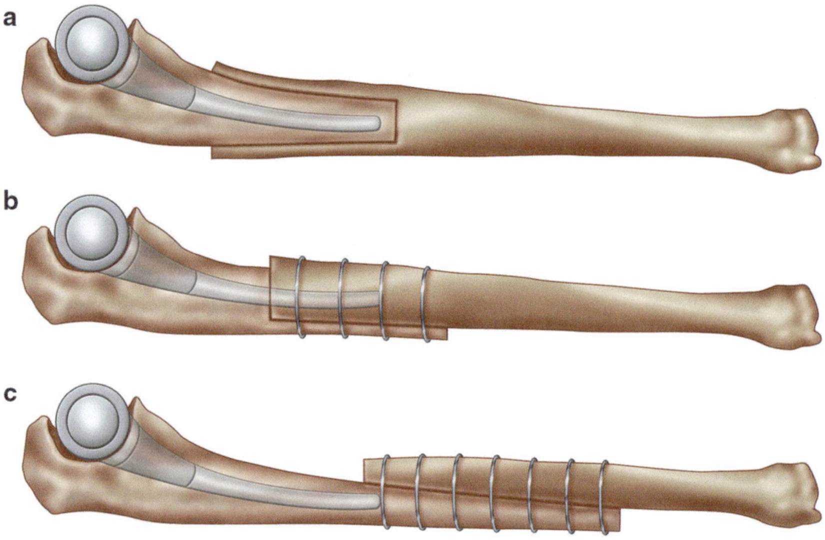

Fig. 13.20 (**a**–**c**) Line drawings of allograft-prosthetic composite (APC) types

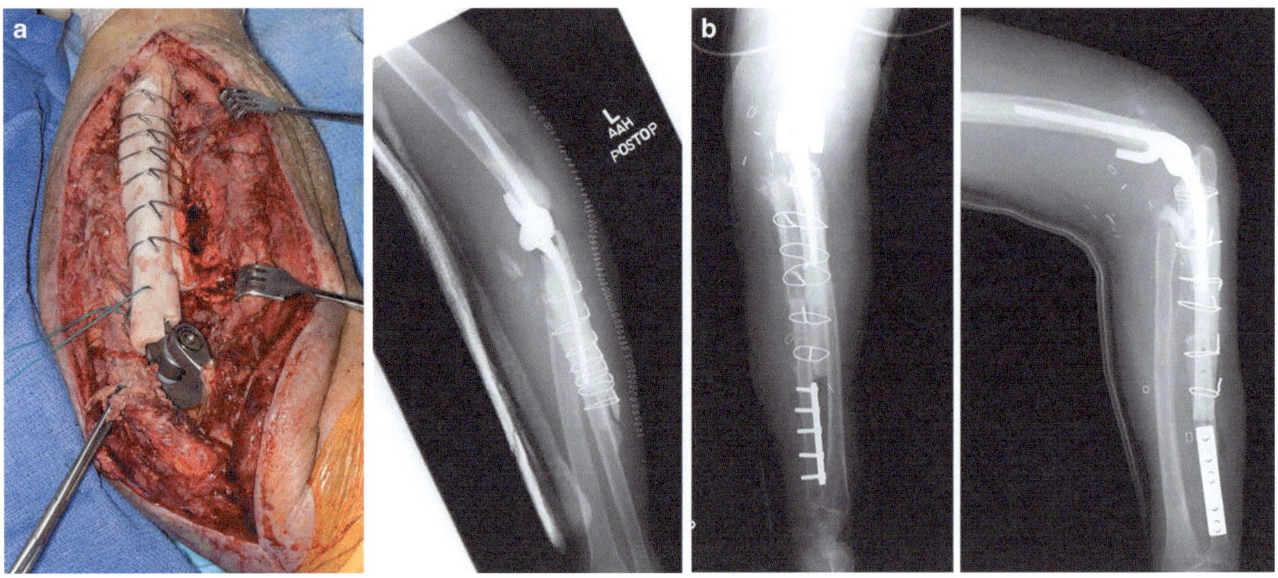

Fig. 13.21 (**a**) Clinical photo and radiograph of extended step cut APC used to reconstruct extensive ulnar deficiency. The braided suture will be used to reattach the triceps mechanism. Note the dorsal extension of the allograft to provide a moment arm to strengthen the reattached triceps muscle. (**b**) AP radiograph of a type c side-to-side APC to reconstruct a deficient ulna (images courtesy of Bernard Morrey, MD)

table, or inserted after the graft is attached. If the proximal ulna is present but patulous, an alternative to impaction grafting utilizes an ulnar APC with a long stem implant extending beyond the end of the allograft. This is intussuscepted inside of the existing ulna, with the stem extending into the intact canal distally. The distal end of the allograft is tapered with a burr to promote an interference fit distally. The distal stem of the implant is cemented into the distal canal. The proximal gaps between the APC and the outer cortex may be packed with morselized cancellous allograft, although this is not always necessary (Morrey, personal communication; 2008 Fig. 13.20a). A second technique is an extended step cut osteotomy with the tip of an extended length implant extending beyond the tip of the allograft. The distal implant is cemented into the native medullary canal and the overlapping bone is approximated with wires or cables. The disadvantages of this technique include increased technical difficulty, minimal ability to adjust the junction, and less surface area for bone healing. The main advantage is diminished bulk (Fig. 13.20b, 13.21a). The final technique is side-to-side application of the APC to the remaining ulnar shaft. The allograft is prepared with the entire ulnar implant within the canal, and the implant cemented in place. Digital pressure over the open end of the distal canal during cementing improves the cement mantle. The flat appositional surface of the APC is approximated to the flat surface of the remaining ulna to maximize the contact area with the host bone and tapered at its distal end. The graft is then approximated with multiple wires or cables, assuring correct rotation. Ulnar length is determined by soft tissue tension and is easily adjusted (Fig. 13.20c, 13.21b).

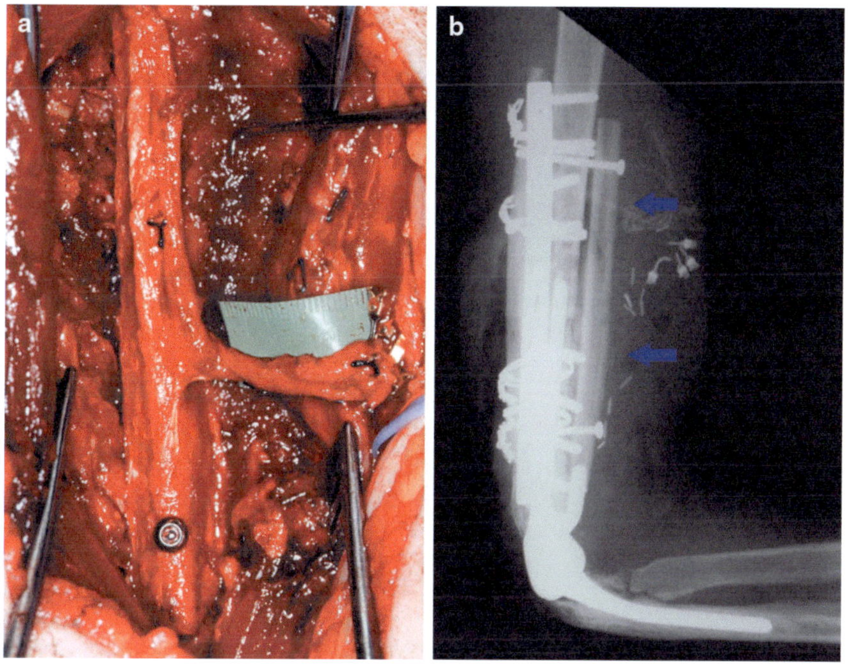

Fig. 13.22 (**a**) The free fibular pedicled graft in place, note screw fixation of graft. Cables or wires should not be used (image courtesy of Allen Bishop, MD). (**b**) Postoperative X-ray of free fibular graft in place (*arrows*) (image courtesy of Allen Bishop, MD)

The application of these techniques for deficiencies of the distal humerus is similar to the ulna.

Pearls

- Previous techniques for fixation of APCs had high complication rates; newer techniques are more promising, although further study with long-term follow-up is required.
- Maximize the amount of bone contact between the allograft and host bone to facilitate graft incorporation.
- The size of the bulk allografts used for the proximal ulna is limited by soft tissue considerations.
- Although the complication rate and reoperation rate are high with the use of APCs, function and pain relief are improved in most patients with these difficult problems.

Other Applications

Vascularized Free Bone Transfers

The use of vascularized free fibular autografts for the treatment of recalcitrant nonunion of long bones is well established [37, 38]. There have been several cases of the use of vascularized free fibular autografts to promote healing at the graft–host junction in revision TEA. This is a rare occurrence, however, and is typically reserved for the failure of conventional grafting techniques. General considerations for the use of a vascularize graft include the following: 1) infection must be addressed if the cause of the nonunion, 2) the implant must be well fixed within the APC (or revised at the same time), 3) the patient must have an adequate soft tissue envelope exists, and 4) available microsurgical expertise. Potential complicating factors include extensive scarring of the surgical bed; compromised vascularity, i.e., diabetes, peripheral vascular disease, tobacco abuse; and lack of microsurgical expertise.

Procedure

The technique for harvesting the free fibula is well described elsewhere and will not be repeated here. The APC/host junction is exposed and the nonunion site prepared. The fracture edges are reopposed if possible or grafted with cancellous autograft if a gap persists. The brachial artery is exposed and prepared for end to side anastomosis. A burr is used to create a longitudinal trough for the fibula to maximize bony contact with the APC and humerus. The periosteum is stripped from the fibula on the opposite side from the pedicle to promote healing; great care is taken to protect the pedicle. The fibula is positioned across the nonunion site, and fixed with a 3.5-mm screw and washer on each side of the nonunion site (Fig. 13.22a, b). Cables are avoided to prevent compression of the pedicle. Postoperative care includes avoidance of nicotine, caffeine, and other vasoconstrictors [39]. The role of platelet inhibitors is not fully established.

Strut Grafts for Pain Associated with Stress Risers

The modulus of elasticity of the implant stem is significantly higher than that of bone, and occasionally, patients develop pain at the tip of the stem. This is more common with small or osteoporotic bone. Patients present with pain, occasionally reactive bone formation (Fig. 13.23a, b), and increased uptake on a three-phase bone scan (Fig. 13.24). These symptoms can be relieved, and a potential stress fracture averted, by the placement of allograft strut grafts spanning the tip of the implant.

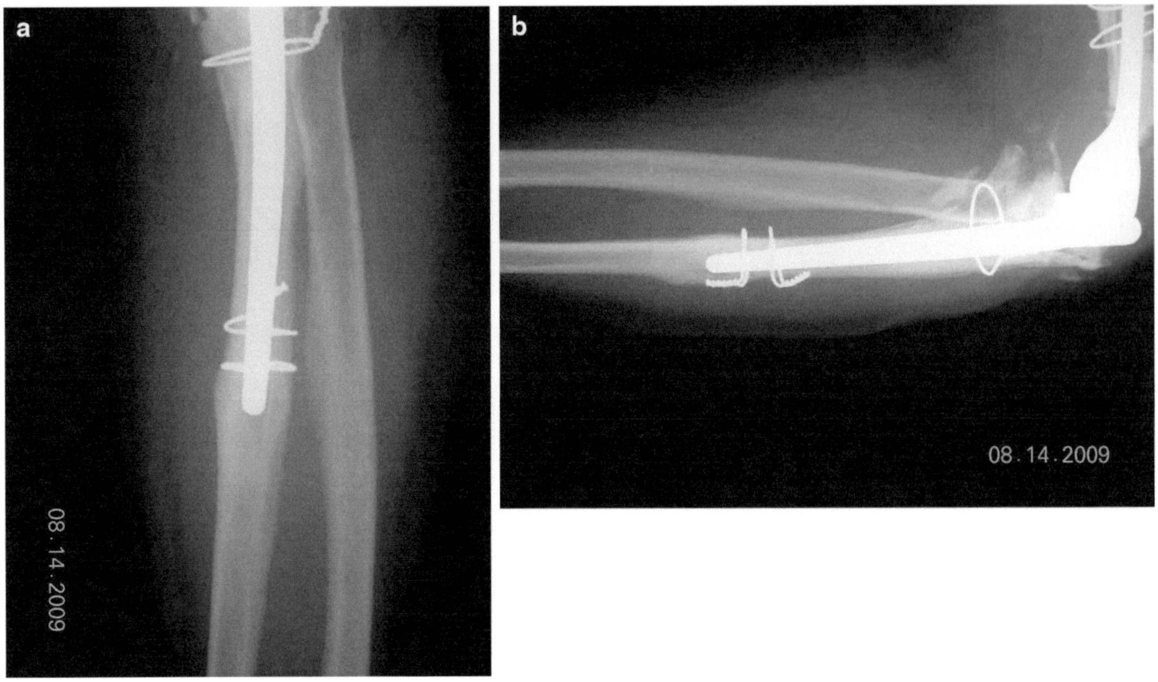

Fig. 13.23 (**a**, **b**) Note the reactive bone formation around the tip of the ulnar implant. This correlates with the patient's aching pain with use

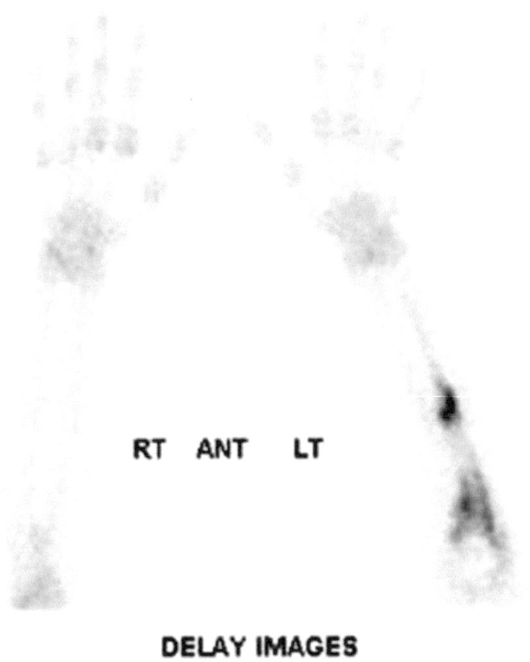

Fig. 13.24 Three-phase bone scan demonstrates increased uptake at the tip of the ulnar implant

Procedure

The shaft of the involved bone, most commonly the ulna, is exposed. The location of the tip of the implant is typically easily identified by reactive periosteum but can be confirmed by the use of X-ray. The periosteum is preserved. One or more allograft bone struts are placed, spanning the shaft at the tip of the stem (Fig. 13.25). The grafts are carefully contoured to maximize contact with the host bone and the ends tapered to minimize bulk and dissipate forces at the end of the graft (Fig. 13.26). Where more than one strut is used, the lengths should be varied. The grafts are attached with wire or cables, avoiding placing the twists or crimp blocks subcutaneously. Gradually, increased use of the arm is allowed based on soft tissue healing.

Pearls

- Pain from stress risers of the ulna or humerus appears to be analogous to the thigh pain identified with THA.
- An initial trial of nonoperative management with activity modification is appropriate, as long as there is not an impending pathologic fracture.
- Multiple narrow struts allow for better contouring to the ulna than few wider struts.
- Respect soft tissue stress from the increased bulk of the grafts.

Complications

- Soft tissue compromise from bone grafts or fixation
- Nerve injury, especially the radial nerve with posteriorly positioned humeral struts

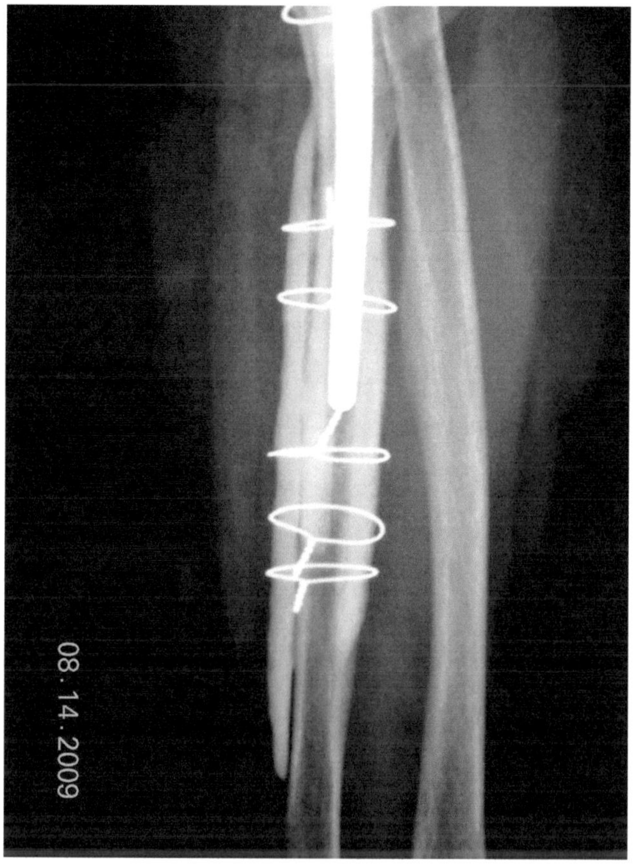

Fig. 13.25 Multiple strut allografts of varying lengths span the tip of the implant and are wired into position

- Impairment of forearm rotation, avoid placement of struts on the lateral ulna
- Graft reabsorption, fracture, or failure of incorporation
- Pain or stress fracture related to stress risers at the end of the bone struts
- Infection

Triceps Deficiency

Introduction

The reported incidence of triceps weakness following TEA ranges from 2 to 29% [12], although the actual incidence is probably underreported. Patients typically do not report weakness with elbow extension, rather a loss of power in closed kinetic chain activities such as cutting meat, pushing the elevator button, or pushing up from a chair. While loss of active extension is not as functionally limiting as loss of flexion, it does impact patient satisfaction postoperatively. Triceps weakness may be a function of surgical approach [40] with Little et al. [41] reporting the lowest rates occurring with techniques which preserve the attachment of Sharpey's fibers to the ulna (triceps turndown) and the highest rate with detachment of the triceps insertion completely. Approaches that preserve the entire triceps mechanism intact have been used in selected situations, such as acute and chronic distal humerus fracture management, and simplify postoperative management. Weakness of the wrist flexors and extensors following resection of the condyles has been postulated with this technique but has not been demonstrated in clinical studies [42]. Several authors have proposed alternative techniques to preserve the triceps without removal of the condyles for constrained TEA placement [40, 43, 44], although experience with these approaches is limited.

Diagnosis

Specific evaluation of the triceps function should be performed at all follow-up visits. The patients often do not complain of this problem. Extension of the elbow joint in a gravity neutral position may still be possible due to the contribution of the anconeus and lateral extensor retinaculum, although extension against gravity or resistance is generally not possible. There may be a palpable defect noted with increased prominence of the humeral component, although more often I have seen a large "bursal" swelling, which is actually pressurization of increased joint fluid distending the loose posterior elbow skin (Fig. 13.27). Additional advanced imaging is generally not necessary and visualization is impaired by metal artifact. Plain radiographs are helpful primarily to determine the status of the olecranon, which may affect the reconstruction technique chosen.

Indications

- *Functionally limiting* lack of elbow extension

Contraindications

- Uncontrolled infection is a contraindication to the use of allograft for extensor mechanism reconstruction.
- Poor medical health.
- Low demand patient/extremity without perceived functional deficit.

Surgical Options

- Repeat direct repair.
- Anconeus rotation flap.
- Allograft reconstruction.

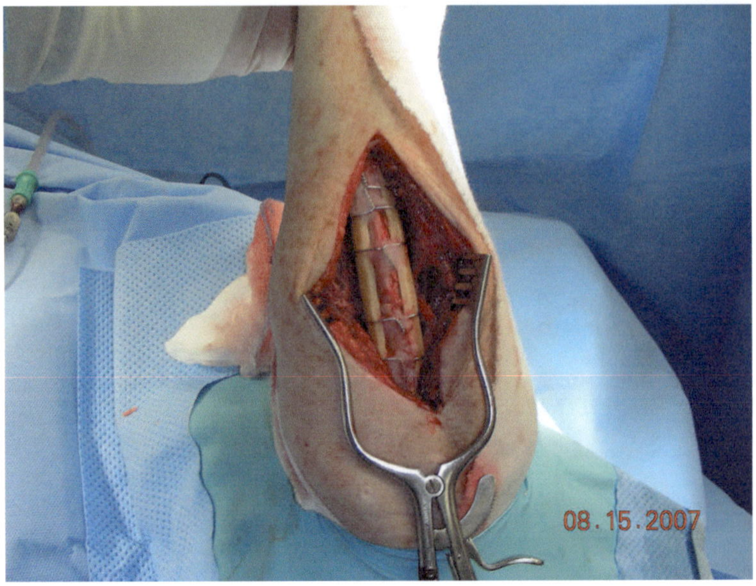

Fig. 13.26 Clinical picture of strut grafts wired in place

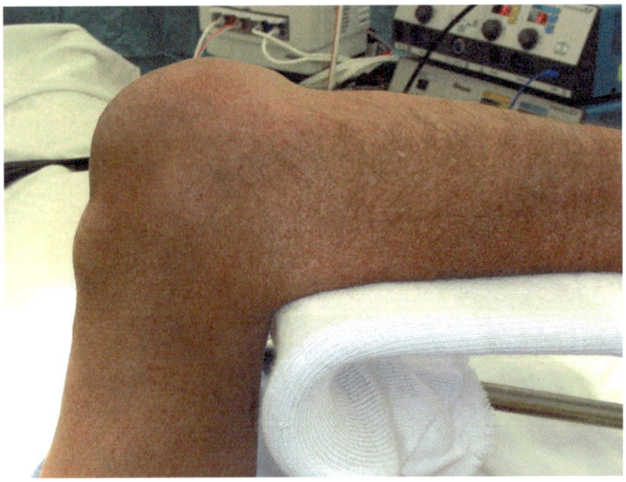

Fig. 13.27 Prominent fluid collection over the olecranon, consistent with triceps detachment

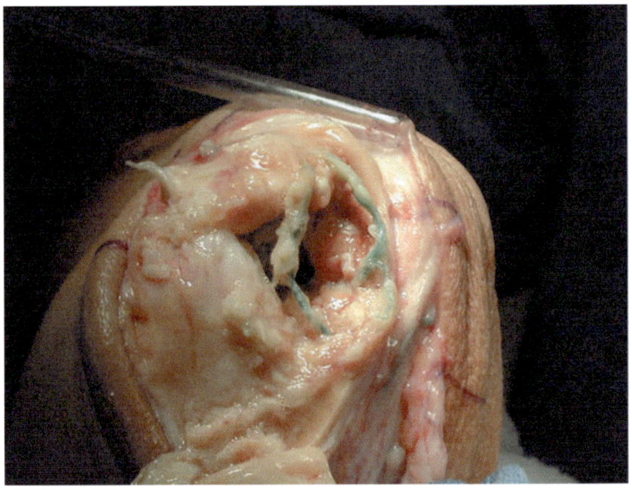

Fig. 13.28 Extensive degenerative changes of the triceps tendon. The suture used to reattach the tendon caused additional damage as it cut though the tissue during failure

Procedure

Repeat Direct Repair

This is rarely a viable option given that the failure mode of the index procedure typically causes further damage to the extensor mechanism (Fig. 13.28). If the primary repair technique has failed and the tissue is still felt to be of adequate quality, repeat direct repair could be considered. A multi-stranded repair utilizing strong (#2 fiberwire or #5 Ticron) sutures woven with multiple tissue-grasping sutures through the intact tendon, and passed though bone tunnels is preferred (Fig. 13.29a–c). The use of one or more suture anchors attached to the posterior surface of the olecranon for tendon attachment is not sufficient and is the technique used in many of the failed triceps repair attempts treated by the author. If there is *any* question about the integrity of the triceps tendon, tissue defect or deficit, or concern about the strength of the bone tunnels, repeat direct primary repair should be abandoned in favor of a reconstructive solution.

Anconeus Rotation Flap

This is an effective reconstructive technique if the central attachment of the triceps tendon has failed or is deficient (occasionally seen in primary repair situations, especially in patients with rheumatoid arthritis). This is more commonly seen with the Bryan–Morrey triceps sleeve approach, or

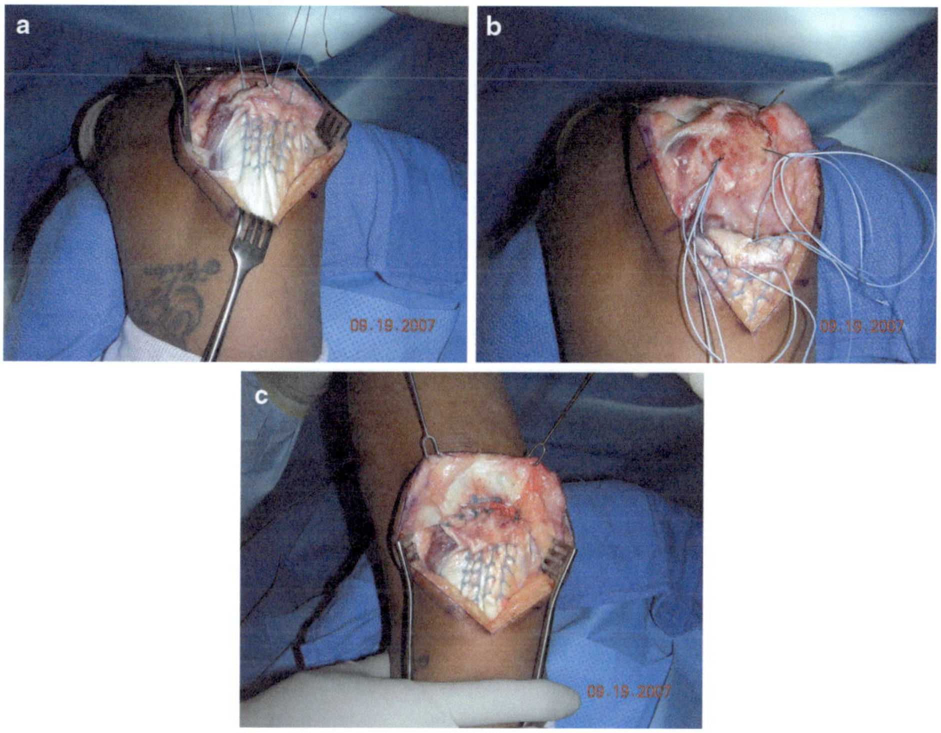

Fig. 13.29 (**a**) Grasping braided nonabsorbable sutures placed in distal triceps tendon. (**b**) Heavy braided suture passed through bone tunnels in the proximal ulna. (**c**) Final repair

triceps split, than with the triceps turndown technique. If the failure mode involves the lateral subluxation of the extensor mechanism volar to the axis of rotation of the ulnohumeral joint, *and* the lateral extensor retinaculum and anconeus are intact, the rotation flap technique can be employed.

Procedure

The patient's previous incision is utilized and the medial and lateral flaps are meticulously protected. Avoid grasping the edges of these flaps with toothed pickups to minimize tissue injury; skin hooks are most appropriate for retraction. The end of the olecranon is often immediately subcutaneous and may be bathed in synovial fluid. Alternatively, there may be amorphous thick scar over the entire area, which requires careful dissection to identify the margins of the extensor mechanism. Kocher's interval is identified between the extensor carpi ulnaris "ECU" and the anconeus. This can be identified by a visible fat stripe, multiple vascular perforators, or the divergence of the muscle fiber orientation. The fascia is incised, and the anterior margin of the anconeus is identified. The muscle is mobilized posteriorly, between the muscle fascia and the periosteum. Proximally, the anconeus continuity is maintained with the lateral triceps, peeling the latter away from the lateral intermuscular septum. The distal attachments of the anconeus are preserved. When this sleeve is fully mobilized, it can be "turned over" from lateral to medial, over the tip of the olecranon, reorienting the line of pull across the olecranon tip and dorsal to the axis of rotation. The flap is secured to the ulna in this position with multiple sutures of nonabsorbable braided material, through bone tunnels. A "cinch" suture, as described by Morrey, should be included to prevent synovial fluid from interfering with soft tissue healing [45]. An arcade of locked grasping sutures placed through the now centralized, lateral triceps tendon, passed through oblique bone tunnels in the olecranon, and tied over the flap can be added for additional support and load sharing during the healing phase. Additional supporting sutures can be added along the medial and lateral intervals to maintain the centralization of the rotation flap. This technique utilizes the anconeus/lateral triceps unit as the extensor motor and restores the extension moment arm of the olecranon.

Achilles Allograft Reconstruction

If the anconeus muscle is deficient or scarred and nonfunctional, or if there is a significant defect in the extensor mechanism, allograft reconstruction is appropriate. An Achilles allograft, with or without attached calcaneus bone, is an excellent choice for size, thickness, strength, and the availability of bone graft. Other allografts have been described [46]; however, the Achilles graft is currently preferred.

The surgical approach is identical to previous techniques. The extent of the deficit is exposed and the scarred, contracted triceps mechanism is mobilized. The ulnar nerve is identified and protected. Often, the deep surface of the triceps

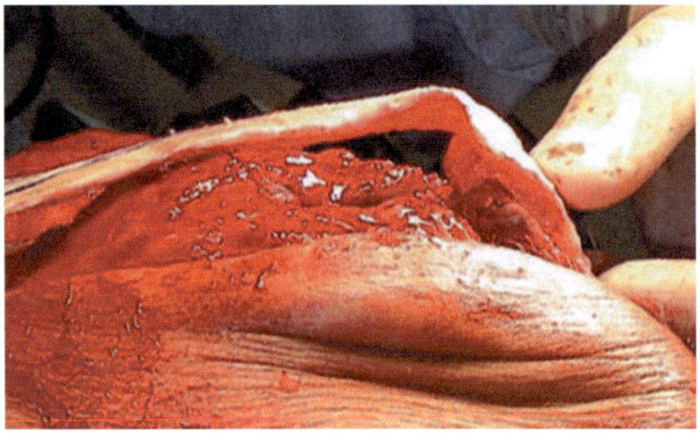

Fig. 13.30 Achilles allograft with calcaneus. The calcaneus is step cut to fit into the proximal ulna and maximize bone contact for healing

muscle is scarred to the posterior humerus and must be released. Care must be taken to avoid injury to the radial nerve in the spiral groove. If there is any question about the location of the radial nerve, it can be identified as it passes across the lateral intermuscular septum, approximately four finger breaths above the elbow, and followed proximally through the spiral groove.

Techniques for allograft tendon attachment to olecranon [12, 45] and allograft calcaneus bone attachment to the olecranon have been described. If there is sufficient olecranon bone stock extending beyond the proximal extent of the ulnar implant to function as a fulcrum, either technique can be used. If the proximal ulna is deficient, the calcaneus allograft should be utilized to elongate the proximal ulna and improve the efficiency of the extensor mechanism (Fig. 13.30). Including a portion of the calcaneus may improve fixation. Several techniques have been described for attaching the calcaneus to the proximal ulna; if the olecranon fragment is large enough, a chevron-shaped wedge can be removed from the proximal ulna, and a matching wedge created from the calcaneus. The calcaneal wedge is secured with a single screw or tension band wire fixation [47]. If the proximal ulna is thin or deficient, the calcaneus can be shaped to envelop the proximal ulna or fit together in a step cut fashion. In this configuration, plate fixation may be more appropriate, although unicortical screws or cables may be required to avoid the ulnar implant (Fig. 13.31a, b). Great care should be taken to avoid notching the ulnar implant when preparing the ulna.

Following stable fixation of the allograft to the proximal ulna, the elbow is placed in 20–30° of flexion. The triceps tendon is pulled as far distal as possible and the graft tensioned proximally. The proximal end of the allograft may be sewn into the triceps tendon with multiple nonabsorbable sutures in an onlay fashion, although splitting the proximal tendon into longitudinal strips (Fig. 13.32) and weaving the strips through the triceps tendon in a Pulvertaft fashion (Fig. 13.33) is much stronger. The woven strips are then sewn in place with multiple nonabsorbable sutures.

Complications

There are few reported series of triceps reconstruction [12, 45, 47]. In the largest reported series, elbow extension against gravity was considered a satisfactory outcome and was achieved in 15/16 elbows. The authors reported no major complications. Failure of healing at the host allograft junction, persistent weakness, and deep infection of the allograft would seem to be the most worrisome complications but are infrequently reported.

Postoperative Care

The elbow is immobilized with a volar splint in a position of near full extension (20–30°) for the first 2–3 weeks. The patient is then placed in a hinged elbow splint allowing motion from 0 to 60° for the next 1–2 weeks. The patient may then increase the flexion stops in the brace by 10–15° per week until full flexion is achieved, usually by week 8. Patients are instructed not to use the extremity for any weight-bearing activities, i.e., cane, walker, etc., until 4 months. Formal strengthening exercises may be initiated if necessary at 6 months postoperatively.

Pearls

- Triceps weakness should be evaluated postoperatively, as patients may not identify this problem. A prominent olecranon "bursa" may indicate underlying triceps detachment. Surgical management for this issue may be appropriate if the deficit is *functionally* limiting.
- Local tissue transposition, such as an anconeus rotation flap is preferable to allograft reconstruction, whenever possible.
- The presence or absence of adequate olecranon bone stock is the most important factor influencing the successful restoration of functional extension.
- Achilles allografts are available with, and without attached calcaneus bone, and are the tissue of choice for allograft reconstruction. The use of an osseotendinous allograft should be very carefully considered in cases of previous infection.
- If the reconstruction is being performed at the time of implant re-implantation, drill necessary holes and place sutures *prior* to implantation of the ulnar implant.
- Place the suture knots along the edge of the ulna, not over the subcutaneous border of the ulna to minimize knot irritation.

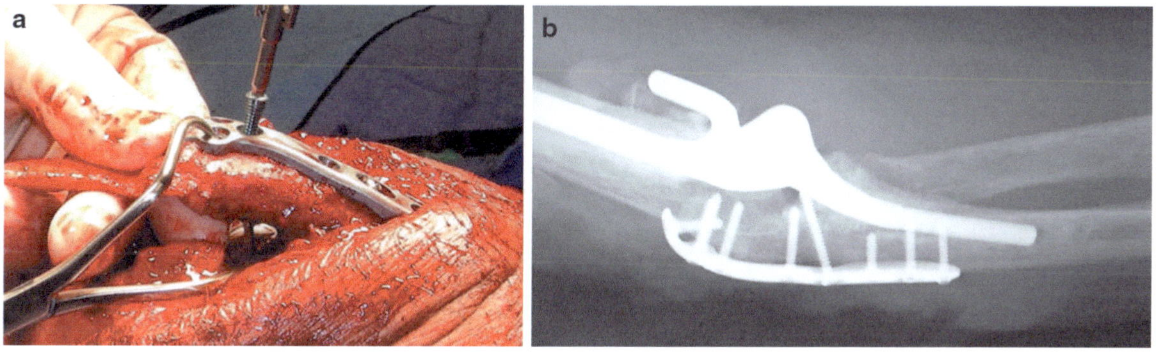

Fig. 13.31 Plate fixation of the allograft bone, (**a**) clinical photo, (**b**) X-ray

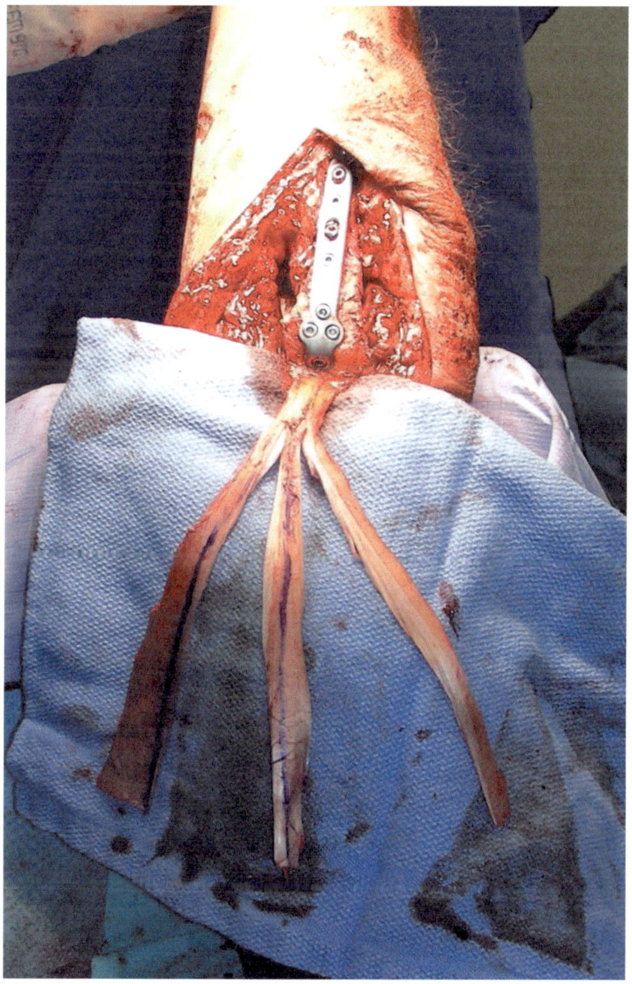

Fig. 13.32 Proximal Achilles allograft split into three tails, to weave into the remaining triceps tendon stump

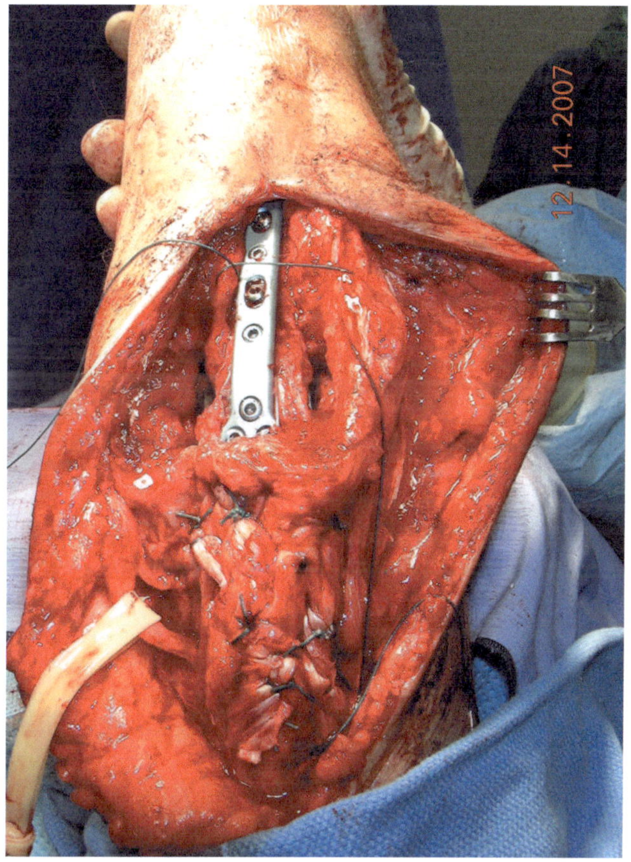

Fig. 13.33 Completed Achilles allograft tendon reconstruction

Salvage Procedures

Elbow Resection Arthroplasty

Peter Evans, MD, PhD

Introduction

An unfortunate consequence of recurrent infection or multiple revision TEA surgery is an elbow without a reasonable opportunity for prosthetic re-implantation and variable amounts of bone loss. This leads to a flail elbow that in some instances precludes basic hand-to-mouth activities of daily living. At other times there is some inherent stability but the range of motion is limited or painful crepitus exists. Elbow resection arthroplasty remains a necessary option for some

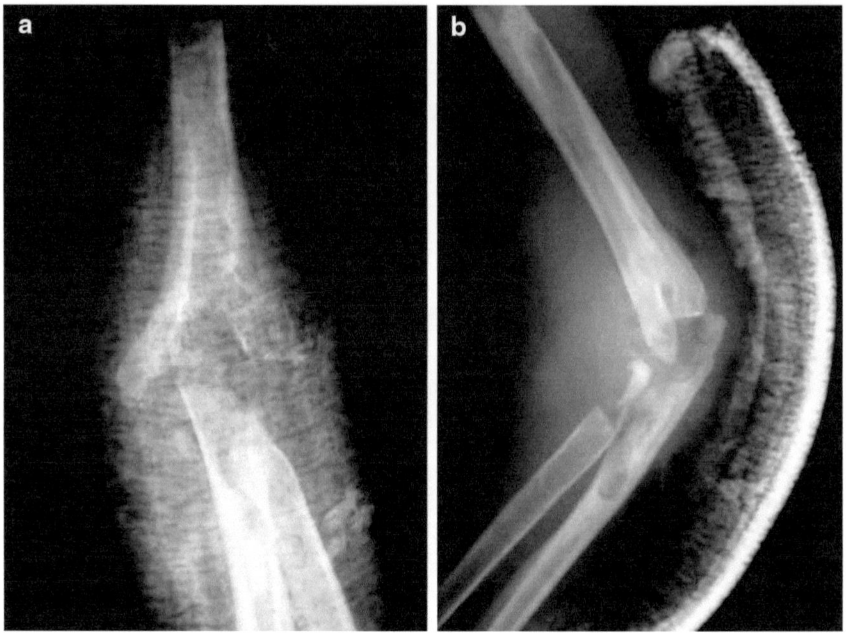

Fig. 13.34 (**a**, **b**) Resection arthroplasty, note retained medial and lateral columns, which help stabilize the articulation. Of the two, the medial is more important (images courtesy of Peter Evans, MD)

patients and an understanding of the surgical options and techniques will help in achieving a better outcome in these difficult cases.

Indications

1. Chronic infection
2. Bone stock incompatible with further reconstructive procedures
3. Patient uncooperative with functional restrictions leading to multiple failed arthroplasties

Resection arthroplasty is most commonly performed as part of a staged elbow reconstruction, but at times it works well enough that patients forgo further reconstruction and the possibility of repeating their previous course of complications. In other cases, it is the logical choice due to poor patient health or a poor bony or soft tissue envelope around the elbow.

Contraindications

- Poor patient health, preventing safe anesthesia

Preoperative History and Considerations

Patients undergoing resection arthroplasty have typically had several operative procedures on the elbow and are aware of the risks involved. However, they should be aware of an increased risk of neurovascular injury with this procedure due to the significant scarring and heterotopic ossification. In particular, the ulnar nerve is at most risk.

Operative Approach

Several options for resection arthroplasty exist and they are typically dictated by the amount of bone remaining and whether there is active infection.

- Simple resection
- Resection plus resurfacing
- Resection plus interposition stabilization
- Cue ball arthroplasty

Simple Resection

Used most commonly, simple resection can be used in any circumstance and is best in cases with active infection. It is most successful functionally when large portions of both the medial and lateral condyle and the olecranon remain. This allows the ulna to engage into the olecranon/coronoid fossa defect (Fig. 13.34a, b).

The surgical approach is posterior followed by isolating the ulnar nerve and ensuring it is released and freed for anterior transposition at the end of the procedure. If extensive proximal dissection is required the radial nerve is isolated between the long and lateral heads of the triceps. The deep elbow exposure is typically via a triceps-on approach, creating windows medially and laterally which typically is enough to disengage an elbow arthroplasty, dislocate and debride by pistoning either the humerus or ulna up through the medial or lateral window. The elbow is thoroughly irrigated and debrided including the bony canals, removing all implants and nonviable tissue.

Closure is done over a drain into the dead space, and the medial and lateral windows closed with #1–0 absorbable polyglactin (Vicryl, Ethicon Inc., Somerville, NJ) suture. If the elbow is highly unstable, #1–0 polydioxanone (PDS, Ethicon Inc.) suture is used to stabilize the ulnohumeral joint. This is achieved by drilling a 3.5 mm transosseous hole from medial to lateral in the proximal ulna at the level of the sublime tubercle and similarly across the humerus at the supracondylar level. Then two to three circuits of suture are passed and tied recreating medial and lateral ligamentous support. The skin is approximated as indicated.

Resection Plus Resurfacing

The procedure is as above but in a patient known to be infection-free. Prior to closure, the articular side of condyles is smoothed and debrided to bleeding bone. A cutis graft, Achilles allograft, or commercial dermal graft (GraftJacket, Wright Medical) is sewn tautly over the debrided side of the condyles and secured with transosseous nonabsorbable sutures which are passed using a straight Keith needle loaded on a power wire driver. Closure as above and PDS suture stabilization is used.

Resection Plus Interposition Stabilization

The procedure as for simple resection, and the patient is infection-free. The procedure has been described recently by Frankle [48] but neither author has experience with the technique. While Frankle indicated its use when the condyles are present, it may have an excellent indication when the condyles are absent.

A bone-patella tendon-bone allograft is prepared with the bone blocks contoured to snugly fit inside the humeral and ulnar canal. The bone blocks can be secured with an interference screw. Closure is as above.

Cue Ball Arthroplasty

The procedure is as for simple resection and useful even when ongoing infection is present. The approach and debridement is as above. Upon closure, several balls of various sizes 4–6 cm are created out of PMMA impregnated with Vancomycin (1 g/bag of PMMA) and inserted into the dead space [49]. Closure is as above. This leads to a mobile, elbow with typically pain-free crepitation.

Pearls

1. Remove all metal, cement, heterotopic bone and nonviable soft tissue and bone.
2. Ensure infection-free status if considering resurfacing or interposition (stage procedures if necessary).
3. Do not close unless relatively good stability exists.
4. Do not initiate motion for 6–8 weeks.

Complications

1. Instability
2. Recurrent infection
3. Nerve injury

Postoperative Care

Wounds are dressed with non-stick gauze, gauze, and a bulky plaster-reinforced long-arm splint with a forearm sugar tong addition in neutral rotation. A 30° external rotation block UltraSling (Don Joy Inc., Vista, CA) can be used to keep the hand pointing forward and avoid varus stress on the elbow during the first 6 week healing phase. The elbow is best placed in a removable long-arm posterior mold thermoplastic splint at 90° of flexion and neutral rotation. After 6 weeks, the patient discontinues use of the sling, and starts range-of-motion exercises and utilizes their splint to immobilize the elbow between exercises. After 3 months, patients discontinue use of the splint but may use a hinged orthosis for vigorous activities. There are no restrictions beyond 6 months.

Conclusion

Resection arthroplasty of the elbow can provide a minimally painful and modestly functional elbow after failure of prosthetic arthroplasty. Care in the selection of procedure and attention to the intraoperative and postoperative details will optimize outcome.

Elbow Fusion

There are few published results in the literature devoted to fusion following failed TEA. What information is available is culled from larger series of elbow fusions for all causes [50], most often after trauma and infection, and single case reports [51]. Multiple surgical techniques have been described, indicating that there is no universally accepted method to best achieve fusion. Despite the paucity of information, elbow arthrodesis may be indicated in select salvage cases.

The function of the elbow is to allow the positioning of the hand in space. It has been well documented that elbow fusion significantly limits the effective "sphere of influence" of the hand [52]. There appears to be no ideal position for elbow fusion to maximize upper extremity function. Authors have suggested positions ranging from 40 to 110°. A position of 60° allows the extremity to be used as a helper hand for bimanual tasks, holding the steering wheel, holding a book, etc. [53]. Intact shoulder and wrist function provide minimal functional compensation for lost elbow flexion [54]. Additionally, the procedure is technically more difficult in the post-arthroplasty patient with diminished bone stock, and the complication rate is high, including nonunion and fracture [55]. Therefore, elbow fusion is generally considered a poor salvage option for failed TEA [56]. Patients generally prefer functional motion to elbow stability. For the patient contemplating elbow fusion, various positions can be simulated with a cylinder cast preoperatively, and the most functional position chosen.

Indications

- Absence of any other viable reconstructive option
- Need for heavy use of the affected limb/young age
- Desire for stability over unstable motion
- Pain relief

Contraindications

Absolute

- Active infection

Relative

- Inadequate bone stock
- Deficient soft tissue envelope
- Adjacent fused joints, or contra lateral elbow fusion

Surgical Technique

There are multiple techniques described, however, they fall into three categories: screw fixation, external fixation, or internal plate fixation. Screw fixation techniques rely on adequate bone stock, which is absent following resection of a failed TEA. Screw fixation is therefore not indicated in this application.

Elbow fusion may be performed at the time of joint removal, or in a staged fashion. In cases of infection, implant removal and joint debridement may be followed by placement of antibiotic beads and provisional external fixation, and converted to definitive internal fixation at a later date. Immediate placement of internal hardware is not recommended in the face of active infection. Plate fixation is preferred by patients over external fixation [53], and may be used for conversion of a resection arthroplasty. Bone loss up to 4 cm is well tolerated and is common in the postresection situation. Supplemental autologous bone graft is used to facilitate healing if there is not good bony apposition. Large, intercalated allografts are avoided if possible. A vascularized free fibula may be required if there is greater than 6–8 cm of bone loss. An adequate soft tissue envelope is required, as wound problems are common. Where possible, previous incisions are utilized to minimize stress on the skin flaps. If required, soft tissue procedures such as pedicle or free flaps are performed prior to the fusion procedure.

The patient is positioned to allow maximal exposure to the elbow joint. A posterior approach is used for external fixation and posterior plating. Both volar and dorsal approaches have been described for anterior plating. Full thickness skin flaps are raised. The ulnar and radial nerves are identified and protected. Posteriorly, the triceps is split in the midline and reflected. The joint space is exposed, debrided, and contoured to provide maximal bone contact in the desired amount of elbow flexion. Autograft is harvested if indicated, and may be supplemented with cancellous allograft or other bone substitute.

External Fixation

Although both full frames and half frames have been described, a unilateral frame applied to the lateral aspect of the elbow is probably sufficient. Large (4 mm or larger) partially threaded pins are placed under direct visualization in the humerus and ulna, and a triangular frame is applied. Provisional fixation with wires or screws can be placed while the fixator is adjusted, and may be left in place, although are usually removed if infection is an issue. Compression is applied along with bone graft at the ulnohumeral junction. If the fixator is placed for stabilization of an infected joint, antibiotic beads are placed throughout the joint at this time. The triceps is approximated over the posterior joint. The ulnar nerve is transposed subcutaneously as indicated. Standard wound closure over a Hemovac drain is performed, unless beads were placed. The pin sites are kept clean and dry; no specific pin site manipulation (ointment, peroxide, etc.) is performed. Placement of a foam sponge around the pin, between the frame and the skin, minimizes motion at the pin–skin interface, and limits pin tract problems. The fusion mass is monitored by serial X-rays and the fixator maintained until the fusion is solid, or until the beads are removed and definitive internal fixation is appropriate.

Plate Fixation

A narrow or broad 4.5 LC-DCP plate is utilized. The plate is bent to the desired flexion angle and applied to the dorsal or volar surface of the humerus and ulna. A minimum of four screws are placed on each side of the fusion, requiring a plate four to six holes longer than the number of screws for posterior application. There are no reports of the use of locking plates for elbow arthrodesis; however, this may be desirable in osteopenic bone. Wound closure is the same as above. Postoperatively, the patient is placed in a splint or cast for 2–4 weeks until the soft tissues have healed. Fusion is monitored by serial radiographs.

Complications

- Nerve injury
- Nonunion
- Wound breakdown/symptomatic hardware
- Stress fracture at the end of the plate

Pearls

- Allow patients considering a fusion to "test drive" various joint angles to determine which is most functional.

- Fusion is a salvage operation which can provide a stable painless joint but may significantly limit extremity function.
- External fixation is indicated in the face of unresolved infection, compromised soft tissue, or other situations in which implanted hardware is undesirable. Rigid internal fixation is usually better tolerated by the patient for the extended time required for solid fusion.
- Radiohumeral arthrodesis has been described [51] for salvage of a failed TEA, however sacrifices forearm rotation as well as flexion/extension, and is not routinely recommended.
- The results of elbow arthrodesis for salvage of failed TEA may be worse than the reported "all cause" literature, due to deficient bone stock and severe osteopenia in this population.

Amputation

Above-elbow amputation for the salvage of a failed TEA is truly the "procedure of last resort." It is used in the situation where the patient has a life-threatening infection caused by a septic elbow arthroplasty, and is too medically unstable to tolerate multiple procedures to attempt to eradicate the infection and restore function. This can occur in patients with end stage renal disease, chemotherapy, AIDS, or other severely immunodeficient hosts. The sole objective of this procedure is to definitively remove the nidus of infection in the most expedient fashion.

Indication

- Life-threatening infection from the TEA

Contraindications

- All other methods to control/eradicate the prosthetic joint infection

Surgical Technique

The controversy regarding transhumeral vs. joint disarticulation is irrelevant in this context. The amputation level is above the level of infection if possible, which typically means above the cement mantle in the humerus. Fish mouth flaps are generally adequate unless the soft tissue is significantly compromised. The procedure is performed without a tourniquet and hemostasis is maintained throughout the procedure. The nerves are identified and transected under tension as proximal as possible. Healthy muscle is transected slightly longer than the bone to allow coverage at the end of the stump. The brachial artery is double suture ligated and divided. The bone is cut with a sagittal saw and irrigation to minimize thermal injury. Sharp bone edges are rounded off with a rasp. The brachialis and triceps muscle bellies are approximated without tension over the end of the stump. Attachment of the muscle to the bone may improve control of the residual limb, however, may not be critical in this indication. Typically, the stump is not definitively closed when performing amputations for infection; however, in this situation, flap contouring and approximation over a suction drain is recommended. The patient may not be stable enough to return to the operating room for repeat washout and definitive stump closure. A large bulky dressing is applied. Postoperative stump wrapping and shoulder range of motion are begun after the drain is removed.

Prosthetic Management

Transhumeral amputation allows for the fitting of an articulated above-elbow (AE) prosthesis. However, patients have a short lever arm to move the prosthesis, rotation of the stump in the socket is a problem, and dynamic elbow motion requires precise scapular control. For these reasons the rate of effective prosthetic use for transhumeral amputees is less than 50% [57], and in this subgroup is much lower. Prosthetic fitting is rarely indicated. Resolution of sepsis, a healed painless stump, and minimal phantom pain are indicators of a successful surgical outcome.

Complications

- Failure to eradicate the source of the infection
- Intraoperative blood loss
- Perianesthetic complications

Pearls

- Measuring the length of the cement column on preoperative radiographs, relative to fixed landmarks, determines the correct level of the bony cut intraoperatively. Do not leave cement behind in the humeral canal.
- Speed matters, these are usually very sick patients and minimizing surgical time is required.
- Prosthetic fitting, while possible, is rarely indicated in these patients.
- This is truly a life over limb salvage procedure, and should be rarely indicated. Careful consideration of the placement of a TEA in a high risk, infirm, or immunocompromised patient is warranted. Early intervention and definitive management, if infection is suspected, will help avoid this devastating salvage operation.

Conclusion

Reoperation after failure of total elbow replacement is complex and multifactorial. A clear understanding of the surgical anatomy, mode of failure, and careful surgical planning is essential to successful revision of these difficult problems. More importantly, careful patient selection, meticulous attention to surgical technique and soft tissue handling, and establishment of appropriate patient expectations and activity limits will minimize the occurrence of many of these problems. Although revision elbow arthroplasty is difficult and the potential complication rates are high, significant improvements can be achieved in the patient's overall function and quality of life.

References

1. HCUP Nationwide Inpatient Sample (NIS). Total elbow replacement. A.f.H.R.a.Q. (AHRQ), Editor; 1998–2006.
2. Fevang BT, et al. Results after 562 total elbow replacements: a report from the Norwegian Arthroplasty Register. J Shoulder Elbow Surg. 2009;18(3):449–56.
3. Shi LL, et al. Semiconstrained primary and revision total elbow arthroplasty with use of the Coonrad-Morrey prosthesis. J Bone Joint Surg Am. 2007;89(7):1467–75.
4. Yamaguchi K, Adams RA, Morrey BF. Infection after total elbow arthroplasty. J Bone Joint Surg Am. 1998;80(4):481–91.
5. Gille J, et al. Single-stage revision of peri-prosthetic infection following total elbow replacement. J Bone Joint Surg Br. 2006;88(10):1341–6.
6. Cheung EV, Adams RA, Morrey BF. Reimplantation of a total elbow prosthesis following resection arthroplasty for infection. J Bone Joint Surg Am. 2008;90(3):589–94.
7. Athwal GS, Morrey BF. Revision total elbow arthroplasty for prosthetic fractures. J Bone Joint Surg Am. 2006;88(9):2017–26.
8. Lee BP, Adams RA, Morrey BF. Polyethylene wear after total elbow arthroplasty. J Bone Joint Surg Am. 2005;87(5):1080–7.
9. Lee BP, Adams RA, Morrey BF. Wear and elbow replacement. In: Morrey BF, Sanchez-Sotelo J, editors. The elbow and its disorders. Philadelphia: Saunders Elsevier; 2009. p. 880–4.
10. Wright TW, Hastings H. Total elbow arthroplasty failure due to overuse, C-ring failure, and/or bushing wear. J Shoulder Elbow Surg. 2005;14(1):65–72.
11. Levy JC, et al. Effectiveness of revision following linked versus unlinked total elbow arthroplasty. J Shoulder Elbow Surg. 2009;18(3):457–62.
12. Celli A, et al. Triceps insufficiency following total elbow arthroplasty. J Bone Joint Surg Am. 2005;87(9):1957–64.
13. Goldberg SH, et al. Modes of wear after semiconstrained total elbow arthroplasty. J Bone Joint Surg Am. 2008;90(3):609–19.
14. Patil N, Cheung EV, Mow CS. High revision rate after total elbow arthroplasty with a linked semiconstrained device. Orthopedics. 2009;32(5):321.
15. Celli A, Morrey BF. Total elbow arthroplasty in patients forty years of age or less. J Bone Joint Surg Am. 2009;91(6):1414–8.
16. Kelly EW, Coghlan J, Bell S. Five- to thirteen-year follow-up of the GSB III total elbow arthroplasty. J Shoulder Elbow Surg. 2004;13(4):434–40.
17. Ramsey ML, Adams RA, Morrey BF. Instability of the elbow treated with semiconstrained total elbow arthroplasty. J Bone Joint Surg Am. 1999;81(1):38–47.
18. Degreef I, Sciot R, De Smet L. Metallosis in revision total elbow arthroplasty. Complications and staging method. Acta Orthop Belg. 2008;74(6):753–60.
19. Marra G, et al. Fracture and nonunion of the olecranon in total elbow arthroplasty. J Shoulder Elbow Surg. 2006;15(4):486–94.
20. Sneftrup SB, et al. Revision of failed total elbow arthroplasty with use of a linked implant. J Bone Joint Surg Br. 2006;88(1):78–83.
21. Gramstad GD, et al. Elbow arthroplasty using a convertible implant. Tech Hand Up Extrem Surg. 2005;9(3):153–63.
22. Furnes A, et al. [Quality control of prosthetic replacements of knee, ankle, toe, shoulder, elbow and finger joints in Norway 1994. A report after the first year of registration of joint prostheses in the national registry]. Tidsskr Nor Laegeforen. 1996;116(15):1777–81.
23. Kraay MJ, et al. Primary semiconstrained total elbow arthroplasty survival analysis of 113 consecutive cases. J Bone Joint Surg Br. 1994;76(4):636–40.
24. Hoddinott C, et al. Determination of bone and fat concentrations following systemic cefamandole and regional cefuroxime administration in patients undergoing knee arthroplasty. J Antimicrob Chemother. 1990;26(6):823–9.
25. Sanchez-Sotelo J, O'Driscoll S, Morrey BF. Periprosthetic humeral fractures after total elbow arthroplasty: treatment with implant revision and strut allograft augmentation. J Bone Joint Surg Am. 2002;84A(9):1642–50.
26. Zook J, Ward Sr WG. Intraosseous radial nerve entrapment complicating total elbow revision. J Arthroplasty. 2001;16(7):919–22.
27. King GJ, Adams RA, Morrey BF. Total elbow arthroplasty: revision with use of a non-custom semiconstrained prosthesis. J Bone Joint Surg Am. 1997;79(3):394–400.
28. Goldberg SH, et al. Thermal tissue damage caused by ultrasonic cement removal from the humerus. J Bone Joint Surg Am. 2005;87(3):583–91.
29. Reilly P, Rees J, Carr AJ. An aid to removal of cement during revision elbow replacement. Ann R Coll Surg Engl. 2006;88(2):231.
30. Morrey BF, Sanchez-Sotelo J. Revision of failed total elbow arthroplasty with osseous deficiency. In: Morrey BF, Sanchez-Sotelo J, editors. The elbow and its disorders. Philadelphia: Saunders Elsevier; 2009. p. 899–910.
31. Figgie III HE, Inglis AE, Mow C. Total elbow arthroplasty in the face of significant bone stock or soft tissue losses. Preliminary results of custom-fit arthroplasty. J Arthroplasty. 1986;1(2):71–81.
32. Hughes RE, et al. Reduction of triceps muscle force after shortening of the distal humerus: a computational model. J Shoulder Elbow Surg. 1997;6(5):444–8.
33. Kamineni S, Morrey BF. Proximal ulnar reconstruction with strut allograft in revision total elbow arthroplasty. J Bone Joint Surg Am. 2004;86(A(6)):1223–9.
34. Bicknell RT, Hughes JS. A new technique for management of ulnar bone loss in revision total elbow arthroplasty using a tuberized tricortical iliac crest autograft: a case report. J Shoulder Elbow Surg. 2008;17(5):e15–8.
35. Brownhill JR, et al. Defining the flexion-extension axis of the ulna: implications for intra-operative elbow alignment. J Biomech Eng. 2009;131(2):021005.
36. Mansat P, Adams RA, Morrey BF. Allograft-prosthesis composite for revision of catastrophic failure of total elbow arthroplasty. J Bone Joint Surg Am. 2004;86(A(4)):724–35.
37. Pho RW, Vajara R, Satku K. Free vascularized bone transplants in problematic nonunions of fractures. J Trauma. 1983;23(4):341–9.
38. Chhabra AB, et al. Treatment of chronic nonunions of the humerus with free vascularized fibula transfer: a report of thirteen cases. J Reconstr Microsurg. 2009;25(2):117–24.
39. Kato T, Bishop AT, Tu YK, Wood MB. Effect of the duration of room-temperature ischemia on function of the vascular endothelium: the role of adrenomedullin in reperfusion injury. J Bone Joint Surg Am. 1997;79(5):647–55.
40. Prokopis PM, Weiland AJ. The triceps-preserving approach for semiconstrained total elbow arthroplasty. J Shoulder Elbow Surg. 2008;17(3):454–8.
41. Little CP, Graham AJ, Carr AJ. Total elbow arthroplasty: a systematic review of the literature in the English language until the end of 2003. J Bone Joint Surg Br. 2005;87(4):437–44.
42. McKee MD, et al. Effect of humeral condylar resection on strength and functional outcome after semiconstrained total elbow arthroplasty. J Bone Joint Surg Am. 2003;85(A(5)):802–7.

43. Pierce TD, Herndon JH. The triceps preserving approach to total elbow arthroplasty. Clin Orthop Relat Res. 1998;354:144–52.
44. Joshi RP, Yanni O, Gallannaugh SC. A modified posterior approach to the elbow for total elbow replacement. J Shoulder Elbow Surg. 1999;8(6):606–11.
45. Sanchez-Sotelo J, Morrey BF. Surgical techniques for reconstruction of chronic insufficiency of the triceps. Rotation flap using anconeus and tendo achillis allograft. J Bone Joint Surg Br. 2002;84(8):1116–20.
46. Wolf JM, McCarty EC, Ritchie PD. Triceps reconstruction using hamstring graft for triceps insufficiency or recurrent rupture. Tech Hand Up Extrem Surg. 2008;12(3):174–9.
47. Morrey BF. Triceps tendon repair and reconstruction. In: Morrey BF, editor. The elbow. Philadelphia: Lippincott, Williams & Wilkins; 2002. p. 193–204.
48. Frankle M. Management of the flail elbow. In: Yamaguchi K, et al., editors. Postraumatic reconstruction of the elbow. Rosemont: American Academy of Orthopaedic Surgeons; 2007. p. 427–33.
49. Graham TJ, Fitzgerald MS. The destroyed elbow. Am J Orthop. 2000;29(9 Suppl):9–15.
50. Koller H, et al. The fate of elbow arthrodesis: indications, techniques, and outcome in fourteen patients. J Shoulder Elbow Surg. 2008;17(2):293–306.
51. Presnal BP, Chillag KJ. Radiohumeral arthrodesis for salvage of failed total elbow arthroplasty. J Arthroplasty. 1995;10(5): 699–701.
52. Morrey BF, Askew LJ, Chao EY. A biomechanical study of normal functional elbow motion. J Bone Joint Surg Am. 1981;63(6): 872–7.
53. Richards R. Elbow arthrodesis. In: Yamaguchi K et al., editors. Advanced reconstruction elbow. Rosemont: American Academy of Orthopedic Surgeons; 2007. p. 421–6.
54. O'Neill OR, et al. Compensatory motion in the upper extremity after elbow arthrodesis. Clin Orthop Relat Res. 1992;281:89–96.
55. Morrey BF. Salvage of the resected joint: revision total elbow arthroplasty. In: Morrey BF, editor. Reconstructive surgery of the joints. New York: Churchill Livingstone; 1996. p. 555–60.
56. Beckenbaugh BD. Arthrodesis. In: Morrey BF, editor. Reconstructive surgery of the joints. New York: Churchill Livingstone; 1996. p. 695–702.
57. Shives TC, Andrews KL. Elbow disarticulation amputation. In: Morrey BF, Sanchez-Sotelo J, editors. The elbow and its disorders. Philadelphia: Saunders Elsevier; 2009. p. 1015–22.
58. Athwal GS, Goetz TJ, Pollock JW, Faber KJ. Prosthetic replacement for distal humerus fractures. Orthop Clin North Am. 2008; 39(2):201–12.

14 Reoperative Options for Compressive Neuropathies of the Upper Extremity

Jason R. Kang and Ranjan Gupta

Abstract

In addressing failed surgery for compressive neuropathies about the arm, it is important to distinguish between what would truly be called recurrence vs. those who have a failure to improve in their symptoms. Evaluation of these patients does require some time in both obtaining a thorough history as well as performing a detailed clinical exam. Electromyographic and neural conduction velocity testing is helpful. In these cases, the surgeon needs to think both proximal and distal; that is, could the symptoms be coming from the neck or could there be areas of further compression proximally or distally about the peripheral nerve? Reoperating on previously operated nerve tissue can be quite stressful as the nerve tissue is frequently less forgiving than other soft tissue structures commonly encountered in the scar bed. The use of a microscope can sometimes be helpful in visualizing the tissue planes and/or nerve tissue. If mechanical reasons are found to explain the patient's continued symptoms, then these points of compression can be surgically addressed if the patient is willing to accept the potential risks of nerve injury and further scarring, which sometimes precludes the patient from improving as much as both doctor and patient were hoping.

Keywords

Carpal • Cubital • Radial • Tunnel • Syndrome • Recurrence

Key Points

- Carpal tunnel syndrome can have true recurrence vs. failure to improve.
- True recurrence is defined as a patient who improved for a period of time (usually 6 months) but then had recurrence of symptoms.
- The other issue with the carpal tunnel surgery is the possibility of incomplete release.
- In cubital tunnel syndrome, failure to decompress all points of compression needs to be considered. Revision surgery usually entails a submuscular transposition (but not always).
- If ulnar neuropathy is present and previous cubital tunnel surgeries failed, one needs to consider possible compression at Guyon's canal.
- Radial tunnel syndrome is a poorly understood process. It can be associated with lateral epicondylitis. It may also be confused with distal biceps tendinopathy.

(continued)

J.R. Kang, BS
Department of Orthopedic Surgery, University of California, Irvine, Orange, CA, USA

R. Gupta, MD (✉)
Department of Orthopedic Surgery, University of California, Irvine, 101 The City Drive South Pavillion III, Building 29A, Orange, CA 92868, USA
e-mail: ranjang@uci.edu

S.F.M. Duncan (ed.), *Reoperative Hand Surgery*,
DOI 10.1007/978-1-4614-2373-7_14, © Springer Science+Business Media, LLC 2012

- Operative treatment for recurrent neuropathies depends on not only immense surgical skill, but also on the diagnostic abilities of the surgeon to try and truly pinpoint the source of the pain, which may or may not be neurogenic in origin.

Introduction

Compressive neuropathies of the upper extremity occur frequently and may require operative treatment. Pathological changes in peripheral nerves result from external mechanical forces of compression with the symptoms described by patients commonly referred to as entrapment syndromes. The most prevalent compressive neuropathy is carpal tunnel syndrome (CTS) and affects up to 10% of the entire population [1]. Although surgical decompression successfully resolves most cases of CTS, as much as 19% of patients receiving carpal tunnel release experience recurring symptoms and 12% of which require reoperation [2]. While the recurrence rates of other upper extremity compressive neuropathies remain underreported, their respective etiologies are unique to each site, and awareness of these differences is critical for successful outcomes in reoperative procedures.

Basic Science and Pathophysiology of Compressive Neuropathies

Treatment of compressive neuropathies has a long-standing history of successful management with surgical intervention. Yet, there remains significant difficulty with both early detection and reversal of late stages of the disease. The finest surgical techniques will not ameliorate the symptoms associated with the motor atrophy present in the later stages of the disease. As such, a deeper understanding of the basic science is required to develop adjuvant therapeutic regimens. The human nervous system is organized into the central and peripheral nervous system (PNS). The central nervous system (CNS) receives, processes, and initiates signals, while the PNS relays signals to and from the environment and CNS. In both systems, the principal cell type is the neuron, which communicates with their targets via long cytoplasmic processes called axons. In the PNS, the peripheral nerves are primarily composed of bundles of axons and their associated Schwann cells. Schwann cells provide protection and trophic support and are found in two phenotypes. Myelinating Schwann cells ensheath large caliber axons in myelin and maintain a one to one relationship with axons. Myelination increases the speed of action potential propagation and allows signals to reach their targets in a timely manner. On the other hand, nonmyelinating Schwann cells associate with numerous axons in structures known as Remak bundles. Remak bundles enclose small caliber C fibers and transmit pain and temperature sensation. Loss of myelination and changes in Remak bundles are common signs of neuropathy in peripheral nerves.

The defining objective feature of compressive neuropathies is the progressive decline in nerve conduction velocity. Chronic nerve compression (CNC) injuries of the median, ulnar, and radial nerves occur in predictable locations in the wrist, forearm, and arm. Overuse and cumulative trauma in areas of restricted anatomical space lead to compression of the nerve. The pathophysiologic changes include slowing of nerve conduction velocity, ischemia, edema, and eventually neuropathy. Only until recently have studies begun to understand these changes at the cellular level.

CNC injuries of peripheral nerves are distinctly different from acute injuries, such as crush and transection. Initially, it was believed that axonal damage during CNC injury triggers Schwann cells dedifferentiation and proliferation. However, studies now indicate that axonal integrity is maintained and free of pathology in CNC injuries [3]. Compressive neuropathies do not show morphometric evidence of Wallerian degeneration, the hallmark of acute peripheral nerve injuries [4]. Furthermore, CNC injuries occur in the absence of inflammation and immune mediated responses, unlike acute injuries [5]. Observational studies have found that CNC injuries lead to subsequent demyelination and remyelination of injured axons [6]. Thinner myelin is formed upon remyelination and this decrease in myelination contributes to the clinical presentation of slowing of the nerve conduction velocity in electrodiagnostic studies. Additionally, studies report that CNC injury induces a switch in Schwann cell phenotype. An increase in number of nonmyelinating Schwann cells and Remak bundles is observed in CNC injuries [4]. These Remak bundles contain an increased number of C fibers correlating to the pain at sites of compression in compressive neuropathies. Lastly, Schwann cells are mechanically sensitive to shear forces and expression of specific surface adhesion proteins are altered in response to hydrostatic pressure [7]. Thus, current research supports that compressive neuropathies are primarily a Schwann cell mediated disease. By further understanding the mechanism of injury response by Schwann cells to mechanical stimulation, molecular therapies can be developed to prevent injury as well as promote regeneration.

Etiology of Recurrent Compressive Neuropathies

Surgical treatments for compressive neuropathies produce successful and satisfactory results in the large majority of cases. However, a significant patient population continues to experience symptoms despite surgical intervention. The symptom complexes encountered after failed surgeries can be classified into categories: persistent, recurrent, and new [8]. In persistent cases, patients experience no period of relief despite surgical treatment. Causes of persistent compressive neuropathies include incomplete release of the entrapped nerve, an alternate site of compression, or incorrect diagnosis. In the latter two cases, other suspected sites of injury must be thoroughly investigated during physical examination to determine if further surgical exploration is required. Truly recurrent compressive neuropathies occur only after patients experience a period of relief for at least 6 months following previous surgery. Recurrent cases occur from reformation of causative structures, fibrous proliferation of scar tissue, alternate sites of compression, or presence of obstructive masses. In new cases, the symptom complex experienced by patients postoperatively is entirely different than those preoperatively and indicates iatrogenic or intraoperative injury of the nerve during the previous surgical procedure.

When treating patients with recurrent compressive neuropathies, surgeons must also consider the possibility of multiple sites of compression along the same nerve and their confounding presentations. As first described by Upton and McComas, double crush syndrome occurs when proximal compression of the nerve increases the susceptibility of the distal portion to pathology [9]. The distal sites of compression often mask the proximal sites of compression, leading to persistent or recurrent symptoms after surgical decompression. In recurrent compressive neuropathies, double crush syndrome should always be considered and ruled out before pursuing reoperation. If suspected, patients require thorough evaluation for conditions such as thoracic outlet syndrome and cervical radiculopathy [10].

Recurrent Compressive Neuropathies of the Median Nerve

Recurrent Carpal Tunnel Syndrome

The most frequently encountered compressive neuropathy in orthopedic clinics is CTS. CTS primarily involves the median nerve, which is derived from the medial and lateral cords of the brachial plexus and composed of nerve roots C6 through C8 and T1. As first described by Sir James Paget in 1863, patients with CTS typically experience gradually worsening symptoms of paresthesia, nocturnal pain, and loss of grip strength [11]. Motor and sensory deficits are typically experienced in the distribution of the median nerve, which includes the radial three and one half digits of the hand. Splinting, activity modification, and glucocorticoid injections are conservative treatments frequently used as first-line therapy. If patients do not experience relief, surgical intervention is indicated.

In the USA, approximately 400,000–500,000 carpal tunnel release procedures are performed per year [12]. Gelberman et al. utilized the wick catheter to measure the hydrostatic pressure within the carpal canal [13]. They established that the normal pressure with the wrist in neutral position was 2.5 mmHg, whereas CTS elevated the intercarpal canal pressure to 32 mmHg. Therefore, the operative strategy is to relieve pressure by surgically dividing the transverse carpal ligament (TCL). This strategy dates back to 1947, where Brain, Wright, and Wilkerson treated six patients by releasing the TCL [14]. The standard approach to decompression is by the open method, but alternative approaches include the limited incision technique as well as variations of the endoscopic approach described by Agee and Chow [15, 16]. In primary procedures, the open method may be favored because the TCL can be fully visualized to ensure complete transection. Complications resulting from the open method are reported in 5–15% of patients and include median nerve injury, neuromas in continuity, and incomplete transection of the TCL [17]. Potential disadvantages of the open method include larger size of incision, increased scar pain, pillar pain, and longer recovery time compared to the endoscopic and limited incisure methods. Although the latter techniques provide smaller scar size and faster recovery times, complications and recurrent CTS have been reported at a higher rate of 2–35% of cases [18]. In secondary CTS, the most frequently encountered cause is incomplete division of the TCL [19, 20]. Other causes include tenosynovitis of the flexor tendon synovial sheaths, scar tissue formation, nerve tethering to the transected TCL flap, and obstructive masses within the carpal canal. Furthermore, reducing technical errors during the primary operation should not be underestimated in avoiding revision surgery [21]. Systemic disorders such as diabetes mellitus, hypertension, and rheumatoid arthritis are other risk factors for recurrent CTS that require consideration when evaluating potential candidates for revision carpal tunnel surgery [22, 23].

Diagnosis of Recurrent Carpal Tunnel Syndrome

The history and physical examination are the foundation for accurate diagnosis of recurrent CTS. Preoperative symptoms must be compared with postoperative symptoms of prior procedures to determine the status of the median nerve. Intraoperative notes from previous surgery are also helpful by indicating the possible cause of recurrent symptoms. Patient complaints will be similar to those found in primary CTS and often include motor and sensory deficits. Paresthesia, numbness, and pain occur in the distribution of the median nerve and usually worsen at night. Severe cases will present with diminished grip strength and atrophy of the thenar muscles. During physical examination, the symptoms are reproducible with percussion over the TCL (Tinel's sign) and prolonged hyperflexion of the wrist (Phalen's sign). Sensory deficits such as decreased two-point discrimination are also measured preoperatively to compare with surgical outcomes. If sensory deficits extend from the hand into the forearm, proximal compression should be suspected.

Electrodiagnostic studies are widely used in evaluating primary cases of CTS; however, their role in recurrent cases is limited. Even after successful decompression, electrodiagnostic studies fail to detect changes or improvements in nerve conduction velocity for up to 6 months [24]. Electrodiagnostic studies are still useful in cases of misdiagnosis and can be performed throughout the upper extremity to rule out compressive neuropathies at alternate or multiple sites. Also, nerve conduction studies may still factor into determining severity and how soon patients require revision procedures.

Imaging modalities have begun to play an increasing role in evaluating recurrent CTS [25]. Magnetic resonance (MR) imaging and ultrasound provide alternative methods of assessing, managing, and postoperatively evaluating the nerve [26, 27]. MR imaging has been successfully used to visualize peripheral nerves and identify obstructive masses or nerve enlargements to a high degree of sensitivity [28]. Furthermore, MR imaging is also sensitive for incomplete division of the TCL and capable of detecting iatrogenic lesions of the median nerve from previous surgery [29, 30]. Because the cost of MR imaging may limit its use, ultrasound provides an economic alternative with comparable results. Ultrasound has been reported to have diagnostic sensitivity of 89% and a specificity of 83% [31]. In compressive neuropathies, imaging modalities are improving and may be particularly useful in addressing the inadequacy of electrodiagnostic studies and evaluating the site of decompression immediately after surgery as these techniques continue to evolve and improve.

It is important to note that published studies provide only a limited scope of recurrent compressive neuropathies. Although the abundance of scar tissue is reported frequently during reoperative carpal tunnel surgeries, the role and significance of scarring on recurrent CTS are not entirely understood [32, 33]. Notably, the level of scar tissue formation in successful open carpal tunnel release procedures is not measured since successful procedures do not involve invasive reexamination of the repair. Also, incomplete division of the TCL can become difficult to discern from postoperative healing of the TCL. As a result, the impact of scar tissue and incomplete division of the TCL in recurrent CTS are not absolute. In some cases, diagnostic injections with lidocaine and/or corticosteroid may aid in sorting out the diagnosis and whether surgery may help.

Surgeons must always counsel patients on their expectations for reoperative procedures. In patients with multiple revision procedures, there is a greater likelihood that symptoms will persist or worsen after reoperation. The reversal of motor deficits is almost always limited. Lastly, secondary factors, such as worker's compensation insurance, have a significant impact on return to work time [34, 35]. These factors must be considered for patients reporting dissatisfaction after several decompression procedures.

Reoperative Options for Carpal Tunnel Syndrome

Revision procedures must address the compression of the nerve in addition to management of the previously failed surgery. Therefore, patients require operative planning personalized to their surgical history and clinical presentation. Regardless of previous surgical approach, the open method is preferred for reoperative CTS (see Fig. 14.1 for carpal tunnel anatomy). An incision begins ulnar to the palmaris longus and ulnar to the scar of the previous site of surgery. While avoiding damage to the median nerve, the new incision is extended beyond the length of the previous incision. In this region, possible anatomical variations of the palmar cutaneous and recurrent branches of the median nerve must be identified and protected. The median nerve must be identified proximally and followed distally past the carpal canal. If the previous incision was placed too far radially, the failed carpal tunnel surgery may also be associated with damage to the palmar cutaneous branch of the median nerve. The resultant neuroma will present with pain and must be exercised. The free nerve ending should be moved to a well-vascularized local tissue bed.

In persistent CTS, the most common indication for reoperation is incomplete division of the TCL [8]. The reported incidence of incomplete TCL division ranges from 0 to 65% [36]. Full visualization and transection of the TCL using the open method will be sufficient, but intraoperative findings will dictate if further treatment of the nerve is required. The surgeon should be aware of variations in median nerve anatomy (see Fig. 14.2). Appropriate measures are used for scar tissue and constrictive fascial bands as encountered. Treatment options will range from dissection under loupe magnification and external neurolysis to nerve coverage with soft tissue flaps.

The operative treatment of truly recurrent CTS is typically more involved, especially in patients with failed open carpal tunnel surgery. Again, the open method previously described is the recommended approach. Nerves found heavily encased in scar tissue require external neurolysis, using a nerve stimulator if necessary. If there are signs of focal swelling characteristic of neuromas in continuity or the nerve is under tension, epineurotomy is often indicated. In contrast, internal neurolysis has not been shown to

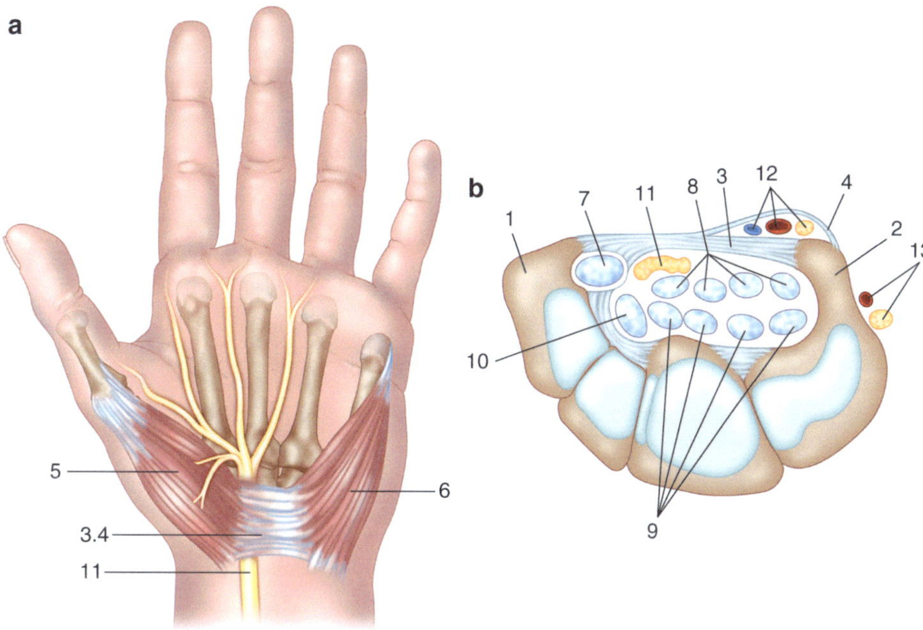

Fig. 14.1 Anatomy of the carpal canal. (**a**) Typical median nerve and hand anatomy at the level of the transverse carpal ligament. (**b**) Carpal tunnel cross sectional anatomy. *1* Trapezium tubercle, *2* hook of the hamate, *3* transverse carpal ligament, *4* palmar carpal ligament, *5* thenar muscles, *6* hypothenar muscles, *7* flexor carpi radialis tendon, *8* flexor digitorum superficialis tendon, *9* flexor digitorum profundus tendon, *10* flexor pollicis longus tendon, *11* median nerve, *12* ulnar artery, vein, and nerve superficial branches, *13* ulnar artery, vein, and nerve deep branches

improve the results of primary carpal tunnel decompression and is not recommended in revision surgery [37, 38]. No studies have been able to prove the efficacy of internal neurolysis in treating recurrent CTS [39]. The success of internal neurolysis varies largely on experience and skill of the surgeon and should only be considered by those trained in microsurgery .

To avoid future recurrences, efforts are made to provide coverage for the median nerve and prevent readherence to the surgical site. Fat pads, muscle transfers, vein wrapping, synovial flaps, and synthetic materials have been previously employed with varying degrees of success [40–42]. Fat grafts from local areas, such as the hypothenar region, provide a well vascularized tissue bed and report excellent results [43]. Fat flaps help restore the pulley function of the TCL and prevent volar displacement of the flexor tendons after transection of the TCL. In a comparison study between the hypothenar fat flap and synovial flap coverage in recurrent CTS, the hypothenar fat flap provided superior results [44]. Patients receiving the hypothenar fat flap coverage experienced improvements in paresthesia, thenar atrophy, and nerve conduction velocity with a satisfaction rate of 73%. Furthermore, Fusetti et al. used the hypothenar fat pad flap where 90% patients reported complete resolution of pain and 80% patients reported return of two-point discrimination to normal levels [45]. Our preferred technique is the pedicled hypothenar fat pad (see Fig. 14.3). After the open incision is made, the incision is extended distally and ulnarly over the hypothenar region. The overlying hypothenar fat pad is lifted in a distal to proximal fashion, leaving the proximal portion attached. Careful dissection and preserving the vascular supply of the tissue are critical. The ulnar segment of the transected TCL is resected and the fat flap is folded over to separate the median nerve from the TCL. The fat pad is pedicaled to the radial wall of the carpal tunnel with sutures. Mathoulin et al. utilized this technique to completely resolve pain in 41 of 45 patients [46]. One disadvantage of using local fat pads is inadequate coverage due to its limited size. Free dermal fat grafts can be used instead; however, vascularity issues of the graft may lead to tissue necrosis and adverse immune responses at the site of coverage. Synthetic materials, such as nerve tubes, can also elicit immunologic responses that irritate the nerve and are not routinely utilized. Muscle transfers of the pronator quadratus, abductor digiti minimi [47], and lumbricles have been employed, but also face issues of vascularity, donor site morbidity, inadequate size, or a combination of these factors. Successful uses of autogenous vein grafts have been reported as well [41]. Reduced pain and sensory disturbances with improved two-point discrimination and electrodiagnostic findings have been achieved in all 19 patients who received this procedure after recurrent CTS.

After revision carpal tunnel surgery, we recommend wrist immobilization for up to 2 weeks. Splinting should be done

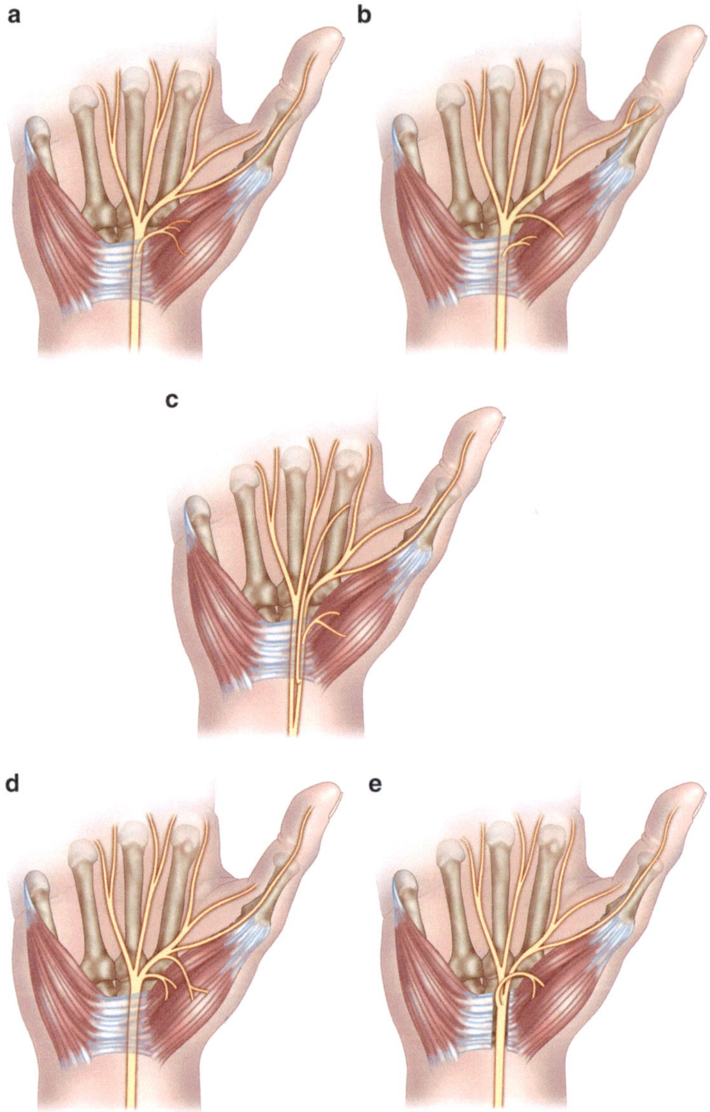

Fig. 14.2 Variations in the median nerve thenar motor branch. Possible variant morphologies include (**a**) extraligamentous (most common) (**b**) extraligamentous with subligamentous accessory branch, (**c**) preligamentous, (**d**) extraligamentous with accessory branch, and (**e**) transligamentous variations

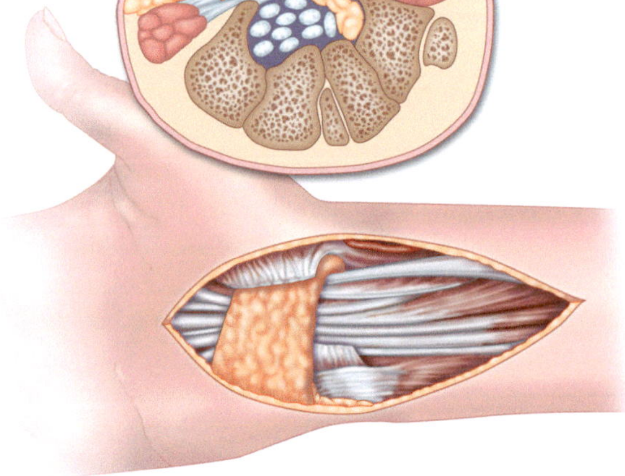

Fig. 14.3 Hypothenar fat flap covering the median nerve and secured to the radial aspect of the carpal canal

with slight 20° dorsi-flexion of the wrist in order to provide the maximal size of the carpal tunnel. Mobilization of fingers is encouraged immediately and aggravating activities such as typing should be avoided for 4 weeks. Formal postoperative therapy is not routinely required. In a study of 150 patients, supervised postoperative therapy did not significantly improve outcomes [48]. Scar pain may persist for up to 6 months. In revision carpal tunnel surgery, some patients will report immediate improvement in motor and sensory functions. However, as mentioned previously, nerve conduction studies may take up to 6 months to return to normal values and in severe cases, patients with irreversible losses in nerve conduction are not uncommon.

The prognosis for patients undergoing reoperative procedures is fair but declines significantly after the primary procedure for carpal tunnel release. Chang and Dellon report that statistically significant improvements are achievable in patients following revision carpal tunnel surgery [49].

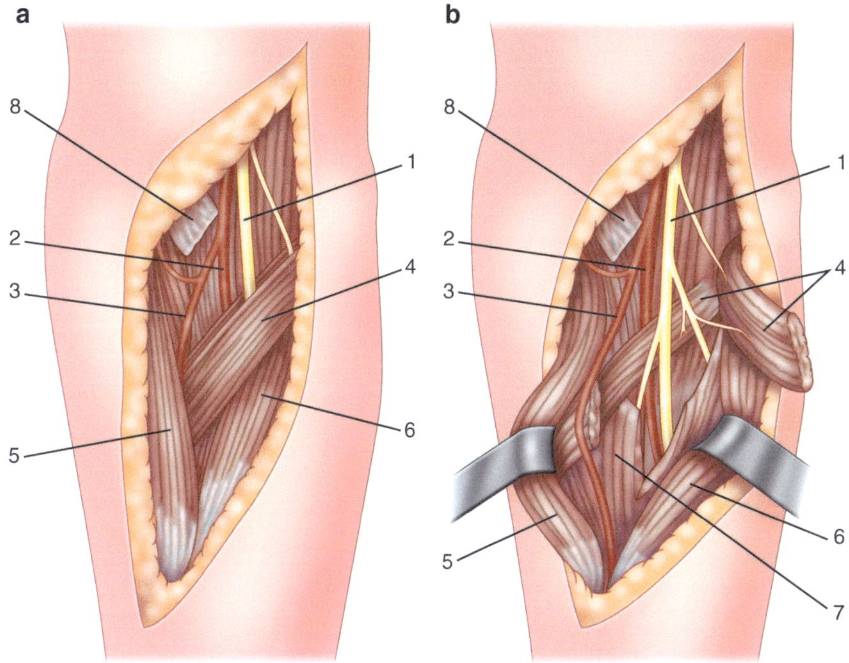

Fig. 14.4 Proximal forearm surgical exposure of the median nerve. (**a**) The bicipital aponeurosis is divided exposing the median nerve at the elbow. (**b**) The humeral head of the pronator teres is sectioned and the flexor digitorum superficialis muscle is split to expose the median nerve. Care should be taken not to injure the anterior interosseous nerve. *1* Median nerve, *2* ulnar artery, *3* radial artery, *4* pronator teres muscle, *5* brachioradialis muscle, *6* flexor carpi radialis muscle, *7* flexor digitorum superficialis muscle, *8* bicipital aponeurosis

Patients with persistent or recurrent symptoms after failed endoscopic release typically have greater improvements compared to those with previous open carpal tunnel surgery [50]. Secondary carpal tunnel surgery has been shown to effectively provide satisfactory results for patients with symptoms such as sensory loss and nocturnal paresthesia, but limited improvement in symptoms such as grip strength [51].

Recurrent Pronator Teres Syndrome

Pronator teres syndrome (PTS) describes entrapment of the median nerve in the proximal forearm (see Fig. 14.4a, b). Patients with PTS experience diffuse pain in the forearm that is associated with increased activity. Pain may also present with numbness and weakness in the distribution of the median nerve and the anterior interosseous nerve and the muscles it innervates may also be involved. The incidence of PTS is rare and conservative treatments, such as avoidance of aggravating activities and corticosteroid injections, successfully resolve most cases of PTS. Patients undergoing primary surgery for PTS have low rates of recurrence. In a study of 39 patients, only 3 failures were reported with the most common cause of recurrent symptoms due to inadequate decompression or wrong diagnosis [52]. Common sites of entrapment occur between the two heads of the pronator teres, lacertus fibrosus, and arch of the flexor digitorum superficialis [53]. Compression of the median nerve can also occur proximally at the supracondylar process of the medial epicondyle. Here the ligament of Struthers may entrap the median nerve as it approaches the pronator teres.

Diagnosis Recurrent Pronator Teres Syndrome

During physical examination, percussion along the course of the median nerve (Tinel's sign) will reproduce symptoms and help localize the site of compression. Symptoms can also be elicited from resisted flexion of the elbow, resisted pronation of the forearm, and resisted flexion of the fingers. Electrodiagnostic studies have not been shown to be useful in detecting PTS or locating the site of compression. As with all cases of primary or recurrent compressive neuropathies, measures must be taken to rule out proximal and distal sites of compression. For example, CTS will be ruled out with normal nerve conduction velocity at the wrist with a negative Phalen's test.

Reoperative Options for Recurrent Pronator Teres Syndrome

Reoperative treatment of PTS involves thorough surgical reexploration of the median nerve. The incision for exploration begins 5 cm proximal to the elbow flexion crease and continues distally until the midpoint of the forearm in a "lazy S" pattern. The median nerve is identified proximally at the supracondylar process and freed of constriction past the arch of the flexor digitorum superficialis. Most secondary cases of

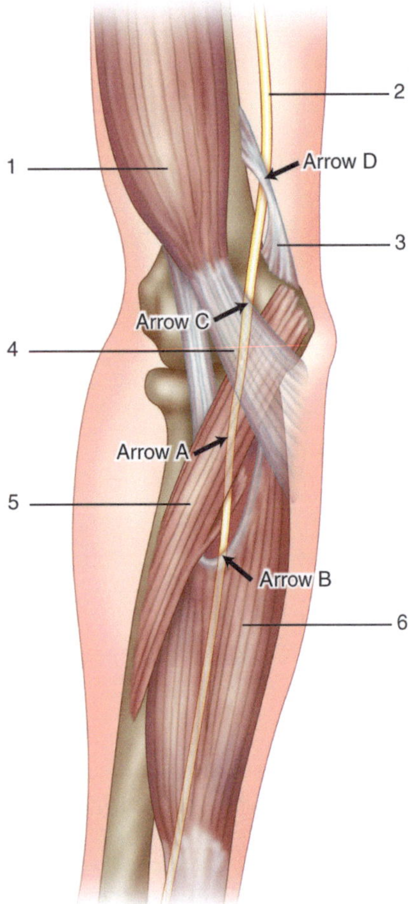

Fig. 14.5 Points of median nerve compression in pronator syndrome. *1* Biceps brachii, *2* median nerve, *3* ligament of Struthers, *4* bicipital aponeurosis, *5* pronator teres muscle, *6* flexor digitorum superficialis muscle. *Arrow A*: compression at the pronator teres muscle, *Arrow B*: compression at the tendinous arch of the flexor digitorum superficialis, *Arrow C*: compression at the bicipital aponeurosis, *Arrow D*: compression at the ligament of Struthers

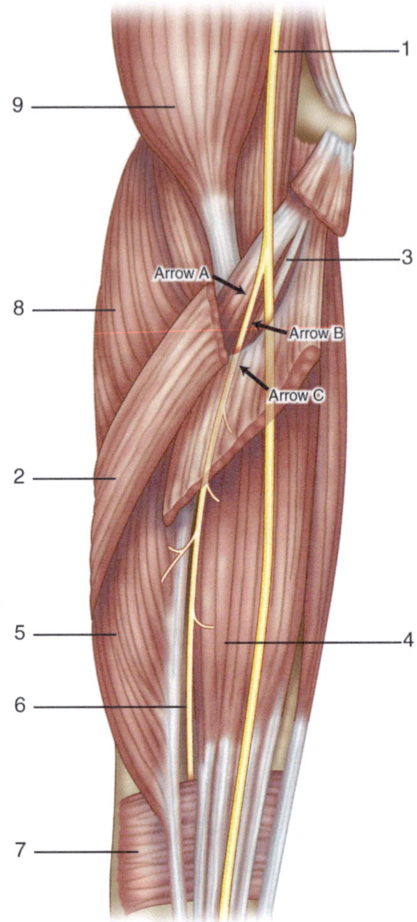

Fig. 14.6 Points of compression in anterior interosseous syndrome. *1* Median nerve, *2* ronator teres muscle, *3* flexor digitorum superficialis muscle, *4* flexor digitorum profundus muscle, *5* flexor pollicis longus muscle, *6* anterior interosseous nerve, *7* pronator quatratous muscle, *8* supinator muscle, *9* biceps muscle. *Arrow A*: compression at the ulnar head of the pronator teres, *Arrow B*: compression at the tendinous edge of the flexor digitorum superficialis, *Arrow C*: compression at an anomalous origin of the flexor pollicis longus

PTS occur due to incomplete release of the entrapped nerve and repeat decompression is often sufficient (see Fig. 14.5). Measures such as external neurolysis for epineurial fibrosis and epineurotomy for neuromas in continuity may be performed based on intraoperative findings.

Recurrent Anterior Interosseous Syndrome

The anterior interosseous nerve is a purely motor branch that arises from the median nerve in the proximal forearm. Entrapment of this nerve is commonly referred to as anterior interosseous syndrome (AIS) or Kiloh–Nevin syndrome, named after those who first described the condition in 1952 [54]. AIS is rare and occurs traumatically or spontaneously. Patients with AIS typically experience diffuse pain in the forearm and difficulty moving the index and middle fingers. Contributing anatomical anomalies include a tendinous origin of the deep head of the pronator teres, an accessory head of the flexor pollicis longus, an accessory tendon of the flexor superficialis to the flexor pollicis longus, and ulnar collateral vessels (see Fig. 14.6) [55].

Diagnosis Recurrent Anterior Interosseous Syndrome

In secondary cases, the physical examination findings are similar to primary AIS. After failed surgical decompression, patients will continue to experience nonspecific pain in the forearm or elbow and weakness of the flexor pollicis longus, pronator quadratus, and the radial half of the flexor digitorum profundis. Common findings include a weak pinch strength and a positive pinch test resulting from an inability to flex the distal interphalangeal joint of the thumb, index finger, and middle finger. In patients with AIS, electrodiagnostic studies of the pronator quadratus could reveal denervation. MR imaging and sonography have also been useful in identifying potential sites of compression on the anterior interosseous nerve [56]. Because AIS occurs traumatically and spontaneously, it is difficult to differentiate whether recurrent symptoms are due to failed surgery or repeat injury to the nerve. Spontaneous cases of AIS can be successfully and effectively treated with nonoperative measures such as rest of the affected limb and nonsteroidal anti-inflammatory medications. Therefore, the literature recommends a waiting period of 2–12 months before considering surgical exploration.

Reoperative Options for Recurrent Anterior Interosseous Syndrome

Decompression in primary cases of anterior interosseous syndrome yields very high success rates [57]. Few cases of recurrent anterior interosseous syndrome have been reported. Persistent AIS is most likely caused by the incomplete release of the anterior interior interosseous nerve. Similar to PTS, the incision begins 5 cm proximal to the elbow flexion crease and continues distally until the midpoint of the forearm in a "lazy S" pattern. The median nerve is identified proximally and explored distally. The anterior interosseous nerve frequently branches from the median nerve between the two heads of the pronator teres. The anterior interosseous nerve should be explored deep to the flexor digitorum superficialis muscle. All sites must be checked for possible anatomical anomalies and entrapment of the nerve. If intraoperative examination reveals a poor prognosis or multiple surgical procedures have failed, tendon transfers can most always be performed with excellent results and minimal loss of donor function.

Recurrent Compressive Neuropathies of the Ulnar Nerve

Recurrent Cubital Tunnel Syndrome

The second most common compressive neuropathy is cubital tunnel syndrome (CuTS). CuTS involves the ulnar nerve, which is derived from the medial cord of the brachial plexus and includes nerve roots C8 and T1. Normally, biomechanical forces and anatomical structures in the elbow region allow the ulnar nerve to glide within the cubital tunnel during flexion of the elbow. However, cumulative trauma and pathophysiologic changes can induce traction and compression injuries during prolonged flexion. Leaning on the elbow during phone use and sleeping with the elbow in flexion are common methods of irritation and eventual damage to the ulnar nerve. Other causes also include fractures of the elbow and obstructive masses. Entrapment of the ulnar nerve can occur at several levels of the elbow region (see Fig. 14.7). As the ulnar nerve courses posterior to the medial epicondyle,

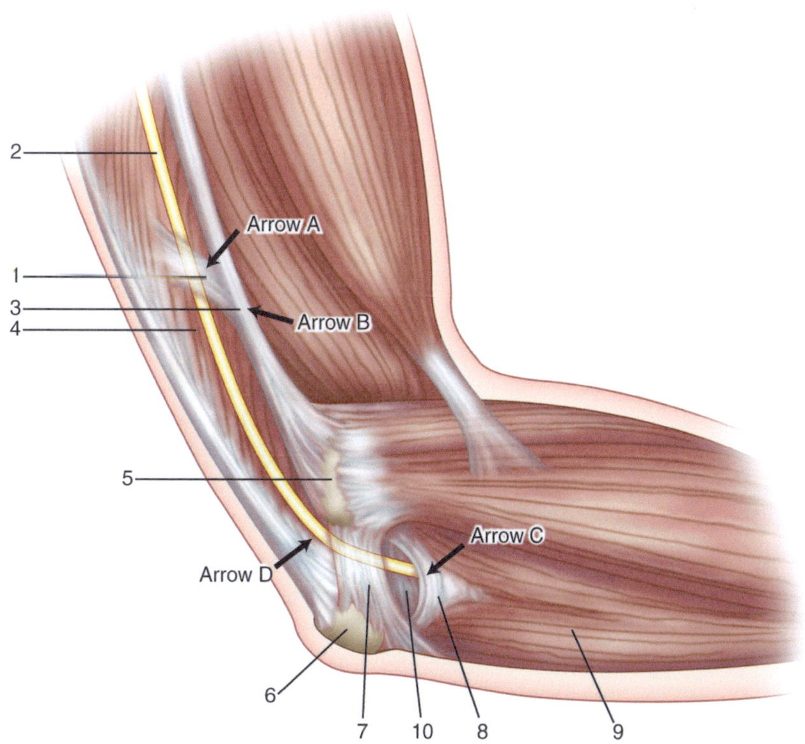

Fig. 14.7 Point of proximal compression in cubital tunnel syndrome. *1* Arcade of Struthers (*Arrow A*), *2* ulnar nerve, *3* medial intermuscular septum (*Arrow B*), *4* medial triceps head, *5* medial epicondyle, *6* Olecranon, *7* epitrochleoanconeus muscle, *8* arcade of the flexor carpi ulnaris (Osbourne's fascia) (*Arrow C*), *9* flexor carpi ulnaris muscle, *10* ulnar collateral ligament, *Arrow D*: the cubital tunnel

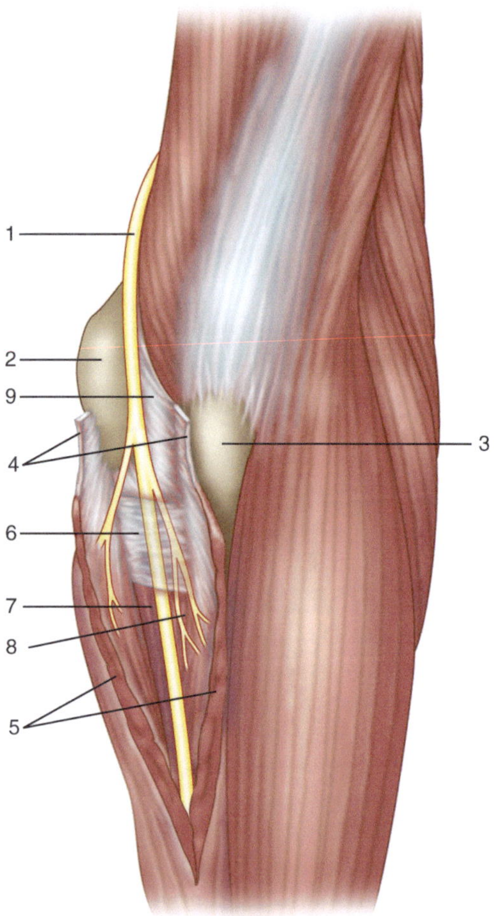

Fig. 14.8 Points of compression just distal to the cubital tunnel. *1* Ulnar nerve, *2* medial epicondyle of the humerus, *3* Olecranon, *4* arcade of the flexor carpi ulnaris, *5* flexor carpi ulnaris muscle, *6* deep flexor aponeurosis, *7* flexor digitorum superficialis muscle, *8* flexor digitorum profundus muscle, *9* ulnar collateral ligament

entrapment can occur within the fibro-osseus ulnar groove known as the cubital tunnel. The ulnar nerve can also become compressed proximal to the cubital tunnel as it courses posterior to the medial intermuscular septum and arcade of Struthers. Another common site of compression is found distal to the cubital tunnel as the nerve continues deep to the common flexor aponeurosis and between the two heads of the flexor carpi ulnaris (see Fig. 14.8). Patients with CuTS experience pain at the elbow with motor and sensory involvement. Common symptoms include including paresthesia, numbness, and weakness in the ulnar one and a half digits. Severe CuTS will present with claw hand and atrophy in the intrinsic and extrinsic muscles of the hand. The severity of symptoms is classified according to the McGowan scale: grade I—minimal lesions, with no detectable motor weakness of the hand, grade II—intermediate lesions, and grade III—severe lesions, with paralysis of one or more of the ulnar intrinsic muscles [58]. Nonoperative treatment options include activity modification, glucocorticoid injections, and neutral splinting of the elbow while sleeping. Indications for surgery include failure to respond to conservative treatments options, progressive decline in motor and sensory deficits, and progressive slowing of nerve conduction velocity.

Surgical treatment for CuTS ranges from simple decompression with external neurolysis to anterior transposition. In mild cases of CuTS, the operative strategy is simple decompression of the nerve and elimination of all points of constriction along the nerve. Traditionally, surgical exploration is performed with an open incision, but recently, studies have described the use of endoscopic methods [59–63]. If anatomic lesions impinge or interfere with the normal course of the ulnar nerve, tension of the ulnar nerve must be reduced with anterior transposition or removal of the offending structure, i.e. the medial epicondyle [64]. The surgical techniques frequently used in these procedures are subcutaneous transposition [65], submuscular transposition [66], intramuscular transposition [67], and medial epicondylectomy [68]. There is no consensus within the field as to which technique provides the best outcomes for primary CuTS. In a meta-analysis study, patient outcomes were evaluated according to the degree of clinical presentation and technique used in the primary procedure [69]. In patients with minimal CuTS, all methods of therapy provided comparable levels of satisfaction. For moderate cases, submuscular transposition was most effective in treating patients. In severe cases of CuTS, none of the techniques provided consistent results and medial epicondylectomy provided the poorest outcomes. Cubital tunnel surgery is the most frequently failed procedure for compressive neuropathies and recurrence rates have been reported to be as high as 58% [70]. However, studies have shown that successful outcomes in revision cubital tunnel surgery can be obtained.

Diagnosis for Recurrent Cubital Tunnel Syndrome

Accurate diagnosis of persistent or recurrent CuTS requires a thorough history and physical examination. Patients typically present with tenderness over the medial aspect of the elbow near the cubital tunnel. Subluxation of the ulnar nerve from the cubital tunnel is also common in symptomatic patients. Pain and paresthesia can be reproduced with the elbow flexion test and percussion over the cubital tunnel (Tinel's sign). Diminished sensory function such as two-point discrimination and vibration sensitivity will also present in the physical exam and should be measured preoperatively. If patients report sensory disturbances or pain at the site of the previous incision, the medial antebrachial cutaneous nerve should be examined in detail to locate a possible lesion. Damage acquired from previous surgery will result in a painful and sometimes palpable neuroma. Excising the neuroma and moving the nerve end to a different location can frequently solve this problem.

There are also several conditions that can mimic CuTS and must be ruled out as possible causes for the patient's symptoms and failed index operation. Cervical radiculopathies, such as thoracic outlet syndrome and cervical spondylosis, may involve the C8 and T1 nerve roots and cause patients to experience CuTS-like symptoms. But unlike true CuTS, the symptoms include sensory pain in dermatomal distributions, reduced blood flow in the upper extremity, and difficulties with overhead activities [71]. Physical examination involves Adson's maneuver, Wright test (hyperabduction of the arm), and Roos stress test. X-rays, MR imaging, electrodiagnostic examination, and blood circulation tests are also helpful in confirming cervical radiculopathies. Additionally, early signs of amyotrophic lateral sclerosis and Guyon's canal syndrome (GCS) present similarly to CuTS and require comprehensive evaluation if suspected.

Electrodiagnostic studies have been effective in confirming clinical findings of CuTS as well as ruling out compressive neuropathies at other locations. Electrodiagnostic studies will show a decrease in nerve conduction velocity over the elbow and are useful in determining how soon patients require operative treatment [72]. Like CTS, nerve conduction is not likely to regenerate quickly after primary procedures. MR imaging may also provide insight into the cause of recurrent symptoms and offer invaluable information in operative planning. MR imaging is sensitive for ulnar nerve dislocation, osteoarthritis, synovitis, muscle atrophy, and causative masses [73]. Alternatively, ultrasound modalities are capable of identifying focal nerve swelling and loss of fascicular patterning in CuTS [74]. Candidates for revision CuTS include those who are experiencing persistent or worsening symptoms after prior surgery, unresponsive to conservative treatment options, and a minimum of 6 months has passed since the previous surgical procedure [75].

Reoperative Options for Recurrent Cubital Tunnel Syndrome

The most difficult aspect of reoperative cubital tunnel surgery involves pathogenic changes that are induced by previously failed surgical procedures. Because of the diversity of techniques used to treat primary CuTS, surgeons must consider the previously used surgical technique, degree of symptom severity, and expectation of outcomes in candidates for reoperative treatment.

If simple decompression was used previously, intraoperative findings may include epineural scarring and fibrosis of the nerve. Measures such as external neurolysis must be performed to free the irritated nerve. The surgeon should also perform full surgical exploration at all common points of compression, which include the arcade of Struthers, medial intermuscular septum, and aponeurosis of the flexor-pronator mass. If there are no pathological changes leading to increased tension of the ulnar nerve, simple decompression may be sufficient. However, if intraoperative findings include compression and traction of the ulnar nerve, transposition of the nerve to a healthy, vascularized bed is indicated.

For previously failed cubital tunnel surgery our preferred approach is the submuscular transposition method (see Fig. 14.9). The submuscular technique described by Learmonth begins with a 6–8 cm incision made in line with the cubital tunnel [66]. The median antebrachial cutaneous nerve injury is at significant risk of injury and must be protected during surgical dissection. The ulnar nerve is identified proximally and freed from the brachial fascia and Osborne's fascia. The medial intermuscular septim is resected if not removed during the prior procedure. The flexor carpi ulnaris fascia and deep flexor-pronator aponeurosis are divided and the nerve is gently removed from its original bed. During transposition, the nerve must be moved into the new host bed with great care. The vascular supply of the nerve is particularly at risk during transposition as well as from external neurolysis. The first branch of the ulnar nerve to the flexor carpi ulnaris must also be protected and may require mobilization. As described by Dellon, Z-lengthening flaps are used when dividing the flexor-pronator fascia and the flaps are elevated while transposing the ulnar nerve anteriorly into the new host bed [76]. The flaps are sutured so the flexor-pronator musculotendinous origin is lengthened. Postoperatively, the elbow is splinted in 90° flexion for 2 weeks. Revision surgery utilizing the submuscular technique has been widely used with success in reoperative procedures. Gabel and Amadio used submuscular transposition to treat 30 patients with failed cubital tunnel surgery and obtained a satisfactory outcome in 22 patients. In a series of 10 patients, Broudy et al. showed improvements in all patients with the submuscular transposition following failed primary procedures [77]. In our experiences, we have found that the submuscular approach provides a better host bed and increased protection for the symptomatic nerve. Patients can expect to be relieved of pain and paresthesias, with limited return in motor function and sensory loss [78].

In patients previously receiving subcutaneous transposition, intraoperative findings may include dense fibrosis and facial bands of constriction at the previous site of surgery. A facial sling is frequently used to prevent subluxation of the nerve and often introduces as point of compression. During reoperation, the nerve should be freed of epineurial fibrosis through standard techniques and submuscular transposition is recommended for moving the nerve into a new host bed. Vogel et al. report that in 18 cases of failed anterior subcutaneous transposition, the most common operative findings were perineural

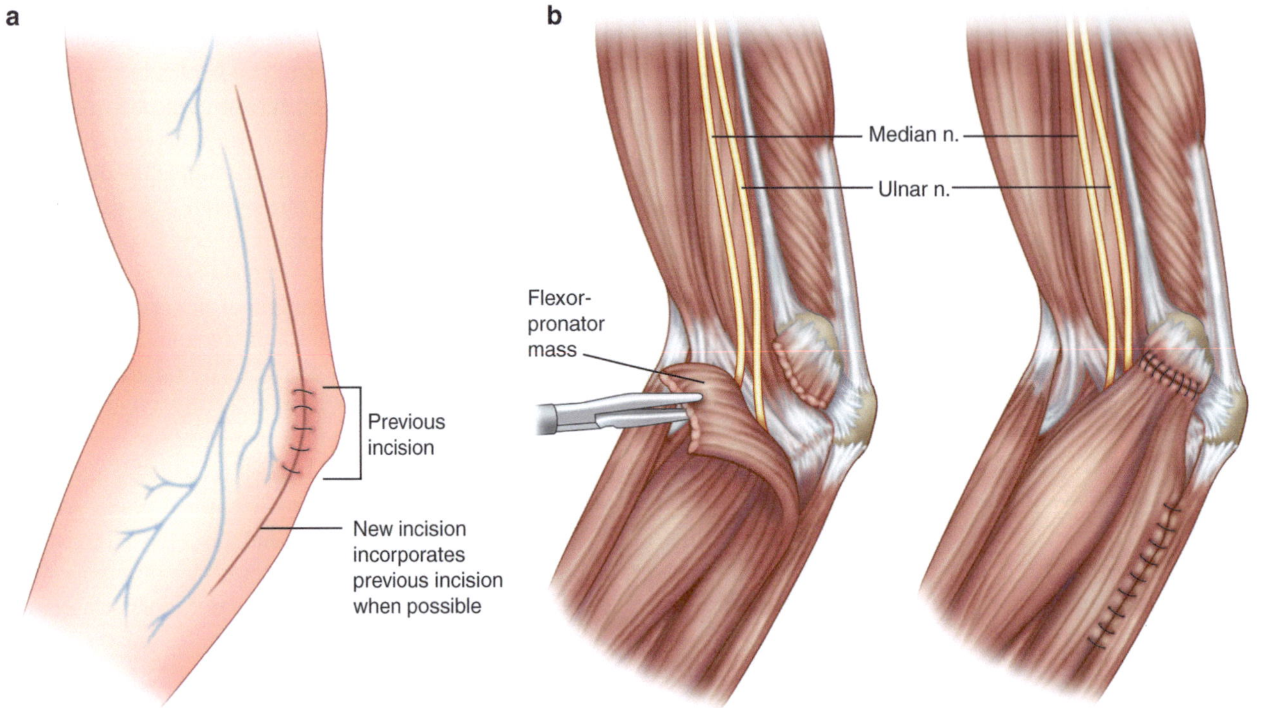

Fig. 14.9 Cubital tunnel revision surgery to a submuscular transposition (**a**) New incision includes previous incision site when possible. (**b**) Division of the flexor pronator mass and submuscular transposition of the ulnar nerve

scarring, retained medial intermuscular septum and common flexor aponeurosis [79]. Utilizing the submuscular transposition during the revision procedure, most patients were partially relieved of pain with a 78% satisfaction rate. In intramuscular transposition, the technique introduces an additional site of compression as the nerve courses within the muscle. Subsequent revision procedures involve addressing issues of fibrosis and moving the ulnar nerve submuscularly. Submuscular transposition may also fail in primary cubital tunnel surgery. This can occur from the nerve being secured too tightly to the new host bed. Reoperation should utilize lengthening of the flexor-pronator musculotedinous origin to remove the causative compression from the submuscular transposition.

Guyon's Canal Syndrome

GCS refers to the distal entrapment of the ulnar nerve at the wrist (see Fig. 14.10). Guyon's canal is formed by the pisiform bone medially, the hook of the hamate laterally, the flexor carpi ulnaris tendinous insertion along with the anterior carpal ligament anteriorly, and the TCL posteriorly. Within or distal to the canal, the nerve bifurcates into a superficial sensory branch and the deep motor branch. The superficial branch supplies sensory innervation to the ulnar one and one half digits. The deep motor branch provides innervation to the hypothenar muscles, interosseous muscles, third and fourth lumbricals, adductor pollicis (AP), and flexor pol-

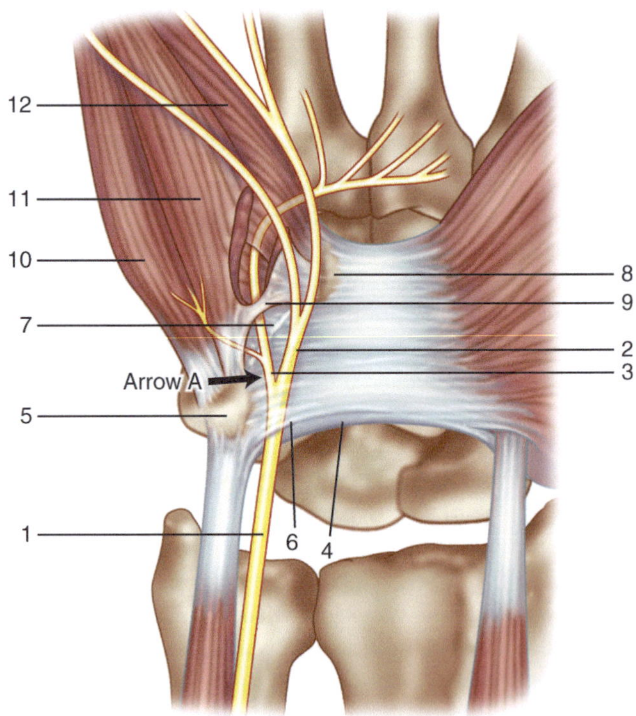

Fig. 14.10 Points of possible constriction in ulnar tunnel syndrome. *1* Ulnar nerve, *2* superficial branch, *3* deep branch, *4* transverse carpal ligament, *5* pisiform, *6* palmar carpal ligament, *7* pisohamate ligament, *8* hook of the hamate, *9* fibrotendinous arcade of the abductor digiti minimi and the flexor digiti minimi brevis, *10* abductor digiti muscle, *11* flexor digiti brevis muscle, *12* opponens digiti minimi muscle. *Arrow A*: compression of the deep branch of the ulnar nerve

licis brevis. The symptoms experienced by patients with GCS can result from sensory, motor, or mixed deficits depending on where the site of compression is located. The most common causes of GCS are due to ganglion cyst compression and chronic compressive trauma.

Diagnosis for Guyon's Canal Syndrome

As mentioned previously, the diagnosis for GCS is often missed because the condition sometimes mimics CuTS. However, a careful history and physical exam, including electrodiagnostic studies at the wrist will be able to reveal GCS [80]. In patients with suspected GCS confirmed by electrodiagnostic studies, we recommend using MR imaging to further identify the cause of compression to aid in operative planning. If the patient experiences recurrent GCS after other compressive neuropathies have been ruled out and conservative therapy has failed, revision surgery is indicated.

Reoperative Options for Guyon's Canal Syndrome

In reoperation procedures for GCS, the incision should allow full visualization of the canal. All obstructive masses must be identified and completely removed. Surgical exploration should be utilized to ensure that the ulnar nerve is free of constriction at all points including the deep motor branch.

Recurrent Compressive Neuropathies of the Radial Nerve

Radial Tunnel Syndrome

Compressive neuropathy of the radial nerve in the proximal forearm is known as radial tunnel syndrome (RTS). The radial nerve is derived from the posterior cord of the brachial plexus and includes nerve roots C5 through C8 and T1. The radial nerve enters the forearm and courses within the radial tunnel formed by the supinator, extensor carpi radialis longus and brevis, and the brachioradialis muscles. Proximal to the radial tunnel, the radial nerve divides into the purely sensory superficial branch of the radial nerve and the motor deep branch of the radial nerve. Therefore, classic RTS is absent of sensory deficits. The most common site of compression is found as the deep branch of the radial nerve pierces the supinator at the arcarde of Frohse (see Fig. 14.11). As the nerve continues distally, it is referred to as the posterior interosseous nerve and can become compressed by several structures. These include the distal border of the supinator muscle, the radial recurrent artery, and fibrous bands distal to the radial head [81]. Biomechanically, passive supination

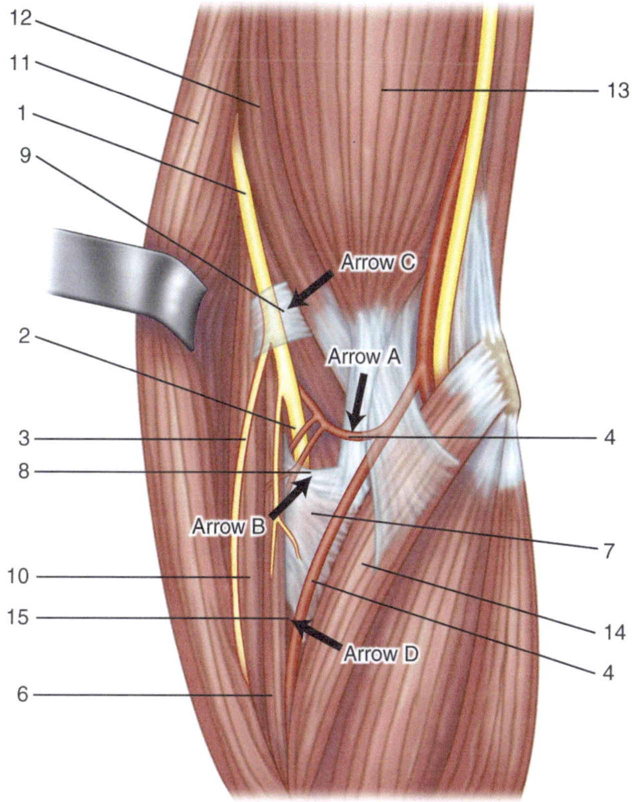

Fig. 14.11 Radial tunnel syndrome site of compression. *1* Radial nerve, *2* deep branch of the radial nerve, *3* superficial radial nerve, *4* radial artery, *5* recurrent radial artery (*Arrow A*), *6* extensor carpi radialis brevis muscle, *7* supinator muscle, *8* arcade of Frohse (*Arrow B*), *9* transverse fibrous band (*Arrow C*), *10* extensor carpi radialis longus muscle, *11* brachioradialis muscle, *12* brachialis muscle, *13* biceps muscle, *14* pronator teres muscle, *15* distal edge of supinator muscle. *Arrow D*: distal border of the supinator

elicits elongation and rotational stress on the posterior interosseous nerve, while passive pronation induces compressive forces [82]. Patients with RTS experience pain and weakness in extensor muscles of the forearm. Also, symptoms are often associated with activities involving repetitive pronation–supination of the forearm. In severe cases, patients may present with wrist drop. Typically, patients are free of sensory deficits because the sensory branch of the radial nerve comes off the radial nerve proximal to the radial tunnel.

Diagnosis for Recurrent Radial Tunnel Syndrome

Patients with secondary RTS present similarly to primary cases. Many patients will experience weakness at the metacarpophalangeal joints of the hand. In severe cases, the hand will radially deviate when the wrist is dorsiflexed and the metacarpophalangeal joints of the hand will not be able to fully extend. Lateral epicondylitis (tennis elbow) can also present similarly to RTS and must be differentiated in all cases. Patients with lateral epicondylitis will present with pain localized to the attachment of the extensor carpi radialis to the lateral epicondyle. Patients with RTS present with an area of tenderness more distally over the supinator muscle in addition to pain and weakness in the extensor muscles of the forearm. Electrodiagnostic studies may detect decreased nerve conduction velocity at the site of compression but are often normal. Nonoperative treatment options should be exhausted before considering reoperation. A strong clinical suspicion based on several physical examinations is required to make this diagnosis.

Reoperative Options for Recurrent Radial Tunnel Syndrome

Persistent cases of recurrent RTS are commonly caused by incomplete decompression during primary procedures. Reoperation typically involves thorough surgical reexploration of the radial nerve, which can be performed by a variety of methods. The anterior (Henry) and posterior (Thompson) approaches are the most commonly used in primary procedures. For reoperation, we prefer a modified anterior approach, which allows for proximal exploration of the radial nerve as well as distal exploration of the posterior interosseous nerve. In patients presenting with signs of proximal compression of the radial nerve, such as wrist drop and mixed sensory and motor deficits, the radial nerve should be explored proximally at the lateral intermuscular septum and lateral head of the triceps [83]. With the patient in the supine or lateral decubitus position, an incision is made between the deltoid and the lateral head of the triceps. The incision is continued between the lateral head of the triceps and the biceps and obliquely crosses the lateral intermuscular septum 10 cm proximal to the lateral epicondyle. If proximal radial nerve compression has been ruled out, the modified anterior approach should be used as follows. The incision begins between the brachioradialis and the biceps and courses distally as it crosses the elbow flexion crease obliquely. The incision is continued along the medial border of the brachioradialis. The lateral antebrachial cutaneous nerve and cephalic vein are protected and the radial nerve is identified between the brachioradialis and brachialis. The radial nerve is followed proximally and distally as decompression is performed at possible sites of constriction. The common points of compression of the posterior interosseous nerve distal to the supinator must be fully explored. Revision procedures may also involve epineurial fibrosis and scarring of the nerve and require treatment by external neurolysis. Postoperative rehabilitation involves immobilization of the elbow in flexion for 3–4 weeks. Therapy and splinting of the wrist and fingers should be continued in the postoperative period [84].

Conclusion

Surgical options for recurrent compression neuropathies of the upper extremity can be quite challenging. Nerve surgery is always fraught with hazard. The surgeon first needs to make sure that the initial diagnosis was correct. This is then followed by evaluating the patient for true recurrence vs. failure to improve. Diagnostic injections may be helpful. There is a role for imaging studies as well as repeat electrical studies. However, ultimately, the decision comes down to what the patient is willing to accept in these sometimes high-risk surgeries. The patient and surgeon need to understand that despite repeat surgery, there may not be any clinical benefit to the patient, short-term or long-term. However, in many cases, this can improve the patient's symptoms and provide them with some relief of their symptomatology.

References

1. AAOS. Carpal Tunnel Syndrome. American Academy of Orthopaedic Surgeons Website. http://orthoinfo.aaos.org/topic.cfm?topic=a00005. Accessed 16 July 2009.
2. Botte MJ, et al. Recurrent carpal tunnel syndrome. Hand Clin. 1996;12(4):731–43.
3. Gupta R, Steward O. Chronic nerve compression induces concurrent apoptosis and proliferation of Schwann cells. J Comp Neurol. 2003;461(2):174–86.
4. Gupta R, et al. Local down-regulation of myelin-associated glycoprotein permits axonal sprouting with chronic nerve compression injury. Exp Neurol. 2006;200(2):418–29.
5. Gray M, et al. Macrophage depletion alters the blood-nerve barrier without affecting Schwann cell function after neural injury. J Neurosci Res. 2007;85(4):766–77.
6. Ludwin SK, Maitland M. Long-term remyelination fails to reconstitute normal thickness of central myelin sheaths. J Neurol Sci. 1984;64(2):193–8.
7. Gupta R, et al. Shear stress alters the expression of myelin-associated glycoprotein (MAG) and myelin basic protein (MBP) in Schwann cells. J Orthop Res. 2005;23(5):1232–9.
8. Tung TH, Mackinnon SE. Secondary carpal tunnel surgery. Plast Reconstr Surg. 2001;107(7):1830–43; quiz 1844, 1933.
9. Upton AR, McComas AJ. The double crush in nerve entrapment syndromes. Lancet. 1973;2(7825):359–62.
10. Flak M, et al. Double crush syndrome evaluation in the median nerve in clinical, radiological and electrophysiological examination. Stud Health Technol Inform. 2006;123:435–41.
11. Paget J. The first description of carpal tunnel syndrome. J Hand Surg Eur Vol. 2007;32(2):195–7.
12. Palmer DH, Hanrahan LP. Social and economic costs of carpal tunnel surgery. Instr Course Lect. 1995;44:167–72.
13. Gelberman RH, et al. The carpal tunnel syndrome. A study of carpal canal pressures. J Bone Joint Surg Am. 1981;63(3):380–3.
14. Brain W, Wright A, Wilkerson M. Spontaneous compression of both median nerves in carpal tunnel. Six cases treated surgically. Lancet. 1947;1:277–82.
15. Agee JM, et al. Endoscopic release of the carpal tunnel: a randomized prospective multicenter study. J Hand Surg Am. 1992;17(6): 987–95.

16. Chow JC. Endoscopic release of the carpal ligament: a new technique for carpal tunnel syndrome. Arthroscopy. 1989;5(1):19–24.
17. Varitimidis SE, Herndon JH, Sotereanos DG. Failed endoscopic carpal tunnel release. Operative findings and results of open revision surgery. J Hand Surg Br. 1999;24(4):465–7.
18. Urbaniak JR, Desai SS. Complications of nonoperative and operative treatment of carpal tunnel syndrome. Hand Clin. 1996;12(2):325–35.
19. MacDonald RI, et al. Complications of surgical release for carpal tunnel syndrome. J Hand Surg Am. 1978;3(1):70–6.
20. O'Malley MJ, et al. Factors that determine reexploration treatment of carpal tunnel syndrome. J Hand Surg Am. 1992;17(4):638–41.
21. Stutz N, et al. Revision surgery after carpal tunnel release—analysis of the pathology in 200 cases during a 2 year period. J Hand Surg Br. 2006;31(1):68–71.
22. Schreiber JE, et al. Common risk factors seen in secondary carpal tunnel surgery. Ann Plast Surg. 2005;55(3):262–5.
23. Stevens JC, et al. Conditions associated with carpal tunnel syndrome. Mayo Clin Proc. 1992;67(6):541–8.
24. Shurr DG, Blair WF, Bassett G. Electromyographic changes after carpal tunnel release. J Hand Surg Am. 1986;11(6):876–80.
25. Jarvik JG, Yuen E, Kliot M. Diagnosis of carpal tunnel syndrome: electrodiagnostic and MR imaging evaluation. Neuroimaging Clin N Am. 2004;14(1):93–102, viii.
26. Mesgarzadeh M, Triolo J, Schneck CD. Carpal tunnel syndrome. MR imaging diagnosis. Magn Reson Imaging Clin N Am. 1995;3(2):249–64.
27. Koenig RW, et al. High-resolution ultrasonography in evaluating peripheral nerve entrapment and trauma. Neurosurg Focus. 2009;26(2):E13.
28. Spratt JD, et al. The role of diagnostic radiology in compressive and entrapment neuropathies. Eur Radiol. 2002;12(9):2352–64.
29. Brahme SK, et al. Dynamic MR imaging of carpal tunnel syndrome. Skeletal Radiol. 1997;26(8):482–7.
30. Silbermann-Hoffman O, et al. Contribution of magnetic resonance imaging for the diagnosis of median nerve lesion after endoscopic carpal tunnel release. Chir Main. 1998;17(4):291–9.
31. Wong SM, et al. Discriminatory sonographic criteria for the diagnosis of carpal tunnel syndrome. Arthritis Rheum. 2002;46(7).1914–21.
32. Hunter JM. Recurrent carpal tunnel syndrome, epineural fibrous fixation, and traction neuropathy. Hand Clin. 1991;7(3):491–504.
33. Amadio PC. Interventions for recurrent/persistent carpal tunnel syndrome after carpal tunnel release. J Hand Surg Am. 2009;34(7):1320–2.
34. Ellis RA, et al. Workers' compensation, return to work, and patient satisfaction after carpal tunnel decompression. Am J Orthop. 2007;36(4):E63–6.
35. Chaise F, et al. Return-to-work interval and surgery for carpal tunnel syndrome. Results of a prospective series of 233 patients. J Hand Surg Br. 2004;29(6):568–70.
36. Cobb TK, et al. Outcome of reoperation for carpal tunnel syndrome. J Hand Surg Am. 1996;21(3):347–56.
37. Mackinnon SE, et al. Internal neurolysis fails to improve the results of primary carpal tunnel decompression. J Hand Surg Am. 1991;16(2):211–8.
38. Steyers CM. Recurrent carpal tunnel syndrome. Hand Clin. 2002;18(2):339–45.
39. Rhoades CE, Mowery CA, Gelberman RH. Results of internal neurolysis of the median nerve for severe carpal-tunnel syndrome. J Bone Joint Surg Am. 1985;67(2):253–6.
40. Pizzillo MF, Sotereanos DG, Tomaino MM. Recurrent carpal tunnel syndrome: treatment options. J South Orthop Assoc. 1999;8(1):28–36.
41. Varitimidis SE, et al. Treatment of recurrent compressive neuropathy of peripheral nerves in the upper extremity with an autologous vein insulator. J Hand Surg Am. 2001;26(2):296–302.
42. Wulle C. The synovial flap as treatment of the recurrent carpal tunnel syndrome. Hand Clin. 1996;12(2):379–88.
43. Strickland JW, et al. The hypothenar fat pad flap for management of recalcitrant carpal tunnel syndrome. J Hand Surg Am. 1996;21(5):840–8.
44. Stutz NM, et al. Clinical and electrophysiological comparison of different methods of soft tissue coverage of the median nerve in recurrent carpal tunnel syndrome. Neurosurgery. 2008;62(3 Suppl 1):194–9; discussion 199–200.
45. Fusetti C, et al. A reliable and simple solution for recalcitrant carpal tunnel syndrome: the hypothenar fat pad flap. Am J Orthop. 2009;38(4):181–6.
46. Mathoulin C, Bahm J, Roukoz S. Pedicled hypothenar fat flap for median nerve coverage in recalcitrant carpal tunnel syndrome. Hand Surg. 2000;5(1):33–40.
47. Spokevicius S, Kleinert HE. The abductor digiti minimi flap: its use in revision carpal tunnel surgery. Hand Clin. 1996;12(2):351–5.
48. Pomerance J, Fine I. Outcomes of carpal tunnel surgery with and without supervised postoperative therapy. J Hand Surg Am. 2007;32(8):1159–63; discussion 1164–5.
49. Chang B, Dellon AL. Surgical management of recurrent carpal tunnel syndrome. J Hand Surg Br. 1993;18(4):467–70.
50. Hulsizer DL, et al. The results of revision carpal tunnel release following previous open versus endoscopic surgery. J Hand Surg Am. 1998;23(5):865–9.
51. Unglaub F, et al. Subjective and functional outcome after revision surgery in carpal tunnel syndrome. Arch Orthop Trauma Surg. 2008;128(9):931–6.
52. Hartz CR, et al. The pronator teres syndrome: compressive neuropathy of the median nerve. J Bone Joint Surg Am. 1981;63(6):885–90.
53. Bilecenoglu B, Uz A, Karalezli N. Possible anatomic structures causing entrapment neuropathies of the median nerve: an anatomic study. Acta Orthop Belg. 2005;71(2):169–76.
54. Kiloh LG, Nevin S. Isolated neuritis of the anterior interosseous nerve. Br Med J. 1952;1(4763):850–1.
55. Kaplan EB, Spinner M. The anterior interosseous nerve syndrome. J Bone Joint Surg. 1969;51A:1677.
56. Dunn AJ, Salonen DC, Anastakis DJ. MR imaging findings of anterior interosseous nerve lesions. Skeletal Radiol. 2007;36(12):1155–62.
57. Mackinnon SE. Compressive neuropathies. In: Green D, editor. Green's operative hand surgery. 5th ed. New York: Churchill Livingstone; 2005.
58. McGowan A. The results of transposition of the ulnar nerve for traumatic ulnar neuritis. J Bone Joint Surg Br. 1950;32-B(3):293–301.
59. Ahcan U, Zorman P. Endoscopic decompression of the ulnar nerve at the elbow. J Hand Surg Am. 2007;32(8):1171–6.
60. Hoffmann R, Meek MF. Endoscopic decompression of the ulnar nerve at the elbow. J Hand Surg Am. 2008;33(4):615; author reply 615–6.
61. Kasdan ML. Endoscopic cubital tunnel release. J Hand Surg Am. 1999;24(3):647.
62. Merolla G, et al. Endoscopic approach to cubital tunnel syndrome. J Neurosurg Sci. 2008;52(3):93–8.
63. Yoshida A, Okutsu I, Hamanaka I. Endoscopic anatomical nerve observation and minimally invasive management of cubital tunnel syndrome. J Hand Surg Eur Vol. 2009;34(1):115–20.
64. Osterman AL, Davis CA. Subcutaneous transposition of the ulnar nerve for treatment of cubital tunnel syndrome. Hand Clin. 1996;12(2):421–33.

65. Curtis B. Traumatic ulnar neuritis: transposition of the nerve. J Nerv Ment Dis. 1898;25:480–4.
66. Learmonth J. A technique for transplanting the ulnar nerve. Surg Gynecol Obstet. 1942;75:792–3.
67. Adson A. The surgical treatment of progressive ulnar paralysis. Minn Med. 1918;1:455–60.
68. King T, Morgan F. Late results of removing the medial humeral epicondyle for traumatic ulnar neuritis. J Bone Joint Surg Br. 1959;41:51–5.
69. Mowlavi A, et al. The management of cubital tunnel syndrome: a meta-analysis of clinical studies. Plast Reconstr Surg. 2000;106(2): 327–34.
70. Dellon AL. Review of treatment results for ulnar nerve entrapment at the elbow. J Hand Surg Am. 1989;14(4):688–700.
71. AAOS. Thoracic Outlet Syndrome. American Academy of Orthopaedic Surgeons Website. http://orthoinfo.aaos.org/topic.cfm?topic=a00336. Accessed 25 Aug 2009.
72. Wein TH, Albers JW. Electrodiagnostic approach to the patient with suspected peripheral polyneuropathy. Neurol Clin. 2002;20(2):503–26, vii.
73. Andreisek G, et al. Peripheral neuropathies of the median, radial, and ulnar nerves: MR imaging features. Radiographics. 2006;26(5): 1267–87.
74. Martinoli C, et al. US of nerve entrapments in osteofibrous tunnels of the upper and lower limbs. Radiographics. 2000;20(Spec No):S199–213; discussion S213–7.
75. Lowe III JB, Mackinnon SE. Management of secondary cubital tunnel syndrome. Plast Reconstr Surg. 2004;113(1):E1–16.
76. Dellon AL. Techniques for successful management of ulnar nerve entrapment at the elbow. Neurosurg Clin N Am. 1991;2(1):57–73.
77. Broudy AS, Leffert RD, Smith RJ. Technical problems with ulnar nerve transposition at the elbow: findings and results of reoperation. J Hand Surg Am. 1978;3(1):85–9.
78. Rogers MR, Bergfield TG, Aulicino PL. The failed ulnar nerve transposition. Etiology and treatment. Clin Orthop Relat Res. 1991; 269:193–200.
79. Vogel RB, Nossaman BC, Rayan GM. Revision anterior submuscular transposition of the ulnar nerve for failed subcutaneous transposition. Br J Plast Surg. 2004;57(4):311–6.
80. Pearce C, Feinberg J, Wolfe SW. Ulnar neuropathy at the wrist. HSS J. 2009;5(2):180–3.
81. Lister GD, Belsole RB, Kleinert HE. The radial tunnel syndrome. J Hand Surg Am. 1979;4(1):52–9.
82. Portilla MAE, et al. The posterior interosseous nerve and the radial tunnel syndrome: an anatomical study. Int Orthop. 1998;22(2): 102–6.
83. Manske PR. Compression of the radial nerve by the triceps muscle: a case report. J Bone Joint Surg Am. 1977;59(6):835–6.
84. Payatakes A, Sotereanos DG. Radial Nerve Injuries. In: Slutsky D, editor. Upper extremity nerve repair—tips and techniques: a master skills publication. Rosemont: American Society for Surgery of the Hand; 2008. p. 399–412.

Secondary Procedures for Failed Tendon Transfers

15

Jennifer Moriatis Wolf

Abstract

Fortunately, in many cases tendon transfers work as planned. However, there can be instances where the initial tendon transfer fails for various reasons. In these cases, the surgeon may be faced with a limited number of options as far as other potential tendon transfers, given the lack of donor tendons already utilized in the previous procedures. Some creative thinking and understanding of the various anatomical considerations will reveal some possibilities. These include harvesting other muscle tendon donor units, soft tissue tensioning procedures as well as joint fusion. These techniques can be considered individually or in combination to help increase the patient's functional abilities of the extremity. These are challenging cases that frequently force the patient and surgeon to engage in some compromises in order to maximize the potential function and this should be explained to the patient in advance. However, in many cases the patients are able to reengage the extremity in a functional fashion. This chapter looks at those options and these challenging reoperative situations.

Keywords

Failed • Tendon • Transfers • Flexor • Extensor • Fusion

Key Points

- In failed tendon transfers, a guiding principle is to look for other sources to power what is missing, without impacting current function.
- Tendon transfers should be done with supple joints.
- The options of carpectomy (to functionally "lengthen" tendons) and arthrodesis (to place the joint in an optimized position for function) should be considered in revision tendon transfers.

J.M. Wolf, MD (✉)
Department of Orthopaedic Surgery, University of Connecticut Health Center, New England Musculoskeletal Institute, 263 Farmington Avenue, Farmington, CT 06030, USA
e-mail: jmwhand@hotmail.com

Introduction

Tendon transfers are utilized in the treatment of nerve palsy or injury, and in the rheumatoid hand or wrist. The use of tendon transfers for spasticity or central nervous system disorders secondary to stroke, cerebral palsy, or spinal cord injury is based on a different set of transfer principles, although some of the salvage procedures are similar. When tendon transfers fail due to rupture, elongation, or scarring, options include the substitution of other muscle-tendon units or joint fusion to place the extremity in an optimized position for function. This chapter evaluates the options for revision of tendon transfers and/or arthrodeses in radial, ulnar, and median nerve palsy as well as in rheumatoid arthritis, and presents some reconstructive strategies for difficult problems. While revision transfers for spasticity are not specifically addressed, many of the salvage procedures overlap.

S.F.M. Duncan (ed.), *Reoperative Hand Surgery*,
DOI 10.1007/978-1-4614-2373-7_15, © Springer Science+Business Media, LLC 2012

Failed Transfers in Radial Nerve Palsy

Introduction

The most commonly used tendon transfer set for radial nerve palsy is the pronator teres (PT) to the extensor carpi radialis brevis (ECRB), the flexor carpi radialis (FCR) to the extensor digitorum communis (EDC), and the palmaris longus to the rerouted extensor pollicis longus (EPL) [1, 2]. If this transfer fails, the options for revision include use of the flexor digitorum superficialis (FDS) tendons of the middle and ring fingers [3].

Chuinard et al. described the FDS transfers as an alternative to the use of the flexor carpi ulnaris tendon for transfer to the wrist and finger extensors, both to provide tendons with greater excursion than the FCU and to avoid sacrifice of its strong wrist flexion action [3]. The middle finger FDS can be transferred to the EDC to replace the FCR action, and the ring finger FDS is used to power the extensor indicis proprius (EIP) and EPL. Transfer of the FDS tendons can be used only in the presence of working flexor digitorum profundus (FDP) tendons to those digits.

Indications for superficialis transfers

- Failed FCR and/or palmaris transfers for finger and thumb extension.
- Intact and functional FDP for transfer.

Contraindications

- Median or ulnar nerve injury.
- Contracture of digits.

Operative Approach: Superficialis Transfers (Figs. 15.1 and 15.2)

– The ring and small finger FDS tendons are approached through separate transverse incisions at the bases of the respective fingers.
– Identify each FDS tendon proximal to the chiasm where it divides and cut each sharply.

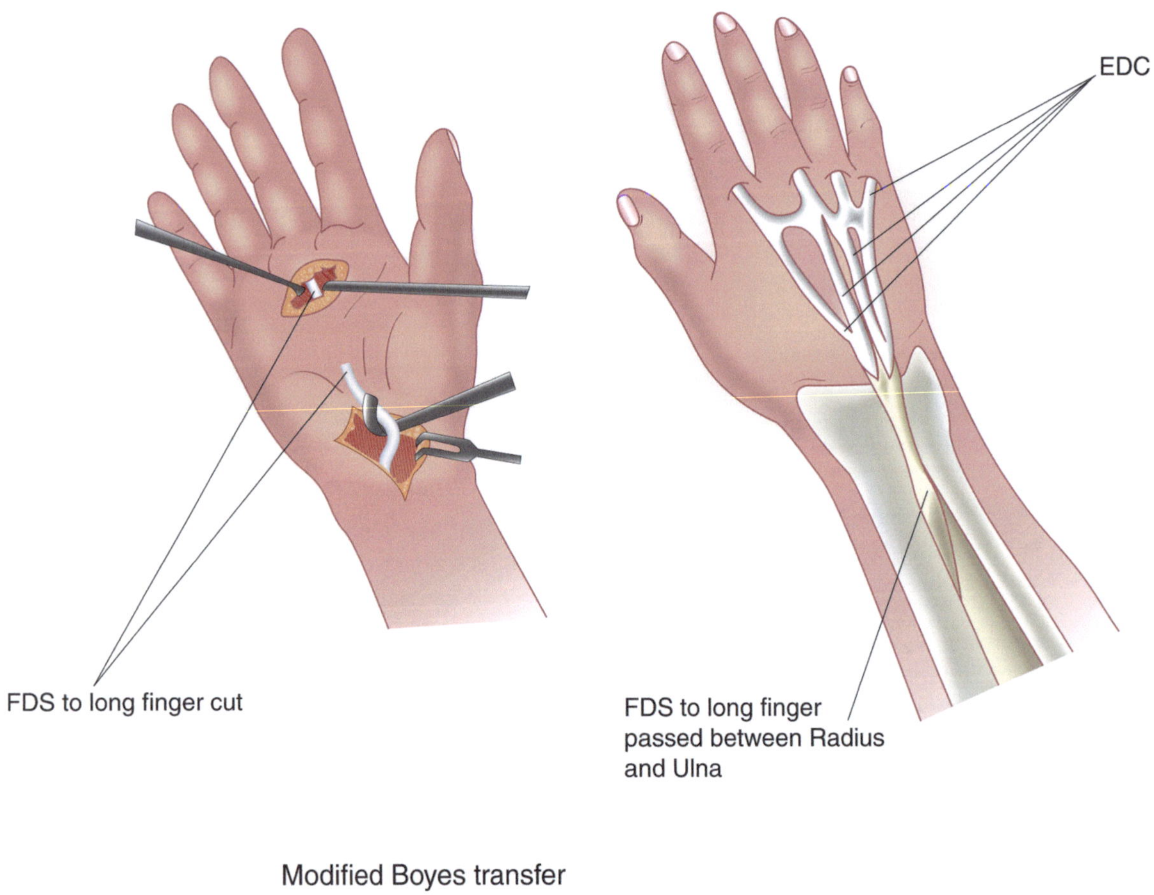

Fig. 15.1 The flexor digitorum superficialis (FDS) from the ring finger (FDS IV) is transferred through the interosseous membrane to the extensor digitorum communis (EDC) and minimi (EDM)

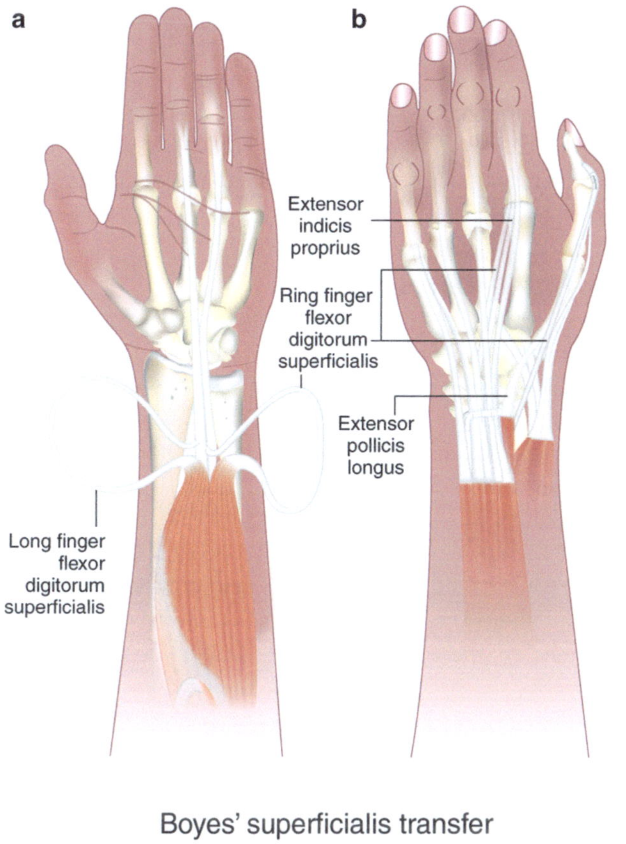

Fig. 15.2 The FDS from the long finger (FDS III) is split and woven into the EPL and EIP

– In the situation of a failed tendon transfer the original forearm incision should be used, generally in the distal third of the forearm. After reopening this incision, the interosseous membrane is identified proximal to the pronator quadratus, taking care to gently retract the median nerve and flexor tendons.
– Identify the anterior interosseous artery and open the membrane on either side of it, careful to preserve the artery. The tendons will be passed through these openings. To prevent adhesions, be sure to open the membrane for at least 1 cm length or more. Alternatively, the tendons can be passed around each side of the forearm, but this risks compression of the ulnar neurovascular bundle and is in a less direct line of pull.
– The dorsal wrist incision (presumably the original incision used) is then opened. The EDC, EIP, and EPL tendons are identified and cleared of scar or adhesions as necessary. Each tendon end should be freshened in preparation for transfer. At this time, tenolysis should be performed if needed.
– Pass the FDS III tendon on the radial side of the profundus tendons, through the radial-sided opening in the interosseous membrane, and the FDS IV tendon through the ulnar side.
– Using 2-0 or 3-0 braided, nonresorbable suture, the tendons are sutured: the FDS III split and woven (using a Pulvertaft weave) [4] into the tendon ends of the EPL and EIP; and the FDS IV woven into the EDC. This can be done by passing the tendon through a slit in the bases of all four tendons and suturing the entire group together, or by preliminarily suturing the EDC tendons transversely to form one tendon end for a weave.
– Tension is set during tendon suture by having an assistant hold the thumb and fingers into a fist and the wrist held in 20–30° of extension. The FDS tendons should be pulled tightly during suturing to increase the tension.

Wrist Extensor Addition

Indications: flexor carpi ulnaris transfer for wrist extension

- If the failed transfer involves the wrist extensors as well (in radial nerve palsy, not posterior interosseous nerve palsy where the wrist extensors are spared due to their proximal innervation).
- FCR *or* the FCU has not been previously sacrificed, but the pronator teres (PT) has already been used, one of the wrist flexors can be transferred to the ECRB tendon as an extensor.

Contraindications

- Previous use of the FCR—it is necessary to leave the patient with one wrist flexor.

Operative Technique (Figs. 15.3 and 15.4)

– The FCU is identified in the distal forearm incision, which is extended to the wrist crease. It is transected just proximal to the pisiform, taking care to protect the ulnar neurovascular bundle beneath it. If the FCR is to be used, the tendon is identified on the radial side of the forearm and freed from its sheath as distally as possible, taking care not to injure the superficial branch of the radial artery.
– If using the FCU for transfer, the muscle belly is debulked generously after opening the fascia to free it up. The FCR, being fairly tendinous in the distal forearm, needs less, if any, debulking. These tendons are usually used for transfer to the EDC tendon and preparation is similar.

- Next, an incision is made over the dorsal forearm, 2 cm distal to the medial epicondyle, and the FCU tendon identified. The overlying fascia is opened and the muscle belly freed in preparation for transfer. Care is taken to avoid deep proximal dissection around the FCU in order to avoid the innervating branches of the ulnar nerve.
- The dorsal wrist is then opened through the (previous) dorsal longitudinal incision and the ECRB identified ulnar to the ECRL. If a previous surgical scar exists, this is excised and tenolysis performed as necessary. The tendon end should be freshened.
- If using the FCU tendon, a large Kelly clamp or tendon passer is passed subcutaneously around the ulnar border of the forearm, taking care to pass *proximal* to the wrist in order to optimize the line of pull for wrist extension. If using the FCR tendon, it is passed, similarly subcutaneously, around the radial border of the forearm. In both instances, tendon passage is performed with gentle pressure to avoid injury to subcutaneous nerves.
- The tension for transfer is set using maximal tension on the donor tendon and the wrist held in 45° of extension, with the tendons optimally secured using a Pulvertaft weave and nonresorbable 2-0 or 3-0 braided suture.

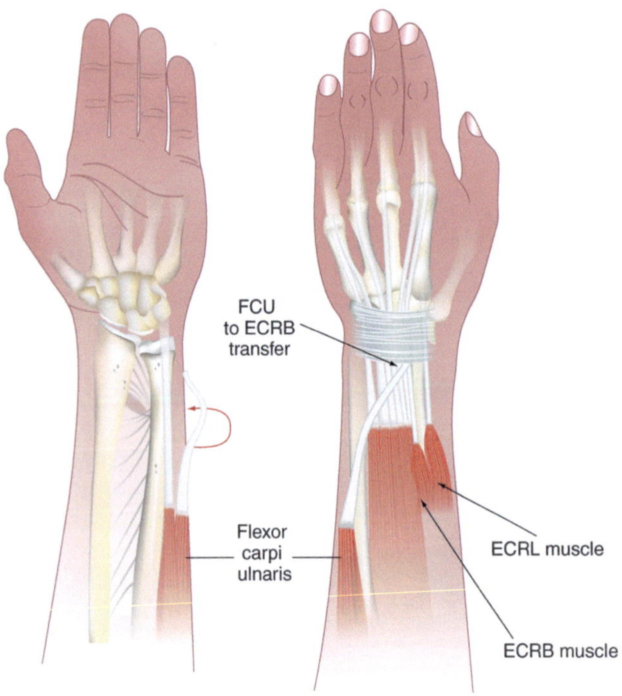

Fig. 15.3 The FCU is routed and woven into the ECRB to restore wrist extension

Optimizing Outcomes

- Perform revision of tendon transfers only after the soft tissues have settled—i.e., there are minimal signs of inflammation.
- Always err on setting the tension of the transfer too tight rather than too loose; tendons frequently stretch out or loosen.
- Use therapy as needed to mobilize the patient and prepare the patient for prolonged rehabilitation, since the situation of previous surgery increases the likelihood of scarring.

Complications and Side Effects

One of the most commonly noted complications of the use of the FCU tendon is radial deviation of the wrist. In a patient with posterior interosseous nerve palsy, use of the FCU is to be avoided because of the strong existing radial wrist extensors and FCR tendon pulling the wrist into radial deviation. If it is absolutely necessary to use the FCU in this situation, the wrist extensor insertion should be transferred ulnarly as suggested by Brand, by reinserting it into the base of the fourth metacarpal [1].

As noted previously, if the tension of transfers is set too loose, the tendons will not work effectively. It is best to set the tension tightly and test the wrist and fingers with tenodesis testing prior to accepting the transfer as final. If, however, excessive loosening occurs, the best solution is to rehabilitate the patient to keep the tendons and joints supple and revise the transfer tension at a later time. Extended splinting or immobilization will not shorten the tendon units and should be discouraged.

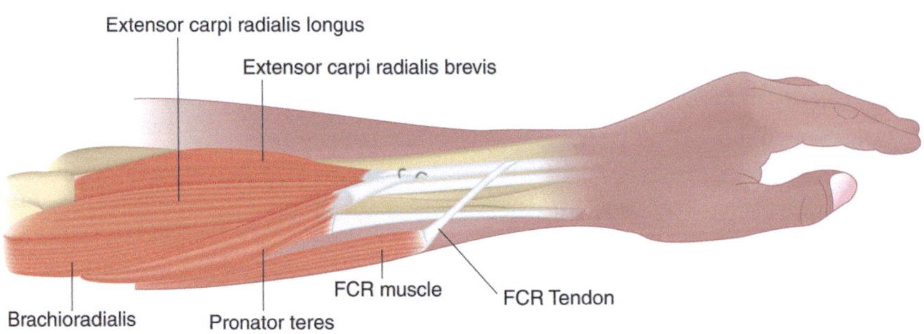

Fig. 15.4 Alternatively the FCR tendon transferred to the ECRB can be used to restore wrist extension

Postoperative Care

After tourniquet deflation, hemostasis, and suture closure, the wrist and fingers are immobilized in a soft dressing and long-arm splint with the forearm pronated at 30°, the wrist extended at 45–50°, and the metacarpophalangeal (MCP) joints flexed minimally, at 5–10°. The proximal interphalangeal (PIP) joints are left free for motion. If the EPL was included in the transfer, the splint is extended out to the tip of the thumb. It is critical to hold the splint in this position until it has completely dried and hardened so the tendons are at the appropriate tension.

While sutures are removed at 10–14 days, the patient is placed back into a similar splint in the same position, and held for a total of 3 weeks postoperatively. At that point, he or she is placed into a short arm splint to extend the wrist to 45° and the MCPs at 0°, with the thumb hyperextended as necessary. This splint is maintained full-time except for therapy, which begins at that point, twice weekly. At 6 weeks, the patient can remove the splint and mobilize more fully, still with therapy supervision for a total of 6 weeks. At 3 months postoperatively, the patient can begin strengthening. Contact sports, heavy labor, and other strenuous activities are deferred for 6 months.

Failed Transfers in Ulnar Nerve Palsy

Introduction

The level of nerve injury is critical in planning revision of failed tendon transfers. With proximal ulnar nerve injury, flexion of the ring and small fingers is decreased and grip strength lost due to the FDP IV and V. Proximal and distal ulnar nerve injury commonly, and more importantly, causes loss of intrinsic power in the hand, with clawing due to hyperextension of the MCP joints and flexion of the PIP joints due to the imbalance of flexor and extensor power at the digit usually mediated by the intrinsics [1]. All must be addressed when treating failed tendon transfers.

The only described motor for strengthening grip through recreation of the FDP power to the ring and small finger is side-to-side transfer of the FDP of the middle finger in the palm to the FDP IV and V. If this fails and it is felt that improved grip is needed, the index FDP can be used, cautioning the patient that power pinch may be impacted.

Indications for FDP transfer
- Need for improved hand grip.
- Supple ring and small finger without contracture.

Contraindications for FDP transfer
- Contractures of the digits.
- Significant palmar scar.
- Concurrent median nerve injury.

Operative Technique (Fig. 15.5)

- An incision is marked at the volar forearm in the distal third.
- The incision is opened and the flexor retinaculum divided carefully for later repair. The median nerve is identified and protected.
- The FDP tendons to the index or middle and ring and small fingers are identified. If previous surgery was performed, scar and adhesions are excised.
- The FDP tendons of the ring and small are then divided and sutured to the FDP donor (either middle, which is optimal, or index) with all the fingers held at the same degree of flexion to equalize the tension and avoid quadriga.

Optimizing Outcomes

- Carefully set the tension to avoid differential tendon pull.
- Splint in flexion to allow tendons to heal.

Complications and Side Effects

Use of the index FDP may decrease the motor to that digit and thus power pinch; this transfer should be used with caution and only if FDP III is not available for transfer.

Volar Static MCP Capsulodesis for Correction of Intrinsic Paralysis

Indications
- Failure of dynamic transfers for clawing correction.
- Supple joints without fixed MCP contracture.

Contraindications
- Heavy laborers.
- Patients with dense global sensory loss (leprosy, multiple nerve injury).

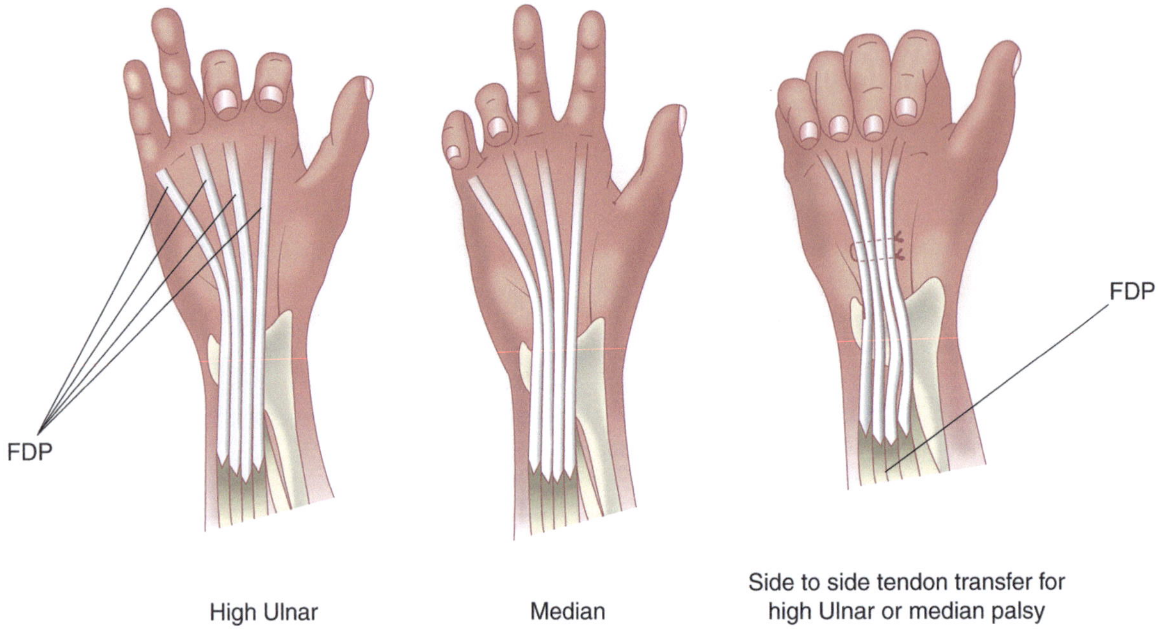

Fig. 15.5 Loss of ulnar innervated FDP IV and V function can be addressed by side to side transfer to the middle finger

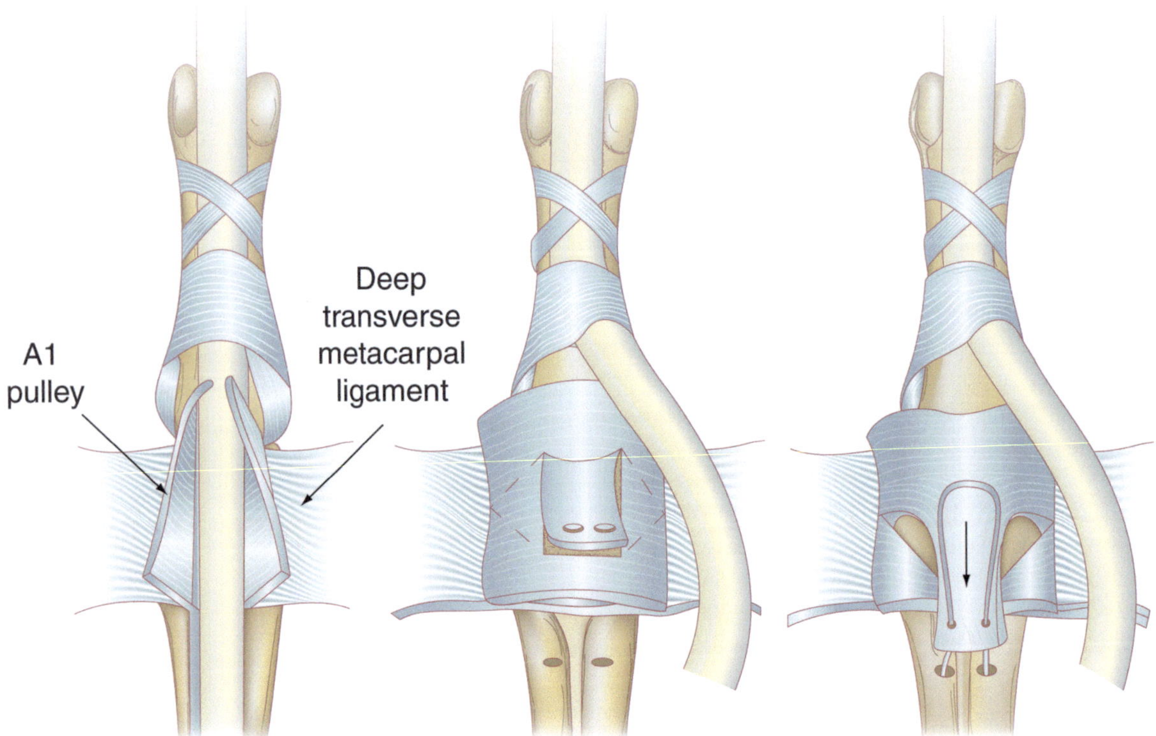

Fig. 15.6 Volar plate advancement technique for correction of clawing. See the text for surgical technique details

Operative Technique (Fig. 15.6)

- A transverse incision is marked over the distal palmar crease. The skin is incised and the A-1 pulley is identified and opened, and the flexor tendons are retracted to expose the volar plate of the MCP joint.
- Two parallel longitudinal incisions are made in the volar plate to form a distally based rectangular flap. Next the base of the volar plate flap is cut transversely and the volar plate released from its metacarpal origin.
- Using either a small drill, K-wire (1.0 mm, 0.054 in.), or a small curved awl, a tunnel is created in the metacarpal

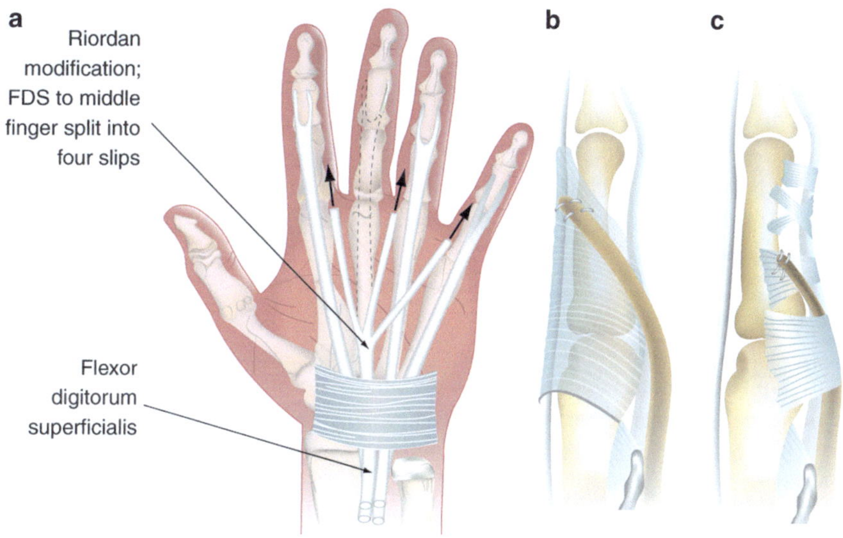

Fig. 15.7 The middle finger FDS tendon can be split into four slips to help correct clawing dynamically. (**a**) FDS split, (**b**) Tendon tail sutured to the lateral band, (**c**) Tendon tail sutured to the A-2 pulley

neck for passage of a small curved needle. Using a 2-0 nonresorbable braided suture, the needle is passed retrograde through the tunnel and the suture then placed into the volar plate flap securely using either a horizontal mattress or Kessler-grasping type technique.

– The MCP joint is then flexed to approximately 45° and the suture tied securely. This is repeated for each digit.

Optimizing Outcomes

- Predrilling the tunnel for suture passage is helpful, especially in patients with good bone stock.

Complications and Side Effects

This capsulodesis is vulnerable to recurrence of deformity if passive hyperextension is an issue. Additionally, flexion contracture of the MCP joints can occur if the volar plate is advanced too proximally. To avoid this, identify the neck of the metacarpal carefully by using a freer elevator or other blunt instrument to palpate the head and neck of the bone at the joint.

Finally, flexor tendon bowstringing can occur if A-1 pulley release is extended. This will decrease flexion of the digits.

Postoperative Care

A bulky dressing is placed, with care taken to avoid excessive interdigital padding, with the wrist in neutral alignment and the MCP joints maintained in flexion of approximately 30°. An extension block splint is placed with the IP joints free. This position is maintained for 4 weeks, at which point the therapist fashions an MCP flexion splint for full-time use for an additional 4 weeks.

Dynamic FDS III transfer for Clawing Deformity

Indications

- Failed static transfers.
- Strong FDP III.

Contraindications

- Weak profundus tendon to middle finger.
- Fixed contractures of the involved joints.

Surgical Technique (Fig. 15.7)

– An incision is made on the volar aspect of the middle finger using a Brunner-type incision to expose the interval between the A-2 and C-2 pulleys. The FDS tendon is identified and sectioned at that level, with one slip to be used for transfer.

– The remaining residual slip is slightly tensioned and sutured to the flexor tendon sheath to act as a tenodesis to prevent swan neck deformity.

– A 1 cm transverse incision is made in the mid palm below the middle finger, and the FDS tendon pulled into this incision and split into four tails.

– An incision is then made in the palm just distal to the level of the distal palmar crease.

– Using a curved hemostat or mosquito clamp, each tendon end is passed from the proximal incision, while remaining volar to the deep transverse metacarpal ligament (DTML), into the distal incision.

– There the tendon end can be sewn using 3-0 or 4-0 nonresorbable suture to either:
  - The proximal phalanx [5].

  - The A-2 pulley [6].
  - The lateral band more dorsally [7].
- *Alternatively*, the tendon end can be passed under the A-1 or the A-1 and A-2 pulleys, retrieved with a straight clamp, and sewn to itself (the Zancolli "lasso" procedure) [8].
- With the wrist in neutral, the MCP joints are flexed to 60° and the tension set when the sutures are placed.

Optimizing Outcomes

- Despite less noticeable clawing in the index and middle fingers, the intrinsic paralysis affects these fingers as well and it is recommended that all four fingers be included in this dynamic transfer.
- Avoid multiple "passes" of clamps and if necessary, make a small incision on the digit to visualize the tendon slip being passed if difficulty is encountered. This is preferable to later tendon adhesions.

Complications and Side Effects

Transfer of the middle finger FDS should be performed only if the FDP III is of sufficient strength to flex the finger. Alternatively, in a distal ulnar palsy the ring finger profundus can be utilized.

In patients with hypermobile joints, this transfer may result in middle finger PIP hyperextension, particularly if the lateral band is used for anchoring the transfer.

Postoperative Care

The wrist is positioned in 5–10° of flexion, with the MCP joints flexed to 90° and the IP joints free for motion. Splinting should be accomplished by a dorsal blocking splint to avoid any stretching out of the transfers early.

The splint is maintained for 3 weeks, after which the patient is placed in a custom MCP flexion splint (MCP joint only) for full time wear except in therapy. Therapy is performed once to twice weekly with the goal to retrain tendon motion. The patient can discontinue the MCP flexion splint at 8 weeks.

Failed Tendon Transfers in Median Nerve Palsy

The primary issue in median nerve injury is loss of functional thumb opposition. Even with complete loss of the median nerve innervations, the dual innervations of the strong flexor pollicis brevis muscle by the median and ulnar nerve often provides adequate thumb opposition. Loss of thumb function is more of an issue with a combined median and ulnar nerve injury.

The most commonly used transfers in median nerve palsy are the extensor indicis proprius (EIP) transfer and the FDS opponensplasty [7, 9, 10]. Other options include the Huber transfer (abductor digiti minimi) and the Camitz (palmaris longus). This section will present the EIP and FDS as alternatives to each other, with the assumption that one procedure failed.

Indications for thumb opponensplasty
Full passive thumb motion.
Expendable donor after loss of original transfer muscle.

Contraindications
First web space contracture.
Capsular contractures of carpometacarpal joint of the thumb.

Surgical Technique: FDS Opponensplasty (Fig. 15.8)

- The ring finger FDS tendon is most commonly used, although the middle finger is an alternative. A transverse volar incision is made over the first annular (A-1) pulley in the palm and the FDS identified and transected just prior to the tendon bifurcation.
- A Brunner-type incision is then made at the volar ulnar forearm over the FCU tendon, and the transected ring finger FDS tendon pulled into this wound. A small strip of distally based FCU tendon is created approximately 3–4 cm proximal to the pisiform to act as a pulley for the FDS tendon transfer. This is sewn into a loop, with the end anchored over the pisiform periosteum, and the FDS passed through this. To anchor the pulley further, it can be sewn to the ECU [11].
- An incision is then made on the dorsum of the thumb over the MCP joint. The ring finger FDS is then passed across the palm subcutaneously and brought out of the thumb incision.
- The FDS is then anchored in one of the following ways, after placing the thumb in full opposition with the wrist in neutral:

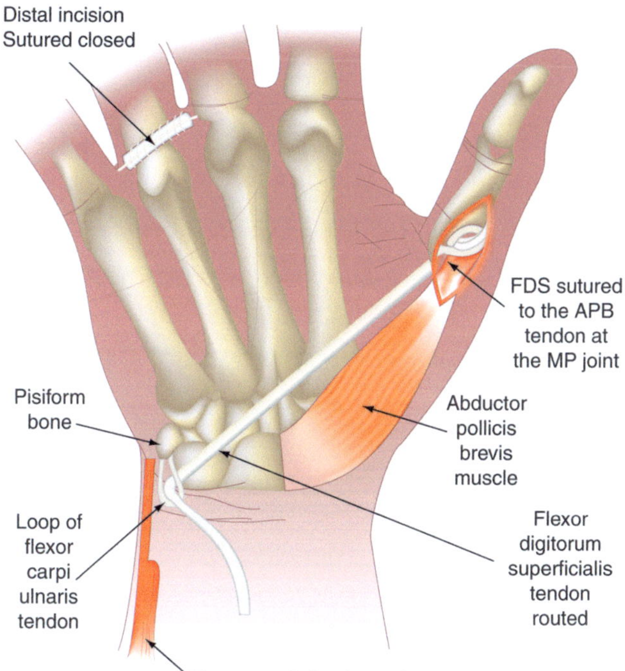

Fig. 15.8 The FDS from the ring finger is routed through a FCU sling and then attached to the APB tendon, which allows for thumb opposition

- To the abductor pollicis brevis (APB) tendon [12].
- Through a drill hole in the base of the proximal phalanx placed dorsal-ulnar to radial-volar, and then sutured to itself or the adjacent periosteum [13].

Optimizing Outcomes

- Taking care to insert the final transfer at the base of the proximal phalanx allows the transfer to also serve to flex the thumb with opposition.

Complications and Side Effects

Swan neck deformity of the donor ring finger can occur with loss of the FDS tendon flexion moment. If this is seen in the early postoperative period, treatment with flexion splinting or custom ring splints to prevent hyperextension of the PIP joint should be done until the joint scars down.

If the superficialis tendon is merely passed around the FCU tendon, the pulley has been noted to migrate proximally over time and becomes less efficient as the line of pull is more longitudinal and not in line with opposition. The above described ECU anchor can prevent this problem.

Postoperative Care

- The wrist and hand are casted in a thumb spica cast with the thumb held in full opposition and the wrist flexed at 30° to relax the transfer.
- The cast is removed at 3 weeks and the patient then placed into a thermoplastic molded thumb spica splint to maintain the wrist in slight flexion and the thumb in full opposition.
- Therapy is begun to initiate tendon retraining at 3–4 weeks.
- The patient is instructed to avoid isolated pinch for 2–3 months except in the context of occupational therapy.

Alternatives: Extensor Indicis Proprius (EIP) Transfer for Opposition

Indications for thumb opponensplasty

- Full passive thumb motion.
- Expendable donor after loss of original transfer muscle.
- High median nerve palsy—FDS tendons unavailable for transfer.

Contraindications

- First web space contracture.
- Capsular contractures of carpometacarpal joint of the thumb.

Operative Technique (Fig. 15.9)

- The EIP tendon is harvested through a longitudinal incision over the index finger MCP joint. The EIP is the most ulnar of the two tendons, and is divided just proximal to the extensor hood.
- Another longitudinal incision is made over the distal third of the forearm and the EIP delivered into this wound. The EIP is pulled out proximal to the extensor retinaculum, preserving the retinaculum if possible. The tendon and musculotendinous junction are then mobilized by cutting all soft tissue attachments to maximize length for transfer.
- Next, a small incision is made over the pisiform at the volar ulnar wrist and the EIP tendon passed subcutaneously to this incision. Care is taken to pass the tendon over the FCU to avoid compression of the ulnar nerve.

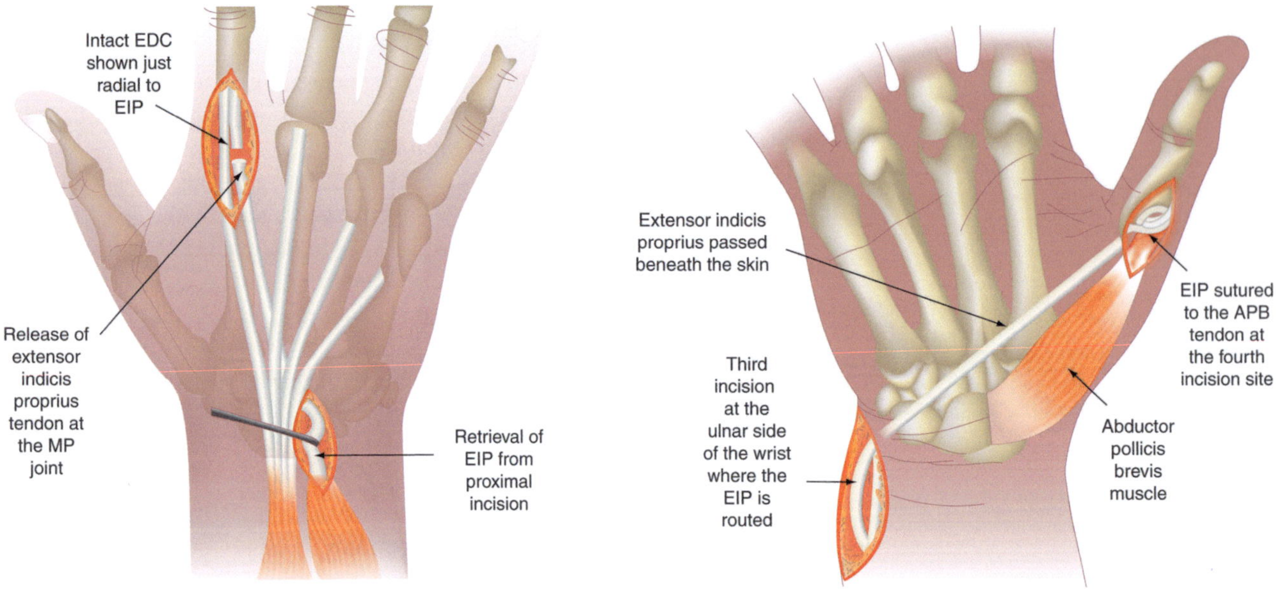

Fig. 15.9 The EIP tendon is released at the level of the MP joint. It is then rerouted around the ulnar aspect of the wrist and attached to the APB tendon

- A small incision is then made on the dorsal radial aspect of the thumb at the MCP joint. The EIP tendon is then bluntly subcutaneously tunneled across the palm and brought out of this incision.
- In a low median nerve palsy, the tendon is sewn to the APB tendon, which is easily exposed in the thumb incision. Tension is set by placing the thumb in full opposition and the wrist in 30° of flexion.
- In a combined median and ulnar nerve palsy, the EIP tendon is anchored to the APB, the MCP joint capsule, and the EPL tendon with the wrist in flexion to allow the tendon end to reach. This transfer restricts thumb IP joint flexion and powers the FPL to flex the MCP joint preferentially [14].

Optimizing Outcomes

- If the surgeon is concerned about length, the EIP length can be increased by harvesting a small piece of contiguous extensor hood, with closure.

Complications and Side Effects

An extensor lag at the index finger can be seen if the extensor hood is not reapproximated after harvest of the EIP tendon [9]. Additionally, it is critical to place the EIP above the FCU in the transfer across the pisiform to prevent ulnar nerve compression.

Postoperative Care

- The wrist and hand are immobilized in a cast for 3 weeks postoperatively, with the wrist flexed and the thumb in maximal opposition.
- The cast is changed to a thermoplastic splint at 3 weeks, with the wrist mildly flexed. The splint is removed 3–4 times daily for tendon gliding and retraining.
- Heavy pinch activity is restricted for 3 months.

Failed Tendon Transfers in Rheumatoid Arthritis

Introduction

The most commonly ruptured tendons in rheumatoid arthritis are the extensor tendons to the wrist, although the flexor side of the hand can also be affected by this disease. On the extensor side of the hand, the caput ulnae syndrome involves volar subluxation of the carpus with prominence of the ulnar head, placing the extensor at risk for rupture due to their tented position over the ulna and often because of arthritic changes of the ulnar head itself. Often the initial surgical treatment of extensor tendon ruptures in rheumatoid patients involves side-to-side transfer, or connection of the distal stump of the ruptured tendon to the adjacent working extensor, in conjunction with synovectomy or other bony procedures. When side-to-side transfers fail, the options for reconstruction of extensor tendon ruptures in the rheumatoid population include the use of the extensor indicis proprius (EIP) or the ring finger FDS tendon [15]. If all the EDC tendons from the index through small are ruptured, the best option is the use of the middle and ring FDS as a transfer to the EDC-2 and 3, and the EDC-4 and 5, respectively. As the FDS transfer technique has been described earlier, the EIP transfer for EDC rupture is the focus of this section.

Indications for EIP transfer to EDC in rheumatoid arthritis
- Failure of side-to-side transfer for attritional tendon rupture.
- Intact EDC to the index finger.
- Plan for concomitant decompression of bony/soft tissue causes of rupture.

Contraindications
- Loss of EDC to the index finger.
- Severe attrition of the donor EIP due to synovitis, which increases the risk of failure.

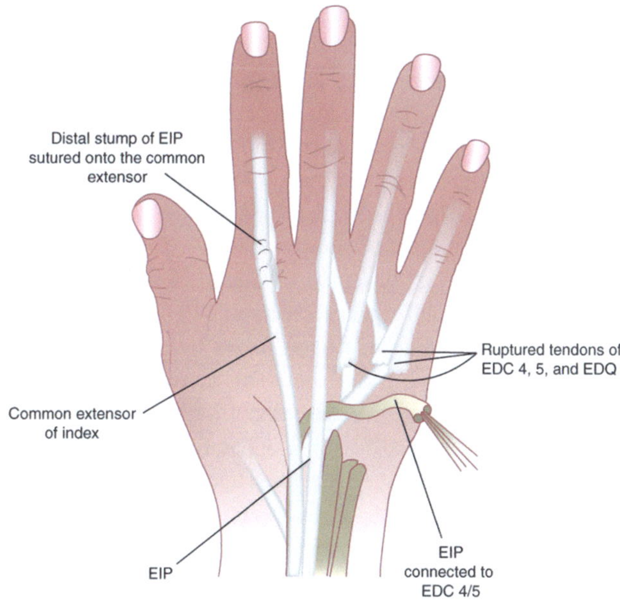

Fig. 15.10 The EIP tendon is transferred to the ruptured ends of the EDC ring and small, and to the ruptured end of the EDQ in order to restore extension

Operative Technique (Fig. 15.10)

- The EIP is identified as the most ulnar tendon at the MCP joint of the index finger through a short longitudinal incision. It is harvested just proximal to its insertion on the extensor hood.
- The EIP is then pulled back into the wrist through a dorsal incision made over the interval between the third and fourth dorsal extensor compartments.
- Through the dorsal wrist incision, the ruptured distal stumps of the EDC tendons are identified and the ends freshened, although care should be taken not to sacrifice length.
- The EIP is transferred, either to the individual tendon, or to both of the EDC to the fourth and fifth fingers. This can be done in combination with FDS tendon transfer. The tendons are sutured using 2-0 or 3-0 nonresorbable sutures.
- Tension is set with the wrist in 30° of extension and the MCPs in 20° extension with the interphalangeal joints fully extended.

Optimizing Outcomes

- It is critical to check the tension of the extensors using the passive tenodesis effect prior to leaving the operating room. It is better to have the tension slightly too tight than too loose, as the tendons may stretch out over time.

Complications and Side Effects

If the EDC to the index finger is attenuated, it is not advisable to harvest the EIP, because this can cause an extensor tendon lag due to the weak EDC to the index. The best alternative is to use a flexor tendon as a donor transfer tendon.

Doing Pulvertaft weaves is generally not as cosmetically acceptable in this population, with very thin skin. An end-to-end or end-to-side suture of the tendon transfer works well and is not as prominent under the skin.

Postoperative Care

- The patient is placed into a splint with the wrist extended approximately 30° and the MCPs extended at 20°.
- This is maintained for 3 weeks, after which time the patient is transitioned to a dynamic extension splint and gradually progressed to further active flexion and dynamic (rubber band) extension.
- Therapy is begun at 3–4 weeks for tendon retraining and range of motion to maintain supple joints.

The Role of Arthrodesis and Carpectomy in Failed Tendon Transfers

Introduction

Creation of bony stability to maintain an optimal position of the extremity for use is another option in failed tendon transfers. Total wrist arthrodesis has been described as an option particularly in flexion deformity due to severe spasticity [16]. Permanent fusion of the wrist can assist in placing it in extension to allow more functional use of the extremity, as long as the finger flexors are not too tight. In patients with rheumatoid arthritis, both limited radiocarpal fusion and total wrist arthrodeses have been described for stabilization, often in association with tendon transfers [15].

Proximal row carpectomy can be used to reduce the tension across wrist and finger flexor and extensor tendons by the relative shortening that occurs with the removal of the scaphoid, lunate, and triquetrum. This can allow improved wrist extension while at the same time causing relative lengthening of the flexor tendon apparatus to avoid further finger flexion deformity. Omer noted that when used in spastic paralysis, the tendency of the remaining carpus for ulnar subluxation was reduced by preserving the distal half of the scaphoid [17].

Indications for total wrist arthrodesis

- Inability to achieve a stable extended position by tendon transfer alone.
- Previous failed transfers for wrist extension.

Contraindications

- Severe osteopenia or osteoporosis—as this increases the risk of nonunion.
- Lack of adequate soft tissue coverage—particularly if a dorsal plate is to be used.

Operative Technique

- The wrist is approached via a dorsal longitudinal incision from the third metacarpal base extending up onto the radial shaft. Full-thickness skin flaps are opened with preservation of the dorsal veins.
- The extensor retinaculum is incised between the third and fourth dorsal compartments and the EPL retracted radially. The second and fourth dorsal compartments are opened and elevated to expose the dorsal distal radius and carpus, as well as the base of the third metacarpal.
- The radiocarpal and midcarpal joints are exposed and all cartilage removed using curettes, osteotomes, and/or small-tipped burrs. Lister's tubercle is removed using a rongeur.
- Cancellous bone graft for fusion can be obtained from several sources: the distal radius, using Lister's tubercle as an entry point for curettes; the proximal ulna; or the iliac crest.
- Bone graft is packed into the radiocarpal and intercarpal spaces and a fusion plate applied. There are specialized wrist fusion plates that can be used for wrist fusion; alternatively, a plate can be shaped to place the wrist in slight extension and ulnar deviation to maximize function and grip [18]. Other fixation options, which are less commonly used, include placing an intramedullary Steinmann pin between the second and third metacarpal web spaces across the carpus into the radius [19].
- The plate is fixed to the distal radial shaft and to the third metacarpal base, using fluoroscopic imaging to ensure plate placement is central. The distal plate is covered with metacarpal periosteum and hand fascia if possible, to minimize extensor tendon irritation.

Optimizing Outcomes

- The plate is placed as proximal as possible on the third metacarpal to allow secure fixation while preventing extensor tendon irritation.
- The use of an oval-shaped 2-mm burr can be helpful in decorticating the more volar aspects of the carpal bones and distal radius.

Complications and Side Effects

Extensor tendon irritation is among the most common side effects of the use of a dorsal plate for wrist arthrodesis, particularly in the rheumatoid or spastic hand with thin skin coverage. This can be minimized by using soft tissue to cover the plate.

Nonunion or delayed union of wrist arthrodesis, while uncommon, can occur. Thorough decortication of cartilage surfaces can minimize this complication. If it occurs, and iliac crest graft was not the original graft source, revision fusion should include the liberal use of iliac crest bone graft, because of its high osteogenic potential.

Postoperative Care

- If necessary, the wound is closed over a drain, typically a small feeding tube, which is removed at 2–3 days postoperatively. A bulky dressing, to allow swelling, and a volar forearm-based splint are applied. Immediate finger range of motion is encouraged.
- At 2 weeks, the sutures are removed and the patient then immobilized in either a circumferential splint or a short arm cast. This is maintained until 6–8 weeks postoperatively,

with activity restrictions and lifting limited to 5 lb for 3 months, or until signs of fusion are seen on a plain radiographs.

Indications for proximal row carpectomy in failed tendon transfer

- Need for shortening the carpus to gain relative length of finger flexors while performing transfers for wrist extension.
- Can be done concomitantly with wrist arthrodesis to position the wrist and give the finger flexors more length.

Contraindications

- Arthritic midcarpal joint.

Operative Technique

- The wrist is approached through a dorsal incision based between the third and fourth dorsal compartments.
- As above, the third compartment is entered and the second and fourth elevated and retracted. The proximal carpal row—the scaphoid, lunate, and triquetrum—is identified. These are removed either en bloc with sharp scalpel dissection and the use of K-wire joysticks placed into the carpal bones, or piecemeal using rongeurs. Either way, it is critical to preserve the volar wrist ligaments.
- After the entire proximal row is removed, the capitate is firmly seated in the lunate fossa. If wrist fusion is to be done in association with a proximal row carpectomy, it is at this point that the cartilage surfaces are denuded.

Optimizing Outcomes

- If proximal row carpectomy is done with the goal of having a mobile wrist, approaching the wrist capsule through a Mayo ligament-sparing capsulotomy is advisable to avoid cutting across the dorsal wrist ligaments [20].

Complications and Side Effects

If the capsular tissue has a high degree of redundancy, subluxation of the distal carpal row on the radius can occur. This can be avoided by tightly imbricating the dorsal wrist capsule to provide stability. While some authors have suggested temporary pinning, this is not generally necessary for stability.

Postoperative Care

- The patient is immobilized in a volar wrist splint while the incision heals, approximately 10–14 days.
- After suture removal, the patient is placed into a removable splint and gentle motion begun. Concomitant tendon retraining can begin at this point with occupational therapy.
- Strengthening is deferred until 3 months postoperatively.

Conclusions

Revision of tendon transfer in the hand and wrist, due to failed previous surgery, can be challenging. The surgeon has to deal with scarring and possible contracture as well as with the need for using a different donor tendon to power what is missing. Knowing the options for primary transfer, the surgeon can often turn to another donor tendon as a revision option. In addition, the use of wrist arthrodesis to place the joint in a functional position can assist in decreasing the number of functions to be replaced by tendon transfer.

References

1. Brand PW. Tendon transfers for median and ulnar nerve paralysis. Orthop Clin North Am. 1970;1:447–54.
2. Tsuge K. Tendon transfers for radial nerve palsy. Aust N Z J Surg. 1980;50:267–72.
3. Chuinard RG, Boyes JH, Stark HH, Ashworth CR. Tendon transfers for radial nerve palsy: use of superficialis tendons for digital extension. J Hand Surg Am. 1978;3:560–70.
4. De Smet L, Schollen W, Degreef I. In vitro biomechanical study to compare the double-loop technique with the Pulvertaft weave for tendon anastomosis. Scand J Plast Reconstr Surg Hand Surg. 2008;42:305–7.
5. Burkhalter WE. Restoration of power grip in ulnar nerve paralysis. Orthop Clin North Am. 1974;5:289–303.
6. Riordan DC. Tendon transfers in hand surgery. J Hand Surg Am. 1983;8:748–53.
7. Bunnell S. Tendon Transfers. In: Boyes JH, editor. Bunnell's Surgery of the Hand. 5th ed. Philadelphia: JB Lippincott; 1970. pp. 409–430.
8. Zancolli EA. Claw-hand caused by paralysis of the intrinsic muscles: a simple surgical procedure for its correction. J Bone Joint Surg Am. 1957;39-A:1076–80.
9. Anderson GA, Lee V, Sundararaj GD. Extensor indicis proprius opponensplasty. J Hand Surg Br. 1991;16:334–8.
10. Burkhalter W, Christensen RC, Brown P. Extensor indicis proprius opponensplasty. J Bone Joint Surg Am. 1973;55:725–32.
11. Sakellarides HT. Modified pulley for opponents tendon transfer. J Bone Joint Surg Am. 1970;52:178–9.
12. Kozin SH. Tendon transfers for radial and median nerve palsies. J Hand Ther. 2005;18:208–15.
13. Jensen EG. Restoration of opposition of the thumb. Hand. 1978; 10:161–7.

14. Riordan DC. Tendon transfers for nerve paralysis of the hand and wrist. Curr Pract Orthop Surg. 1964;23:17–40.
15. Papp SR, Athwal GS, Pichora DR. The rheumatoid wrist. J Am Acad Orthop Surg. 2006;14:65–77.
16. Hayden RJ, Jebson PJ. Wrist arthrodesis. Hand Clin. 2005;21: 631–40.
17. Omer GE, Capen DA. Proximal row carpectomy with muscle transfers for spastic paralysis. J Hand Surg Am. 1976;1:197–204.
18. Jebson PJ, Adams BD. Wrist arthrodesis: review of current technique. J Am Acad Orthop Surg. 2001;9:53–60.
19. Viegas SF, Rimoldi R, Patterson R. Modified technique of intramedullary fixation for wrist arthrodesis. J Hand Surg Am. 1989;14:618–23.
20. Berger RA, Bishop AT, Bettinger PC. New dorsal capsulotomy for the surgical exposure of the wrist. Ann Plast Surg. 1995;35: 54–9.

Surgical Options for Failed Replantation

16

S.C. Tay and Alexander Y. Shin

Abstract

Replants can be one of the most challenging and technically difficult procedures that the hand surgeon will face. Failure of replantations can occur both interoperatively as well as postoperatively. Interoperatively, there are mechanisms to try and reduce vasospasm as well as reduce thrombosis. These principles are important postoperatively as well. If a replant has been doing well and then changes in the immediate postoperative period, exploration may be warranted. In these cases, sometimes a reversed interpositional vein graft will help. Other techniques including further shortening, subcutaneous pocketing, and retrograde/antegrade arterial drainage techniques can be utilized. In the cases where the replant is not salvageable, revision to an amputation will be needed. If the replant has been unsuccessful interoperatively, then a primary amputation is very reasonable option. Otherwise if the replant fails late or for other reasons the surgeon can wait and perform the amputation secondarily after demarcation. As far as reconstructive options for failed replantation, many patients may choose no further surgery. However, other osteoplastic reconstructions, flap surgeries, or toe to hand transfers can be performed. Each case is very unique, but this chapter will hopefully give the reader some guidelines and a better feeling on how to treat these unfortunate and difficult injuries.

Keywords

Failed • Finger • Digit • Replant • Technique

Key Points

- Replantation is a sequential multistage procedure.
- The proper execution of this staged replantation procedure, in the proper sequence, is the key to keeping the rate of replantation failures low.
- Failures of replantations can occur intraoperatively or postoperatively. Management of failures at each stage is discussed separately.
- Many replantation failures can be resuscitated with a combination of local and general nonsurgical maneuvers. These measures are based on concepts of increasing flow rate across the anastomosis, reducing

(continued)

S.C. Tay, MD, MS
Department of Hand Surgery, Singapore General Hospital, Outram Road, Singapore 169608

A.Y. Shin, MD (✉)
Division of Hand Surgery, Department of Orthopedic Surgery, Mayo Clinic College of Medicine, 200 First Street SW, Rochester, MN 55905, USA
e-mail: shin.alexander@mayo.edu

S.F.M. Duncan (ed.), *Reoperative Hand Surgery*,
DOI 10.1007/978-1-4614-2373-7_16,

vasospasm, reducing thrombophilia, as well as ensuring the absence of hypovolemia and hypothermia.

- Exploration is indicated when replant resuscitation is not successful.
- Surgical options for the management of failed replantations include reversed interpositional vein grafting, proximal/heterodigital artery transfer, further bone shortening, arteriovenous anastomosis techniques, postoperative bleeding techniques, subcutaneous pocketing, and retrograde antegrade arterial drainage techniques.
- Management of segmental injuries and no-reflow phenomenon is discussed.
- If a replant has been deemed to be not salvageable, revision of amputation will be required. As far as possible, it should be performed primarily. In some situations, it can be performed secondarily, after the replant has demarcated itself.
- Depending on the level of the amputation, the revision of amputation can range from simple bone shortening procedures to achieve primary closure, to ray amputation procedures.
- Reconstructive procedures following failed replantations can range from no further surgeries to osteoplastic reconstructions, flap surgeries to finger pollicizations or toe transfer procedures.

Introduction

Replantation is a sequential multistage procedure with microsurgery performed at the end after a long surgery, frequently in the middle of the night. The stages of replantation are as follows:

1. Excisional debridement and identification of structures.
2. Bone work which includes adequate bone shortening and fixation.
3. Tendon repairs.
4. Microsurgical repair or reconstruction of arteries, veins, and nerves.
5. Skin closure and dressings.

The multistage process of replantation cannot be overemphasized. The success of the replantation rests on the successful and careful completion of the preceding stages. If excisional debridement is not adequately performed, the surgeon will subsequently encounter difficulties in identifying healthy vessels and will also have problems when performing the anastomosis.

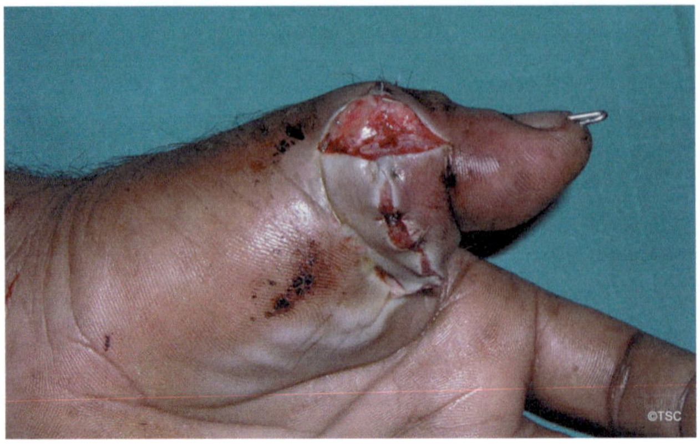

Fig. 16.1 Mid-lateral split incisions should never be closed as the replant will swell postoperatively. The mid-lateral split wounds will decrease in size gradually as the swelling decreases. They can be skin grafted after 1 week or left to heal secondarily if small

We recommend that sharp debridement of injured tissues be performed as the first important stage of replantation. This will remove all injured and crushed tissues leaving clean, healthy tissues at the level of the amputation. This will greatly facilitate identification of structures, in particularly the dorsal and volar veins, as well as ensure that the vascular structures that are available for anastomosis are in good condition. A careful initial excisional debridement and irrigation will also reduce the chances of late replantation failures from infection.

Bone shortening is the next key step in replantation surgery. Depending on the level and the mechanism of amputation, and the configuration of the bony injury, as well as the amount of soft tissue debridement performed in the preceding stage, the amount of bone shortening ranges from a couple of millimeters, up to 10 mm or more. The main objective of bone shortening is to shorten enough to achieve primary tension-free apposition of the vascular structures without the need for a vein graft and to achieve adequate soft tissue cover of the anastomosis. Once the replantation surgeon has set himself up well with the proper and meticulous execution of the first two stages, the following stages of replantation will occur smoothly and the chance of success will be high.

The final stage of replantation is skin closure and dressings. Swelling of the replant is to be expected postoperatively. Hence, the mid-lateral split incisions should be left open and not be closed (Fig. 16.1). Transverse wounds can be closed taking care not to damage the underlying vascular anastomoses. Vessel and nerve anastomoses should be covered by appropriate skin closure, ensuring they are not too constricting. Dressings should not be compressive or constricting. Gauze, tulle-graz, and crepe dressings should not be applied in a continuous circumferential manner.

Replantation is a sequential multistage process and deficiencies at any stage could increase the chance of failure, which can occur intraoperatively, immediately postoperatively at the surgical recovery, or after replantation when the patient is in the ward.

Failure of replantation is defined as loss of viability of the replanted part. This can be due to an arterial or venous problem. Arterial problems are characterized by pallor, poor capillary refill, decreased temperature of the replant, and poor tissue turgor. Venous problems are characterized by purplish congestion of the replant, excessively brisk capillary refill, decreased temperature, and increased tissue turgor. On pricking the replant, dark or red venous blood will appear. In a replant with an arterial problem, pricking typically will not yield any blood.

More often, the replant will run into venous problems, which if left untreated, will eventually result in arterial thrombosis. Arterial or venous problems can be intrinsic or extrinsic to the vessel. Intrinsic causes include technical problems at the anastomosis resulting in vascular thrombosis. Extrinsic causes include, but are not limited to, external compression from postoperative swelling or tight dressings, and generalized vasoconstriction. Eventually, extrinsic causes can also result in vascular thrombosis.

Indications and Contraindications: Summarize in Box Before Detailed Text

Surgical management of failed replantation includes exploration in the event that nonsurgical measures are not successful in restoring vascularity to the replant. Clearly, exploration should be more indicated in replants which are expected to have a higher chance of success and less indicated in replants with a lower chance of success. Towards that end, replants that have sustained significant injury or which are severely contaminated to the point that effective debridement is not possible, will have lower priority for exploration. Patients who are not fit for further anesthesia or surgery are not candidates for exploration regardless of how ideal the replant is for exploration.

Chronic smokers or patients with peripheral vascular diseases are less likely to have a successful replant [1]. Although replantation or exploration is definitely not a contraindication, the presence of significant peripheral vascular disease in combination with a replant that is failing following a well-performed replantation procedure may be a relative contraindication for exploration.

Preoperative History and Considerations

The following points are important considerations in the preoperative history that will assist in the management of a failing replantation. These are as follows:

1. Patient's age
2. Patient's occupation and sociocultural background
3. Medical history
4. Smoking history
5. Mechanism of amputation
6. Ischemia time

Factors such as age, medical history, and smoking status will determine the suitability of the patient for further prolonged anesthesia and surgery. The above factors will also suggest the health of the vessels in the amputated part. In addition, the state of preservation of the amputated part is indicated by the mechanism of injury. In a sharp guillotine injury, the tissues are likely to be well preserved distal to the narrow zone of injury (Fig. 16.2). In an extensive crush or

Indications

Restoration of arterial inflow and/or venous outflow into replanted part.

Contraindications

Medically unfit patient who is unable to undergo further surgery or anesthesia.

Presence of significant gangrene or infarct in the replantation.

Significant injury of the replant.

Severe contamination of the amputation.

Uncontrollable infection of the replant.

Relative Contraindications

Chronic smokers with evidence of peripheral vascular disease.

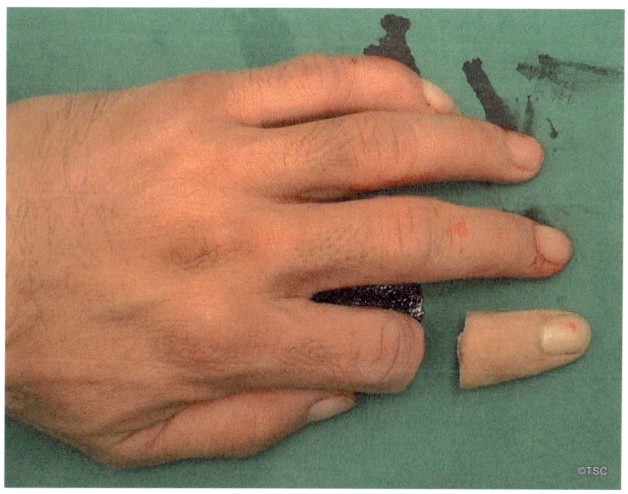

Fig. 16.2 A guillotine amputation injury of the index finger: The amputated part is otherwise well preserved

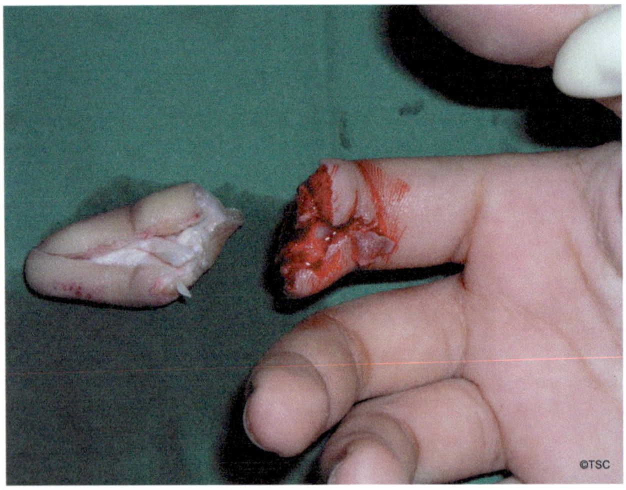

Fig. 16.3 A crushing amputation injury: Note the extent of the burst laceration and bruising on the side of the amputate indicating extensive soft tissue injury of the amputated part

avulsion injury, extensive damage is expected to be present (Fig. 16.3). The patient's occupation and sociocultural background are also important factors for consideration on the amount of effort to be put into salvaging the failing replant.

In a young, healthy, nonsmoking executive with a strong desire for preservation of a "whole body" image, and a well-preserved amputated part, reexploration and salvage would be more likely indicated. In an elderly farmer with significant medical and smoking history, who has sustained an avulsion amputation, reexploration and salvage would be less indicated.

Ischemic time is also of obvious importance. The longer the ischemic time, the higher the likelihood of failure, and thus *the less likely that surgical intervention will salvage the amputated part.*

Operative Approach: Step by Step with Details

Failure of replantation can occur intraoperatively or postoperatively. Postoperative failures can present in the surgical recovery or in the wards. Management of an intraoperative failure will differ from management of a postoperative failure. As such, we discuss them separately.

Intraoperative Failure of Replantation

This is the situation where the replant fails to "pink-up" when the microclamps and tourniquet are released after completion of the arterial anastomosis. This could be due to one of three factors: (1) thrombosis at the anastomosis due to technical errors, (2) poor arterial inflow from the proximal artery due to undetected proximal damage or vasospasm, or (3) blockage of the distal artery by a clot or failure of the distal arterial circulation.

Even if the replantation is performed under general anesthesia, it is recommended that an indwelling interscalene catheter be placed for continuous brachial plexus block to reduce vasospasm [2, 3].

Typically, at the completion of the arterial anastomosis, the anesthetist is instructed to start intravenous antithrombotics. This could include intravenous Dextran 40 to run at 1 pint every 12 h for the first day, and intravenous heparin 5,000 IU push [4]. The microclamps are then gently removed and an inspection of the anastomosis can be performed. If the anastomosis is satisfactory and there are no leaks, a passive patency test can be performed while the tourniquet is still inflated (Fig. 16.4). It is termed a passive patency test, as it is performed while the tourniquet is still inflated. This is performed by gently indenting the bottom of the anastomosed vessel with the side of a forceps and gliding it in a proximal to distal direction while watching the filling of the lumen. If the anastomosis is good, there will be prompt filling of the vessel lumen when the forceps passes the anastomosis. If the passive patency test is satisfactory, the next step is to deflate the tourniquet. The anastomosis can be checked to ensure no leaks and the active patency test can be performed. This involves gently occluding the vessel lumen downstream of the completed anastomosis, by emptying the lumen distal to the occlusion and by sweeping a gently closed forceps for a few millimeters downstream before occluding the lumen distally. If the anastomosis is good, it will pass the active patency test with prompt filling of the emptied segment of vessel, when the proximal forceps is opened.

If the anastomosis is not mechanically viable, there will either be delayed or no filling of the lumens in both the passive and the active patency tests. In such a situation, the anastomosis should be immediately checked and if necessary, revised. If the anastomosis passes the above tests, the replant can be checked to see if it "pinks up."

Intraoperative Replant Resuscitation

Local Maneuvers

If the replant does not "pink up" after a suitable interval, "resuscitation" of the replant should be started. The first steps involve the topical application of warmed normal saline and a topical vasodilator such as lignocaine (1 or 2%), papaverine, or magnesium sulfate [5]. The replant should be kept warm using gauze or towels soaked in warm water or saline. Other local measures include manually performing proximal to distal massaging of the arterial inflow in the anatomical region proximal to the replant. For a finger replant, this

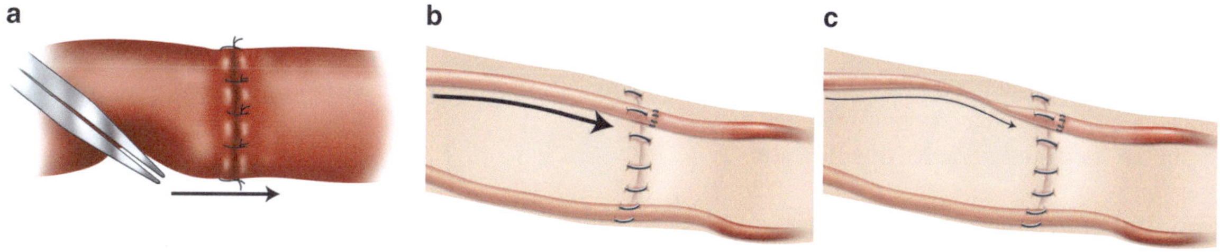

Fig. 16.4 Passive patency test is performed with the microclamps removed but the tourniquet still inflated. This is a technique for preliminary testing of the anastomosis before the tourniquet is released. (**a**) the vessel is gently swept with a microforceps to push the vessel contents across the anastomosis. (**b**) the contents of the vessel easily pass the anastomosis, and (**c**) the vessel returns to normal when the forcep is removed

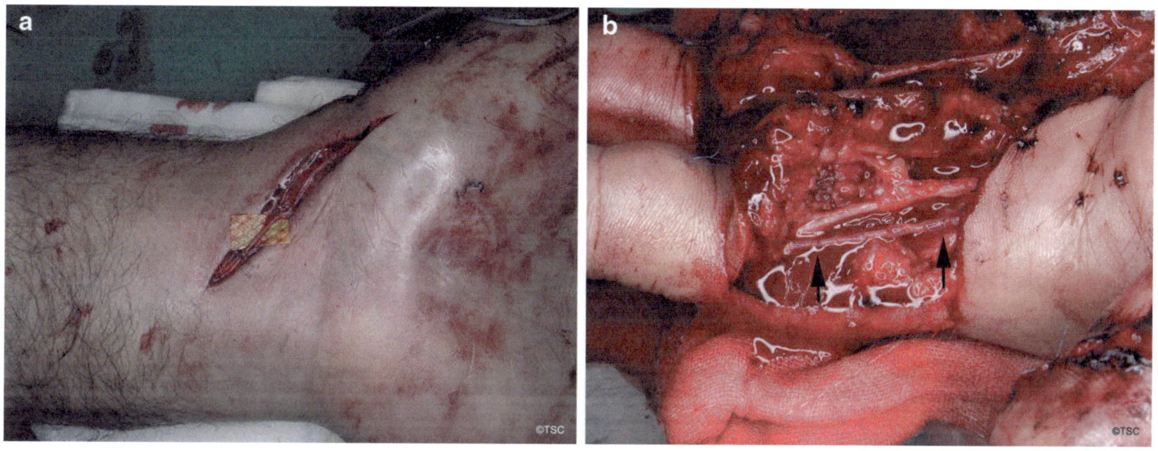

Fig. 16.5 (**a**) Harvesting a long vein graft from the volar wrist. (**b**) An interpositional reversed vein graft of appropriate length and caliber. The ends of the vein graft are depicted by the positions of the *black arrowheads*

would involve massaging the palm area where the common digital artery of the replant would lie. The aim is to attempt to increase the arterial pressure head.

General Maneuvers

The anesthetist should be informed to reverse any hypotension and to ensure adequate hydration of the patient. Hypothermia, if present, should be corrected and the patient should be warmed up and the core temperature kept within the normal range. Hypothermia may be an important cause of vasoconstriction in prolonged surgeries.

Revision of Anastomosis

If after 30–45 min, the replant is still not "pinking up," then the problem may not be due to vasospasm. There are three possible causes at this point, which are mentioned previously: (1) Technical errors at the anastomosis. This will be evident with the presence of thrombosis at the anastomosis. (2) Poor arterial inflow due to undetected damage. This may be suggested by poor refill in the proximal artery. (3) Blockage of the distal artery by a clot or failure of the distal arterial circulation.

If it is the first two causes, then the anastomosis will have to be taken down and revised. The mid-lateral incisions may have to be extended so as to afford better exposure of the proximal and distal artery. The proximal artery will need to be resected more proximally until a good and sustained arterial pressure head is demonstrated. At this point, if there is inadequate vessel length for direct anastomosis, a reversed vein graft from the volar wrist should be harvested.

Reversed Interpositional Vein Graft

Care must be taken to select an appropriately sized vein and to ensure that it is neither too long nor short (Fig. 16.5). If the vein graft is too large, it will balloon up when the anastomosis is completed. If it is too long, it will be become tortuous. A vein graft that is too short will result in excessive tension at the anastomosis and will be at high risk of failure. After the vein has been harvested, it must be reversed. The proximal anastomosis is usually performed first, followed by the distal anastomosis. If the graft is too long, it should be shortened before the distal anastomosis is started. Care should also be taken to ensure that the vein graft is also not twisted along its length.

In some situations where there is a concomitant skin defect over the vascular defect, a free flow through flap may be harvested, which would help solve the problem [6–10]. These flaps may contain an artery or a vein, and they can be heterodigital or harvested from the volar forearm.

Heterodigital or Proximal Artery Transfer

An alternative surgical option to an interposition reversed vein graft is to look for a proximal artery to vascularize the replant. This artery can be harvested from an adjacent finger, provided that its harvest does not jeopardize the vascularity of the donor finger. Although this method avoids the need to perform two arterial anastomoses, it can be tedious, especially if a long length of the arterial pedicle needs to be dissected. We thus recommend this option only for levels of amputation limited to the proximal finger. This technique can also be applied for ring avulsion injuries where a long segment of vein graft would otherwise be required for venous and/or arterial reconstruction. A proximal arterial or venous transfer from an adjacent digit can be harvested and utilized, thus avoiding the need to harvest a vein graft and the requirement for two microanastomoses [11, 12].

In some situations of thumb avulsion, a proximal artery transfer can be performed in conjunction with a vein graft. In these cases, the superficial radial artery is connected to the thumb digital artery via a vein graft [13].

Bone Shortening

Another method to achieve primary arterial anastomosis without the use of a vein graft is to perform additional bone shortening. This can be considered, particularly if bone shortening was initially inadequate, or not performed. However, this would require all the tendon repairs and bone work to be undone. The surgeon would have to balance this option of undoing virtually the entire surgery, against the benefit of performing a primary arterial anastomosis without an interposition vein graft.

Arteriovenous Anastomosis

There have been a number of reports where arteriovenous anastomoses were used to salvage replantations of the fingers and thumbs [14–20]. Two types of arteriovenous anastomoses have been described in replantation surgery, afferent [15, 17–20] and efferent [14, 16].

Afferent arteriovenous anastomoses are so called because they carry arterial blood *towards* the replant. An afferent arteriovenous anastomosis is created when a proximal artery is connected to a vein distally (Fig. 16.6). The connection can be direct or via a vein graft. Afferent arteriovenous anastomoses are performed when conventional arterial anastomoses are unsuccessful, or when there is no artery in the amputated part suitable for conventional arterial anastomosis. Afferent arteriovenous anastomosis has been described

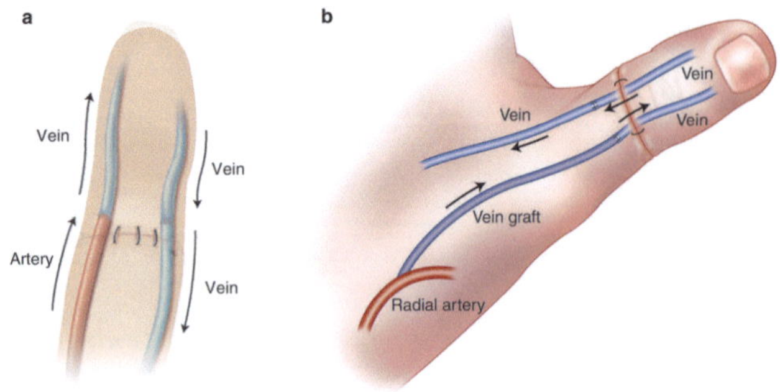

Fig. 16.6 (**a**) Afferent arteriovenous anastomosis. Arterial inflow is brought into the replant via a distal vein. Venous outflow is through a conventional venous anastomosis. (**b**) Another version of an afferent arteriovenous anastomosis, via a vein graft, bringing arterial blood from the radial artery to a dorsal vein on the replanted thumb. Venous drainage is again through conventional venous anastomosis

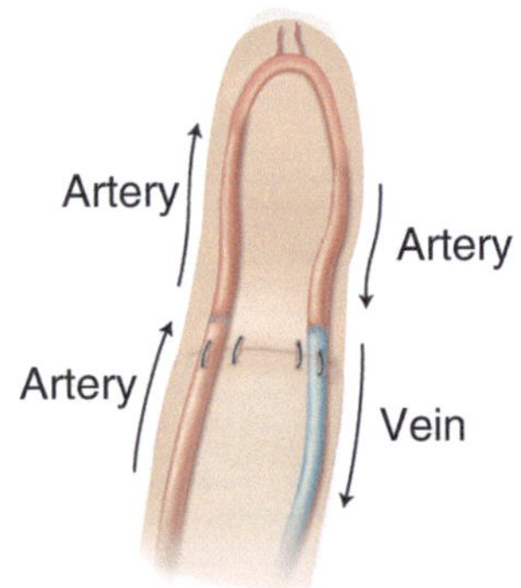

Fig. 16.7 An efferent arteriovenous anastomosis for venous outflow from the replant. Arterial inflow is via conventional arterial anastomosis

between volar digital artery to dorsal veins, volar digital artery to volar veins, and for the thumb, radial artery to dorsal vein via a long vein graft. At least one conventional venous anastomosis should be performed to allow blood outflow as afferent arteriovenous anastomoses are associated with significant venous congestion. If no venous anastomosis can be performed, postoperative bleeding using fishmouth incisions and/or leeches should be instituted. Replants salvaged with afferent arteriovenous anastomosis tend to suffer significant congestion with abnormal color for the first week with the color returning to normal by the end of the first or second week. Although none of the reported cases failed completely, seven of the ten reported cases had partial or superficial necrosis of the replant [15, 17, 18, 20–22].

An efferent arteriovenous anastomosis can be performed in the event that no veins can be identified in the replant. In such a situation, if the contralateral volar digital artery has excellent backflow, it can be anastomosed to a vein in the proximal segment, directly or via a vein graft (Fig. 16.7). Obviously, replants with an efferent arteriovenous anastomosis

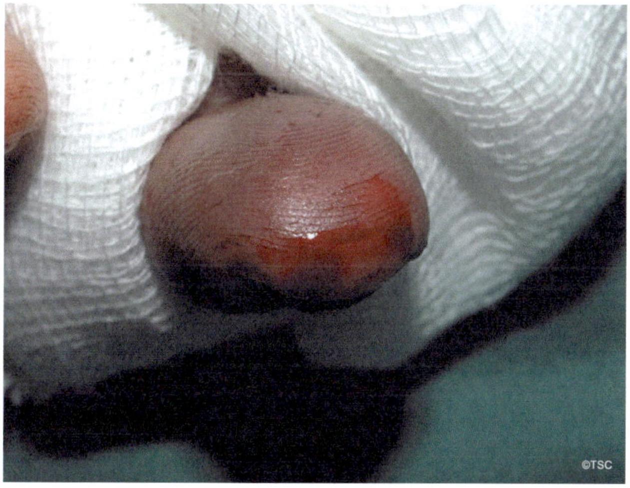

Fig. 16.8 Fish-mouth incision for postoperative bleeding to relieve venous congestion

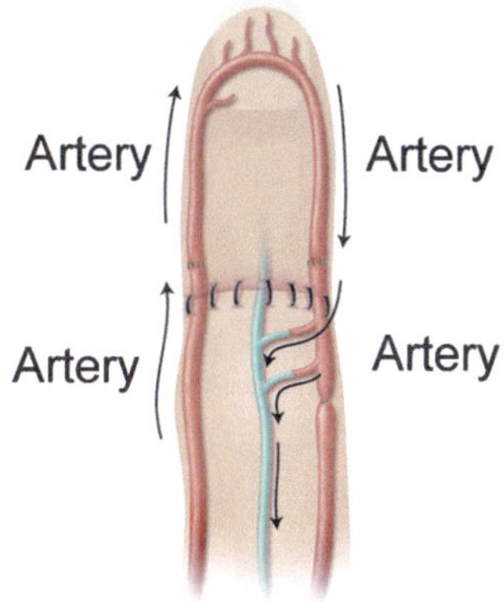

Fig. 16.9 Retrograde antegrade arterial drainage. In this schema, the larger digital artery is ligated proximally after completion of both arterial anastomoses. This converts the larger arterial into a conduit for return of blood from the replant. This is initially retrograde; subsequently, it enters the dorsal branches of the digital artery in an antegrade manner before draining into the dorsal venous system of the finger

should have at least one conventional arterial anastomosis for arterial inflow to the replant. Based on Suzuki's report of five successful cases, the efferent arteriovenous anastomosis appears to be a viable option to be considered if a venous-venous anastomosis is not possible [14]. Some early postoperative congestion was reported in Smith's series of three cases; otherwise, all the eight reported replants survived with no mention of any necrosis [14, 16].

Post-Op Bleeding

If no vascular anastomosis can be performed for venous drainage, the replant would then need to be bled in the postoperative period for 4–5 days through regular pin-pricks, milking of the replant [20], bleeding through a fish-mouth incision [20, 23, 24] (Fig. 16.8), leech therapy [25, 26], or chemical leech where heparin is injected subcutaneously into the replant [27]. If external bleeding is performed, care must be taken to monitor the patient's hemoglobin and vascular status.

Subcutaneous Pocketing

If it is a fingertip replantation and no vascular reconstruction is possible, one can consider removing the nail, deepithelializing the entire replant, and placing it in a subcutaneous pocket in the palm or in the abdomen for periods of 1–3 weeks [28–31]. Success rates ranging from 58% to more than 90% have been reported. One should make sure that the replant has been well debrided to avoid placing a potentially contaminated reattached amputate into the palm or abdomen.

Retrograde Antegrade Arterial Drainage

If both arteries can be repaired in a fingertip replantation, but no veins can be found, one option is to ligate the larger digital artery some distance proximal to the anastomosis to force it to function as a vein. Care must be taken to ensure that the dorsal branches of the larger artery are present and functioning distal to the ligation (Fig. 16.9). The idea behind this method is to stop the arterial inflow into the larger digital artery so that it now functions as an outflow conduit for arterial blood coming in from the contralateral smaller digital artery. Blood returning in the larger digital artery will then flow through it in a retrograde manner across the anastomosis proximal to the level of amputation. Here, it will flow in an antegrade manner into the dorsal arterial branches which will eventually drain into the venous system. Zhang et al. reported 96% success in his series of fingertip replantation using this method for venous reconstruction [32]. It appears that this concept for venous reconstruction may even be applied to more proximal digital replantations in the rare situations where no dorsal or volar veins are available for venous anastomoses.

Segmental Arterial Injury

If the arterial anastomosis is working well with sustained flow of blood across the anastomosis, but the replant is still not "pinking-up," one should exclude a more distal vascular injury. This situation is most likely to occur in avulsion or degloving type of injuries. If the intervening segment of artery is healthy and there is sufficient length after resection, the surgeon can perform a second primary anastomosis of that digital artery. However, it is more likely that the intervening vessel has some injury and there would be insufficient length to perform a second primary arterial anastomosis. In this situation, it would be prudent to take down the proximal anastomosis, remove the intervening arterial segment and replace it with a reversed interpositional vein graft from the original proximal anastomosis to the level of the second injury. The principle is to limit the number of anastomosis within the reconstructed digital artery to two.

If the segmental arterial injury of the digital artery is not reconstructable for any reason, the amputated part can be removed at this stage and a revision of amputation performed.

No-Reflow Phenomenon

A no-reflow phenomenon is due to failure of the distal microcirculation with intravascular aggregation and leakage, in conjunction with cellular swelling [33, 34]. It cannot be addressed by any microsurgical maneuver. It is characterized by the following:

1. Technically correct anastomosis
2. Healthy vessels the site of the anastomosis
3. No distal segmental injury
4. Good proximal-to-distal filling of artery 5–10 mm proximal and distal to anastomosis
5. Failure of the replant to "pink-up"

There are three options at this stage. The first is to remove the replant and perform a primary revision of amputation since the likelihood of replant survival is low. Another option is to keep the replant as it is, and monitor it postoperatively, while keeping the patient on antithrombotics and in a warm room. When the replant has demarcated, a secondary revision of amputation can then be performed.

The third option is experimental and involves the use of intra-arterial infusion of fibrinolytic agents to dissolve the microthrombi. The agents reportedly used include but are not limited to urokinase, tissue plasminogen activator, lidocaine, and/or enoxaparine [35–40]. These agents are often infused through a proximal large artery such as the radial artery. There are potential risks of bleeding, arterial injury, and anaphylactic reactions associated with the use of these agents. The surgeon has to weigh the risks against the benefits of the replant. The reader is advised to refer to the individual reports for details of usage.

Postoperative Failure of Replantation

The failure occurs when the patient has left the operating room and is either in recovery, or in the ward. A failure at this stage does not always require an immediate return to the operating room. This is because constrictive dressings or postoperative swelling of the replant are possible causes of failures. Before an order is issued for a return to the operating room, the replant should again be resuscitated. The chances of success of resuscitation are obviously higher if the failure is detected early. This is most likely if the replant is well monitored [41–43]. The postoperative resuscitation of replant can be divided in local and general maneuvers.

Postoperative Replant Resuscitation

General Maneuvers

The surgeon, in conjunction with the anesthetist, should check the following:

1. Patient is normovolemic and normotensive. Intravenous fluids may have to be increased.
2. Patient is not hypothermic. If so, the patient should be warmed with blankets or the room made warmer.
3. Patient is not in pain. If so, the anesthetist should administer appropriate parenteral analgesics.
4. Check that intravenous antithrombotics have been started and running at the appropriate rate.
5. Interscalene block is working and the infusion is running. If there is no interscalene block, consider having one inserted. This will help with pain control and reduce vasoconstriction from excessive sympathetic output [3].

Local Maneuvers

1. Local heat can be applied to the replant to encourage vasodilation. This can be in the form of a heat lamp (Fig. 16.10) or an ambient control device (Fig. 16.11).
2. The dressing should be checked. The dressing can be too tight and be a source of external compression on the replant and the vascular structures. This can be further exacerbated by postoperative swelling of the replant. Depending on the time interval from the replantation surgery, the dressing may be soaked or caked with blood. A blood soaked dressing will be heavy and be a source of compression too. A dressing caked with blood will be stiff and unaccommodating. Whatever the case may be, it is highly recommended that the dressing be removed as it can be difficult on inspection to exclude the above. If removal of the dressing alleviates the vascular problem, then a new dressing can be applied taking care to ensure that is not constricting.
3. Release of sutures. The mid-lateral incisions should never be sutured. If they have been sutured, they should be immediately released. Sutures along the transverse wounds should be inspected and if deemed to be a source of compression should also be released.
4. Venous failure. If the failure is due to a venous outflow problem, pulp massage in conjunction with elevation can be performed to increase the venous pressure head across the venous anastomosis. If this does not work, postoperative bleeding can be started using the methods previously mentioned under postoperative bleeding. Our first choice is elevation in conjunction with fish-mouth incision, topical heparin, hourly bleeding, and pulp massage. Leech therapy can be substituted for bleeding at a later stage.
5. Arterial failure. Proximal artery massage and putting the extremity in a more dependent position may be attempted.

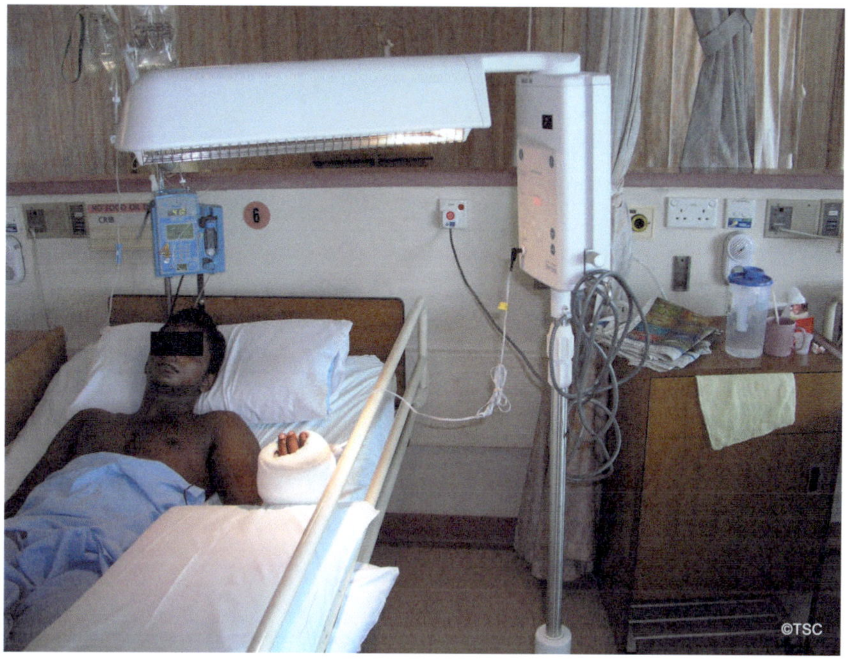

Fig. 16.10 Heat lamp keeping a replant of a finger warm. The heat dissipation is more diffused. In tropical climates, it can be uncomfortable for the patient

If the replant does not respond to the above replant resuscitation measures after 30 min to 2 h, the replant will require a return to the operating room for exploration as soon as possible. The need to explore may be more indicated if the replantation process was otherwise quite smooth and the failure was unexpected. It is recommended not to wait more than 6 h after replant failure to perform the exploration.

Exploration of Failed Replant

If an interscalene block is in place and working, general anesthesia may not be necessary and sedation may be all that is necessary [2]. A sterile arm tourniquet should be applied if the exploration is expected to take more than 4 h. This is to allow the surgeon to completely remove the tourniquet during the tourniquet rest-times without having to redrape the patient. This will ensure that there is no residual tourniquet effect after tourniquet deflation.

Sutures should be released and the skin flaps gently elevated. If there is excessive swelling of the replant, the surgeon should consider extending the mid-lateral incisions as releasing incisions to further relieve the compression. This should preferably be performed under magnification to avoid damaging the artery. Extension of mid-lateral incisions also has the additional benefit of affording better exposure of the vascular structures.

Depending on whether the failure is arterial, venous, or both, the anastomoses are checked in an appropriate sequence.

If there is thrombosis in the anastomosis, then it is likely a technical problem and the anastomosis will need to be revised. This involves taking down the anastomosis, resecting back to healthy vessel ends, making sure that there is adequate proximal pressure head and that the vessel lumens are clear, before performing the anastomosis. If there is inadequate vessel length for tension-free anastomosis, a reversed interpositional vein graft will be required. Consideration can also be given to performing additional bone shortening, or to look for an alternate proximal artery as discussed previously. Other options for venous reconstructions are as mentioned above and will include arteriovenous anastomosis, retrograde antegrade arterial drainage (RAAD), postoperative bleeding techniques, or subcutaneous pocketing. If it turns out to be a no-reflow phenomenon, the options are as previously discussed.

Revision Amputations and Beyond

Revision amputations are best performed primarily, as the emotional impact on the patient will be less. If a secondary revision amputation is performed, it is usually within the first week after the replant has declared and demarcated itself.

In general, for revision amputations, the bone should be shortened just sufficiently to allow tension-free closure of the skin flaps. For failed incomplete amputations, opportunistic use of fillet flaps should be considered as these can assist with skin coverage for revision amputations (Fig. 16.12). During revision amputations, care should be taken to section the digital nerves under distal traction so that the neuromas will form at a location proximal to the cutaneous scar (Fig. 16.13). There is experimental data that bipolar electrocautery applied to the transected end of the digital nerve may reduce the rate of neuromas formation [44].

For failed distal replantations with sufficient nail bed left, digit length and cosmesis can be preserved by performing

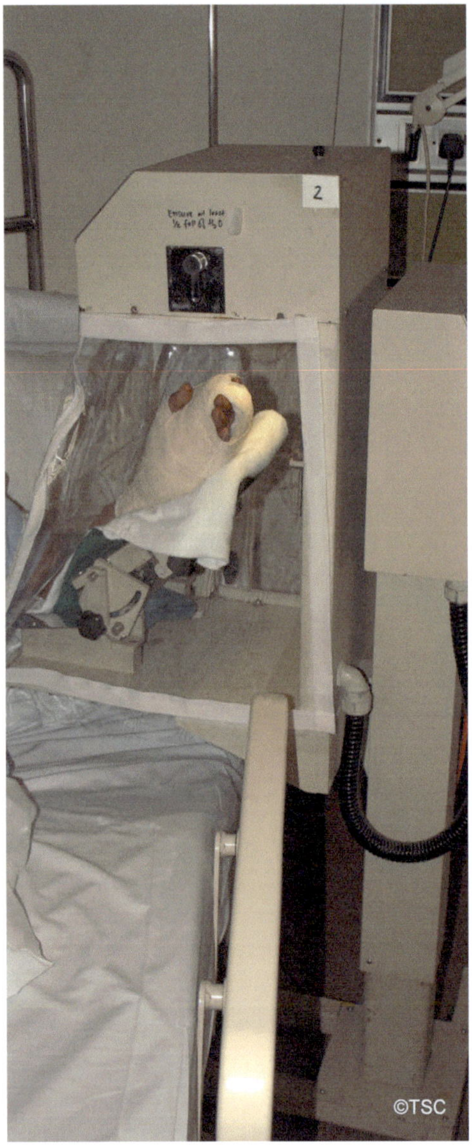

Fig. 16.11 Ambient control device. Only the patient's hand is kept within the device. The temperature and the amount of elevation of the hand can be adjusted. As the heat is kept within the device, patient comfort is greatly improved

some form of local flap coverage. This includes VY-plasty, cross-finger flaps, and thenar flaps. For failed amputations of the thumb distal to the interphalangeal joint, flap options to preserve thumb length are classically limited to sensory flaps such as Littler's neurovascular island flap [45], innervated cross-finger flap [46–49] and innervated first dorsal metacarpal artery flaps [50, 51]. Noninnervated flaps can also be used. The evidence does not appear to support the extra effort spent in performing an innervated flap. Most series report a return of two-point discrimination in the range of 5–9 mm for noninnervated flap transfers [52–55]. Options for noninnervated flaps include the traditional cross-finger flap, heterodigital arterialized flaps [56, 57], and first dorsal metacarpal artery flap.

For failed replantations distal to the distal interphalangeal joint with insufficient nail bed for finger tip preservation, we recommend that the revision amputation be performed at the level of the distal interphalangeal joint with care taken to rongeur off the volar and lateral condylar prominences so as to avoid having a finger tip with a "cobra-head" deformity (Fig. 16.14). Whatever remnant cartilage should be preserved, as it is believed to reduce inflammation [58]. The extensor and flexor tendon ends should be inspected and their cleanliness established. They should not be stitched together as this would limit finger flexion. The digital nerves should be managed in the same way as previously described. If there is insufficient skin cover, the amputation can be performed at the neck of the middle phalanx.

For failed replantations distal to the insertion of the flexor digitorum superficialis, the middle phalanx can be preserved. For failed replantations proximal to the insertion of the flexor digitorum superficialis, the remaining middle phalanx will have no active flexion control, and preservation becomes more of a cosmetic rather than a functional concern.

For failed replantations at the proximal phalanx level, the bone should be shortened sufficiently for skin closure. The remaining proximal phalanx will have active control through the intrinsic muscles of the hand.

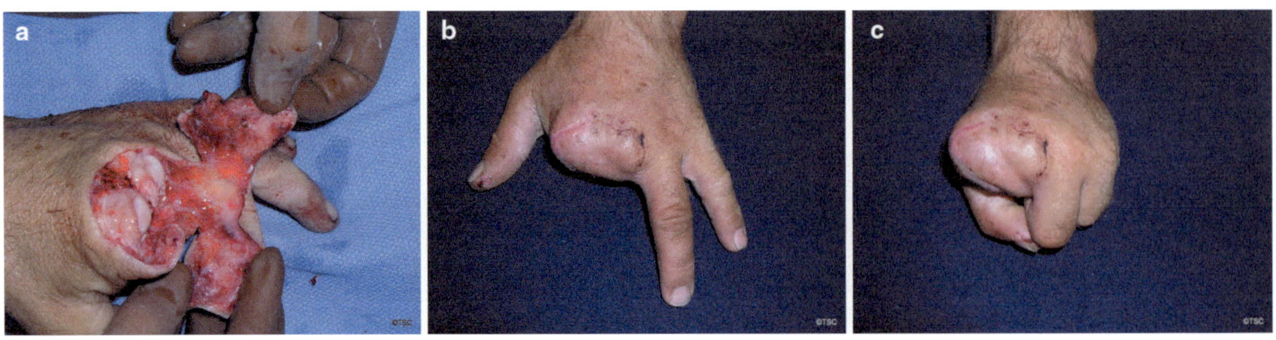

Fig. 16.12 (**a**) Fillet flap harvested from a mangling injury of the index and middle finger. (**b**) The eventual fillet flap required was smaller. It healed primarily and provided robust coverage of the amputation. (**c**) Functional outcome. Metacarpophalangeal disarticulation in this situation was better as it preserved hand span for a more stable grip

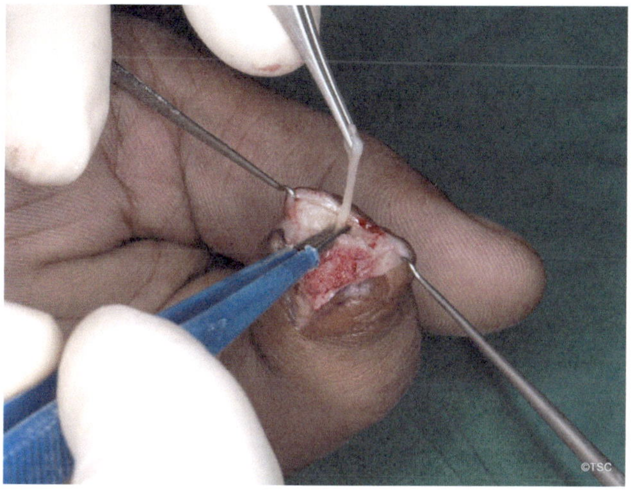

Fig. 16.13 The digital nerve while under traction, receives a 10 s duration of bipolar electrocautery at its base before the neurectomy is performed just distal to the segment of nerve cauterized

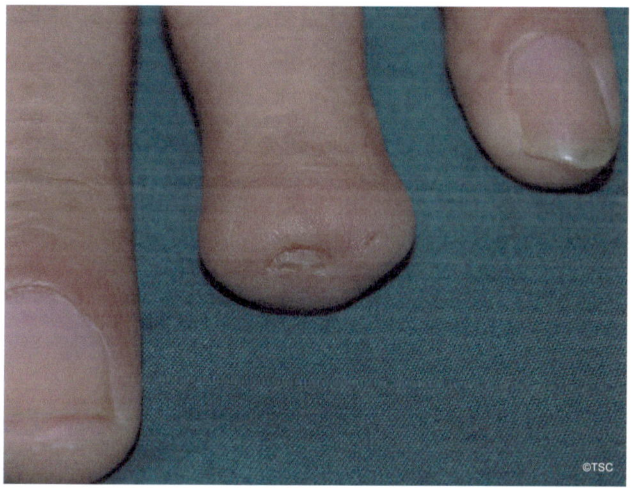

Fig. 16.14 Cobra-head deformity after terminalization or revision amputation at the distal interphalangeal level. This is due to failure to remove the lateral prominences of the condyles of the middle phalanx. Also note the remnant nail indicating incomplete removal of the germinal and sterile nail matrix

For failed replantations near or at the metacarpophalangeal joint, particularly for the middle and ring fingers, functional problems such as dropping small objects through the defect may occur. In these situations, one may have to consider prosthetic replacement or a more proximal ray amputation to close up the defect. For the border digits (namely, the index and little finger), consideration can be made to perform a disarticulation at the metacarpophalangeal joint instead of a ray amputation if it is felt that preservation of hand span for stability of grasp is more important.

For failed thumb amputations proximal to the interphalangeal joint, toe transfer procedures may be indicated [59, 60]. In such situations, care must be taken to preserve length in the bone, nerves, arteries, and tendons to facilitate the toe transfer procedure. Other options for thumb reconstruction include osteoplastic reconstruction, osteoplastic reconstruction in combination with toe transfer [61], and index finger pollicization [62–64].

For failed multiple finger replantation left with a metacarpal hand, various combinations of toe transfer procedures may be offered to reconstruct a hand with a chuck grip function. In such situations, if there is insufficient skin coverage, it is recommended that a pedicled groin flap be performed, instead of further skeletal shortening [59, 65–69].

Conclusion

The replantation surgeon must remember that replantation is a multistage sequential procedure. Although most surgeons fear the final stage of microsurgery, in reality, the success of replantation often rests on the successful performance of the first two stages which consists of adequate excisional debridement and adequate bone shortening and fixation.

Replantation failures can occur intraoperatively or postoperatively. In both instances, the replant can be resuscitated with a combination of local and general maneuvers which are largely nonsurgical.

Surgical options for failed replantation are as follows:

1. Revision of anastomoses.
2. Exploration.
3. Reversed interpositional vein grafts.
4. Proximal or heterodigital arterial transfer.
5. Further bone shortening.
6. RAAD.
7. Arteriovenous anastomosis.
8. Postoperative bleeding techniques.
9. Subcutaneous pocketing techniques.
10. Experimental techniques, such as intra-arterial fibrinolytics.
11. Revision amputations—primary or secondary.
12. Reconstructive options with local or regional flap coverage, osteoplastic thumb reconstructions, pollicizations, and various toe transfer techniques.

References

1. Waikakul S, Sakkarnkosol S, Vanadurongwan V, Un-nanuntana A. Results of 1018 digital replantations in 552 patients. Injury. 2000; 31(1):33–40.
2. Matsuda M, Kato N, Hosoi M. Continuous brachial plexus block for replantation in the upper extremity. Hand. 1982;14(2):129–34.
3. Berger A, Tizian C, Zenz M. Continuous plexus blockade for improved circulation in microvascular surgery. Ann Plast Surg. 1985;14(1):16–9.
4. Conrad MH, Adams WP. Pharmacologic optimization of microsurgery in the new millennium. Plast Reconstr Surg. 2001;108(7): 2088–96; quiz 2097.

5. Swartz WM, Brink RR, Buncke HJ. Prevention of thrombosis in arterial and venous microanastomoses by using topical agents. Plast Reconstr Surg. 1976;58(4):478–81.
6. Wong M, Kiat DTM, Sebastin SJ, Tan TC, Peng YP. Heterodigital vascular island flap for simultaneous resurfacing and revascularization of digits. Ann Plast Surg. 2009;62(1):34–7.
7. Wong CH, Teoh LC, Lee JYL, Yam AKT, Khoo DBA, Yong FC. Free digital artery flap: an ideal flap for large finger defects in situations where local flaps are precluded. Ann Plast Surg. 2008;60(3): 254–9.
8. Koch H, Moshammer H, Spendel S, Pierer G, Scharnagl E. Wrap-around arterialized venous flap for salvage of an avulsed finger. J Reconstr Microsurg. 1999;15(5):347–50.
9. George P, Dejesus RA. Venous flow-through flap reconstruction following severe finger wound infection: case report. J Reconstr Microsurg. 2009;25(4):267–9.
10. Inoue G, Maeda N, Suzuki K. Resurfacing of skin defects of the hand using the arterialised venous flap. Br J Plast Surg. 1990;43(2):135–9.
11. Adani R, Castagnetti C, Busa R, Caroli A. Transfer of vessels in the management of thumb and ring avulsion injuries. Ann Acad Med Singapore. 1995;24(4 Suppl):51–7.
12. LeBlanc R, Bindra R. Ipsilateral heterodigital artery transfer for finger revascularization. Tech Hand Up Extrem Surg. 2008;12(3):180–2.
13. Cao X, Cai J, Liu W. Avulsive amputations of the thumb: comparison of replantation techniques. Microsurgery. 1996;17(1):17–20.
14. Suzuki Y, Ishikawa K, Isshiki N, Takami S. Fingertip replantation with an efferent A-V anastomosis for venous drainage: clinical reports. Br J Plast Surg. 1993;46(3):187–91.
15. Inoue G, Tamura Y. The use of an afferent arteriovenous fistula in digit replantation surgery: a report of two cases. Br J Plast Surg. 1991;44(3):230–3.
16. Smith AR, Sonneveld GJ, van der Meulen JC. AV anastomosis as a solution for absent venous drainage in replantation surgery. Plast Reconstr Surg. 1983;71(4):525–32.
17. Chen KT, Chen YC, Mardini S, Wei FC. Salvage of an avulsion amputated thumb at the interphalangeal joint level using afferent arteriovenous shunting. Br J Plast Surg. 2005;58(6):869–72.
18. Fukui A, Maeda M, Inada Y, Tamai S, Sempuku T. Arteriovenous shunt in digit replantation. J Hand Surg Am. 1990;15(1):160–5.
19. Koshima I, Soeda S, Moriguchi T, Higaki H, Miyakawa S, Yamasaki M. The use of arteriovenous anastomosis for replantation of the distal phalanx of the fingers. Plast Reconstr Surg. 1992;89(4): 710–4.
20. Yabe T, Muraoka M, Motomura H, Ozawa T. Fingertip replantation using a single volar arteriovenous anastomosis and drainage with a transverse tip incision. J Hand Surg Am. 2001;26(6):1120–4.
21. Germann G, Raff T, Schepler H, Wittemann M. Salvage of an avascular thumb by arteriovenous flow reversal and a microvascular "kite" flap: case report. J Reconstr Microsurg. 1997;13(4):291–5.
22. Theile DR, Berger AC, Wilson YT, Tham SK. Afferent arteriovenous anastomosis for thumb replantation: a case report. Microsurgery. 1994;15(11):808–10.
23. Yamano Y. Replantation of the amputated distal part of the fingers. J Hand Surg Am. 1985;10(2):211–8.
24. Sadahiro T. A fish mouth incision for congestion in replantation of the amputated finger experimental and clinical studies (author's transl). Nihon Seikeigeka Gakkai Zasshi. 1979;53(4):411–28.
25. Golden MA, Quinn JJ, Partington MT. Leech therapy in digital replantation. AORN J. 1995;62(3):364–6. 369, 371.
26. Whitlock MR, O'Hare PM, Sanders R, Morrow NC. The medicinal leech and its use in plastic surgery: a possible cause for infection. Br J Plast Surg. 1983;36(2):240–4.
27. Barnett GR, Taylor GI, Mutimer KL. The "chemical leech": intra-replant subcutaneous heparin as an alternative to venous anastomosis. Report of three cases. Br J Plast Surg. 1989;42(5):556–8.
28. Sawabe K, Suzuki S, Miyata A, Kitayama T, Ishikawa K. Application of the palmar pocket method for total nail reconstruction without vascular anastomoses. Ann Plast Surg. 2005;54(6):673–5.
29. Arata J, Ishikawa K, Soeda H, Sawabe K, Kokoroishi R, Togo T. The palmar pocket method: an adjunct to the management of zone I and II fingertip amputations. J Hand Surg Am. 2001;26(5):945–50.
30. Lin TS, Jeng SF, Chiang YC. Fingertip replantation using the subdermal pocket procedure. Plast Reconstr Surg. 2004;113(1):247–53.
31. Kim KS, Eo SR, Kim DY, Lee SY, Cho BH. A new strategy of fingertip reattachment: sequential use of microsurgical technique and pocketing of composite graft. Plast Reconstr Surg. 2001;107(1):73–9.
32. Zhang X, Wen S, Wang B, Wang Q, Li C, Zhu H. Reconstruction of circulation in the fingertip without vein repair in zone I replantation. J Hand Surg Am. 2008;33(9):1597–601.
33. May JW, Chait LA, O'Brien BM, Hurley JV. The no-reflow phenomenon in experimental free flaps. Plast Reconstr Surg. 1978;61(2): 256–67.
34. Urbaniak JR, Seaber AV, Chen LE. Assessment of ischemia and reperfusion injury. Clin Orthop Relat Res. 1997;334:30–6.
35. Hashim HA, Atiyeh BS, Hamdan AM, Musharrafieh RS. Local intravenous thrombolysis with recombinant tissue plasminogen activator for salvage of forearm replantation. J Reconstr Microsurg. 1996;12(8):543–6.
36. Stassen JM, Lü G, Andréen O, Nyström E, Nyström A. Intraoperative thrombolytic treatment of microarterial occlusion by selective rt-PA infusion. Plast Reconstr Surg. 1995;96(5):1215–7.
37. Krapohl BD, Siemionow M, Zins JE. Effect of tissue-plasminogen activator on leukocyte-endothelial interactions at the microcirculatory level. Plast Reconstr Surg. 1998;102(7):2388–94.
38. Atiyeh BS, Hashim HA, Hamdan AM, Musharafieh RS. Local recombinant tissue plasminogen activator (rt-PA) thrombolytic therapy in microvascular surgery. Microsurgery. 1999;19(6):265–71.
39. Huang CT, Li JK, Zhu JK, Lu XQ, Li QY. High-dose urokinase for thrombolysis following replantation of severed limbs or fingers. Di Yi Jun Yi Da Xue Xue Bao. 2004;24(12):1431–4.
40. Oufquir A, Bakhach J, Panconi B, Guimberteau JC, Baudet J. Salvage of digits replantations by direct arterial antithrombotic infusion. Ann Chir Plast Esthet. 2006;51(6):471–81.
41. Kiyoshige Y, Tsuchida H, Watanabe Y. Color monitoring after replantation. Plast Reconstr Surg. 1996;97(2):463–8.
42. Bakri K, Moran SL. Monitoring for upper-extremity free flaps and replantations. J Hand Surg Am. 2008;33(10):1905–8.
43. Ruopsa N, Kujala S, Kaarela O, Ohtonen P, Ryhanen J. Wireless infrared thermometer in the follow-up of finger temperatures. J Hand Surg Eur Vol. 2009;34(4):526–9.
44. Tay SC, Teoh LC, Yong FC, Tan SH. The prevention of neuroma formation by diathermy: an experimental study in the rat common peroneal nerve. Ann Acad Med Singapore. 2005;34(5):362–8.
45. Littler JW. The neurovascular pedicle method of digital transposition for reconstruction of the thumb. Plast Reconstr Surg. 1953;12(5):303–19.
46. Cohen BE, Cronin ED. An innervated cross-finger flap for fingertip reconstruction. Plast Reconstr Surg. 1983;72(5):688–97.
47. Gaul JS. Radial-innervated cross-finger flap from index to provide sensory pulp to injured thumb. J Bone Joint Surg Am. 1969; 51(7):1257–63.
48. Cohen BE. Innervated cross-finger flap. Plast Reconstr Surg. 1984;73(5):859.
49. Hastings H. Dual innervated index to thumb cross finger or island flap reconstruction. Microsurgery. 1987;8(3):168–72.
50. Muyldermans T, Hierner R. First dorsal metacarpal artery flap for thumb reconstruction: a retrospective clinical study. Strategies Trauma Limb Reconstr. 2009;4(1):27–33.
51. Tränkle M, Sauerbier M, Heitmann C, Germann G. Restoration of thumb sensibility with the innervated first dorsal metacarpal artery island flap. J Hand Surg Am. 2003;28(5):758–66.

52. Woon CYL, Lee JYL, Teoh LC. Resurfacing hemipulp losses of the thumb: the cross finger flap revisited: indications, technical refinements, outcomes, and long term neurosensory recovery. Ann Plast Surg. 2008;61(4):385–91.
53. Nicolai JP, Hentenaar G. Two-point discrimination in cross-finger flaps. Handchir Mikrochir Plast Chir. 1983;15(4):241–4.
54. Nicolai JP, Hentenaar G. Sensation in cross-finger flaps. Hand. 1981;13(1):12–6.
55. Nishikawa H, Smith PJ. The recovery of sensation and function after cross-finger flaps for fingertip injury. J Hand Surg Br. 1992;17(1):102–7.
56. Tay SC, Teoh LC, Tan SH, Yong FC. Extending the reach of the heterodigital arterialized flap by vein division and repair. Plast Reconstr Surg. 2004;114(6):1450–6.
57. Teoh LC, Tay SC, Yong FC, Tan SH, Khoo DBA. Heterodigital arterialized flaps for large finger wounds: results and indications. Plast Reconstr Surg. 2003;111(6):1905–13.
58. Whitaker LA, Graham WP, Riser WH, Kilgore E. Retaining the articular cartilage in finger joint amputations. Plast Reconstr Surg. 1972;49(5):542–7.
59. Coskunfirat OK, Wei FC, Lin CH, Chen HC, Lin YT. Simultaneous double second toe transfer for reconstruction of adjacent fingers. Plast Reconstr Surg. 2005;115(4):1064–9.
60. Wei FC, Chen HC, Chuang CC, Chen SH. Microsurgical thumb reconstruction with toe transfer: selection of various techniques. Plast Reconstr Surg. 1994;93(2):345-51; discussion 352.
61. Lin CH, Mardini S, Lin YT, Lin CH, Chen CT, Wei FC. Osteoplastic thumb ray restoration with or without secondary toe transfer for reconstruction of opposable basic hand function. Plast Reconstr Surg. 2008;121(4):1288–97.
62. Muzaffar AR, Chao JJ, Friedrich JB. Posttraumatic thumb reconstruction. Plast Reconstr Surg. 2005;116(5):103e–22.
63. Ishida O, Taniguchi Y, Sunagawa T, Suzuki O, Ochi M. Pollicization of the index finger for traumatic thumb amputation. Plast Reconstr Surg. 2006;117(3):909–14.
64. Lister G. The choice of procedure following thumb amputation. Clin Orthop Relat Res. 1985;195:45–51.
65. Wei FC, el-Gammal TA, Lin CH, Chuang CC, Chen HC, Chen SH. Metacarpal hand: classification and guidelines for microsurgical reconstruction with toe transfers. Plast Reconstr Surg. 1997; 99(1):122–8.
66. Ma HS, Abdalla el-Gammal T, Wei FC. Current concepts of toe-to-hand transfer: surgery and rehabilitation. J Hand Ther. 1996;9(1):41–6.
67. Wei FC, el-Gammal TA. Toe-to-hand transfer. Current concepts, techniques, and research. Clin Plast Surg. 1996;23(1):103–16.
68. Wei FC, Yim KK. Single third-toe transfer in hand reconstruction. J Hand Surg Am. 1995;20(3):388–94; discussion 395.
69. Tsai TM, Jupiter JB, Wolff TW, Atasoy E. Reconstruction of severe transmetacarpal mutilating hand injuries by combined second and third toe transfer. J Hand Surg Am. 1981;6(4): 319–28.

Reoperative Issues Following Upper Extremity Injuries

17

George S.M. Dyer and David Ring

Abstract

This chapter presents some interesting cases encompassing some of the psychosocial aspects regarding reoperative surgery, specifically in the traumatic situation. As reviewed in the first chapter, reoperative surgery does require more counseling, time, and patience in explaining and discussing options with the injured patient. This chapter, in developing some cases, allows the reader to understand more fully some of the personal issues affecting these patients; and how in some cases further surgery or reoperative surgery may not be in the patient's best interest. This chapter serves to hopefully further hone the reoperative surgeon's judgment skills in discerning who may and may not benefit from more surgery.

Keywords

Mangled • Extremity • Expectations • Surgical • Social

Introduction

Some of the most difficult challenges a surgeon can face are those presented by the patient who has had previous surgery that failed:

- The previous surgery may have "used up" the best surgical option for a given problem—the most appropriate donor tendon, the chance for optimal fixation in virgin bone, or simply an unscarred field through which to make a surgical approach.
- The patient is disappointed in the result of their last operation and may even have been made worse by it.
- The patient has already endured pain, as well as tangible and intangible losses from not having used the limb. They are likely to approach another surgery with some degree of fear and mistrust.

Despite these challenges reoperative surgery on the upper limb can be extremely rewarding. The keys to success are to listen carefully to the patient's hopes and expectations regarding outcome, to be humble and honest in counseling the patient on what is possible to do, and to carefully plan an efficient operation or series of operations that will/may achieve the patient's realistic goals.

Patient Evaluation, Counseling, and Operative Planning

Patient evaluation begins with understanding the history of the patient's injury or condition, and the previous intervention. Take a methodical history including all that you can learn about the patient's status and function *before* their injury, and also before their intervention (or before each intervention if there have been several). A time-worn axiom bears repeating: you are unlikely to make a patient better than their age, general fitness and life circumstances had left them before the saga of their current condition began.

G.S.M. Dyer, MD
Department of Orthopedic Surgery, Harvard Medical School and Brigham and Women's Hospital,
Boston, MA, USA

D. Ring, MD, PhD (✉)
Massachusetts General Hospital, Yawkey 2100, 32 Fruit Street,
Boston, MA 02114, USA
e-mail: Dring@partners.org

S.F.M. Duncan (ed.), *Reoperative Hand Surgery*,
DOI 10.1007/978-1-4614-2373-7_17, © Springer Science+Business Media, LLC 2012

Next is understanding in detail the patient's current status. Are they able to work? If not at their customary profession then can they work at all? Is the limb in question the primary reason for not working or are there other factors? Although there is good evidence that attitudes toward work and whether the patient blames his job for his injury are predictors of return to work [1], it is also clear that factors such as good counseling regarding outcomes can speed return to work [2]. Issues of litigation and secondary gain may have less influence over return to work than is sometimes thought [3].

Ask about pain, motion, and limits to activities of daily living. How about leisure activity? Everything from loss of manual hobbies to sexual dysfunction is linked to limitation of hand use [4]. A detailed physical exam is useful, including sensory and motor function, joint motion and stability, vascularity, as well as tenderness and visual deformity. Children born with congenital differences can be comfortable with their appearance. But for adults, who consider themselves disfigured by an injury or condition, do not underestimate the importance of how the limb *looks* in determining the patient's overall acceptance of it.

Understand Expectations

It is important to understand the patient's expectations. How will they appraise the result? In parallel, the surgeon should be realistic with his or her own expectations and promises to the patient. It can be helpful to ask the patient to list what they hope for in terms of outcome in very specific terms. For example if they cite a hobby, activity of daily living, or work function they would like to resume, try to break that activity down into its component parts to clarify and specify the improvements that will be necessary to do it. Distinguish impairment from disability and identify any psychological barriers to accomplishing specific tasks that should be possible based on the given disease and objective impairment. Develop and discuss a realistic, achievable plan for meeting the patient's expectations, given the realities of their history and current status.

The results of reoperative hand surgery are best when there is a shortcoming of diagnosis or treatment that is amendable to treatment. Such shortcomings are an unavoidable aspect of the practice of medicine; they are experienced by the most careful surgeons and the most thoughtful patients. In hand surgery, the more discrete the problem, and the more predictable the surgical treatment, the better the results. The patient and surgeon each need to weigh the likelihood of benefit against the likelihood of harm and make a shared decision regarding whether to operate again.

Here is another way to conceptualize the elements of this tradeoff. Much as a surgeon can calculate a Mangled Extremity Severity Score (MESS) [5], as a combination of soft tissue and other elements of the injury, it is possible to imagine a similar construct when considering a repeat or revision operation. The concept of a "Reoperative Extremity Severity Score," although not designed for quantitative use or as a threshold, may help frame the elements of an informative discussion with the patient.

Reoperative Extremity Severity Score

Technical Feasibility of Surgical Correction

- Minor abnormality (e.g., simple scar contracture amenable to z-plasty, straightforward malunion)
- Moderate abnormality (more than one original injury, significant downstream effects of simple original problem)
- Major abnormality (multiple muscle groups or skeletal elements affected)
- Severe abnormality (e.g., multiple nerve palsies, no donors for transfer, or large-volume bone loss)

Complicating Factors

- Minor previous complications (e.g., resolved prior infection)
- Moderate (e.g., wound infection, transient nerve palsy)
- Major (e.g., active deep infection, recalcitrant CRPS, permanent nerve injury)

Patient Psychosocial Barriers

- Psychological appropriate distress (depression/anxiety) expected with disease/impairment
- Exaggerated fears, denial, recrimination
- Grossly inappropriate understanding (e.g., pain catastrophizing, heightened illness concerns, pain medication addiction)
- Organic mental illness (psychotic disorder, e.g., schizophrenia)

Patient Circumstance Assets/Liabilities

- Good personal support network, clear understanding of risks and benefits, self-efficacy, adaptive/resilient, motivated/determined. Likely able to persist with difficult or lengthy rehab
- Adequate understanding but will require significant external support to complete rehab and recovery (e.g., needs rides to rehab, perfect compliance is possible but unlikely)
- Poorly equipped to manage recovery (personally isolated, has another major illness or a chemical addiction)
- Major barrier to recovery (e.g., homelessness)

Each domain includes a spectrum from mild to more severe involvement. This framework may also help to weight the intangible aspects against the concrete ones.

Patient Examples

These example patients are intended to provide discussion points for how reoperative hand surgery might be approached. They were selected to encompass several important areas of surgical planning: deficits of bone length, loss of articular surfaces, recalcitrant nonunion, stiffness, instability, and soft tissue coverage. These are not intended as "how-to" guides for specific patient management. We intend to emphasize the preoperative discussion of options with the patient, and aspects of the operative and postoperative management.

Patient 1

A 24-year-old man presented 2 years after a high-energy fall to an outstretched hand during military service that resulted in a displaced fracture of the waist of the scaphoid. The initial treatment was reduction and percutaneous screw fixation, performed at another facility. After a period of 6 months, he presented to a second surgeon with a clearly established nonunion without apparent avascular necrosis of the proximal pole fragment. According to that surgeon's notes and records, some flexion deformity was seen in the scaphoid but the joint surfaces remained well preserved and so that surgeon elected to attempt a nonunion repair using a dorsal vascularized bone graft based on the 1,2 intercompartmental supraretinacular artery and revision screw fixation. That operation failed to achieve union.

At the time of presentation to one of us he was 26 and he had been disabled from work by wrist pain for 4 years. Although there were slight early signs of arthrosis in the scaphoid facet of the radius and in the scaphoid itself, the lunate facet and the proximal capitate were both well preserved. His objective for this surgery was to be free of pain and to be able to resume work as a computer technician. His greatest concern was that he might require more operations or procedures. He was on his third doctor, due to circumstances rather than doctor shopping.

We discussed additional surgery to try to maintain the anatomy of the wrist by gaining union of the scaphoid as well as salvage procedures to reconstruct the wrist. This patient had a humpback deformity and two prior unsuccessful surgeries. Continuing to seek union seemed inconsistent with his stated goal of "being done having operations on this wrist." Since the lunate, the capitate, and the lunate facet of the radius were all well preserved, the salvage options included proximal row carpectomy or a partial carpal arthrodesis. While both types of procedures are reported to have reasonable results, intercarpal arthrodesis is associated with more short-term complications because of the requirement for implants or wires, and a risk of nonunion.

The surgeon and patient discussed the advantages and disadvantages of these options in detail. A shared decision was made to proceed with proximal row carpectomy.

He was last seen 1 year after surgery. He had returned to work. He was pleased with his pain relief. The surgery met his expectations and achieved his goals for "being done with operations on the wrist." On the other hand his motion was worse than he had hoped it would be—only about 40% of normal.

Patient 2

A 43-year-old man presented 1 year after an injury working at home on a craft project with a table saw when all five digits of his left hand were injured. He had dorsal combined injuries (skin, extensor tendon, bone and joint) to the index through small finger at the level of the proximal interphalangeal joints and a thumb tip injury. All the fingers had at least one intact artery, the flexor tendons were intact, and only the ring finger had nerve injuries. Initial management was staged, culminating in arthrodesis of the proximal interphalangeal joint of the long finger. The index proximal interphalangeal joint has minimal motion and advanced arthrosis.

Nine months after injury, his goal was to improve writing with his left hand. He thought he might be able to write better if he had more flexion at his index and long finger PIP joints. During recovery he had learned to write with his right, nondominant hand, but he found it inadequate for his work as a technical consultant. He felt that even a 20° arc of motion would improve his function.

In a series of three scheduled appointments over a 5-month period, we discussed at length the options for reconstructing his hand his proximal interphalangeal joints: including autogenous articular grafting, free tissue transfer such as a vascularized toe, or prosthetic arthroplasty. Autogenous hemi-hamate autograft was less appropriate in this case because of the extent of bone loss. Autograft joint transfers or vascular transfer of the PIP joint of a toe to a finger was distasteful and did not appeal to the patient because of donor-site morbidity. Arthroplasty with silicone spacer implants or resurfacing implants such as the pyrolytic carbon implant generally achieves good pain relief but only minimal improvement in motion. The long-term problems with these implants are not well understood.

On balance it appeared a takedown of the long finger PIP fusion and PIP arthroplasty in that joint would yield the most functional improvement and was the only option acceptable to the patient that might achieve his goal of slight additional motion. A simple summary of the data above was discussed in detail. He understood that this would be a less certain procedure than arthroplasty of the index PIP for

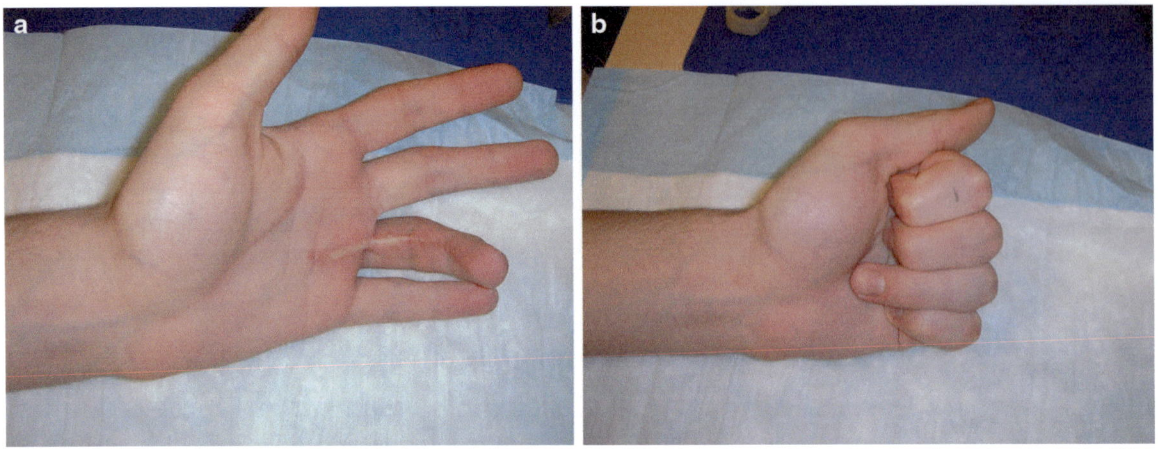

Fig. 17.1 A 16-year-old young man presented with his mother after operative repair of a jersey finger (FDP avulsion to the ring). (**a**) He has scar contractures of the MP and PIP joints. (**b**) And no active DIP flexion

posttraumatic arthritis [6]. He was reluctant to have a silicone arthroplasty out of concern it would fracture and require eventual revision [7]. A shared decision was made to proceed with pyrocarbon implant arthroplasty of the PIP joints of the index finger to relieve pain and the long finger to improve motion.

He elected to proceed with the surgery and regained a 20° arc of motion in his long finger that he felt greatly improved his writing, and substantial pain relief in the index finger. He was highly satisfied with his outcome.

Patient 3

A 16-year-old young man presented with his mother for evaluation of his right dominant ring finger. Two months prior to presentation, he underwent operative treatment for FDP avulsion sustained in a football game via the classic "jersey finger" mechanism. Trying to tackle another player he had grabbed the jersey and felt a pop as the player pulled away.

His presenting complaint was of MP, PIP, and DIP flexion contractures as well as absent flexion of the DIP. On examination he had a longitudinal incision with scar thickness and resultant flexion contractures (Fig. 17.1). He has normal FDS function and no FDP function.

On the one hand, there is good news, given that the flexion contractures are easily addressed with z-plasties. It feels good for both patient and surgeon that another operation can be offered with a high probability of improving the finger with limited and acceptable risks and a quick recovery period.

On the other hand, the jersey finger—a difficult problem in general—is probably best considered a lost cause. The surgeon and the family must therefore accept the situation, and accept the fact that the patient had two surgeries and ended up no better than had he declined the initial surgery. These are delicate issues and dealing with any bitterness, denial, or unrealistic expectations can be challenging and stressful.

Fortunately, this patient and his mother were appreciative that predictable improvement was offered, understanding of the difficulties involved and the beneficence of his caretakers, and prepared to accept his situation. The z-plasties were straightforward, produced a straight finger with no DIP flexion and full PIP and MP motion, and the patient and his mother were satisfied.

Patient 4

A 38-year-old woman fractured her right dominant distal radius in a fall bicycling. She had open reduction and internal fixation with a volar locking plate. She regained good finger and forearm motion, but the plate was bothersome to her. It was decided to remove the plate 2 months after the original surgery. It turned out that the fracture was not completely healed. The fracture had shortened and was angulated volarly (Fig. 17.2).

She presented with her wrist supported in a splint. Out of the splint there was an obvious deformity of the wrist. The incision was well healed. There were no nerve problems and the fingers were not stiff.

In this case, the obvious solution was to reapply the plate. The key points of discussion were the need to keep the plate in place for a minimum of 1 year, and the possible need for an osteotomy if the bone was healed, or bone graft if it was not. There was a high probability of success with reoperation, but the key point was to prepare the patient for the difficulties of the recovery period—the need to keep the plate in most importantly.

She elected to proceed and accepted the need to keep the plate in for at least a year no matter what. At surgery there

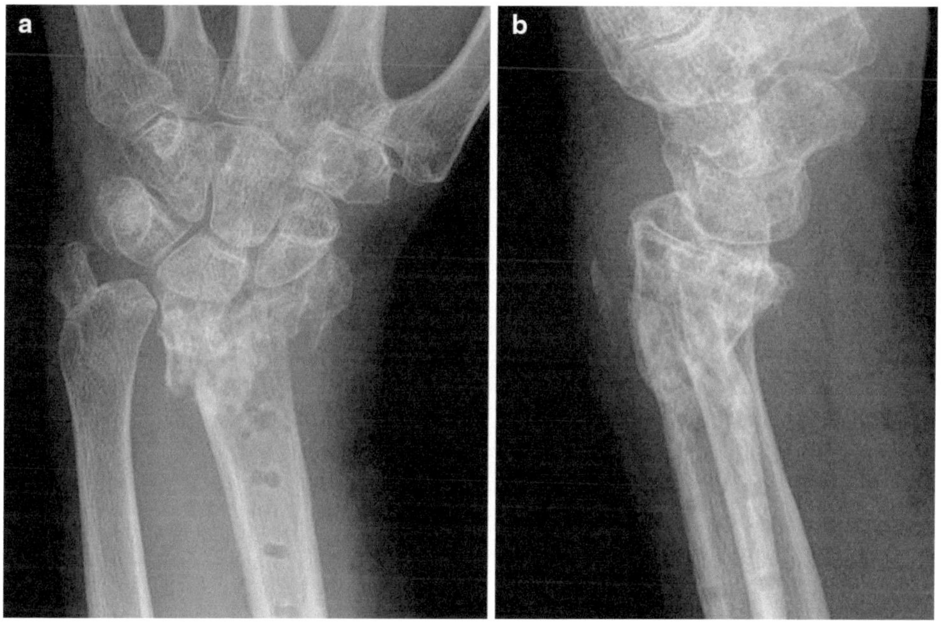

Fig. 17.2 (**a**, **b**) Posteroanterior and lateral radiographs 1 month after plate removal show a volar mal/nonunion of the distal radius

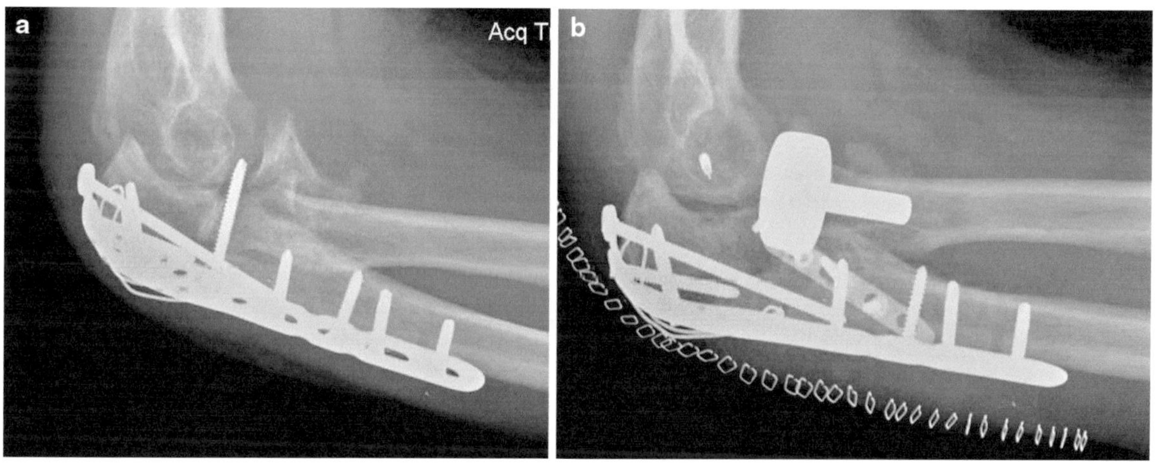

Fig. 17.3 A 60-year-old man had a fracture-dislocation of the elbow. (**a**) After two surgeries elsewhere he still had subluxation of the elbow. (**b**) Reconstruction consisting of reduction and fixation of the coronoid, replacement of the radial head, and reattachment of the lateral soft tissues restored alignment, but this surgery was complicated by infection

was a malunion. Osteotomy and plate application restored good alignment. One year after the fracture, she has a healed fracture with good alignment, full digit and forearm motion, and two-thirds normal wrist flexion and extension.

Patient 5

A 60-year-old healthy male presented 4 weeks after a fall from a standing height. He had a posterior olecranon fracture-dislocation involving fractures of the radial head and coronoid process. The elbow remained unstable after the first surgery, prompting a second surgery. On presentation to the second surgeon, he had persistent subluxation, and loss of fixation of the coronoid process (Fig. 17.3a).

The patient was understandably frustrated and pessimistic. This had been particularly difficult on top of his baseline anxiety and depression. Fortunately, he understood the complexity of his injury and appreciated the efforts of the other treatment team on his behalf. He was resigned to additional surgery, primarily because he is healthy and active and desires optimal elbow function.

For the second surgeon, the difficulty is not only stepping into a frustrating and suboptimal evolution, and adopting the care of an injury that would lead to severe elbow impairment even under optimal circumstances, but also the fact that multiple operations this early after injury are associated with increased risks of infection, wound problems, and heterotopic ossification, not to mention the fact that scarring, prior fixation, loose fixation, and other aspects of prior surgery will increase the difficulty and the risks of a second surgery.

There were felt to be good targets for improving the status of this elbow including replacement of the radial head to restore radiocapitellar contact, reattachment of the origin of the lateral collateral ligament and the common wrist and digital extensors to the lateral epicondyle, and, most importantly, improved fixation of the large coronoid fracture with a medial plate and screws. The risks of infection, wound problems, heterotopic bone, and failure to achieve these goals were outlined in detail. In addition, a new medial dissection in a scarred field would place the ulnar nerve at substantial risk. Consent was obtained for external fixation, with attendant risks such as radial nerve palsy. The risks of not operating were also reviewed, and the patient and surgeon both felt that reoperation was the best option in spite of the risks and complexity involved.

At surgery, no infection was encountered and the original olecranon plate was adequate and not loose. The fractured radial head was resected and replaced with a metal prosthesis. The origins of the LCL and the common wrist and digital extensors were reattached to the lateral epicondyle with suture anchors. The ulnar nerve was transposed, and a medial plate and screws were applied to the medial aspect of the coronoid using the split between the flexor carpi ulnaris for access. The elbow was stable and no external fixation, pinning, or immobilization of the elbow was needed (Fig. 17.3b).

Active-assisted exercises of the fingers, forearm, and elbow were initiated within a few days. Shoulder abduction (varus stress) was avoided. The reduction remained concentric on control radiographs.

Two weeks after surgery, the wound continued to drain non-purulent drainage. The wound was otherwise benign and the patient was afebrile. The patient was taken back to the operating room for a debridement and irrigation. Although no purulence or devitalized tissue was encountered, cultures grew *Staphylococcus aureus*. The patient was admitted for parenteral antibiotics, and arrangements for home antibiotics were prepared including a peripherally inserted central catheter and sensitivities on the organism in order to confirm antibiotic choice. This occurred during a holiday weekend, and the patient felt very anxious and found it difficult to remain in the hospital.

After 6 weeks of parenteral antibiotics, oral suppression was initiated. Six months later, the antibiotics were withheld for 2 weeks and then the medial plate and screws and the radial head prosthesis were removed. The coronoid was healed and there were no signs of deep infection. The cultures were negative. Postoperative radiographs showed concentric reduction of the elbow.

He has a 100° arc of ulnohumeral motion, near full forearm motion, full wrist and digit motion, and he is neurovascular intact. There is some pain in the elbow with forceful activities. Overall, he is happy with the result, based on the perspective of how things might have gone and he is very appreciative of his care. Although the course was challenging and stressful, it was ultimately very rewarding for patient and surgeon alike.

Patient 6

A 45-year-old woman presents with complaints of lateral elbow pain persistent after 18 months. She strongly associates this with her work throwing mail in a post office. Prior treatment consisted of five corticosteroid injections, splinting, pain medication, stretching and strengthening exercises and other modalities under the supervision of an occupational therapist, and surgery. She still has pain and is looking for additional intervention to improve her situation.

The best available evidence supports a conception of her illness as one of the many transient and benign enthesopathies of middle age, however, that runs counter to her beliefs and gut feelings, which have been reinforced by her providers thus far. Serial injections teach a patient that treatment is necessary and that the doctor plays a crucial role in the resolution of the illness. In other words, the use of ineffective treatments (corticosteroids have been shown to be no more effective than placebo injection) medicalizes and pathologizes what is probably most accurately considered a rite of passage through middle age. As you speak with this patient it becomes clear that she feels her only hope is additional surgery. If you tell her that reoperation is unlikely to help, you risk leaving her hopeless, which is one of the worst human feelings.

Her husband accompanies her to the appointment, and they are open about the stress this has placed on their marriage. Her employer has been very understanding. At first worksite modifications and limited duty were provided, and now she is on short-term disability; however, she has been informed that they cannot hold her position indefinitely and she will lose her job soon if she cannot return. She uses words and phrases like "excruciating," "I can't bear it," and "just cut the arm off" when describing her illness and she becomes tearful when you convey empathy ("Wow," "I really admire how well you've dealt with this"; "this must be really hard on you").

When you ask permission to address the topic, she is open to hearing about the ways that nociception can cause distress, increase pain intensity, and create disability due to automatic thoughts (intuition, gut feelings) that represent the normal physiology of pain and the human response to perceived threat. She fervently ascribes (lots of head nodding) to all three of the top automatic human thoughts in response to nociception: (1) that the pain indicates ongoing damage or prevention of healing; (2) that the pain will be permanent; and that (3) she will never be able to enjoy activities that are important to her as long as the pain persists. She is reassured to know that these are a reflection of her normal and healthy "wiring" and a product of her intelligent, pattern-forming, rationalizing human brain.

She understands the analogy of the fire alarm that goes off when you're cooking and that once the absence of danger is ensured, it's appropriate to remove the battery from the fire alarm until the smoke/grease clears because the alarm at that point is a false alarm. The fact that it went off is a reassuring proof that the system is in good working order, but once the danger is past the alarm is more of a hindrance or nuisance than a help. She understands that magicians don't fool us because we are stupid—it's the opposite, they use our intelligence to get us rationalizing and believing that we know how the trick is done, then they do it in some other way and the illusion is complete. Magicians fool us from our strengths, not our weaknesses. We should not be ashamed of being fooled, we should not feel that we are flawed—quite the contrary. This analogy provides an opportunity to discuss the stigma often associated with the cognitive and emotional aspects of illness, captured in the phrase, "are you saying it's all in my head"?

She sees opportunity in your explanation that these "top 3" responses to nociception are misconceptions or overstatements that arise because we have evolved to be protective and "overcall" the danger. She also understands the power of gut feelings and how difficult they can be to "shake." The analogy of waking up from a nightmare and feeling bad long after she has realized that it was just a dream makes sense to her. She is both detail-oriented and vigilant. She places a great deal of faith in her intuition: she tends to "go with her gut" and thinks it's risky to question it, as in her assessment "it has always been right."

The surgeon is careful to point out that much of what an expert says may be counterintuitive. There is no expectation that the patient will agree with or understand everything that science and expertise have to offer. Being explicit and mindful of this helps to avert any tendency for the doctor–patient relationship to become adversarial: the patient's gut feeling will "win"—they will leave feeling and believing much the same as they did when they walked in and the "expert" can only "plant seeds" of alternative gut feelings that the patient may be able to cultivate into new opportunities.

The value of changing the goal from cure to improved function, comfort and quality of life is raised. Resistance to this is expected and natural. Again—just planting a seed. Improved function, comfort, and quality of life are very realistic goals, no matter what happens to the pain.

Finally, the treatment options are introduced without going into detail: (1) a second surgery; (2) a course for building the skills that are needed to understand and manage gut feelings to optimize comfort, function, and quality of life; and (3) the conservative approach including splints, ice/heat, pain medications, injections, therapy, etc. At this point, follow the patient's preferences. Provide slight additional detail regarding any options she inquires about and wait for her to express greater interest. With three options on the table, it will feel less threatening to hear the downsides or limitations of any specific option. For instance, the surgeon may not have confidence in a second surgery meeting the patient's expectations and the patient may feel that they have exhausted all conservative measures; but there is always the skill-building course to fall back on. It's important to wait for the patient to "buy in" to the skill-building course, which is a more appealing way of conveying the concept of cognitive behavioral therapy—a scientifically well-supported method of optimizing automatic thoughts and behaviors in response to symptoms to maximize health and wellness [8].

The patient inquired about the skill building and was open to giving it a try. After four sessions or "parts of the 12-part course," she had a better understanding of her gut feelings and where they come from, was more appreciative of the value of questioning them, and had made some progress in changing them. She felt confident to return to work in spite of continued pain. She felt optimistic about the future, and her former protectiveness and vulnerability were not noted in her speech or body language. She was very grateful to the surgeon that she was able to get well without additional surgery.

Final Thoughts

The decision to operate again magnifies the complexities present during the original decision for operative treatment. Our culture often loses sight of the fact that surgery is controlled injury: after all it's done with a knife. The patient is vulnerable to the hope that surgery can restore the limb to its prior status without impairment and solve all of his or her problems—including psychological distress, maladaptive coping, difficult life circumstances (difficult employment circumstances, relationship problems, etc), legal and work disputes, etc. The surgeon wants to help and the only option familiar to him or her may be operative treatment: the appropriate cliché here is, "to a hammer everything appears as a nail."

As this chapter demonstrates, the keys to effective reoperative hand surgery are to understand the entirety of the illness experience; to identify predictable, evidence-based targets for surgical intervention; to provide other sources of hope in case reoperation is not the best option or in case it doesn't meet the patient's goals; to make sure that the patient is considering their options from an empowered and informed rather than a vulnerable and desperate perspective; and to make a shared decision with the patient.

References

1. Rusch MD, Dzwierzynski WW, Sanger JR, Pruit NT, Siewert AD. Return to work outcomes after work-related hand trauma: the role of causal attributions. J Hand Surg Am. 2003;28(4):673–7.
2. Wong JY. Time off work in hand injury patients. J Hand Surg Am. 2008;33(5):718–25.
3. Grunert BK, Matloub HS, Sanger JR, Yousif NJ, Hettermann S. Effects of litigation on maintenance of psychological symptoms after severe hand injury. J Hand Surg Am. 1991;16(6):1031–4.
4. Grunert BK, Devine CA, Matloub HS, Sanger JR, Yousif NJ. Sexual dysfunction following traumatic hand injury. Ann Plast Surg. 1988;21(1):46–8.
5. Rosenthal RE. The mangled extremity syndrome (MES): a severity grading system for multi-system injury of the extremity. J Trauma. 1986;26(6):579.
6. Bravo CJ, Rizzo M, Hormel KB, Beckenbaugh RD. Pyrolytic carbon proximal interphalangeal joint arthroplasty: results with minimum two-year follow-up evaluation. J Hand Surg Am. 2007;32(1): 1–11.
7. Takigawa S, Meletiou S, Sauerbier M, Cooney WP. Long-term assessment of Swanson implant arthroplasty in the proximal interphalangeal joint of the hand. J Hand Surg Am. 2004;29(5): 785–95.
8. Vranceanu AM, Barsky A, Ring D. Psychosocial aspects of disabling musculoskeletal pain. J Bone Joint Surg Am. 2009;91:2014–8.

Reoperative Tenosynovitis

18

Steven C. Haase and Kevin C. Chung

Abstract

Recurrent tenosynovitis about the hand and wrist fortunately is an uncommon problem. For stenosing tenosynovitis, the usual culprit for continued symptoms is incomplete release. At this point, the appropriate surgery is to repeat the release and make sure that there are no further constricting points about the flexor tendon sheath. Of course, the A2 pulley needs to be preserved and protected, but the A0 and A1 pulleys should be thoroughly released. The other condition discussed is deQuervain's tenosynovitis. The most common reason for failure of this surgery is a hidden slip of tendon in a separate compartment that was not released. Other potential causes include tendon subluxation about the radial styloid. Reoperative options in these scenarios include decompressing all of the tendons and making sure no tendons are left in any separate compartments. For tendon subluxation, a slip of the brachioradialis tendon can be used to reconstruct the retinaculum. Ultimately, if the patient still has symptoms that cannot be completely explained, but continue to appear to be deQuervain's tenosynovitis, a slip of tendon can be resected, thereby decreasing the cross-sectional area going through the first dorsal compartment. In general, the harder part of these cases is trying to reassure the patient that despite what is normally viewed as an "easy" surgery, technical challenges do occur and fortunately in most cases reoperative surgery in these situations does provide improvement in the patient's symptomatology.

Keywords

Tenosynovitis • deQuervain's • Trigger • Finger • Tendinosis

S.C. Haase, MD, FACS (✉)
Section of Plastic Surgery, University of Michigan Health System, 2130 Taubman Center, 1500 E. Medical Center Drive, SPC 5340, Ann Arbor, MI 48109, USA
e-mail: shaase@med.umich.edu

K.C. Chung, MD
Department of Surgery, University of Michigan Health System, Ann Arbor, MI, USA

S.F.M. Duncan (ed.), *Reoperative Hand Surgery*,
DOI 10.1007/978-1-4614-2373-7_18,

Key Points

- Medical management of systemic problems must be coordinated with surgical treatments to help prevent recurrence.
- Consider corticosteroid injections as a diagnostic/therapeutic measure.
- Avoid steroid injection for deQuervain's in people of color because of potential depigmentation.
- When mired in scar tissue, work from known to unknown.
- Do not struggle; make a larger incision if needed.
- Preserve and protect the A2 pulley.
- Treat superficial radial nerve branches with respect.
- Do not overlook joint stiffness associated with tenosynovitis.
- When patients do not improve as expected, investigate carefully.
- Be specific with instructions for activities after surgery; avoid overactivity that can increase inflammation.

Introduction

The broad range of terms that help us describe pain associated with tendons can be confusing to hand surgery professionals, let alone the lay public. It is helpful at the beginning of this chapter to discuss the various terms being used in the literature (see Table 18.1).

Tendinitis (or, informally, *tendonitis*) literally means inflammation of a tendon or tendons. Although the term is often used imprecisely, it should be restricted to pathologic conditions involving tendon inflammation (such as Achilles tendinitis or patellar tendinitis). *Tendinosis*, on the other hand, refers to a damaged or degenerating tendon without implying the presence of inflammation. This condition may also be called chronic tendinitis or chronic tendinopathy.

Tenosynovitis, which is the focus of this chapter, refers to inflammation of the synovial lining of the tendon sheaths. Semantically, if the pathologic condition involves the tendon sheath, then the proper term is tenovaginitis (tendon + sheath + inflammation), e.g., stenosing tenovaginitis for trigger fingers or deQuervain's tenovaginitis for inflammation of the first dorsal compartment tendon sheath. An example of tenosynovitis is the invasive synovitis associated with rheumatoid arthritis. Other less common types of tenosynovitis can be associated with infection, deposits of crystalline or proteinaceous material, and other entities.

Table 18.1 Tendon terms and appropriate definition

Term (synonyms)	Definition
Tendinitis (tendonitis)	Inflammation of tendon
Tendinosis (chronic tendinitis, chronic tendinopathy)	Damage to tendon (without signs of inflammation)
Tenosynovitis (tenovaginitis)	Inflammation of the synovial lining of tendon sheaths
Tendon entrapment (stenosing tenovaginitis)	Fibrous, often noninflammatory, thickening and narrowing of tendon sheaths

The focus of this chapter is on reoperative surgery for tenosynovitis and tendon entrapment. These reoperations are uncommon for most hand surgeons, but are sometimes required to treat recurrence or complications arising after the index surgery. Within this chapter, we present some strategies to help avoid complications, prevent recurrence, and perform effective reoperation when necessary.

Rheumatoid Tenosynovitis

Tenosynovitis of the hand and wrist develops in most patients with rheumatoid arthritis. This process can originate within the synovial linings of the tendons themselves or in an adjacent joint. The process usually produces a fairly painless mass that tracks with the involved tendons (Fig. 18.1). It may affect both the flexor tendons [1] and/or the extensor tendons [2, 3]. Although this sort of synovitis is often managed medically, especially with immunomodulating drugs, occasionally surgery is required for persistent, refractory synovitis that endangers joints and tendons. Because of the painless nature of the tenosynovitis in rheumatoid disease, the often rather large masses on the dorsum of the wrist are ignored by the patient until they rupture one or more extensor tendons. In our experience, recurrence of synovitis after surgical treatment in the rheumatoid wrist is fairly uncommon, especially if the patient is being properly medically managed. Nonetheless, when a patient presents with multiple tendon ruptures due to recalcitrant tenosynovitis, reconstruction can sometimes be complicated.

Crystalline Tenosynovitides

Gout is the end result of hyperuricemia, which leads to deposition of urate crystals in joints and soft tissues. The intense inflammatory reaction to this crystalline material leads to the characteristic pain, swelling, and erythema seen

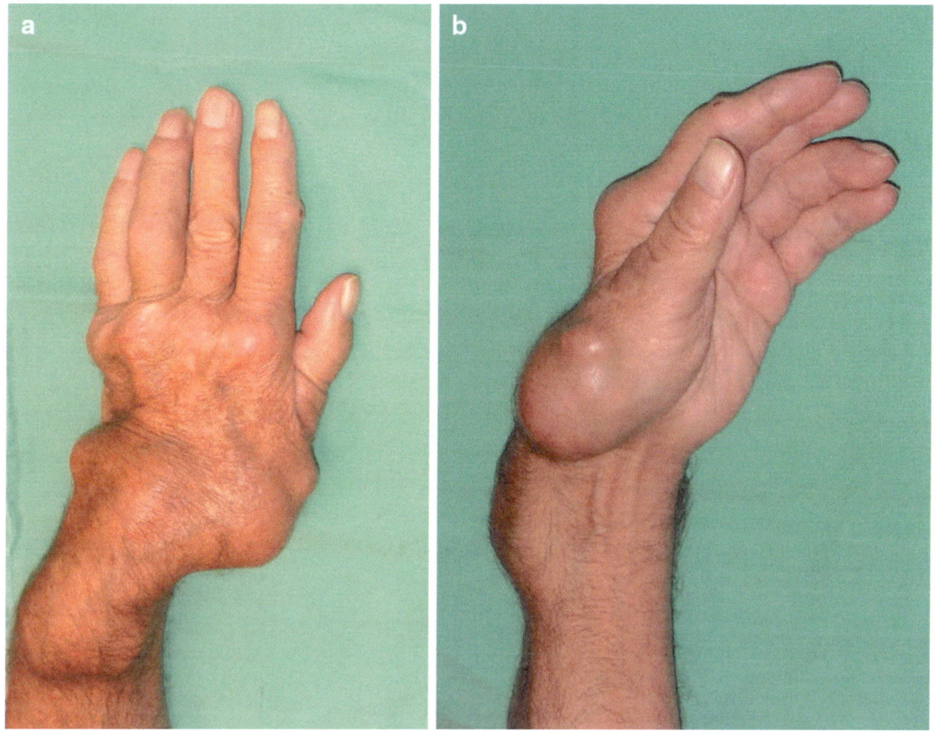

Fig. 18.1 (a, b) Extensive rheumatoid tenosynovitis in a 59-year-old male

in this disease, which can easily be mistaken for septic arthritis or rheumatoid disease. Aspiration of involved joints usually confirms the diagnosis, by visualizing the negatively birefringent crystals under a polarizing microscope.

Although gout commonly affects the joints of the hand, its effect on tendons is less common [4]. Still, tendon nodules or thickenings can occur, presenting as nerve compression, flexion contracture, or tenosynovitis; tendon rupture from gout is exceedingly rare. Treatment involves excision of the gouty material and diseased synovium. Medical management is important in controlling this disease and preventing recurrence after surgical treatment.

Other types of crystalline tenosynovitis are fairly uncommon. Calcific tendinitis, pseudogout, and hydroxyapatite deposition have all been described in the literature as occasionally affecting the hand. These are treated very similar to gout, requiring medical management of their respective systemic problems, as well as excision or debridement of the irritating crystalline material.

Infectious Tenosynovitis

Acute suppurative tenosynovitis due to bacterial infection is a diagnosis that is usually easy to recognize, and prompt surgical drainage should be curative. Chronic tenosynovitis due to a more indolent infection may masquerade as one of the above-mentioned diseases, and defies diagnosis until biopsy and special cultures are performed. Typical causative agents are tuberculosis, atypical mycobacteria [5], gonococci, and fungi [6].

Amyloidosis

Although this disease can result from a rare genetic condition, it is more commonly seen in dialysis patients. Excess protein (β_2-microglobulin) accumulates and becomes deposited in bone and soft tissue. Deposition along tendons and other structures in the hand can lead to carpal tunnel syndrome, trigger fingers, and occasionally tendon rupture. This disease presents with chronic swelling along the course of the affected tendons, without inflammatory signs of pain, warmth, or erythema. Surgical removal is the only effective treatment for these deposits; recurrence after excision is uncommon [7].

Sarcoidosis

Sarcoidosis is a systemic inflammatory disorder in which granulomatous lesions involve multiple organ systems, including bone, joint, and/or tenosynovial involvement in a minority of cases. Systemic corticosteroid medications can be used to manage the inflammation, but tenosynovectomy is also commonly required for successful treatment of associated tenosynovitis [8].

Tendon Entrapment

The most common types of tendon entrapment are trigger finger (or trigger thumb) and deQuervain's disease [9]. These entities are notable for a distinct lack of inflammatory findings within the tenosynovium. Rather, a fibrosis and thickening of the tendon sheath seems to be the underlying cause.

Trigger digits that do not respond to corticosteroid injection [10] are typically treated with a release of the A1 pulley. This results in the resolution of triggering in the vast majority of cases. Caution should be taken when dealing with a rheumatoid arthritis patient experiencing triggering. These patients require tenosynovectomy to relieve their symptoms, and the classic teaching indicates that the A1 pulley should be preserved to restrain the flexor tendons from deviating ulnarly [11].

Analogous to this, *deQuervain's disease* is typically relieved by release of the first extensor compartment at the level of the wrist. Abductor pollicis longus typically has multiple tendon slips within its retinacular sheath, and it is not uncommon to find a subdivision within this compartment encasing the diminutive extensor pollicis brevis tendon (Fig. 18.2). It is often the failure to release this additional subcompartment that leads to persistent or recurrent symptoms following a deQuervain's release [12].

Stenotic tendinopathies can affect many other tendons at the level of the wrist. *Intersection syndrome* presents with painful symptoms about 4 cm proximal to the wrist crease where the abductor pollicis longus and extensor pollicis brevis tendons cross over the radial wrist extensors [13]. Release of the second extensor compartment retinaculum is typically curative; recurrence is rare. Entrapment of extensor carpi ulnaris occasionally requires surgical treatment for relief of this common cause of ulnar-sided wrist pain. Recurrence after treatment of this, or the other rarer forms of tendon entrapment (flexor carpi radialis, extensor pollicis longus, etc.), is unlikely.

Indications and Contraindications

Indications for reoperation

Rheumatoid arthritis
- Recurrent synovial hypertrophy
- Tendon rupture

Crystalline, deposition, or septic tendinopathy
- Recurrent swelling, pain, neuropathy, or stiffness

Tendon entrapment
- Recurrent triggering, pain, or stiffness
- Bowstringing or subluxation

Contraindications for reoperation
- Medically unstable patient (absolute contraindication)
- Uncontrolled pain syndrome
- Suspicion of factitious disorder
- Obvious secondary gain issues

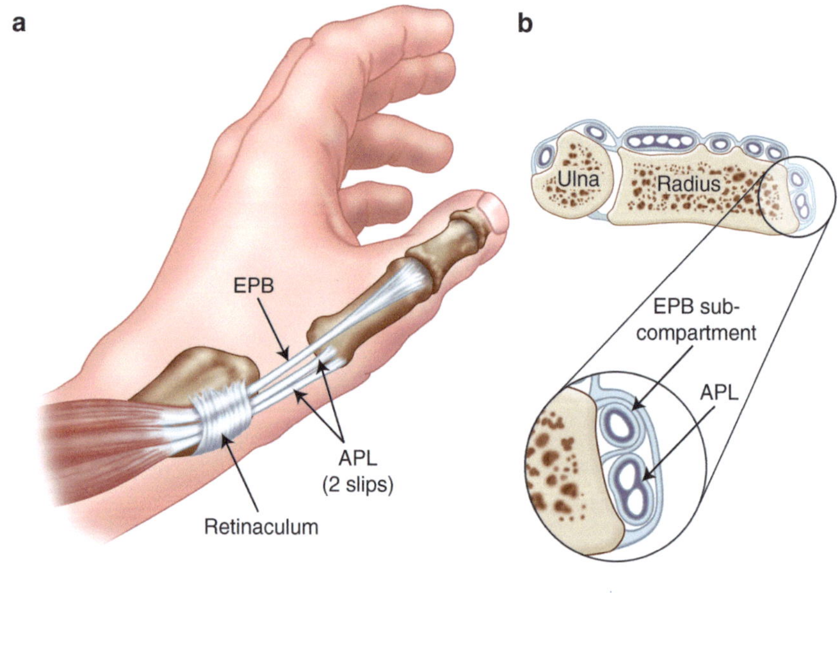

Fig. 18.2 (**a**) The first extensor compartment includes the abductor pollicis longus (APL) and extensor pollicis brevis (EPB) tendons. (**b**) The EPB tendon is often located within a separate subcompartment

A patient presenting with recurrent symptoms or complications after tenosynovitis surgery should be examined carefully. Mild residual symptoms or minor recurrences may respond to corticosteroid injection. More significant cases with return of pain, loss of function, or obvious technical complications should be considered for reoperation.

Recurrence of rheumatoid tenosynovitis is uncommon with proper medical management, but these patients may present with new masses, or with complications related to unrecognized or incompletely treated disease (i.e., tendon ruptures). Patients with functional limitations due to tendon rupture are candidates for reconstruction, but this is not a surgical emergency. Careful planning is warranted to ensure the best functional result.

As with rheumatoid disease, medical management is usually helpful in preventing recurrence of tenosynovitis related to gout and chronic infection as well. Patients with return of symptoms, especially when associated with functional impairment, should be considered for reoperation before they develop difficult joint stiffness or irreversible soft tissue damage from their disease. Of course, patients with suspected acute infection (or superinfection) should not have surgery delayed.

Trigger digit recurrence is uncommon, but new triggering in adjacent digits can lead to pain and stiffness mimicking recurrence. Careful examination should be able to discern the difference. Other complications such as flexion contracture or bowstringing have been reported. The latter is usually due to inadvertent division of the A2 pulley. If functionally significant, this might require pulley reconstruction.

A unique situation occurs for pediatric trigger fingers. Unlike the thumb trigger in which A1 pulley release will predictably solve the triggering problem, trigger fingers in the pediatric patient are often caused by more distal problems from the A1 pulley. In many of these cases, the trigger can be caused by a nodule over the flexor tendons at the flexor digitorum superficialis decussation [14]. Opening up the decussation site is often curative.

Contraindications to reoperation would include those patients who are medically unfit for surgery due to other health problems. Also, patients with complex regional pain syndrome (formerly called reflex sympathetic dystrophy) should have an attempt at controlling their neuropathic pain with medication or nerve blocks before proceeding with another surgical insult.

Finally, patients presenting with "recurrence" without any objective evidence of disease should be evaluated with scrutiny. If it appears there are unusual secondary gain issues, or if there is behavior consistent with a factitious or spurious disorder, hand surgeons should tread carefully. Sometimes a trial of splinting, hand therapy, or even casting can be a helpful test to measure a difficult patient's compliance, motivations, and truthfulness.

Preoperative History and Considerations

Although we all strive to be thorough in our surgical practices, careful preoperative evaluation is even more important on reoperative cases. The patient's complaints should be carefully recorded in detail, so the exact nature of the problem can be easily recalled weeks or months later. Documentation of active and passive motion, grip strength, sensibility, and other objective measures are critical. Physical findings can also be recorded objectively with photographs.

When contemplating reoperation on tenosynovitis, it is important to consider that perhaps something was missed the first time. For this reason, in addition to routine radiographs to evaluate joint and bone involvement, we strongly recommend additional imaging in most cases. Our initial diagnostic test of choice is usually a dynamic musculoskeletal ultrasound exam. This test can demonstrate in real-time imaging of recurrent triggering and other forms of stenotic tendon entrapment. It can diagnose tendinitis, tendinosis, and other abnormal tendon anatomy. Finally, it allows us to determine the exact location and extent of recurrent tenosynovitis [15]. If an ultrasound exam is suboptimal or not available, or if it raises additional questions that cannot be easily satisfied, an MRI exam should be considered [16].

Recurrence of tenosynovitis may be due to improper medical management. If surgery can be delayed without leading to a less functional outcome, referring the patient for a trial of appropriate medical management should be considered before embarking on reoperation.

Because most of these tenosynovitis procedures have a fairly low rate of complications or recurrence, one must always consider the individual patient's potential for secondary gain, as it applies to their particular situation. Suspicion should be raised if reported symptoms and objective exam do not correlate well. It may be helpful to have such patients work in a one-on-one fashion with an experienced hand therapist for a predetermined length of time. The therapist has the ability to observe the patient over a longer time period, and they are often able to discern factitious disorders from genuine diseases from that unique perspective. At the very least, this will provide a second set of examinations that can be compared with your own if reoperation is being considered.

The following procedures are presented as examples of reoperative tenosynovitis surgery. The principles illustrated here can be applied to many similar situations.

Reoperative Rheumatoid Tenosynovitis

Operative Approach

Approach to the patient with extensor tendon ruptures (Fig. 18.3a) due to recalcitrant tenosynovitis is via a longitudinal linear or "lazy-S" incision. Retinacular flaps are elevated (or reelevated) and synovectomy is performed. Tendon transfers can then be performed for any ruptures that are identified (Table 18.2; Fig. 18.3b, c). When flexor digitorum superficialis tendons must be transferred, we prefer a subcutaneous path for the transfer, rather than through the interosseous membrane. In our experience, this allows for better tendon gliding, and fewer problems with adhesions.

Optimizing outcomes

- Incorporate previous incisions whenever possible; extend previous incisions when necessary.
- See Table 18.2 for suggestions regarding extensor tendon reconstructions.
- For FDS transfers to reconstruct extensor ruptures, use a subcutaneous tunnel rather than cross the interosseous membrane.
- Tendon transfers should be tensioned with the fingers in full extension, since some loosening and stretching will occur during the healing/rehabilitation process.

Complications

With any reoperation for tenosynovitis, the risk of recurrence, delayed healing, tendon rupture, nerve irritation, and infection should be discussed preoperatively with the patient. Tendon transfers that lose tension over time ("stretch out") may require reoperation for tightening.

Postoperative Care

Splinting requirements will vary dramatically with the different types of surgery, but typically at least 2 weeks is required; extensor tendon transfers are splinted for 4 weeks in extension before starting a postoperative rehabilitation protocol.

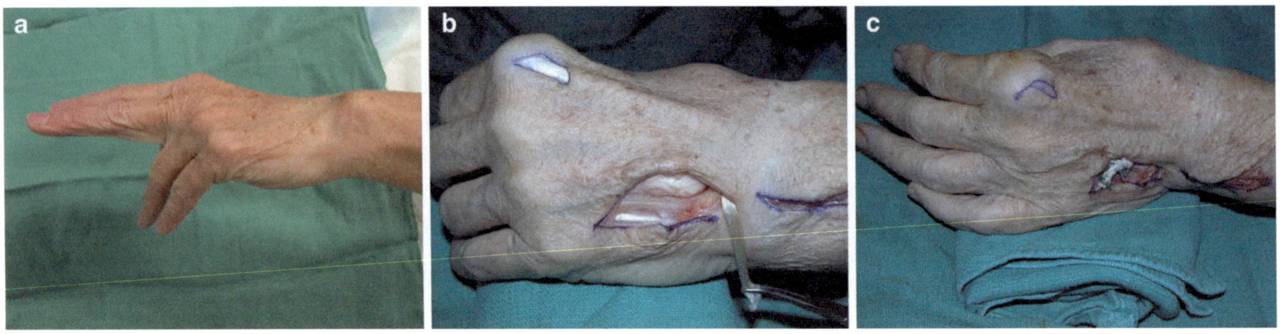

Fig. 18.3 (**a**) A seventy-six-year-old female who presented with dorsal wrist tenosynovitis and loss of extension of her ring and small fingers. (**b**) The extensor indicis proprius (EIP) tendon was selected for reconstruction. (**c**) The EIP tendon is woven into the distal ends of the ring and small finger extensor tendons

Table 18.2 Preferred tendon rupture reconstructions

Tendon(s) ruptured	Preferred reconstruction
Small finger extensor(s)	Attach distal end of small finger extensor end-to-side to ring finger extensor
Ring and small finger extensors	Transfer EIP tendon to power both the ring and small finger extensors
Middle, ring, and small finger extensors	Attach distal end of middle finger extensor end-to-side to index finger extensor
	Transfer EIP tendon to power both the ring and small finger extensors
Index, middle, ring, and small finger extensors	Transfer flexor digitorum superficialis (FDS) tendon of middle finger to power both the middle and index finger extensors
	Transfer FDS tendon of ring finger to power both the ring and small finger extensors

Reoperative Septic Tenosynovitis

Operative Approach

Patients with atypical infections leading to chronic tenosynovitis may require long-term medical treatment and, over the course of time, more than one tenosynovectomy for their disease (Figs. 18.4 and 18.5). Previous incisions should be incorporated whenever possible. Extending incisions into unscarred territory is often helpful so that neurovascular bundles can be easily identified in areas where scarring is minimal. Reoperations on the flexor tendon system should carefully preserve the pulleys whenever possible, especially A2 and A4, to prevent bowstringing. Pulley reconstruction should be undertaken in cases where pulleys have been destroyed by the infectious process.

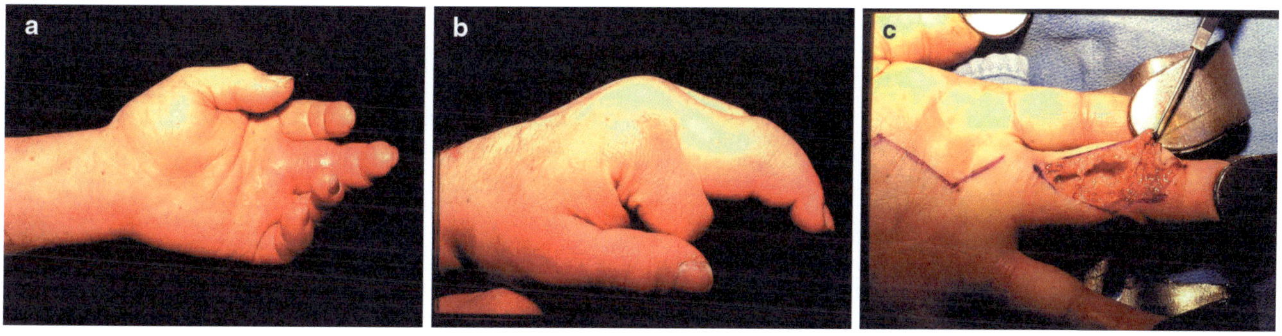

Fig. 18.4 (**a**, **b**) A forty-year-old male presented with chronic tenosynovitis of the left middle finger. (**c**) Initial surgical exposure to remove disease and obtain a tissue sample. Laboratory results showed infection with *Mycobacterium terrae* complex

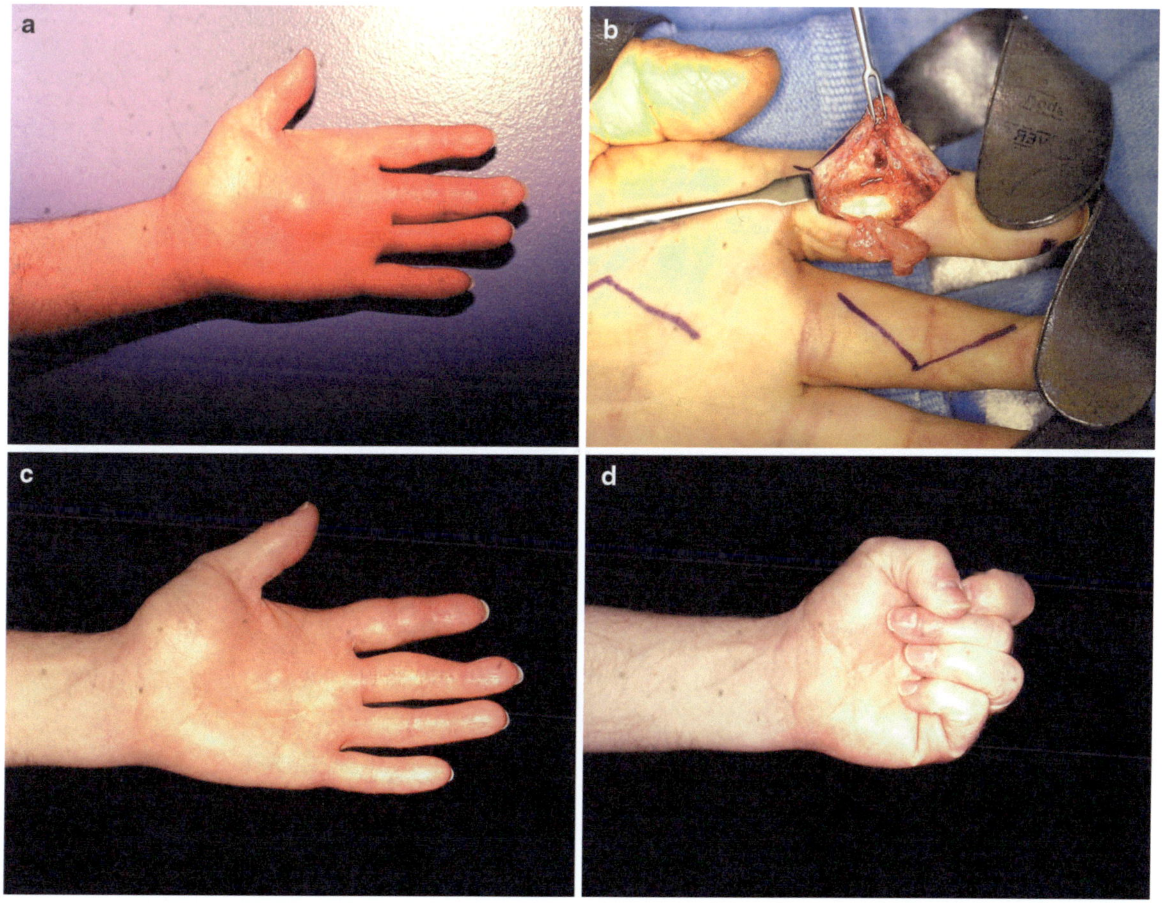

Fig. 18.5 (**a**) Despite optimal medical treatment, he presented many months later with an enlarging palm mass and flexor tendon nodules of the index and middle fingers that limited his finger motion. (**b**) Operative exposure required to excise recurrent tenosynovitis. (**c**, **d**) Final results, showing very good range of motion

Optimizing outcomes

- Make sure patients have been compliant with prescribed medical therapy.
- Utilize Bruner-style incisions liberally on volar surfaces; extend into unscarred tissue to more easily identify neurovascular bundles.
- Preserve the A2 and A4 pulleys when operating on flexor tendons.
- Send tissue for microbiological and pathological evaluation to reaffirm the diagnosis with each debridement/debulking.

Complications

Recurrence is certainly possible due to the indolent nature of this disease. Medical therapy may require months to complete, and compliance can therefore play a critical role in recurrence. Patients need to be encouraged to follow through with appropriate medical therapy even if they are enjoying good hand function after tenosynovectomy.

Postoperative Care

Splinting can be used to rest the hand and maintain good position, but should not continue full-time for very long. These patients should be mobilized to preserve joint motion as soon as their postoperative pain/swelling allow, usually within 3–4 days of surgery.

Reoperative deQuervain's Disease

Operative Approach

The existing scar will need to be incorporated into a longer incision for better exposure (Fig. 18.6a, b). The dorsal sensory nerve should be carefully identified proximal to the surgical site, where it can be found in an area free from scar. If a patient has a significant neuropathic component to their pain, complete neurolysis should be performed to release the nerve from scar tissue. The nerve can be wrapped with a vein to provide a barrier against recurrent scarring (Fig. 18.6c, d).

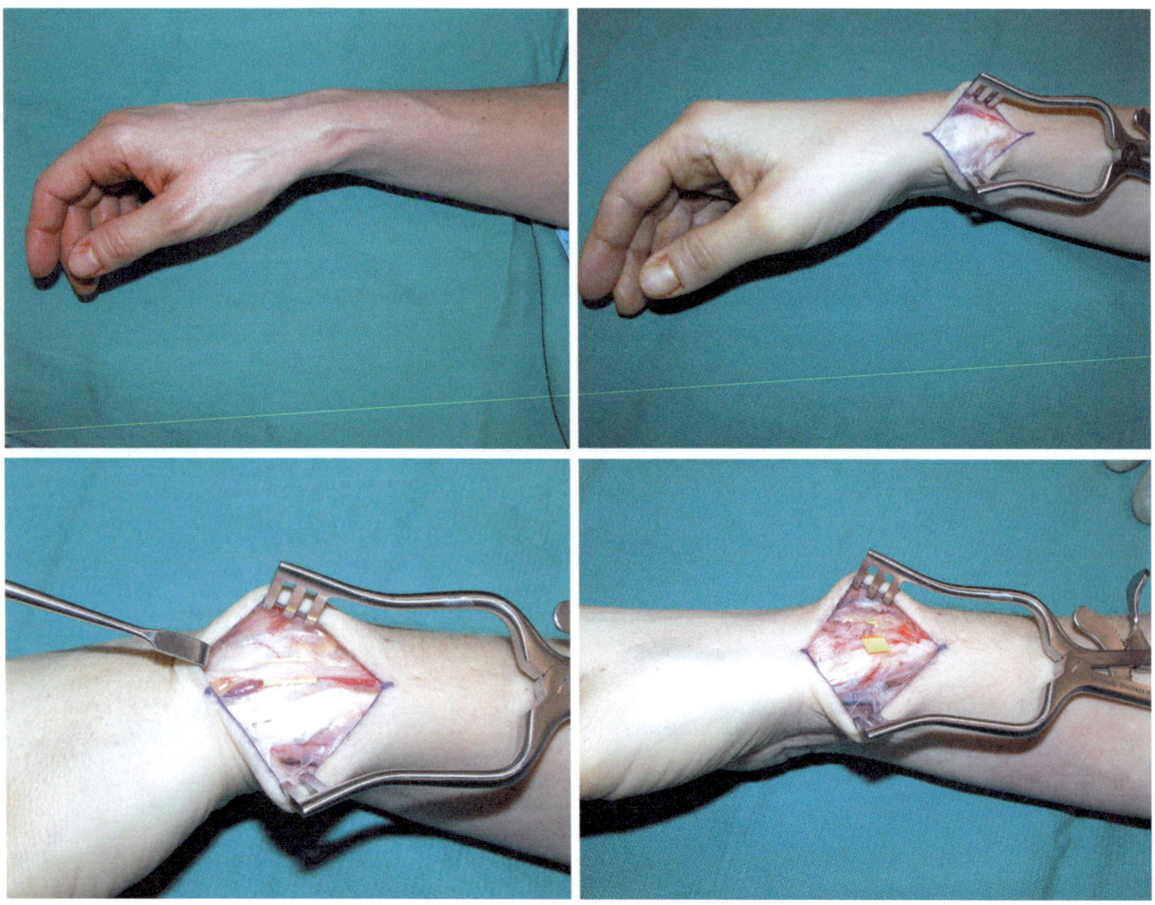

Fig. 18.6 (**a**, **b**) A forty-year-old female with persistent neuropathic pain after deQuervain's release. (**c**, **d**) Superficial branch of the radial nerve is identified, dissected free from scar tissue, and wrapped with a vein conduit for protection

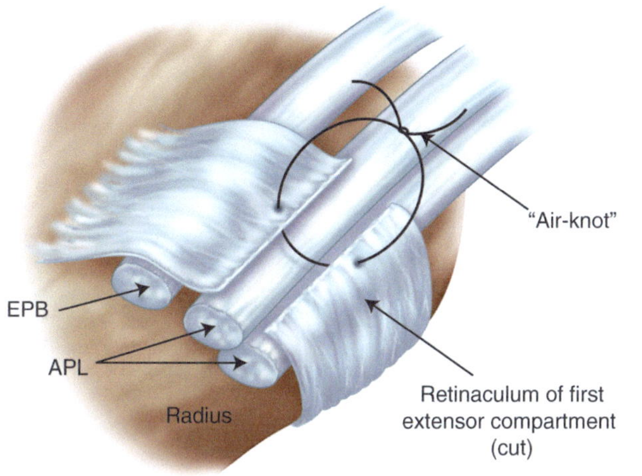

Fig. 18.7 Loosely restraining the cut retinaculum with an "air-knot" of 4-0 absorbable suture can help eliminate postoperative tendon subluxation after deQuervain's release

If subluxation or "snapping" of the tendons over the radial styloid occurs postoperatively, it usually gets better on its own within several weeks. If it persists, the problem can be corrected by using a portion of the adjacent retinaculum to provide a loose "sling" for the first compartment tendons. A technique we have used to prevent symptomatic subluxation after deQuervain's release is to place a loose suture (4-0 absorbable monofilament) between the halves of the retinaculum after confirming complete release (Fig. 18.7). This temporary suture is deliberately left loose, so there is no tendon entrapment, but seems to provide just enough support in the early healing phase to prevent uncomfortable subluxation.

Optimizing outcomes

- Incorporate previous incisions whenever possible; extend previous incisions when necessary.
- Take care to protect the superficial branch of the radial nerve.
- Make sure EPB is released from its separate subcompartment, if present.
- Consider placing an "air-knot" between the halves of the retinaculum to prevent tendon subluxation/snapping in the early postoperative period.

Complications

Complications unique to this operation include tendon subluxation or snapping over the radial styloid. This usually improves with time. Nerve irritation or injury, when it occurs, is much more difficult to manage. Patients may benefit from referral to a specialty pain clinic if nerve irritation or pain persists postoperatively, or if complex regional pain syndrome is suspected.

Postoperative Care

Splinting is routine for the very early postoperative period, but gentle mobilization should be started within a week to eliminate adhesions between tendon, nerve, and surrounding tissues.

Other Considerations

One of the complications that can occur from first dorsal compartment release is volar subluxation of the tendons. This risk can be minimized by trying to maintain the volar portion of the retinaculum. It may also be minimized by postoperative splinting or casting. However, when it does occur there are some reconstructive options. As previously mentioned, most of these are usually asymptomatic, but if the patient is symptomatic various options have been described. There is retinacular reconstruction utilizing a piece of the extensor retinaculum, and this has been described by Ramesh and Britton [17]. The brachioradialis tendon has also been utilized as a method of retinacular reconstruction and this is described by McMahon et al. [18]. The editor has firsthand experiencing utilizing this technique, and it has been relatively successful in preventing further subluxation problems. More recently El Rassi et al. [19] have described a technique. It consists of lengthening the first dorsal compartment without disrupting its continuity and without using a suture. Any repeat surgery should also look for any potentially unreleased slips, as previously mentioned. If there has been a complete release but it still appears that there is evidence of deQuervain's, resection of one of the slips of the APL tendon can be performed with minimal loss of biomechanical function and usually improved symptoms by decreasing the volume of tendons going through the tunnel.

Conclusion

In our experience, recurrence of tenosynovitis requiring reoperation should be quite uncommon. When the need arises to reexplore one of these patients, the surgeon should approach each case with thoughtful consideration and planning. Reoperative surgical cases are never "textbook" cases and should be undertaken with general principles in mind, but also with particular attention to the details of the individual case.

References

1. Ferlic DC. Rheumatoid flexor tenosynovitis and rupture. Hand Clin. 1996;12(3):561–72.
2. Williamson SC, Feldon P. Extensor tendon ruptures in rheumatoid arthritis. Hand Clin. 1995;11(3):449–59.
3. Wilson RL, DeVito MC. Extensor tendon problems in rheumatoid arthritis. Hand Clin. 1996;12(3):551–9.
4. Fitzgerald BT, Setty A, et al. Gout affecting the hand and wrist. J Am Acad Orthop Surg. 2007;15(10):625–35.
5. Mateo L, Rufi G, et al. *Mycobacterium chelonae* tenosynovitis of the hand. Semin Arthritis Rheum. 2004;34(3):617–22.
6. Cucurull E, Sarwar H, et al. Localized tenosynovitis caused by *Histoplasma capsulatum*: case report and review of the literature. Arthritis Rheum. 2005;53(1):129–32.
7. Fitzpatrick DC, Jebson PJ, et al. Upper extremity musculoskeletal manifestations of dialysis-associated amyloidosis. Iowa Orthop J. 1996;16:135–8.
8. Carlson JA, Wei-Lee H, et al. Sarcoidal granulomatous tenosynovitis of the hands occurring in an organ transplant patient. J Cutan Pathol. 2007;34(8):658–64.
9. Ahuja NK, Chung KC. Fritz de Quervain, MD (1868-1940): stenosing tendovaginitis at the radial styloid process. J Hand Surg Am. 2004;29(6):1164–70.
10. Peters-Veluthamaningal C, van der Windt DA, et al. Corticosteroid injection for trigger finger in adults. Cochrane Database Syst Rev. 2009;(1):CD005617.
11. Ryzewicz M, Wolf JM. Trigger digits: principles, management, and complications. J Hand Surg Am. 2006;31(1):135–46.
12. Ilyas AM, Ast M, et al. De Quervain tenosynovitis of the wrist. J Am Acad Orthop Surg. 2007;15(12):757–64.
13. Hanlon DP, Luellen JR. Intersection syndrome: a case report and review of the literature. J Emerg Med. 1999;17(6):969–71.
14. Bae DS, Sodha S, et al. Surgical treatment of the pediatric trigger finger. J Hand Surg Am. 2007;32(7):1043–7.
15. Backhaus M. Ultrasound and structural changes in inflammatory arthritis: synovitis and tenosynovitis. Ann N Y Acad Sci. 2009;1154(1):139–51.
16. McQueen FM. The MRI view of synovitis and tenosynovitis in inflammatory arthritis: implications for diagnosis and management. Ann N Y Acad Sci. 2009;1154:21–34.
17. Ramesh R, Britton JM. A retinacular sling for subluxing tendons of the first extensor compartment. A case report. J Bone Joint Surg Br. 2000;82(3):424–5.
18. McMahon M, Craig SM, Posner MA. Tendon subluxation after de Quervain's release: treatment by brachioradialis tendon flap. J Hand Surg Am. 1991;16(1):30–2.
19. El Rassi G, Bleton R, Laporte D. Compartmental reconstruction for de Quervain stenosing tenosynovitis. Scand J Plast Reconstr Surg Hand Surg. 2006;40(1):46–8.

Reoperative Brachial Plexus Surgery

19

Douglas M. Sammer and Susan E. Mackinnon

Abstract

This chapter provides a very nice outline and summary of options in treating the patient who has experienced no recovery or only partial recovery after a brachial plexus injury. These options are broken down into those that help hand function, elbow function, and shoulder function. Common reoperative procedures to improve the function of a patient with a brachial plexus injury that has not healed from the initial procedures include tendon transfers, joint fusions, and, in some circumstances, sensory nerve transfers in order to maximize the patient's ability to gain some function with the extremity. In extreme cases, where a patient is having severe chronic pain, as well as in some other unique situations, the option of amputation can be entertained. Expertise in brachial plexus surgery is difficult for the individual hand surgeon to gain unless he or she is at a major referral center. However, fusions and tendon transfers may be within the typical hand and upper extremity surgeon's repertoire. This chapter outlines these reconstructive options for this difficult and challenging clinical situation.

Keywords

Brachial • Plexus • Fusion • Tendon • Transfers

Key Points

- Because the motor end plates of the target muscles have undergone fibrosis by the time the original brachial plexus operation fails, rarely is reoperation on the brachial plexus or peripheral motor nerves indicated.
- Brachial plexus reoperative surgery consists of secondary operations such as tendon transfers, arthrodeses, and sensory nerve transfers.
- Surgery for failed brachial plexus reconstruction can be divided into operations for shoulder function, operations for elbow function, and operations for hand function.

D.M. Sammer, MD
Department of Plastic and Reconstructive Surgery, University of Texas Southwestern Medical School, Dallas, TX, USA
e-mail: douglas.sammer@utsouthwestern.edu

S.E. Mackinnon, MD (✉)
Department of Surgery, Washington University School of Medicine, 660 South Euclid Avenue, Campus Box 8238, St. Louis, MO, 63110, USA
e-mail: mackinnons@wudosis.wustl.edu

S.F.M. Duncan (ed.), *Reoperative Hand Surgery*,
DOI 10.1007/978-1-4614-2373-7_19, © Springer Science+Business Media, LLC 2012

Introduction

Primary brachial plexus surgery should ideally be completed within 6 months from the time of injury. Because of the long distances required for nerve regeneration, and ongoing motor end-plate fibrosis, if primary reconstruction is performed more than 9 months after injury, the chance of meaningful functional recovery is decreased. If primary brachial plexus surgery fails, secondary surgeries such as arthrodeses and tendon transfers may help improve function. In most cases, because of motor end-plate fibrosis, repeat surgery on the brachial plexus or peripheral nerves is contraindicated. One exception is that distal sensory nerve transfers, which are not time-sensitive in nature, can provide benefit to some patients whose primary surgery has failed.

When evaluating a patient for secondary surgery such as tendon transfers, it is helpful to categorize the problem into broad anatomic zones, including failure of shoulder function, failure of elbow function, and failure of hand function. Unfortunately, in some cases, patients with failed brachial plexus surgery will have very few functioning muscle-tendon units to serve as donors for tendon transfer and subsequently have few options for improving function. Fortunately, patients often do not have a complete failure of their primary brachial plexus surgery. In many instances, some aspects of the nerve reconstruction succeed, while others do not. This leaves the patient with patchy or limited areas of persistent functional loss, a situation in which the surgeon has numerous options for secondary reconstruction.

Indications and Contraindications

1. An adequate amount of time must be allowed to pass prior to considering the original operation a failure.
2. Patients must have demonstrated a high level of motivation and compliance after their original surgery to be considered for tendon or muscle transfers.
3. Patients with severe chronic neuropathic pain in the extremity may be poor candidates for reoperation.
4. Inability to attend multiple therapy sessions postoperatively is a contraindication to tendon transfers.
5. The joints must be passively supple prior to performing a tendon transfer.

Before embarking on secondary reconstruction for failed brachial plexus surgery, the surgeon must ensure that enough time has passed to allow nerve regeneration. During this time period, the surgeon should assess patient compliance and motivation. Noncompliance or lack of motivation is a contraindication to further surgery, as a high level of compliance is required after tendon transfers. Chronic neuropathic pain should also be considered a relative contraindication to further surgery. Unfortunately, another common problem is lack of resources. Patients who undergo secondary brachial plexus surgery, and in particular tendon transfers, will require multiple therapy visits postoperatively for optimum results. Finally, it is crucial to treat contractures, operatively or nonoperatively, prior to performing tendon transfers.

Preoperative History and Considerations: Shoulder

The primary reconstructive goals for the shoulder after brachial plexus injury are restoration of abduction and external rotation. Another crucial and often disregarded issue is painful shoulder subluxation. Primary operations to restore shoulder function include intraplexal nerve grafting or more often nerve transfers from extraplexal sources, such as the spinal accessory to suprascapular nerve transfer. If primary nerve surgery fails, patients may exhibit a lack of abduction, external rotation, or both and may have painful glenohumeral inferior subluxation.

Shoulder arthrodesis is an option and does address painful glenohumeral subluxation. Although glenohumeral motion is lost after arthrodesis, some active motion is achieved through scapulothoracic rotation and lateral flexion of the spine. However, there are a number of drawbacks. Complications such as nonunion, infection, and fracture are common and occur in as many as a third of patients [13]. To have optimal function after shoulder arthrodesis, the serratus anterior and other muscles in the shoulder area must be working, and this is often not the case in patients with brachial plexus injuries [7, 14].

Shoulder-level tendon transfers can sometimes be used to improve shoulder function in patients who fail to develop active glenohumeral motion or who continue to have persistent inferior glenohumeral subluxation after primary brachial plexus surgery. Often, few periscapular muscles are available and adequate for use as donors for tendon transfer. Fortunately, the trapezius is often functional. Depending on whether the spinal accessory nerve has been used in a transfer, and whether all or part of the trapezius is denervated, all or part of the trapezius may be used for transfer [11]. We have recently used a partial injury to the accessory nerve in an end-to-side fashion to reconstruct the suprascapular nerve in order to maintain trapezius function [12].

The most commonly performed transfer is the trapezius transfer. Even in patients who have undergone prior spinal accessory to suprascapular nerve transfer, the upper portion of the trapezius muscle continues to function normally and remains a suitable donor muscle-tendon unit for tendon transfer [2]. Results, while not perfect, can be good. In some studies, reduction of inferior shoulder subluxation occurs in 80% or more of patients. Some degree of shoulder abduction (averaging 40°) may be achieved after surgery [8, 10]. However, it should be noted that in patients with severe brachial plexus injuries that result in a completely flail shoulder, restoration of glenohumeral abduction is not as good. It should also be noted that this transfer does not improve external rotation. Elhassan et al. have described a new trapezius transfer, employing the middle and inferior portions of the trapezius, which attempts to improve external rotation [5]. Achilles tendon allograft is required to elongate the trapezius tendon, which is transferred to the infraspinatus tendon insertion. This is a promising transfer for restoring external rotation, a motion critical for positioning the hand out in front of the patient for activities.

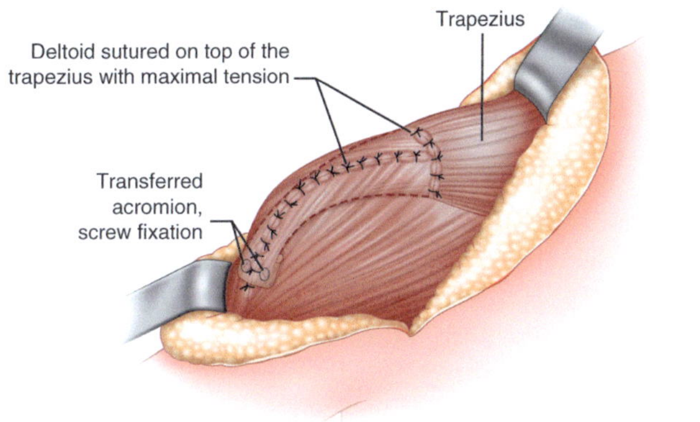

Fig. 19.1 Final appearance of the trapezius transfer. The deltoid is mobilized medially as far as possible and sutured over the trapezius, covering the transferred acromion

Operative Approach: Trapezius Transfer

The patient is placed in the lateral decubitus position. An anterior-posterior incision is made across the shoulder, just medial to the deltoid. Often, preexisting scars require a modification of the incision and are incorporated into the incision design. Dissection is carried down to the muscle, and skin flaps are elevated at the level of the muscle, exposing the trapezius and deltoid muscles. The clavicle is exposed anteriorly, and the scapular spine and acromion are exposed as well. The deltoid will appear atrophic, consistent with prolonged denervation. The trapezius should appear healthy and contractile. Using electrocautery and lateral traction, the deltoid is elevated in a medial to lateral direction, releasing it and lifting it from its origins on the lateral aspect of the clavicle and the lateral aspect of the scapular spine and acromion. Care should be taken to preserve the insertion of the trapezius on the acromion. Using an oscillating saw, an osteotomy is made in the acromion, releasing it from the clavicular spine, while preserving the coracoclavicular ligament. The coracoacromial and acromioclavicular ligaments are necessarily divided to allow mobilization of the acromion. Using electrocautery, the atrophic deltoid is then divided along its fibers longitudinally at its midline, until the proximal lateral humerus is exposed. To prepare the humerus for insetting of the acromion, the cortex of the humerus just inferior to the greater tuberosity is decorticated with a high-speed bur or with an osteotome and mallet. The shoulder is abducted 90°, and the acromion with attached trapezius is advanced toward the decorticated surface. Medial to lateral mobilization of the trapezius is performed and is required to achieve adequate advancement of the trapezius. The acromion should be advanced as far as possible inferiorly along the humerus and should reach below the greater tuberosity. Once advanced, the shoulder is abducted while maintaining reduction of the glenohumeral joint, and the acromion is secured with two 6.5-mm cancellous screws. Fluoroscopy is used to check screw position. The position of acromial insertion is important. If it is placed anterior to the lateral midline, it will result in unwanted internal rotation. It is important to insert it laterally, slightly posterior to the midline, to prevent increased internal rotation. The deltoid is then sutured to the trapezius as medially as tension will permit, using 0-0 Vicryl mattress sutures (Fig. 19.1). The wound is irrigated, two closed-suction drains, one anterior and one posterior, are placed below the skin flaps, and the skin is closed. The shoulder is immobilized in 80° of abduction. Postoperatively, finger, wrist, and elbow range of motion is encouraged, with continued immobilization of the shoulder. Immobilization continues for 6 weeks. Radiographs are obtained to confirm bony union and to confirm position of the acromion. The shoulder is gradually permitted increasing adduction and active abduction is initiated with therapy.

Optimizing Outcomes: Trapezius Transfer

- The acromion should be fixated posterior to the lateral midline of the humerus to prevent unwanted internal rotation.
- Postoperative radiographs should be obtained at 6 weeks after surgery to confirm healing prior to mobilization.
- Ensure that the glenohumeral joint is reduced when tensioning the transfer.

Complications and Side Effects: Trapezius Transfer

Because of the large "dead space," hematoma or seroma can occur. Meticulous hemostasis, the use of fibrin glue, and the placement of two drains help to minimize this. Fracture of the acromion during screw placement can occur and is minimized by harvesting an adequate acromial fragment. If initial screw fixation is not secure, a washer on the near cortex of the acromion can be used to achieve secure fixation of the acromial fragment to the humerus. It is important to place the acromion posterior to the lateral midline in order to avoid inducing internal rotation. Placement anterior to the midline will result in undesirable internal rotation at the glenohumeral joint. It is important to ensure that the glenohumeral joint is reduced when abducting the shoulder and insetting the acromion. If this is not performed, the tension on the transfer will not be adequate. Postoperatively, the abduction splint can cause pressure sores if not padded correctly. Attention should be paid to adequately padding contact pressure points. After rehabilitation, persistent painful subluxation is an indication for arthrodesis.

Postoperative Care: Trapezius Transfer

Postoperatively, finger, wrist, and elbow range of motion is encouraged, with continued immobilization of the shoulder. Immobilization continues for 6 weeks. Radiographs are then obtained to confirm healing. The shoulder is gradually permitted increasing adduction, and active abduction is initiated with therapy.

Preoperative History and Considerations: Elbow Function

Loss of elbow flexion severely limits the function of the upper extremity. If the patient cannot position the hand in space for performing tasks, the usefulness of a normally functioning hand is markedly diminished. The most common indication for tendon transfers to restore elbow flexion is a brachial plexus injury in which primary nerve surgery has failed. It is also not unusual for a patient to regain some elbow flexion after primary brachial plexus surgery, only to discover that this incomplete recovery is inadequate for daily activities. If brachial plexus surgery does not result in M4 or greater function, then a tendon transfer to augment the strength of elbow flexion can be considered. In general, elbow extension is less important for hand positioning because it can be compensated for by gravity. Although elbow extension is less important for upper extremity function than flexion, some tasks may be difficult without active extension. Examples include pushing up from a sitting position, powering a wheelchair, or lifting an object over the head. However, in brachial plexus patients with failed primary surgery, the surgeon should focus on restoring elbow flexion rather than extension. We have had success with nerve transfers for triceps function as a primary nerve operation, but would always prioritize elbow flexion.

Multiple tendon transfers have been described for elbow flexion. The pectoralis major, latissimus dorsi, and triceps muscles each may be transferred to the biceps. The Steindler flexorplasty, which we consider the workhorse for restoration of elbow flexion, involves the proximal transposition of the origin of the flexor-pronator mass, increasing its moment arm across the elbow and converting it to an elbow flexor [9]. Other transfers, such as the sternocleidomastoid transfer described by Bunnell, are of primarily historical interest [1].

For a successful outcome, the forearm flexors and pronator teres must be innervated and sufficiently strong to power elbow flexion. The Steindler flexorplasty works best in patients who have some degree of preoperative Steindler effect (augmentation of elbow flexion strength, or maintenance of elbow flexion position by forceful wrist and/or finger flexion, with pronation). This scenario is common after upper trunk injuries, and we have found the Steindler flexorplasty to be a useful operation for restoring or augmenting elbow flexion in these patients. It should also be remembered that although not strictly contraindicated, a Steindler flexorplasty will limit the feasibility of future tendon transfers for hand function.

The Steindler flexorplasty is not an option in patients with complete brachial plexus palsy, with poor grip strength, or who lack a Steindler effect. Furthermore, in patients with complete brachial plexus palsy, the pectoralis, triceps, or latissimus transfers are not feasible either because these muscles have been denervated by the injury. In these situations, we prefer a free functioning gracilis or free functioning contralateral latissimus transfer. The status of recipient vessels is an important consideration prior to performing a free gracilis transfer. In most cases, the thoracoacromial trunk is used as a recipient artery. If there has been significant trauma to the area or if the patient has had prior surgery in the area, as is often the case, a preoperative angiogram should be obtained to confirm the patency of the thoracoacromial trunk. If the patient uses tobacco, cessation should begin 6 weeks prior to surgery and should be confirmed preoperatively with a urine cotinine test.

Many extraplexal nerves, including the contralateral C7, may serve as a recipient nerve. Often, the spinal accessory or the intercostal nerves are used. Although nerve grafting should be avoided, in some situations an extraplexal nerve must be elongated by cable grafts which are directed to the site of future coaptation with the gracilis. If nerve grafting is required, it should be performed at a preliminary stage prior to free functioning muscle transfer. In order to minimize the denervation time of the transferred muscle, the surgeon should wait for the advancing Tinel's to reach the distal end of the graft prior to performing the free functioning muscle transfer.

A final consideration is the stability of the glenohumeral joint. Because the free muscle crosses the shoulder, when it contracts it expends a portion of its motion reducing the glenohumeral subluxation, resulting in decreased elbow flexion. To maximize elbow flexion, glenohumeral instability should be addressed prior to free muscle transfer.

Operative Approach: Steindler Flexorplasty

The patient is positioned supine. The extremity is placed on an arm board and is prepped onto the chest. A proximal sterile tourniquet is used during the case and is crucial to a successful operation. A curved incision is made over the medial arm and forearm, centered over the medial epicondyle and extending 10 cm above and below the elbow. In the forearm, the incision should curve along the course of the pronator teres, and in the arm, it curves toward the anterior midline. Skin flaps are elevated at the level of the muscular fascia, preserving the medial antebrachial cutaneous nerve. The ulnar nerve is identified just proximal to the cubital tunnel and is dissected in a similar fashion to an ulnar nerve transposition. Motor branches distal to the medial epicondyle are preserved. Next, the median nerve is identified proximally in the arm. The median nerve is dissected proximal to distal into the proximal forearm. Motor branches must be preserved. The first branch encountered, arising from the anterior aspect of the nerve, is a branch to the pronator teres. Once the median and ulnar nerves have been freed (Fig. 19.2), a medial epicondylectomy is performed with a sagittal saw. The epicondyle fragment should be 2–2.5 cm in diameter and 5 mm thick at its center portion. Care should be taken to avoid injury to the medial collateral ligament of the elbow. The medial epicondyle is then retracted distally, and the flexor-pronator muscle bellies are elevated off of the anterior surface of the elbow and the anterior surface of the ulna. During this process, the motor branches from both the median and ulnar nerves are preserved. If the joint capsule is violated, it is irrigated and repaired with a 3-0 Vicryl. The periosteal attachment of the muscles bleed readily, and this area requires attention when hemostasis is being achieved. The dissection is performed as far distally as required to allow proximal transposition of the medial epicondyle by 5–7 cm (Fig. 19.3). The elbow is flexed to 120–130° to allow maximal proximal transposition (Fig. 19.4). While protecting the median nerve and brachial artery, the atrophic brachialis muscle is divided longitudinally exposing the anterior surface of the humerus. The periosteum is incised longitudinally at the site of inset and raised with a periosteal elevator. A high-speed bur or osteotome and mallet are used to decorticate the anterior surface of the humerus in preparation for insetting the epicondyle. The epicondyle should be transferred to the anterior, not medial, surface of the humerus in order to maximize supination and prevent pronation contracture. Fixation is performed with a 3.5-mm cortical screw. The medial epicondyle drill hole is overdrilled, and the epicondyle is lagged to the humerus using a washer to prevent the screw head from fracturing the fragment. During this portion of the operation, the median nerve must be retracted laterally. The surgeon must pay close attention to this retraction and minimize it, as excessive retraction can result in median nerve injury. Screw length is confirmed with fluoroscopy. The tourniquet is deflated, hemostasis is obtained, and the skin is closed over a closed-suction drain. The elbow is splinted in 120° of flexion with the forearm supinated.

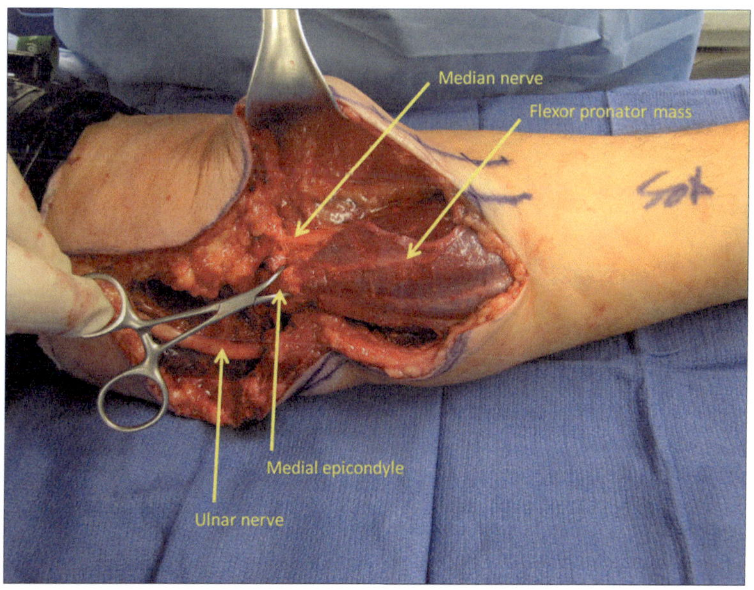

Fig. 19.2 The median and ulnar nerves have been identified and dissected out, and the medial epicondyle is ready for epicondylectomy

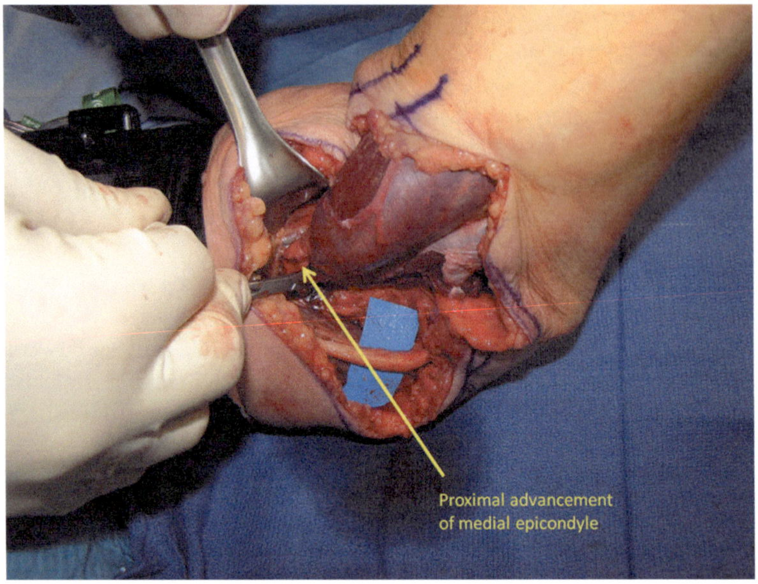

Fig. 19.3 After epicondylectomy, the medial epicondyle can be advanced proximally

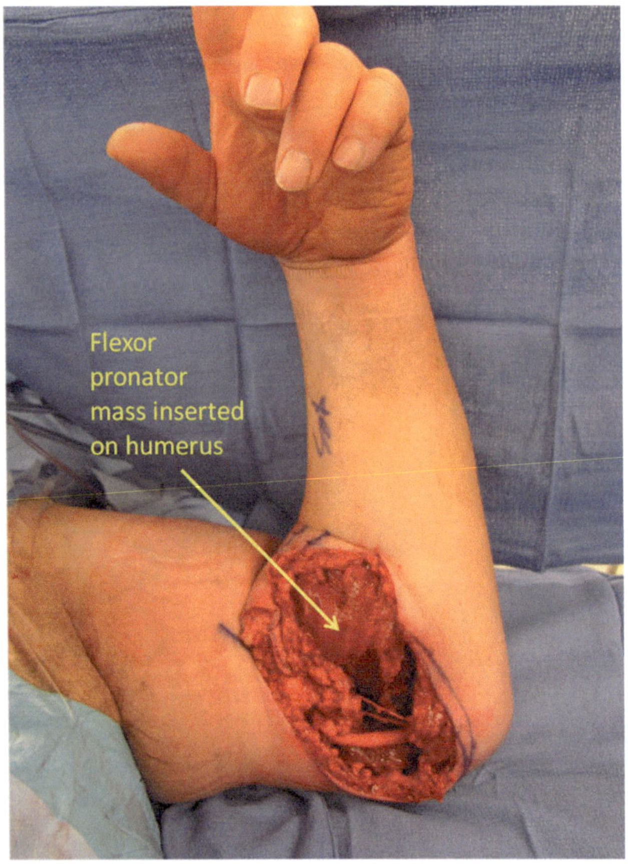

Fig. 19.4 The medial epicondyle has been secured to the humerus, and the elbow naturally rests in 100° of flexion

Optimizing Outcomes: Steindler Flexorplasty

- Patients should have demonstrated preoperative Steindler effect for best outcomes.
- To minimize pronation contracture, the epicondyle fragment should be secured to the anterior surface of the humerus.
- Although a tourniquet may impede the proximal-most dissection, a high sterile tourniquet will make most of the dissection easier, and the operation faster.
- The elbow should be immobilized in 120° of flexion with the forearm supinated, for 6–8 weeks postoperatively or until evidence of bony healing.
- No attempt should be made to overcome the resultant flexion contracture of 30–50°.
- Because this operation relies on successful bony union, smoking is a relative contraindication.

Complications and Side Effects: Steindler Flexorplasty

Preoperatively, one important consideration is the fact that performing a Steindler flexorplasty may limit the ability to perform forearm-level tendon transfers for hand function. Although we have performed forearm-level tendon transfers successfully after a Steindler flexorplasty, one should consider other options for elbow flexion if these are a future possibility.

During surgery, the bloodiest part of the dissection involves elevating the flexor-pronator mass off of the anterior surface of the ulna. Meticulous hemostasis is required here to prevent hematoma. In terms of positioning the medial epicondyle, it should be placed as proximally as possible, a minimum of 5 cm proximal to its original location and ideally 7 cm or more. This provides the best moment arm for elbow flexion. Additionally, an anterior or slightly anterolateral location for the insertion on the humerus prevents pronation contracture. Immobilization with the forearm supinated helps prevent this as well. Finally, during the preparation of the humerus and transposition and fixation of the medial epicondyle, somewhat prolonged lateral retraction on the median nerve is required. This retraction should be very gentle, using a broad retractor, and as brief as possible to prevent injury to the median nerve.

Postoperative Care: Steindler Flexorplasty

The elbow is splinted in 120° of flexion for a minimum of 6–8 weeks and until bony union is achieved. Once healing is demonstrated radiographically, progression of active motion is initiated with therapy. Passive elbow extension is not allowed, and no attempt is made to overcome the flexion contracture at the elbow that invariably results. Patients should be counseled preoperatively that an elbow flexion contracture of 30–50° is expected. This flexion contracture increases the moment arm of the transferred muscles across the elbow and is beneficial. Therapy begins with active elbow flexion with gravity eliminated, by drawing the forearm toward the body across a smooth surface such as a table. This is followed by active motion against gravity and then with increasing resistance. Initially, patients should focus on simultaneous grip, pronation, and elbow flexion in order to activate the transferred muscles. Eventually, this maneuver will not be necessary to activate the transfer. It may take a year or more for motion and strength to plateau.

Operative Approach: Free Functioning Gracilis Muscle Transfer for Elbow Flexion

The operation is best performed with two teams, one at the lower extremity and one at the upper extremity. The operation begins with exposure of the recipient nerve and vessels, and the harvest of the gracilis should not start until the recipient nerve and vessels are exposed and confirmed to be acceptable for the transfer. In order to minimize ischemia time, the recipient vessels and nerve should be prepared under the operating microscope and should be ready for microsurgery prior to dividing the gracilis pedicle. In addition, the sites for proximal and distal inset of the gracilis, as well as the subcutaneous tunnel in the arm, should be prepared prior to dividing the gracilis pedicle. The recipient site incision will vary somewhat, depending upon the recipient vessels and nerves to be used and depending upon preexisting incisions. Skin flaps are elevated, and the lateral one fourth of the clavicle and the acromion are exposed. A series of suture anchors with 0-0 or 2-0 Ethibond are placed into the clavicle and acromion. Usually, at least two or three anchors can be placed in the acromion, and two or three can be placed in the adjacent lateral portion of the clavicle. In the antecubital fossa, an incision is made for exposure of the biceps tendon. The incision begins 3–4 cm proximal to the elbow flexion crease, on the medial side of the arm, and continues distally toward the flexion crease along the posterior border of the biceps. It then curves laterally and crosses the antecubital fossa at the elbow flexion crease and then is extended distally for 3–4 cm along the lateral border of the forearm. Skin flaps are elevated. The lacertus fibrosus is divided and repaired at the time of closure. Tenotomy scissors are used to dissect down to the biceps brachii muscle, which lies just lateral to the brachial vessels. The muscle is followed distally, with retraction on the brachioradialis laterally and on the pronator teres medially. Care is taken to protect the brachial artery and median nerve. The tendon is identified travelling toward the radial tuberosity just distal to the radial head. The tendon is dissected out circumferentially, and a Penrose drain placed around it to aid in later identification and retraction. A subcutaneous tunnel is then developed between the shoulder incision and the antecubital incision. Although this can be done bluntly, it is easily accomplished under direct visualization by using a small Deaver retractor or malleable band for retraction and an extended-tip electrocautery for dissection just superficial to the muscular fascia.

After confirming the adequacy of the recipient vessels and nerve, the second team begins the harvest of the gracilis. The gracilis is harvested in a distal to proximal direction, through three incisions. First, a 3-cm longitudinal incision is made over the distal tendon at its insertion on the medial surface of the tibia. The fascia of the sartorius is elevated, exposing the tendons of the gracilis and the semitendinosus (the gracilis tendon inserts superior to the semitendinosus tendon). The gracilis tendon is dissected circumferentially and is isolated with a Penrose drain. The tendon is retracted, tenting the tendon and muscle in the distal aspect of the thigh, helping to identify the course of the gracilis. A 4-cm longitudinal incision is then made in the distal thigh over the gracilis, a few centimeters proximal to the knee, at the level of the musculotendinous junction. The entire tendon is freed circumferentially through the two incisions. A 15-cm proximal incision is made next, extending longitudinally along the course of the proximal gracilis and ending proximally at the groin crease.

Retraction on the distal tendon helps identify the gracilis, which can be difficult in obese patients. It should be noted that although a skin paddle can be elevated for monitoring, we use an implantable Doppler and therefore do not routinely transfer a skin paddle. Through the two thigh incisions, the superficial surface of the gracilis is exposed, defining the anterior and posterior borders along its entire length. The pedicle to the gracilis arises from the medial femoral circumflex artery and enters the deep surface of the muscle obliquely, approximately 10 cm distal to its origin at the public tubercle. The motor nerve to the muscle, the obturator branch, is identified proximal to the vascular pedicle and enters the muscle approximately 2 cm proximal to the artery. To identify the nerve and vessels, dissection with tenotomy scissors is performed in the interval between the adductor longus and the anterior border of the gracilis. Once the vascular pedicle and nerve have been identified and preserved, proximal and distal dissection circumferentially around the muscle can proceed. Proximal dissection of the muscle is carried to the pubic tubercle, and fascia is left on the muscle proximally to aid in insetting. Once the muscle has been completely dissected, the vascular pedicle is dissected all the way to its take-off from the profunda femoris. Multiple small arterial and venous branches must be ligated with microvascular clips and divided. The obturator nerve is dissected 10 cm proximally. When the recipient site is ready, the gracilis is divided at its origin proximally, and its tendon is divided distally. Finally, the nerve and vascular pedicle are divided and the muscle transferred to the recipient site. One surface of the vessel is marked longitudinally with a marking pen in order to identify and avoid torsion after the pedicle has been divided.

The proximal end of the gracilis is inset at the clavicle and acromion via the preplaced suture anchors. It is then passed through the subcutaneous tunnel. The microvascular anastomosis of the donor vessels with the thoracoacromial artery and cephalic vein are performed, followed by nerve coaptation under the operating microscope. If the intercostal nerves are used, the neurorrhaphy should be performed with the shoulder abducted to make sure that there is no postoperative tension on the neurorrhaphy. Finally, the gracilis tendon is transferred to the biceps tendon in the antecubital fossa incision. Using a tendon weaver, a Pulvertaft weave consisting of three passes is performed and is secured with 0-0 or 2-0 horizontal mattress sutures (Fig. 19.5). The transfer is set at maximum tension with the elbow at 30–40° of flexion.

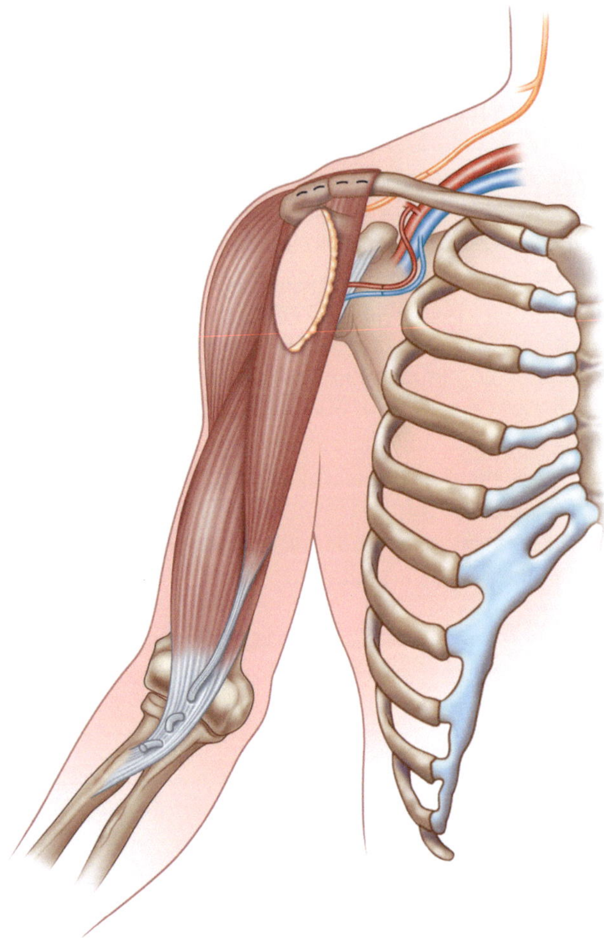

Fig. 19.5 Final inset of the free functioning gracilis muscle

- Although not ideal, if an interpositional graft is required, its distal end should be banked, and the muscle transfer not performed until an advancing Tinel's reaches the distal end of the graft.
- The recipient nerve and vessels should be identified, dissected out, and assessed for adequacy before making an incision on the thigh.
- The recipient site should be fully prepared, including placement of suture anchors, creation of subcutaneous tunnel, exposure of biceps tendon, and preparation of vessels and nerve, with microscope and instruments ready, prior to dividing the pedicle to the gracilis.
- Ischemia time should be less than 1 h.

Optimizing Outcomes: Free Functioning Muscle Transfer for Elbow Flexion

- Full passive elbow range of motion should be present before surgery.
- An acceptable extraplexal motor nerve must be available as a source of axons for neurotization of the gracilis.

Complications and Side Effects: Free Functioning Muscle Transfer for Elbow Flexion

The most feared complication is flap failure. Because the flap is buried, monitoring can be difficult. One option is to elevate a buoy flap based on the musculocutaneous perforators from the gracilis. However, we prefer an implantable Doppler monitor to allow monitoring of the flap. Any evidence of vascular compromise is an indication for immediate return to the operating room for exploration. Difficulties with vascular anastomosis can be prevented with a preoperative arteriogram. Smoking cessation is required 6 weeks prior to surgery and should be confirmed preoperatively with a urine cotinine test.

Postoperative Care: Free Functioning Muscle Transfer for Elbow Flexion

Patients are kept well hydrated, and a Foley catheter is maintained for the first 24 h for evaluation of volume status. Patients are kept NPO the first night after surgery, in case emergent take-back is required. Smoking, nicotine patches, and nicotine of any type are avoided. Caffeine should be avoided. Pain control is achieved with patient-controlled analgesia. The room temperature is maintained at 80°F. Patients are kept in the intensive care unit, or in the flap step-down unit for the first 48 h, and are examined every hour. After 48 h, they are transferred to the regular floor and are discharged within 4–5 days. The elbow is splinted in 90° of flexion, with the forearm supinated for 6 weeks; after which, mobilization is initiated that includes passive flexion and extension to 30°. Passive extension beyond 30° of flexion should not be permitted until a number of months have passed. Immediately after surgery the patient should practice activating the recipient nerve. After 3–4 months, depending upon the length of the donor nerve (the obturator nerve), the patient will be able to voluntarily elicit contractions in the gracilis. Formal therapy should be initiated at this point, involving retraining and strengthening.

Preoperative History and Considerations: Hand Function

Recovery of hand function is often disappointing in patients with brachial plexus injuries. Unfortunately, some patients with complete or near-complete brachial plexus injuries fail to recover any useful hand function and end up with an insensate and motionless hand. In this situation, double free functioning muscle transfers are performed as described by Doi et al. [3, 4].

In patients with partial plexus injuries, there may be enough functioning muscle-tendon units in the forearm to permit a combination of tendon transfers and arthrodesis to restore some hand function. If a functioning sensory nerve or nerves are present, sensory nerve transfers may be performed to improve sensibility in the hand. Because of the highly variable nature of brachial plexus injuries and subsequent recovery, it is not possible to describe a single algorithm for tendon or nerve transfers in these patients. In general, the surgeon must create a plan that is customized to the individual deficits, functioning muscle-tendon units, and sensory nerves of each patient. However, some common patterns of injury and functional loss exist.

Upper plexus injuries involving C5 and C6 are common. An injury limited to C5 and C6 usually does not result in a significant loss of hand motor function. Forearm supination and radial wrist extension are lost but can often be compensated for. These patients also experience a loss of critical sensibility in the thumb and index fingers. However, if the upper plexus injury extends to involve C7, the patient experiences more significant deficits in the hand. Wrist and finger extension are lost, resulting in a motor deficit similar to high radial nerve palsy. Sensory losses involve the long finger in addition to the index and thumb.

In the case of an isolated C5, C6 injury, in which sensibility in the long finger is present, the third web portion of the median nerve is transferred to the digital nerves of the first web space. When the injury extends to include C7, motor reconstruction is similar to that of radial nerve palsy, with the additional requirement for restoration of median nerve distribution sensibility. A typical reconstructive plan would include pronator teres (PT) to extensor carpi radialis brevis (ECRB), flexor carpi radialis (FCR) to extensor digitorum communis (EDC), and palmaris longus (PL) to extensor pollicis longus (EPL) tendon transfers. To restore sensibility to the crucial first web space distribution, a sensory nerve transfer is performed in which the common digital nerve to fourth web space is transferred end-to-end to the digital nerves of the first web space. Less critical second web space sensibility is restored by transferring the common digital nerve to the second web space to the proper digital nerve to the ulnar border of the small finger in an end-to-side fashion. These transfers result in restoration of sensibility in the first and second web distributions, while preserving sensibility to the critical ulnar border of the small finger.

Although much less common than upper trunk injuries, isolated lower plexus injuries result in a greater degree of hand dysfunction. Injuries limited to C8 and T1 result in a complete loss of intrinsic function and significant but variable loss of finger flexion. If the injury extends to include C7, finger extension is lost as well. The brachioradialis (BR) remains intact, and the radial wrist extensors and FCR usually remain intact and can be used as donors for tendon transfers. In addition to the motor deficits, sensibility on the ulnar border of the hand as well as the small ring and long fingers is absent. The extent of injury and the resultant clinical deficits can be quite variable, and tendon transfers should be customized to the unique functional losses of the patient. If the lower plexus injury extends to include C7, an extensor carpi radialis longus (ECRL) to combined flexor digitorum profundus (FDP) tendons, BR to flexor pollicis longus (FPL), and finger extensor tenodeses are performed. This set of transfers maintains wrist motion and restores rudimentary grasp [6]. It should be noted that a reasonable alternative to extensor tenodesis is to perform a wrist arthrodesis, thereby allowing the FCR to be transferred for active finger extension. For sensory function, if third web sensibility is intact, the third web portion of the median nerve is transferred end-to-end to the sensory portion of the ulnar nerve, and the DCU is transferred end-to-side to the remaining sensory portion of the median nerve. However, if C7 has been injured, third web sensibility may not be intact. In this situation, the sensory portion of the ulnar nerve and the DCU are transferred end-to-side into the remaining functional sensory portion of the median nerve.

Because the combination of required tendon transfers and arthrodeses is highly variable, and because these are standard techniques that are well described in the literature, the surgical techniques for each tendon transfer and arthrodesis are not described in this chapter. Below, the surgical techniques for the sensory nerve transfers mentioned above are described.

Operative Approach: Sensory Nerve Transfers for Upper Plexus Injuries

In patients with isolated C5, C6 injuries who do not have an injury to C7, long finger sensibility is often preserved (Fig. 19.6). In this situation, the common digital nerve to the third web space is transferred to the nerves to the radial border of the thumb and to the nerves to the first web space. First, an extended carpal tunnel release exposure is made. A longitudinal carpal tunnel incision is made in the palm 6 mm ulnar to the thenar depression. This is extended 6–8 cm into the distal forearm, with a zigzag at the wrist flexion crease. The carpal tunnel incision in the palm is also extended distally in a zigzag fashion to the distal palmar flexion crease. Tenotomies are used to spread through the subcutaneous fat in the palm. The superficial palmar fascia is divided longitudinally with a 15-blade, and dissection is continued down to the transverse carpal ligament (TCL). The TCL is divided longitudinally just radial to the hook of the hamate with a 15-blade, and the distal and proximal release of the TCL is

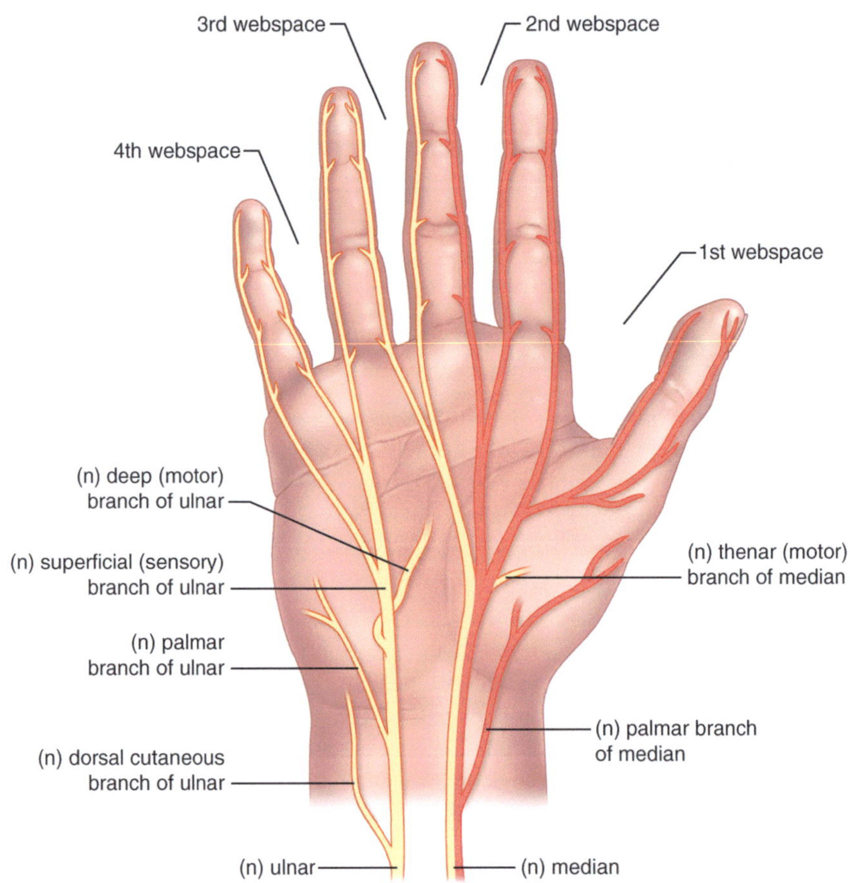

Fig. 19.6 Demonstration of the sensory deficit in a C5, C6 brachial plexus injury. *Red* coloration indicates loss of sensibility, and *yellow* coloration indicates intact sensibility

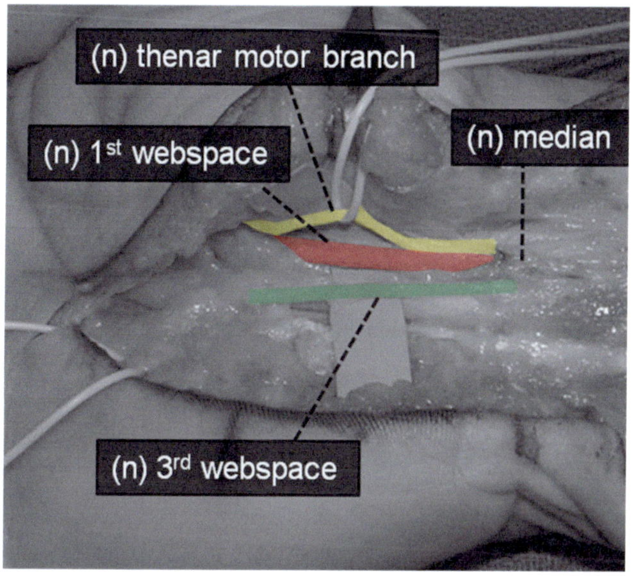

Fig. 19.7 The median nerve has been dissected out, and its components separated, including the recurrent motor branch, sensory portion to the first web space, and sensory portion to the third web space

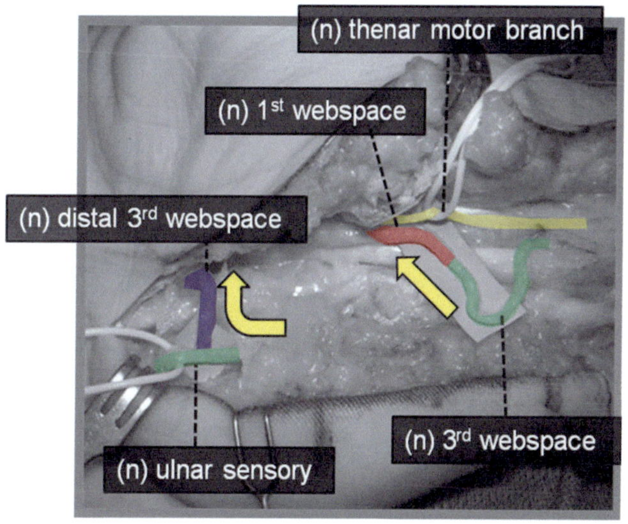

Fig. 19.8 The functioning portion of the median nerve to the third web space has been transferred end-to-end to the portion of the median nerve to the first web space. In addition, the distal stump of the third web portion of the median nerve has been routed toward the sensory portion of the ulnar nerve, when an end-to-side coaptation will be performed

completed under direct visualization using tenotomy scissors. Proximally, the antebrachial fascia is divided under direct visualization, just radial to the ulnar neurovascular bundle. The ulnar nerve is not released or dissected out unless for some other indication. The branches of the median nerve to the radial border of the thumb and to the first web space are identified and dissected out distally and then neurolysed proximally into the distal forearm, separating them from the remainder of the median nerve. The common digital nerve to the third web space is identified distally and is neurolysed proximally as well (Fig. 19.7). The common digital nerve to the third web space is then divided distally, and the branches to the thumb and first web space are divided proximally, allowing a tension-free transfer. Under the operating microscope, the common digital nerve to the third web space is coapted end-to-end to the nerves to the radial border of the thumb and to the first web space (Fig. 19.8).

We have recently begun to include an additional procedure with all sensory nerve transfers. The distal end of the donor sensory nerve is susceptible to painful aberrant reinnervation by pain fibers from surrounding functioning nerves. To prevent this, the distal stump of the divided donor sensory nerve is transferred end-to-side to an adjacent or nearby functioning sensory nerve. For example, in the case of the transfer for isolated C5, C6 injury, the distal stump of the common digital nerve to the third web space is sutured end-to-side to the common digital nerve to the fourth web space (or the sensory portion of the ulnar nerve) to prevent painful aberrant reinnervation of the third web space. Figure 19.9 demonstrates the final sensory transfers for isolated C5, C6 injury.

For restoration of sensibility in C5–C7 brachial plexus injuries, sensory nerve transfers from the ulnar to the median nerve are performed. The same extended carpal tunnel incision described above is made, and the median nerve is exposed as described above. A Guyon's canal release is performed, dividing all bands volar the ulnar nerve, beginning proximally and moving distally. The ulnar neurovascular bundle is retracted ulnarly, and the deep motor branch is identified diving deep to the fibrous hypothenar origin. The deep motor branch is released as well by dividing the fibrous hypothenar origin overlying the deep motor branch. The common digital nerve to the fourth web space is identified and is dissected distally beyond its bifurcation. The proper digital nerves arising from the common digital nerve to the fourth web space are then divided at the level of the distal palmar flexion crease and are retrieved proximally. In order to increase its mobility, the common digital nerve is then neurolysed proximally. Using straight microdissecting scissors, care is taken to separate it from the proper digital nerve to the ulnar border of the small finger and from the deep motor branch. Usually, not much proximal neurolysis is required to complete the transfer without tension. Next, the proper digital nerve to the ulnar border of the small finger is also dissected out into the midpalm and identified with a vessel loop. Next, exploration and identification of the median nerve branches is performed. The branch to the radial border of the thumb, the branches to the first web space, and the common digital nerve to the second web space are identified. These sensory branches are then neurolysed in a distal to proximal direction, separating them from the fascicles to the

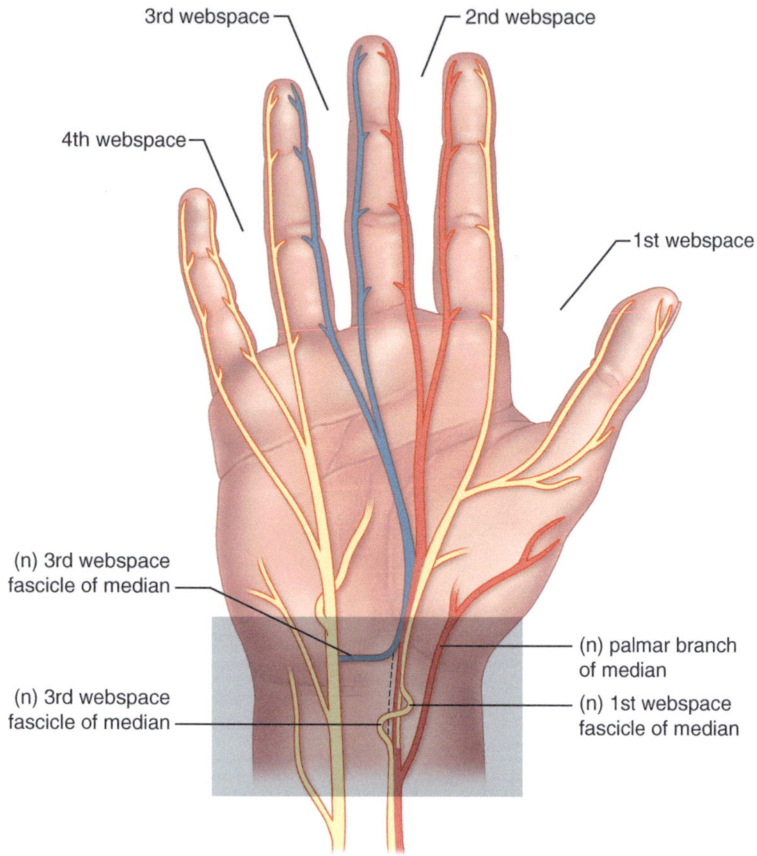

Fig. 19.9 The final arrangement of the sensory transfers for C5, C6 palsy are diagrammed

third web space and from the fascicles to the recurrent motor branch. This is facilitated by identifying the branches distally and then working proximally. Neurolysis is continued into the distal forearm. Once neurolysis is complete, the nerve to the radial border of the thumb, the nerves to the first web space, and the common digital nerve to the second web space are divided in the forearm and are turned distally.

Under the operating microscope, the common digital nerve to the fourth web space (or the two proper digital nerves arising from the bifurcation) is coapted end-to-end to the nerves to the first web space and to the nerve to the radial border of the thumb. Next, the common digital nerve to the second web space is brought over to the intact proper digital nerve to the ulnar border of the small finger. An epineural window is made in the ulnar digital nerve, without axonal injury, and an end-to-side coaptation of the common digital nerve to the second web space is made to the proper digital nerve to the ulnar border of the small finger. Finally, the distal stump of the common digital nerve to the fourth web space is coapted end-to-side to the proper digital nerve to the ulnar border of the small finger to prevent painful aberrant reinnervation of the fourth web space.

It is crucial to perform sensory nerve transfers in a tension-free manner. The nerves should lie loosely and redundantly in their new locations. This is achieved by adequate neurolysis and adherence to the principle of dividing the donor distal and the recipient proximal. After achieving hemostasis, an adhesion barrier (hyaluronate/carboxymethyl cellulose) is applied to the wound covering the transferred nerves. The skin incision is closed and the hand is splinted for comfort. If no tendon transfers were performed, patients can begin ROM within 5–7 days.

Operative Approach: Sensory Nerve Transfers for Lower Plexus Injuries

Patients with lower plexus injuries have a loss of ulnar-sided sensibility, with intact median nerve sensory function, but with variable sensibility in the long finger (Fig. 19.10). Transfers from the median nerve to the ulnar nerve are performed. The same incision and release of the carpal tunnel and Guyon's canal are performed as described above. In the forearm, the antebrachial fascia is divided just radial to the

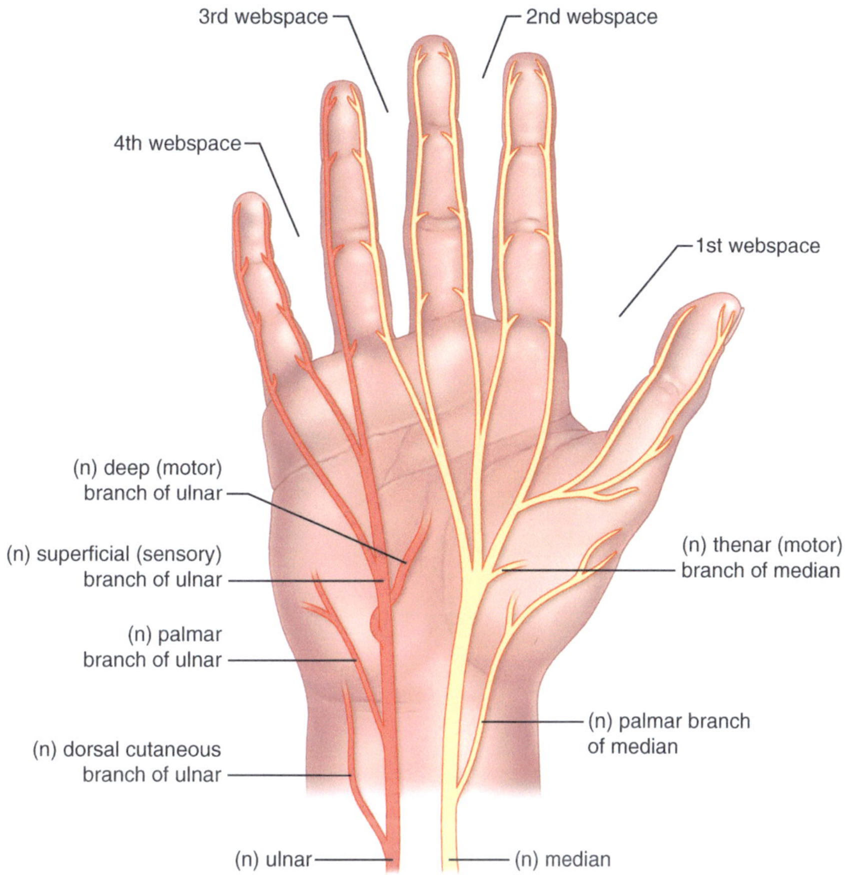

Fig. 19.10 Demonstration of the sensory deficit in a lower plexus injury. *Yellow* coloration indicates intact sensory function, and *red* coloration indicates absent sensory function. It should be noted that sensibility in the third web space and to the long finger is variable

ulnar neurovascular bundle. The flexor digitorum superficialis (FDS) tendons are retracted radially, and the FCU is retracted ulnarly with a blunt self-retaining retractor. Flexion of the fingers and slight flexion at the wrist facilitates retraction. The ulnar nerve is visualized and dissected free along the length of the forearm incision, including the DCU. The DCU is then neurolysed for 3–5 cm proximal to its take-off point using straight microdissecting scissors, separating it from the rest of the ulnar nerve. Intraneural plexi are divided as necessary. Next, the deep motor branch is identified at Guyon's canal. The motor branch is neurolysed proximally, separating it from the sensory portion of the ulnar nerve up to the DCU take-off. A vessel loop is then passed around the motor portion of the nerve for identification. The DCU is divided as proximally as possible and turned distally. The sensory portion of the ulnar nerve is also divided proximally and turned distally, leaving the motor portion of the ulnar nerve intact. Next, the median nerve is prepared. If third web sensibility is preserved (C7 is intact), the third web space portion of the median nerve is used as the donor (Fig. 19.11). The third web portion of the median nerve is identified in the distal forearm by identifying a cleavage plane separating the radial 2/3 and the ulnar 1/3 of the nerve. The cleavage plane, which can be identified by gentle pressure with the tip of a

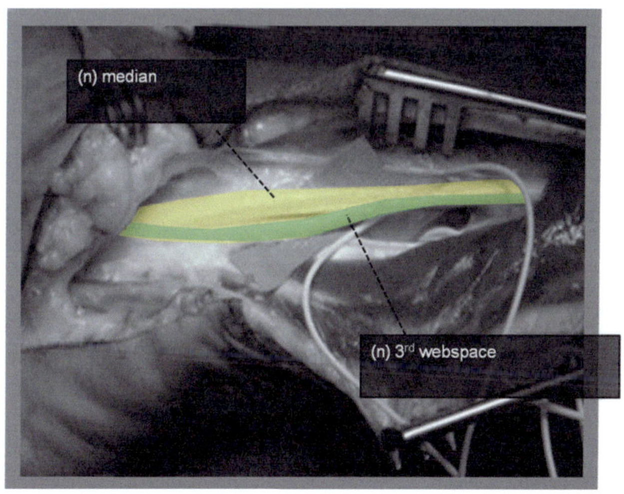

Fig. 19.11 The third web portion of the median nerve has been neurolysed and separated from the remainder of the median nerve

jeweler's forceps, is often marked by a longitudinal vessel. The third web portion of the median nerve is divided at the level of the wrist flexion crease and is neurolysed proximally enough to allow easy transposition to the sensory portion of the ulnar nerve (Fig. 19.12). Under the operating microscope,

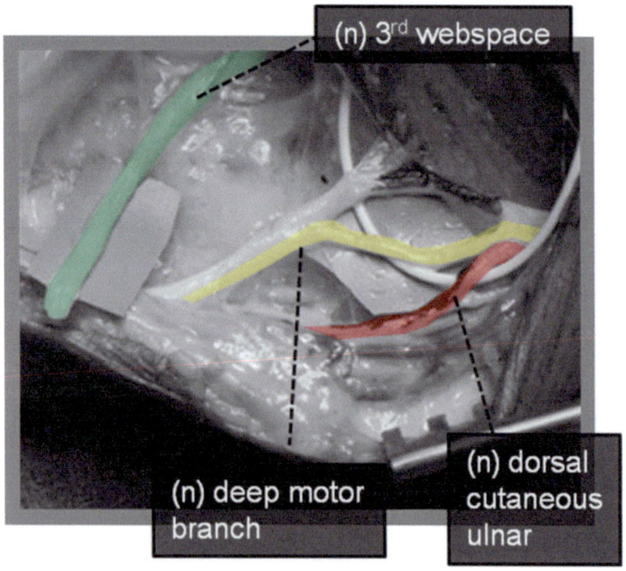

Fig. 19.12 The third web portion of the median nerve has been divided distally and turned toward the ulnar nerve. The ulnar nerve has been neurolysed, separating its sensory and motor components

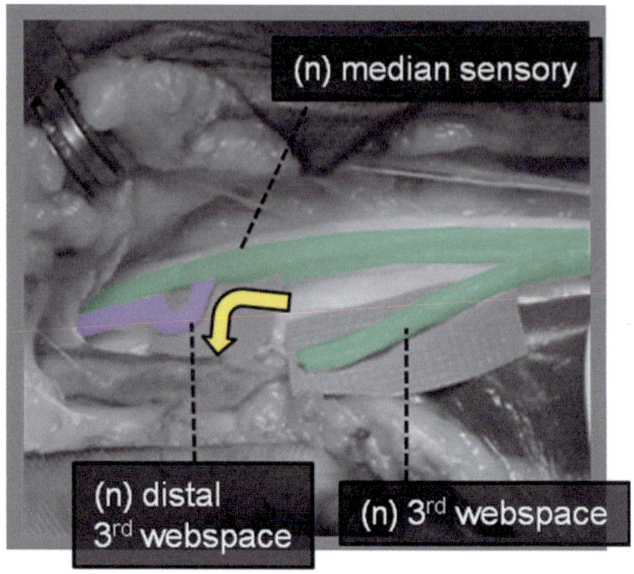

Fig. 19.14 Demonstration of end-to-side coaptation of the distal stump of the third web portion of the median nerve back into the remaining sensory portion of the median nerve, with the purpose of avoiding aberrant painful innervation of the third web space

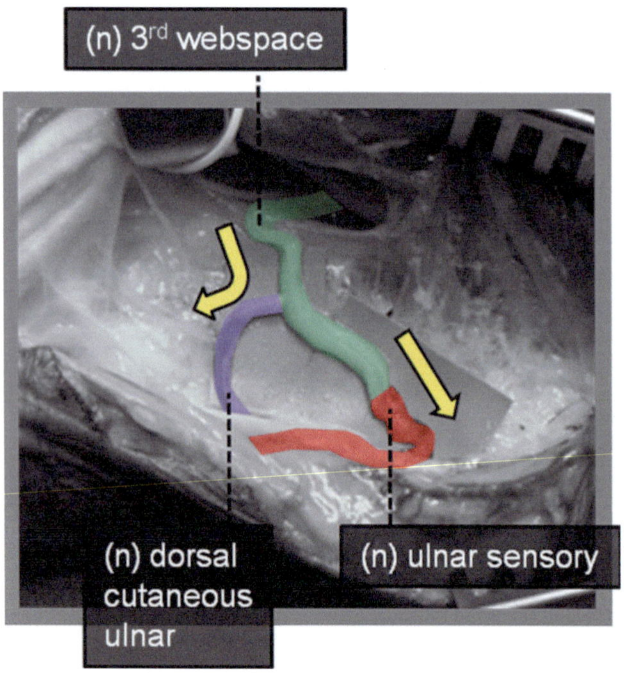

Fig. 19.13 Photograph demonstrating the end-to-end coaptation of the third web portion of the median nerve to the sensory component of the ulnar nerve. The dorsal cutaneous branch of the ulnar nerve has been coapted end-to-side to the third web portion of the median nerve

an end-to-end coaptation of the third web portion of the median nerve to the sensory portion of the ulnar nerve is performed. An epineural window is made in the sensory portion of the median nerve, and the DCU is transferred end-to-side to the median nerve (Fig. 19.13). In addition, the distal stump of the third web portion of the median nerve is neurolysed for a short distance distally, and turned back into the remaining sensory portion of the median nerve, and sutured end-to-side. This is done in order to restore some sensibility to the third web donor site and to prevent painful aberrant reinnervation of the third web space (Fig. 19.14). Figure 19.15 demonstrates the completed transfers.

In some cases, the third web portion of the median nerve is not functional, but patients retain sensory function in the first web space and radial border of the thumb. In this case, the DCU and sensory portion of the ulnar nerve can both be transferred end-to-side to the functioning sensory portion of the median nerve.

Optimizing Outcomes: Sensory Nerve Transfers in the Hand

- The transfers should be performed in a tension-free fashion, and the nerves should lay loose and redundant in their new locations.
- The donor nerve is divided distal, and the recipient nerve is divided proximal (donor distal, recipient proximal).
- An adhesion barrier (hyaluronate/carboxymethyl cellulose) is applied to the transfers prior to skin closure to reduce adhesions.
- Unless tendon transfers are performed simultaneously, movement is initiated at 5 days to prevent adhesions.

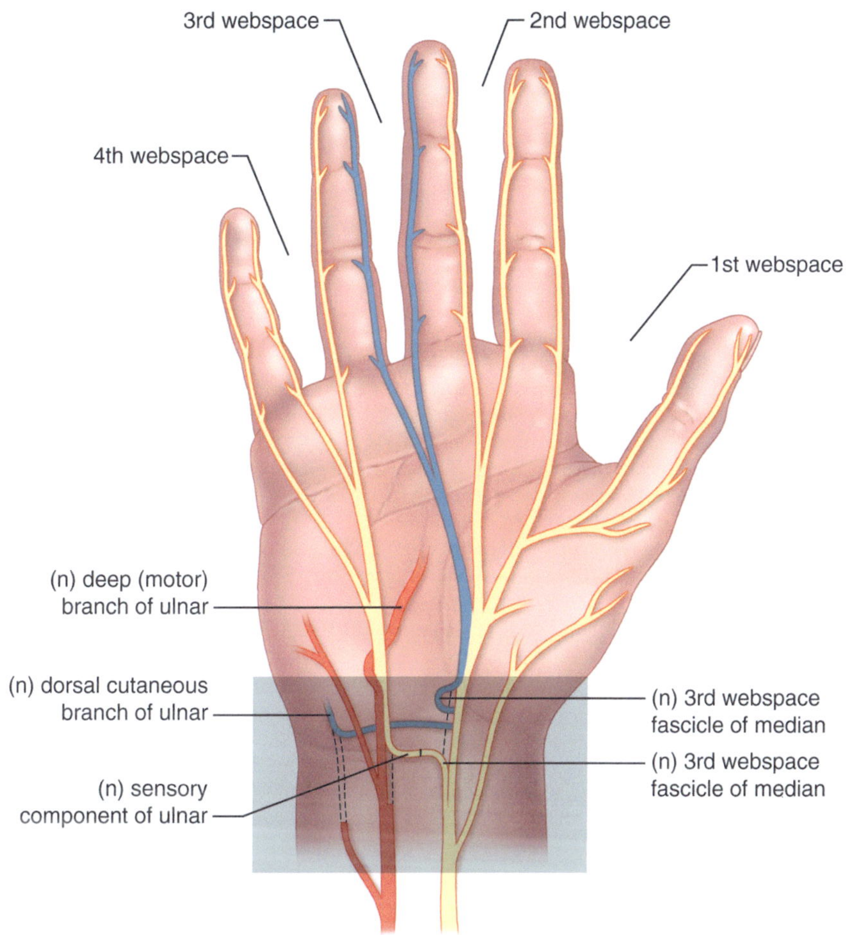

Fig. 19.15 Diagram of the sensory transfers performed for restoration of sensibility in the ulnar distribution

Complications and Side Effects: Sensory Nerve Transfers in the Hand

Failure of the transfer is usually due to excess tension on the coaptation. The transfer is not worth doing unless it is done in such a way that there is no tension on the transfer at all. The transferred nerves should lie with redundancy in the wound bed and should have no kinking or impingement. The key is to divide the donor nerve as distally as possible and the recipient nerve as proximally as possible. The donor nerve is then dissected or neurolysed proximally, and the recipient nerve is dissected or neurolysed distally. With the above-described operations, plexus formation is minimal, but any plexi that limit a tension-free transfer should be divided.

If not addressed, the distal stump of the donor sensory nerve can become reinnervated by pain fibers from surrounding functioning nerves. This painful aberrant reinnervation of the donor nerve can be prevented by performing an end-to-side transfer of the distal stump of the donor nerve to an adjacent functioning sensory nerve and should be performed in all sensory nerve transfers when possible.

Postoperative Care: Sensory Nerve Transfers in the Hand

As long as the transfers are redundant and there is no tension on the nerves, only a brief period of immobilization for comfort (5–7 days) is required.

Conclusion

When initial brachial plexus surgery fails, repeat surgery on the brachial plexus or on peripheral motor nerves is not indicated because of motor end-plate fibrosis. However, in most patients, secondary reconstructive options exist. In order to simplify evaluation and organize treatment, secondary surgery is divided into surgery for shoulder, elbow, and hand function. Secondary shoulder surgery relies upon the trapezius transfer to reduce painful subluxation and improve abduction. Surgery for elbow function consists of the Steindler flexorplasty or a free functioning muscle transfer, depending upon whether good hand function is present.

In the hand, tendon transfers are individualized to the unique pattern of motor loss and remaining functioning muscle-tendon units, and sensory nerve transfers are used to restore sensibility in critical areas.

References

1. Bunnell S. Restoring flexion to the paralytic elbow. J Bone Joint Surg Am. 1951;33-A(3):566–71, passim.
2. Comtet JJ, Herzberg G, Naasan IA. Biomechanical basis of transfers for shoulder paralysis. Hand Clin. 1989;5(1):1–14.
3. Doi K, Muramatsu K, Hottori Y, Watanabe M. Reconstruction of upper extremity function in brachial plexopathy using double free gracilis flaps. Tech Hand Up Extrem Surg. 2000;4(1):34–43.
4. Doi K, Sakai K, Ihara K, Abe Y, Kawai S, Kurafuji Y. Reinnervated free muscle transplantation for extremity reconstruction. Plast Reconstr Surg. 1993;91(5):872–83.
5. Elhassan B, Bishop A, Shin A. Trapezius transfer to restore external rotation in a patient with a brachial plexus injury. A case report. J Bone Joint Surg Am. 2009;91(4):939–44.
6. Goubier JN, Teboul F. Management of hand palsies in isolated C7 to T1 or C8, T1 root avulsions. Tech Hand Up Extrem Surg. 2008;12(3):156–60.
7. Hawkins RJ, Neer 2nd CS. A functional analysis of shoulder fusions. Clin Orthop Relat Res. 1987;223:65–76.
8. Kotwal PP, Mittal R, Malhotra R. Trapezius transfer for deltoid paralysis. J Bone Joint Surg Br. 1998;80(1):114–6.
9. Mayer L, Green W. Experiences with the Steindler flexorplasty at the elbow. J Bone Joint Surg Am. 1954;36-A(4):75–89; passim.
10. Monreal R, Paredes L, Diaz H, Leon P. Trapezius transfer to treat flail shoulder after brachial plexus palsy. J Brachial Plex Peripher Nerve Inj. 2007;2:2.
11. Narakas AO. Muscle transpositions in the shoulder and upper arm for sequelae of brachial plexus palsy. Clin Neurol Neurosurg. 1993;95 Suppl:S89–91.
12. Ray WZ, Kasukurthi R, Yee A, Mackinnon SE. Functional recovery following an end to side neurorrhaphy of the accessory nerve to the suprascapular nerve: case report. Hand (N Y) 2009.
13. Ruhmann O, Schmolke S, Bohnsack M, Flamme C, Wirth CJ. Shoulder arthrodesis: indications, technique, results, and complications. J Shoulder Elbow Surg. 2005;14(1):38–50.
14. Saha AK. Surgery of the paralysed and flail shoulder. Acta Orthop Scand. 1967;Suppl 97:5–90.

20 Reoperative Medial and Lateral Epicondylitis Surgery

Nicholas E. Rose

Abstract

Reoperative surgery for failed previous medial or lateral epicondylitis surgery can be quite challenging. One key concern is making sure that other structures are not actually the cause of persistent symptoms. In the case of medial epicondylitis, it is important to assess for possible medial antebrachial cutaneous nerve (MABCN) injury, ulnar neuropathy, or medial collateral ligament damage. These can sometimes be a source of continued symptomatology despite expertly performed medial epicondylitis surgery. One of the newer techniques for addressing failed or recurrent medial epicondylitis is medial epicondyle denervation surgery. This chapter delves into the surgical detail of this procedure. Similarly, for lateral epicondylitis, it is important to rule out evidence of persistent radial tunnel syndrome, radial capitellar joint plica or synovial fistula, as well as any damage to the lateral collateral ligament. In cases of true failed lateral epicondylitis surgery, a lateral epicondyle denervation surgery can be performed. This can be helpful in the patient who has had multiple previous surgeries. The other issue in treating patients with these conditions is trying to set a reasonable level of expectations regarding outcomes. This chapter details some of the newer techniques for treating these challenging clinical problems.

Keywords

Elbow • Tendon • Antebrachial • Epicondylitis • Denervation

Introduction

Medial and lateral epicondylitis are the two most common overuse injuries of the elbow. Both conditions represent enthesopathies, a disorder occurring where tendons and ligaments attach to bone. The term "epicondylitis" is somewhat of a misnomer, implying that an inflammatory pathologic process is taking place. A more appropriate term is "tendinosis" as inflammatory cells are rarely encountered in the condition. The pathology for both conditions is a tendonous microtearing followed by an incomplete reparative response, as evidenced by the chronic inflammatory cells typically encountered in pathologic analysis.

N.E. Rose, MD (✉)
California Orthopaedic Specialists,
360 San Miguel Drive, Suite 701, Newport Beach, CA 92660, USA
e-mail: nickrosemd@yahoo.com

Medial epicondylitis, often referred to as "golfer's elbow", is the most frequent cause of medial elbow pain, though it is only about 10% as common as lateral epicondylitis. Lateral epicondylitis, commonly referred to as "tennis elbow", is the most frequent overuse injury of the elbow, affecting approximately 2% of the population.

Elbow epicondylitis involves pathological alteration in the muscultendinous origins at the lateral or medial epicondyle. The central focus of pathology in medial epicondylitis is the flexor–pronator origin at the anterior medial epicondyle. Lateral epicondylitis is a result of angiofibroblastic degeneration at the common extensor origin, most often the extensor carpi radialis brevis (ECRB).

Regardless of the etiology of medial or lateral epicondylitis, nonoperative measures have been reported to be successful in up to 90% of patients [1]. Furthermore, surgery success rates for medial and lateral epicondylitis have been reportedly

S.F.M. Duncan (ed.), *Reoperative Hand Surgery*,
DOI 10.1007/978-1-4614-2373-7_20, © Springer Science+Business Media, LLC 2012

as high as 90% and as low as 40% regardless of the specific technique used. The overall reliability and success rate of operative procedures for medial and lateral epicondylitis make the need for reoperation very uncommon. In light of these factors, very little has been written about subsequent management of cases where operative intervention has failed. The purpose of this chapter is to provide a basis for determining the cause of failed operative treatment for medial and lateral epicondylitis and also to provide a foundation for further management. Specifically, we have focused on identifiable causes of failure that may be successfully addressed with a secondary surgical procedure.

Medial Epicondylitis

Summary Box (Medial Epicondylitis)

1. Evaluate the ulnar nerve and obtain electrodiagnostic studies as indicated, as ulnar neuropathy can be present in up to 60% of cases.
2. Clinical examination of the ulnar nerve should also include an assessment for subluxation. If ulnar nerve subluxation is present, the surgeon should consider performing an anterior submuscular or subcutaneous ulnar nerve transposition in concert with a medial release.
3. Evaluate the medial collateral ligament (MCL), as medial instability is a common cause of medial elbow pain, particularly in younger athletes engaged in chronic valgus activities.
4. When giving cortisone injections to the common flexor origin, great care must be given to avoid the ulnar nerve, particularly when subluxation is present. Placing the elbow in no more than 45° of flexion during the injection can help avoid this complication.
5. Careful dissection posterior to the medial epicondyle should be performed as damage to the origin of the anterior oblique ligament (AOL) portion of the MCL may occur in this area and lead to iatrogenic medial instability.
6. The medial conjoint tendon (MCT) serves as a surgical landmark in medial epicondylitis surgery and allows the surgeon to avoid injury to the AOL.

Introduction

Medial epicondylitis (golfer's elbow in layman's terms) is an overuse injury affecting the flexor–pronator muscle origin at the anterior medial epicondyle of the humerus. It is the most common cause of medial elbow pain, but is only 10–20% as common as lateral epicondylitis. Other causes of medial elbow pain include ulnar nerve compression within the cubital tunnel, ulnar nerve subluxation or dislocation, MCL instability, and snapping triceps syndrome.

The etiology of medial epicondylitis is a repetitive use of the flexor–pronator muscles of the elbow, typically the pronator teres and flexor carpal radialis origin. The pronator teres originates from the superoanterior medial epicondyle as well as from the MCT, a structure sometimes referred to as the accessory AOL. The flexor carpi radialis (FCR) also has a small medial epicondylar origin as well as an origin off the distoulnar aspect of the MCT. The MCT serves as a surgical landmark in medial epicondylitis surgery and allows the surgeon to avoid injury to the AOL.

Contractile loading at the medial elbow, both concentric and eccentric, associated with repetitive forearm pronation and wrist flexion contributes to the degenerative process occurring in the flexor–pronator origin. Microtears develop in the tendon and the tendinosis that results is primarily the result of failure of the damaged tendon to heal. Microscopic examination of the pathologic tissue shows granulation tissue, fibrovascular and fibrocartilaginous tissue, tendon microfragmentation, calcification, and sometimes necrosis.

Preoperative History and Considerations

Patients with medial epicondylitis typically present with medial sided elbow pain. The pain is aggravated by activities that entail repetitive or forceful pronation. It tends to occur in the third to fifth decade and is twice as common in males. Ulnar neuropathy is associated with the condition in up to 25–60% of cases and must be ruled out on clinical examination. If elbow "popping" is a presenting complaint, one must rule out a snapping medial head of the triceps or ulnar nerve subluxation as an etiology.

A comprehensive examination of the neck and shoulder should be performed, as referred pain from these areas can be a source of medial elbow pain. Examination of the elbow reveals localized tenderness over the common flexor origin. Ulnar neuropathy and medial instability must be ruled out in each patient. The elbow should also be assessed for possible ulnar nerve subluxation. If ulnar nerve pathology is suspected, electrodiagnostic evaluation is indicated but electromyography can be normal in up to 50% of cubital tunnel cases. Valgus stability must be evaluated, as medial instability is a common cause of medial elbow pain, particularly in overhead throwing athletes.

Though imaging studies are of limited value, radiographs can rule out other etiologies of elbow pain such as osteoarthritis or osteochondritis dissecans. Medial epicondylar calcification is present in 10–20% of cases. Other imaging studies are of limited value. MRI typically does not play a useful role in the evaluation and treatment of this condition, though signal changes in the common flexor origin are commonly found. MRI findings include thickening and increased T1 and T2 signal intensity of the common flexor tendon and soft tissue edema around the common flexor tendon.

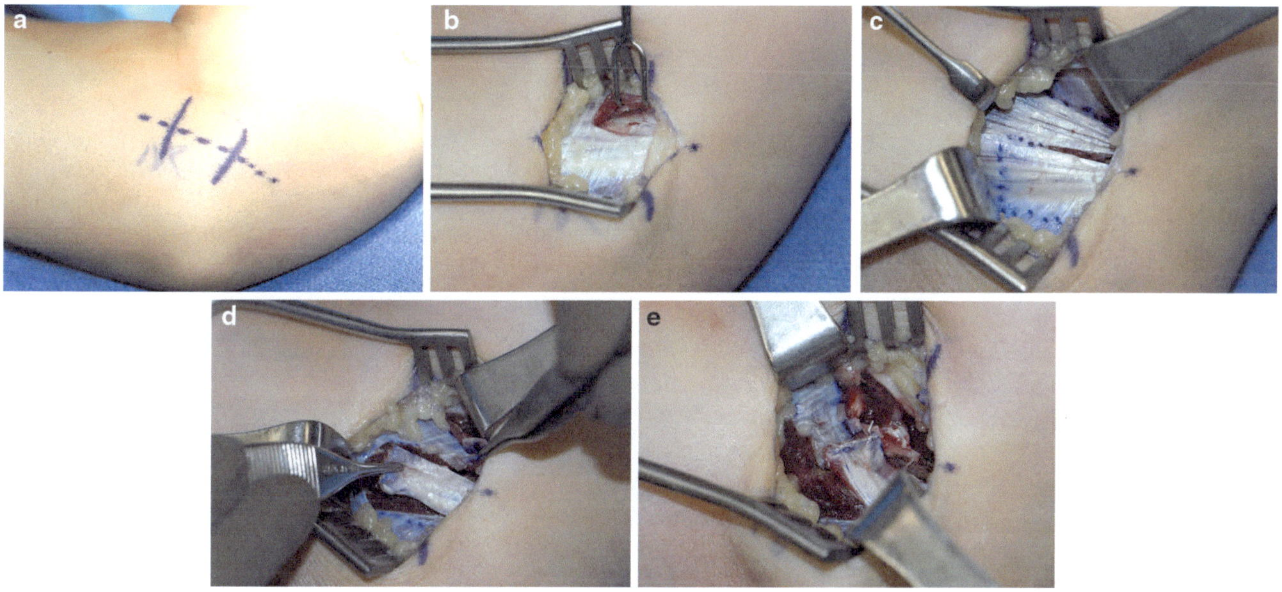

Fig. 20.1 (**a**) Longitudinal incision along the medial epicondyle. (**b**) Degenerative nidus within the MCT. (**c**) Marking out the Z-plasty of the common flexor origin. (**d**) The incised tendon prior to lengthening. (**e**) Completion of the Z-plasty

Indications and Contraindications

Nonoperative measures for medial epicondylitis should be exhausted before surgical intervention is considered. These measures include patient education, physical therapy, countertraction strapping, and nonsteroidal anti-inflammatory medications (NSAIDS). Wrist bracing can also be considered. Physical therapy consisting of local modalities (ultrasound, electrical stimulation, and iontophoresis) along with a conditioning, stretching, and strengthening program can be beneficial as well.

Corticosteroid injections should consist of equal volume local anesthetic and corticosteroid for a total volume of 2 mL injected in the area of maximal tenderness on the anterior aspect of the medial epicondyle. Care must be taken to avoid intraneural ulnar nerve injection, particularly in patients with evidence of ulnar nerve subluxation, as this can have devastating consequences. This complication can be avoided by injecting the common flexor origin with the elbow placed at no more than 45° of flexion. When ulnar nerve subluxation is present, injection should be performed with the elbow near full extension.

If ulnar neuropathy is present, patients are instructed to avoid activities involving prolonged or repetitive elbow flexion and also avoid leaning on the elbow and placing direct pressure on the ulnar nerve. Nighttime extension bracing can also be beneficial.

Autologous blood injections for medial epicondylitis have had mixed results and further studies are warranted to confirm its efficacy. Suresh et al. used ultrasound guidance to inject a mixture of autologous blood and local anesthetic into the common flexor origin with satisfactory results in 17 of 20 patients. They showed that the combined action of dry needling and autologous blood injection under ultrasound guidance appears to be an effective treatment for refractory medial epicondylitis as demonstrated by a significant decrease in VAS pain and a fall in the modified Nirschl scores [2].

Surgery is considered in patients who have failed nonoperative management. The main indication for surgery is failure to respond to the nonoperative measures for a minimum of 6 months. Typically, this includes persistent symptoms despite two or three corticosteroid injections. Progressive ulnar pathology is also an indication for surgery and should be addressed surgically with ulnar nerve decompression with or without anterior transposition.

Operative Approach

Surgery for medial epicondylitis consists of a medial release with medial epicondylar debridement. In the presence of ulnar neuropathy, the ulnar nerve needs to be addressed with either a decompression or decompression combined with anterior transposition.

Under tourniquet control, a 3–4-cm longitudinal incision is made just anterior to the medial epicondyle (Fig. 20.1a). Dissection is carried through the skin and subcutaneous tissue with care taken to identify and protect branches of the MABCN. In isolated medial release cases without ulnar nerve pathology or subluxation, the ulnar nerve does not need to be exposed from its location posterior to the medial epicondyle, but the surgeon should be aware of its location throughout the case. The flexor–pronator fascia is identified and the pronator teres and FCR origins are elevated off the medial epicondyle, leaving a 2-mm rim of superficial fascia attached to the medial epicondyle for later repair. The pronator teres and FCR are elevated off the MCT to allow identification of the degenerative nidus (Fig. 20.1b). This nidus is typically found within the origin of the MCT. Care is taken to distinguish the MCT from the AOL; this is easier distally where the two structures are more distinct. Proximally, a 3- to 4-mm section of the MCT that includes the degenerated nidus is resected taking great care not to encroach upon the AOL. The flexor–pronator origin is then reattached to the previous 2-mm cuff of tissue left attached to the medial epicondyle. Alternatively, the author's preference is to perform a Z-plasty of the common flexor origin by raising proximally and distally based flaps that are then sewn end-to-end to complete the release and "reset" the tension in the common flexor origin (Fig. 20.1c–e). This option is also desirable when ulnar nerve pathology is present, as the sewn fascial ends can serve as a loose bridge maintaining the ulnar nerve in the anteriorly transposed position.

Optimizing Outcomes

- Take care to identify and protect the MABCN.
- When detaching the pronator teres and FCR off the medial epicondyle, leave a 2-mm cuff of superficial fascia attached to the medial epicondyle for later repair.
- Distinguish the MCT from the AOL to avoid damage to the AOL and subsequent instability.
- If ulnar nerve pathology is evident perform ulnar nerve decompression with anterior transposition.
- Consider Z-plasty of common flexor origin to "reset" tension on tissues.

Postoperative Care

The extremity is placed in a long arm splint with the elbow at 90° and the forearm neutral, leaving the wrist and hand free. Hand and wrist movement is encouraged immediately post-op. Active elbow exercises are started 2–3 days post-op and a removable splint is continued for 1 week post-op. The patient is allowed to resume normal activities of daily living during the first week after surgery. Wrist and forearm range of motion exercises without resistance are started 1 week after surgery. At 3 weeks gradual resistance strengthening exercises including wrist resistance exercises with one pound weights are started. Patients wear a countertraction brace during these strengthening exercises for 2–3 months after surgery while performing their activities of daily living. The countertraction strap is continued thereafter for sports and more strenuous work activities for an additional 3 months. Tennis players may resume easy strokes at 6 weeks post-op while golfers may start chipping and putting 4 weeks post-op. Return to full strength use in competitive athletes and manual laborers typically occurs at 6 months post-op. Patients may opt to continue prophylactic use of the countertraction strap thereafter.

Complications and Side Effects

Medial Antabrachial Cutaneous Nerve Damage

The medial antabrachial cutaneous nerve (MABCN) travels in the subcutaneous tissue in the medial arm. Just proximal to the medial epicondyle, it divides into an anterior and posterior branch. The posterior branch courses directly over the flexor–pronator origin to travel to the posterior medial aspect of the forearm. Damage to the MABCN during primary medial epicondylitis surgery can result in a painful neuroma and is a frequent cause for persistent elbow pain following medial release surgery.

Patients will frequently present with medial elbow pain associated with hyperesthesia or hypoesthesia at the medial forearm. On examination, a Tinel's along the course of the MABCN will confirm the diagnosis.

Ulnar Neuropathy

In patients with isolated medial epicondylitis, exposure of the ulnar nerve is typically unnecessary unless a subluxing ulnar nerve is noted preoperatively. Nevertheless, some patients may develop postoperative ulnar nerve symptoms, either as a result of subclinical cubital tunnel syndrome becoming symptomatic after surgery or development of scar tissue causing ulnar neuropathy postoperatively.

Medial Colateral Ligament Damage

The MCT serves as a surgical landmark in medial epicondylitis surgery and allows the surgeon to avoid injury to the AOL. The MCT originates from the anterior inferior medial epicondyle and immediately posterior to the proximal 4–5 mm of the MCT is the AOL. Over the proximal 50% of the AOL, the two structures are contiguous but over the distal 50% the structures are surgically distinguishable. Therefore, any dissection of the MCT posterior to the medial epicondyle risks damage to the AOL, as it violates the origin of the AOL and places the patient at risk of developing postoperative medial instability.

Medial Antebrachial Cutaneous Nerve Damage

Introduction

The MABCN, also known as the medial cutaneous nerve of the forearm, is a sensory nerve whose distribution includes the medial aspect of the forearm from the elbow to the wrist. It originates from the medial cord of the brachial plexus and

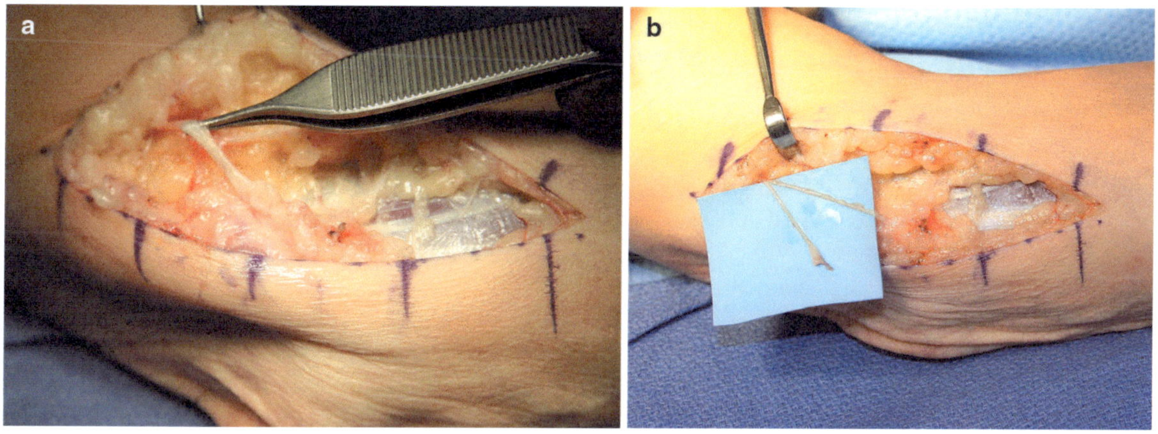

Fig. 20.2 (**a**) Careful dissection of the MABCN. (**b**) Neuroma from previous transection; neuromas should be excised when possible

is composed primarily of nerve fibers from the ventral rami of C8 and T1. After passing through the axilla deep to the pectoralis insertion and anterior to the latissimus dorsi, it lies medial to the axillary artery then medial to the brachial artery as it courses through the arm. It then pierces the deep fascia with the basilic vein becoming cutaneous in the mid-portion of the arm. It then divides into an anterior and a posterior branch. The anterior branch, typically the larger of the two, then continues distally along the anteromedial aspect of the forearm, supplying the skin of the anteromedial forearm as distally as the wrist. The posterior branch courses anterior to the medial epicondyle curving posteriorly to reach the dorsal portion of the medial forearm. It continues distal to the wrist supplying the overlying skin.

Though either of the two branches can be damaged with medial epicondylitis surgery, it is usually the posterior branch that is at most risk. Damage to the nerve typically involves either a simple stretch-type neuropraxia, a partial transection of the nerve, or complete transection. A partial or complete transection can result in a neuroma-in-continuity or neuroma, respectively.

Preoperative History and Considerations

Patients who sustain injuries to the MABCN typically develop persistent medial elbow pain along with sensory disturbance in the medial forearm. Patients will describe burning or sharp pain in the medial aspect of the elbow along with sensitivity in the area of the incision site, often complaining of discomfort when the area is contacted, such as when resting the elbow on an armrest.

Physical examination reveals a painful Tinel's in the area of the MABCN along with dysesthsias or paresthesias in the distribution of the nerve in the medial forearm. Patients with simple neuropraxia injuries may show improvement in their symptoms over the course of several weeks, but patients with persistent symptoms should be considered for surgical exploration.

Indications and Contraindications

Patients with persistent symptoms unresponsive to nonoperative measures should be considered for surgery. It is important to instruct patients that the goal of the surgery is to eliminate the painful neuroma on the medial aspect of the elbow and that they likely will still be left with some degree of numbness in the medial forearm. It is imperative that patients be informed that the goal of the surgery is to eliminate the pain associated with the neuroma and that restoration of normal sensation in the medial forearm is unlikely.

Operative Approach

In the preoperative holding area, the area of maximum Tinel's is identified and marked with a permanent marker, noting the angulation of the elbow when the mark is made. The patient is placed in the supine position and the procedure is performed under tourniquet control. The original incision is utilized but often will need to be extended proximally. It is imperative that the MABCN be identified proximally, allowing the surgeon to dissect from normal to abnormal tissue, as identification of the transected MABCN in thickened scar can often be difficult. Often, either the anterior or posterior branch (more typically the latter) will be encased in scar tissue, and gentle dissection is necessary to dissect the nerve free from this tissue (Fig. 20.2a). In the best-case scenario, the MABCN will be found to be intact and simple neurolysis will suffice. At times a neuroma-in-continuity will be encountered and under microscopic dissection the area of neuroma-in-continuity may be spliced out and direct repair of the nerve may be performed. In this case, it is imperative that the surgeon completely excise all neuroma scar tissue and transect enough of the nerve to allow anastamosis of normal nerve tissue. Failure to do so can result in persistent neuroma-in-continuity and therefore persistent symptoms. However, in the majority of cases a complete transection will be encountered along with a neuroma. (Fig. 20.2b) The neuroma is excised. Assuming that only one of the two branches is damaged, the surgeon often must gently dissect proximally to separate the posterior branch from the anterior branch to allow maximum excursion of the damaged nerve to allow for adequate transposition. The triceps fascia is then split and the nerve ending is buried deep within the triceps. The wound is then closed in layers.

Optimizing Outcomes

- In the preoperative holding area, have the patient identify the area of maximal Tinel's and mark this area with a permanent marking pen.
- Identify the MABCN proximally so that dissection can proceed from normal to abnormal nerve tissue.
- Mobilize the MABCN adequately in a proximal direction so that ample nerve can be buried into the triceps musculature with minimal tension. If necessary, gentle intraneural neurolysis will allow separation of the anterior and posterior MABCN branches to allow adequate transposition of the involved branch.

Complications and Side Effects

As with any nerve surgery, further nerve damage is a possible consequence of MABCN neuroma excision and transposition. Displacement of the transposed nerve from its triceps bed is a rare complication but should be considered should persistant pain and Tinel's be encountered postoperatively.

Postoperative Care

Following MABCN neuroma and transposition, the patient is immobilized in a long arm posterior splint with the elbow at 90° and the wrist and hand free for 7–10 days to allow the transposed MABCN to settle into the triceps musculature. Physical therapy is then initiated consisting of active and passive ROM along with desensitization and strengthening exercises. Return to regular activities is allowed 4 weeks post-op.

Persistent or Postoperative Ulnar Neuropathy

Introduction

Ulnar neuropathy is a common etiology for medial-sided elbow pain. Typically, it is associated with dysesthesias extending into the ring and small finger, particularly at night. On physical examination, a positive elbow flexion test and positive Tinel's and compression tests of the ulnar nerve should alert the physician of possible ulnar nerve pathology. As mentioned above, if the clinician suspects ulnar nerve involvement, EMG/NCV studies should be included in the patient's diagnostic workup, keeping in mind the relatively high false negative rate of these studies in patients with cubital tunnel syndrome as these studies are not always sensitive enough to detect mild nerve compression [3]. When only portions of the nerve fibers are compressed during early stages, i.e., mild nerve compression, electrodiagnostic studies can be normal. Nevertheless, some patients may develop postoperative ulnar nerve symptoms, either as a result of subclinical cubital tunnel syndrome becoming symptomatic post-op or development of scar tissue causing ulnar neuropathy postoperatively (Fig. 20.3).

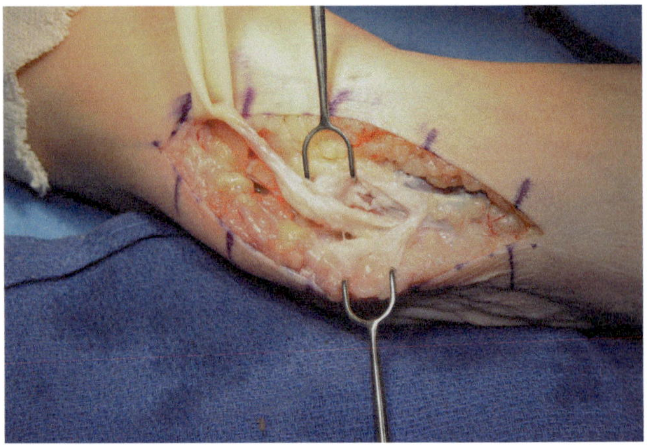

Fig. 20.3 Careful dissection of scarred ulnar nerve

Preoperative History and Considerations

Patients who develop ulnar neuropathy in the postoperative period will typically complain of persistent medial elbow pain along with paresthesias in the ulnar nerve distribution of the hand. This can be the result of either ulnar neuropathy that was subclinical in the preoperative period or new onset ulnar neuropathy developing in the postoperative period, possibly as a result of scar tissue or traction injury during surgery. Rarely, intraoperative injury to the ulnar nerve should also be considered. As with all patients presenting with dysesthesias in the hand, the physician must examine the neck and entire upper extremity to localize the source of the patient's neuropathy. On examination, patients will typically demonstrate a positive Tinel's and compression test along with a positive elbow flexion test. Dysethesias in the ulnar distribution of the hand will often be present. Electrodiagnostic studies can be beneficial in evaluating the ulnar nerve, but may not be conclusive.

Indications and Contraindications

Patients with postoperative nerve pathology should be followed and monitored closely. In cases of intraoperative neuropraxia, symptoms will often improve with conservative management over several weeks or months. If electrodiagnostic studies confirm ulnar neuropathy in the postoperative period, repeat studies can be considered down the line, but are usually unnecessary. Should ulnar nerve symptoms persist or worsen and become unresponsive to nonoperative measures, one should consider surgical exploration of the ulnar nerve with possible anterior transposition.

Operative Approach

The patient is placed in the supine position and the procedure is performed under tourniquet control. A generous incision along the posteromedial aspect of the elbow is utilized to adequately expose the ulnar nerve. Care is taken to identify and protect branches of the MABCN. The ulnar nerve is identified proximally at the medial border of the triceps and followed distally. This will allow the surgeon to dissect from normal to scarred nerve tissue. Proximally, the Arcade of Struthers is identified and released. The medial intermuscular septum is identified and the plexus of veins posterior to this structure is protected. The distal 5 cm of the medial intermuscular septum is excised to prevent tenting of the transposed nerve over this structure. Dissection of the nerve is carried distally to Osborne's fascia. Great care is taken in dissecting the nerve around the previous medial epicondyle surgical site. Osborne's fascia is released and the multiple ulnar nerve branches to the flexor carpi ulnaris musculature are preserved. An anterior subcutaneous, intramuscular, or submuscular transposition is performed depending on surgeon preference. As mentioned above, if medial release surgery is being performed in concert with ulnar nerve anterior transposition, the surgeon may consider a common flexor origin Z-plasty, raising proximally and distally based fascial flaps that are then sewn end-to-end to act as a loose bridge maintaining the ulnar nerve in the anteriorly transposed position (Fig. 20.1c, e).

Optimizing Outcomes

- Localize ulnar nerve proximally in order to carry dissection from normal to abnormal nerve tissue.
- Take great care when dissecting ulnar nerve around the medial epicondyle as adherence of the nerve scar tissue at the medial epicondyle may be present.
- When ulnar neuropathy is noted preoperatively in conjunction with medial epicondylitis, the surgeon should consider raising proximally and distally based flexor–pronator fascial flaps, sewing the flaps end-to-end to function as a loose bridge maintaining the ulnar nerve in the anteriorly transposed position.
- If significant scar tissue is present at the common flexor origin from previous medial release, the surgeon should consider submuscular transposition to avoid placing the ulnar nerve in a scarred bed.

Complications and Side Effects

As with any nerve surgery, persistant ulnar nerve symptoms may be encountered. When ulnar nerve surgery is performed following previous medial release surgery, postoperative scarring may occur resulting in worsening ulnar neuropathy. To help prevent this complication, the surgeon should be wary of a scarred common flexor origin. In the presence of a scarred common flexor origin, submuscular ulnar nerve transposition should be considered.

Postoperative Care

The patient is placed in a long arm posterior splint with the elbow at 90° and the wrist neutral for 3–4 days. The splint is then removed and the patient is sent to therapy for range of motion and nerve gliding exercises. The patient may use a sling for comfort for 2–3 weeks post-op. Strengthening of the common flexor muscles is initiated at 6 weeks post-op.

Medial Instability

Introduction

Medial instability is a common cause of medial elbow pain, particularly in the throwing athlete. The MCL of the elbow consists of three parts: the anterior bundle, the posterior bundle, and the transverse ligament (Fig. 20.4). The anterior bundle is the most discrete component, while the posterior bundle is often simply a thickening of the posterior elbow capsule. The transverse ligament contributes little or nothing to elbow stability.

Throwing exposes the medial elbow to high tensile forces and the lateral elbow to high compressive forces. Valgus stability to the elbow is provided by the MCL, ulna/trochlear articulation, the flexor–pronator muscle mass, and the radiocapitellar articulation. Repetitive valgus stresses to the elbow occur during the late cocking and acceleration phases of throwing and can often lead to MCL injury, ulnar neuritis, and posteromedial olecranon impingement. The physician should assess medial stability in all patients presenting with medial-sided elbow pain.

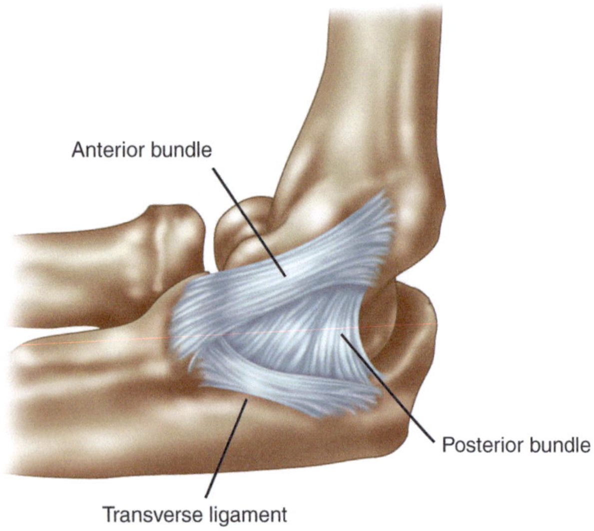

Fig. 20.4 Anatomy of the MCL complex

Patients, particularly throwing athletes, with persistent medial elbow pain following medial release surgery should be closely evaluated for MCL incompetence. This can be the result of unrecognized preoperative medial instability or, more rarely, can result from intraoperative damage to the MCL. As medial release surgery involves dissection of the common flexor origin, the loss of this structure's medial stabilizing role should also be considered.

Preoperative History and Considerations

Patients with medial instability will present with persistent medial elbow pain. This can be difficult to distinguish from normal postoperative medial elbow pain encountered in patients following medial release surgery. However, if medial pain persists or worsens, particular in the throwing athlete, MCL insufficiency should be considered. Often, medial elbow pain or new symptoms may occur when the patient or athlete returns to throwing and the patient will typically present with pain in the late cocking and acceleration phases of throwing—occasionally associated with a popping sensation. Pitchers may report loss of pitch velocity. Paresthesias in the ring and small finger may be reported.

On physical examination, patients will have medial tenderness and a positive valgus and moving valgus stress test. The milking maneuver may also illicit medial instability. Plain radiographs will typically be unremarkable. MRI arthrogram is the procedure of choice to evaluate the MCL, as a standard MRI will typically show postoperative changes in the MCL following medial release surgery.

Indications and Contraindications

Unless gross valgus instability is present, nonoperative measures including rest from throwing and physical therapy with stretching, flexor–pronator strengthening and modalities should be considered as a first treatment option. Should symptoms persist in spite of nonoperative measures, MCL reconstruction should be considered. The modified Jobe technique is the gold standard for MCL reconstruction with a reported success rate as high as 93% in terms of allowing throwing athletes to return to athletic competition [4]. Alternately, the docking technique is a modification of the Jobe technique that simplifies passage, tensioning, and fixation of the graft.

Operative Approach

Jobe Technique

The patient is placed in the supine position and the procedure is performed under tourniquet control. A 5-cm longitudinal incision is made centered over the medial epicondyle and branches of the MABCN are identified and protected. A muscle-splitting approach is created by incising the raphe of the flexor carpi ulnaris. The flexor muscle mass is separated from the MCL with a periosteal elevator. The MCL is visualized and inspected as a valgus stress is placed on the elbow at 30° of flexion. Converging tunnels are then made in the ulna anterior and posterior to the sublime tubercle utilizing a 3.5-mm drill, leaving a minimum 5-mm bridge between the drill holes. An angled curette is utilized to connect the drill holes.

Attention is then directed to the medial epicondyle. The anatomic origin of the anterior bundle of the MCL is located and a 4.5 mm drill hole is made without penetrating the posterior cortex of the humerus. The anteriorsuperior epicondyle is then exposed and a 3.2-mm drill is utilized and directed distally to communicate with the original drill hole made at the anterior origin of the MCL. The original 4.5-mm drill hole is then utilized as a starting hole and a second tunnel is created by directing a 3.2-mm drill proximal and posterior, creating two proximally diverging tunnels in the medial epicondyle. In this fashion, two tunnels separated by 1 cm that connect to the primary humeral tunnel at the origin of the MCL are created.

The palmaris longus is then harvested from the ipsilateral forearm using a single wrist incision and tendon stripper or alternatively through multiple small transverse incisions along the volar aspect of the forearm. This graft is passed through the ulnar tunnels and medial epicondyle in a figure-8 configuration (Fig. 20.5). Tension is applied to the graft with

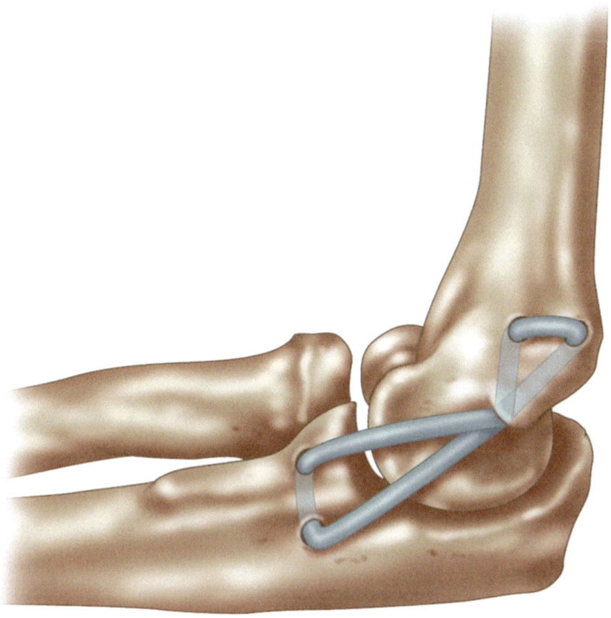

Fig. 20.5 Diagram showing the classic Jobe MCL reconstruction with isometric graft placement

the elbow held in varus, 60° of flexion and the forearm in supination. The graft is sutured to the remnants of the MCL to augment the reconstruction while proximally the graft is sutured to the periosteum and medial intermuscular septum. The elbow is then placed through a full range of motion to ensure that the ligament is isometric. The flexor–pronator fascia is then repaired over the graft and the skin is closed once meticulous hemostasis is obtained.

Docking Technique

The docking technique is a modification of the Jobe technique. Exposure is identical to the Jobe technique mentioned above. The starting point for the humeral tunnel, as in the Jobe technique, is at the anatomic insertion of the native MCL. A 4 mm burr or drill is utilized to create a tunnel 15 mm deep. Two small exit tunnels are then created proximally in the medial epicondyle in a diverging manner, separated from one another by 10 mm. Suture loops are placed in the humeral tunnels to allow passage of the graft. The palmaris longus tendon graft is then placed through the ulnar tunnel in an anterior to posterior manner. A No. 1 braided nonabsorbable stitch is placed through the ends of the graft in a Krackow fashion. Using suture loops, both limbs of the palmaris longus graft are then placed through their respective tunnels and tensioning of the graft is performed through the superior humeral drill holes. The graft is tensioned by tying the sutures over the bony bridge with the elbow at 90° of flexion with elbow varus and forearm supination forces applied.

Optimizing Outcomes

- Great care must be taken to identify the true location of the anatomic origin of the anterior bundle of the MCL in order to ensure an isometric graft.
- Limited dissection of the flexor–pronator origin should be performed in order to maintain its role as a secondary medial stabilizer of the elbow.
- Minimal handling of the ulnar nerve optimizes outcome.
- Great care must be taken in creating medial epicondyle and ulnar tunnels to avoid fracture of the bridge connecting the tunnels.

Complications and Side Effects

The flexor–pronator mass plays an important role as a dynamic secondary valgus stabilizer of the elbow. Excessive muscular dissection of the flexor–pronator mass can affect this structure's role as a dynamic medial stabilizer of the elbow.

As with any dissection about the medial aspect of the elbow, ulnar nerve complications may occur. Earlier MCL reconstruction techniques recommended submuscular ulnar nerve transposition as part of the procedure. However, later modifications recommend a muscle-splitting approach without transposition of the ulnar nerve. Improved outcomes have been reported with minimizing dissection of the flexor–pronator mass and minimal handling of the ulnar nerve [4].

Intraoperative fracture of the bony bridge between the ulnar and/or humeral tunnels can occur. Should this be encountered, the surgeon should consider the technique of interference screw fixation. The technique of interference screw fixation has been evaluated in cadavers and graft fixation strength was noted to be 95% that of intact MCLs subjected to valgus loads [5].

Persistent medial instability may occur if the graft is not appropriately placed and tensioned at surgery. Great care must be taken to identify the true location of the anatomic origin of the anterior bundle of the MCL in order to ensure isometric graft placement. Correct positioning of the elbow and forearm during tensioning of the graft can also optimize outcomes.

Postoperative Care

The elbow is immobilized at 90° in a long arm posterior splint for ten days. A hinged elbow brace is then applied and range of motion exercises are initiated. The hinged elbow brace is discontinued at 4–6 weeks post-op. Strengthening exercises are initiated at 6 weeks post-op. Valgus stress is avoided for 4 months post-op. A program for gradual return to throwing is then started of 4 months post-op. Throwing in competition is permitted at 1 year post-op.

Medial Denervation

Introduction

For both medial and lateral epicondylitis, pain perception is mediated by an afferent nerve. Wilhelm was the first to describe the innervation of the lateral humeral epicondyle and found that in lateral epicondylitis, pain perception from the lateral humeral epicondyle is mediated by the posterior branch(es) of the posterior cutaneous nerve of the forearm (PCNFA) [6]. Dellon described the innervation of the medial humeral epicondyle and identified this nerve in a cadaveric study using 20 specimens [7]. He identified the nerve to the medial humeral epicondyle to be present within the intermuscular septum when this septum was resected during anterior submuscular ulnar nerve transpositions. In his cadaveric studies, Dellon noted that in one pair of specimens, a branch from the ulnar nerve in the axilla joined the branch from the radial nerve. In six fresh cadavers, bilateral dissections identified the source of this nerve as the radial nerve in the axilla. It courses adjacent to the ulnar nerve in the upper arm, then moves laterally to be superficial to (or within) the medial intermuscular septum. The nerve terminates in the periosteum of the medial humeral epicondyle at the origin of the flexor–pronator muscle mass (Fig. 20.6). This small nerve plays a role in afferent pain signals in patients with medial epicondylitis. It can also be damaged with dissection in the area of the medial intermuscular septum during medial release or ulnar nerve surgery, particularly in the latter where a portion of the medial intermuscular septum is removed. Therefore, an injury to this nerve may be considered a complication of either of these surgeries, just as an injury to the MABCN during these surgeries is a known complication. There is, however, a difference between the two pain syndromes. An injury to the MABCN is associated with pain in the subcutaneous tissue anterior to the medial humeral epicondyle along with dysesthesias in distal skin of the forearm. In contrast to this, an injury to the nerve to the medial humeral epicondyle will result in tenderness directly on this bone with no associated dysesthesias. Both nerves can be injured in the same patient.

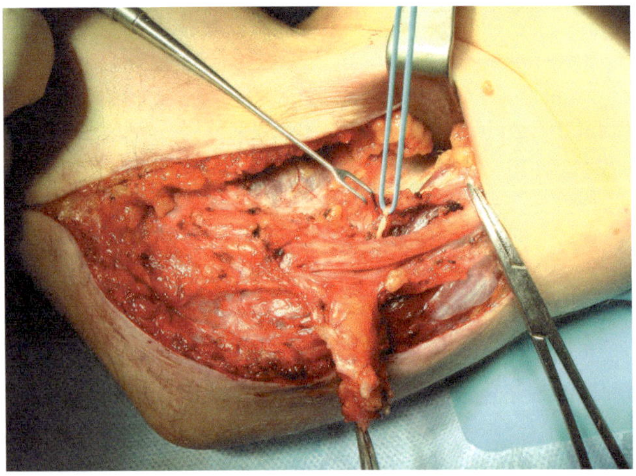

Fig. 20.6 Nerve terminating in the periosteum of the medial humeral epicondyle at the origin of the flexor–pronator mass

Preoperative History and Considerations

Patients with continued medial sided elbow pain following medial release surgery may be experiencing persistent pain as a result of damage to this small nerve branch innervating the medial epicondyle. This should especially be considered in patients with persistent tenderness over the medial epicondyle. In patients with persistent medial elbow pain and medial epicondyle tenderness, the surgeon may consider proceeding with medial denervation surgery, with resection of the small nerve to the medial epicondyle. Resection of this nerve can also be considered in concert with other procedures performed following initial medial release surgery, including ulnar nerve anterior transposition, MABCN neuroma resection, and medial stabilization surgery.

Wilhelm described a procedure for treatment of recalcitrant tennis elbow by denervating the lateral epicondyle [8]. It has been hypothesized that part of the "success" of many of the lateral release procedures is due to the inadvertent denervation of the lateral humeral epicondyle. The mechanisms causing medial epicondylitis are thought to be similar to those that cause lateral epicondylitis. Dellon et al. proposed denervation of the medial humeral epicondyle in patients who have failed to respond to the traditional approach for medial epicondylitis as well as in patients with pain following ulnar nerve transposition in which this nerve may have been injured by the division or resection of the medial intermuscular septum [7]. Denervation of the medial humeral epicondyle can also be considered in patients with persistent medial epicondyle pain following elbow fracture or dislocation.

While a diagnostic nerve block would demonstrate relief of the pain being transmitted from the nerve to the medial humeral epicondyle, a nerve block would probably also block the ulnar nerve, creating undue anxiety in the patient and risking damage to the ulnar nerve. This is in contrast to the workup for the lateral denervation procedure for lateral epicondylitis, where a preoperative diagnostic injection is tremendously useful.

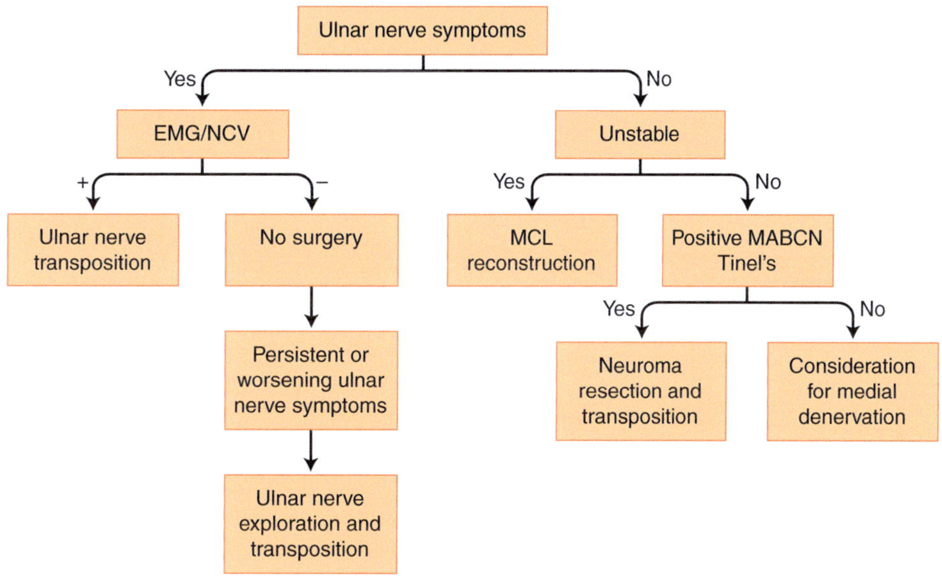

Fig. 20.7 Surgical algorithm for the management of patients who have failed surgical management of medial epicondylitis

Indications and Contraindications

- Persistent medial elbow pain following medial release surgery or ulnar nerve surgery.
- Persistent medial epicondyle tenderness with no associated paresthesias.
- May be performed in concert with ulnar nerve transposition, MCL reconstruction, and MABCN neuroma resection.

Operative Approach

The extremity is prepped and draped in the usual sterile manner. The procedure is performed under tourniquet control. A longitudinal incision is made along the medial aspect of the elbow. Dissection is carried through the skin and subcutaneous tissues with care taken to identify and protect branches of the MABCN. The ulnar nerve is identified at the medial aspect of the triceps and protected throughout the procedure. The medial intermuscular septum is identified and the plexus of veins posterior to this structure is protected. The small nerve of interest is identified coursing adjacent to the ulnar nerve in the upper arm, then moving laterally to be superficial to, or within, the medial intermuscular septum, terminating in the periosteum of the medial humeral epicondyle at the origin of the flexor–pronator muscle mass (Fig. 20.6). The nerve to the medial humeral epicondyle is then transected distally and the proximal end of the nerve is implanted into the medial head of the triceps muscle. The wound is irrigated and closed in layers.

Optimizing Outcomes

- Identify and protect the MABCN throughout the procedure.
- Identify and protect the ulnar nerve during the procedure.
- Protect the plexus of veins posterior to the medial intermuscular septum, as this can be a source of persistent bleeding following the procedure.
- Identify the nerve to the medial epicondyle within the intermuscular septum.
- Adequately mobilize the nerve in order to develop sufficient excursion to allow it to be transposed into the medial head of the triceps.

Postoperative Care

Following medial denervation surgery, the patient is placed in a soft dressing and is instructed to use a sling for comfort. Immediate range of motion exercises are initiated and the patient is allowed to return to their activities of daily living. Heavy lifting and athletic activities are allowed at 4 weeks post-op.

Conclusion

A surgical treatment algorithm for patients with persistent symptoms following medial release surgery is shown in (Fig. 20.7). When a distinct etiology for persistent symptoms is identified (ulnar nerve pathology, medial instability, MABCN neuroma) and symptoms persist despite nonoperative measures, surgery should be considered as outlined in the algorithm. When the exact etiology of persistent medial elbow pain is less clear, conservative management should be pursued. In the latter category of patients, medial denervation surgery, with its low morbidity and minimal recovery period, can be considered when medial elbow pain persists in spite of nonoperative measures.

Lateral Epicondylitis

Summary Box (Lateral Epicondylitis)

- Most frequently occurs at the ECRB origin.
- Nonoperative management often successful in up to 90% of cases.
- The measurement of grip strength with elbow in full extension is a useful objective tool to diagnose lateral epicondylitis, as grip strength in these patients decreases as one moves from a position of elbow flexion to a position of elbow extension.
- Pathology involves angiofibroblastic degeneration. No acute or chronic inflammatory cells are found.
- 80–90% resolution 1 year after onset, regardless of treatment.

Introduction

Lateral epicondylitis (tennis elbow) is more common than the medial by a ratio reportedly ranging from 4:1 to 7:1 [9]. It affects 2% of the population with its peak incidence in the third, fourth, and fifth decade of life. Lateral epicondylitis is the most common cause of lateral-sided elbow pain. Other causes include elbow arthritis and posterolateral elbow instability.

The primary structure involved in lateral epicondylitis is the ECRB tendon origin. In up to 50% of cases, the anterior edge of the extensor digitorum communis (EDC) may be involved as well. The condition results from activities that increase the stress of the wrist and finger extensor muscles and therefore increase tendon loads in the ECRB and EDC. As a result, these muscles sustain contractile overloads, either concentrically or eccentrically, that ultimately result in microtears in the tendon substance, leading to tendon degeneration of the ECRB and occasionally the EDC origin. Poor musculoskeletal fitness is also felt to play a role in its etiology.

As with medial epicondylitis, there is an absence of inflammatory cells, as pathologic analysis of the ECRB origin tends to reveal fibrovascular degeneration along with total distortion of collagen. Therefore, lateral epicondylitis is a degenerative process rather than an inflammatory process. Regan et al. performed microscopic evaluation of pathologic lateral epicondylitis tissue and confirmed the absence of acute and chronic inflammation in all cases they evaluated [10]. In normal tendons, collagen fibers are ordered in parallel fashion. Adjacent blood vessels are present in the connective tissue septae but do not invade the collagen bundles. With tendinosis, this normal orderly arrangement is disturbed as fibroblasts and vascular granulation-type tissue invade the collagen bundles, a process referred to as angiofibroblastic degeneration. Hyaline degeneration is also evident on hematoxylin and eosin stains. The tendon itself develops microtears and becomes hypercellular and degenerated. These microscopic changes combine to give the ECRB origin the characteristic gray, edematous appearance noted at surgery. Studies have shown that the degree of angiofibroblastic degeneration closely correlates with the duration of clinical symptoms [11].

Preoperative History and Considerations

Patients with lateral epicondylitis typically present with burning pain in the lateral aspect of the elbow that radiates down the forearm. Pain tends to occur with reaching out to lift and is greater when lifting with the elbow extended than flexed. Commonly, patients will also experience elbow pain with the use of a computer mouse.

Once again, a comprehensive examination of the neck and upper extremity should be performed to rule out possible sources of referred pain to the elbow. On examination, a significant drop in grip strength measured with the elbow extended as compared to grip strength measured with the elbow flexed is diagnostic for lateral epicondylitis. On average, the affected arm averages 50% of the strength of the healthy arm in extension [12]. There usually is maximal tenderness at a point 5 mm distal and anterior to the lateral epicondyle. Lateral-sided elbow pain is elicited by the examiner with resisted wrist and finger extension. Typically, there is increased pain with elbow extension. Kalainov and Cohen reported three cases of posterolateral rotatory instability of the elbow associated with lateral epicondylitis [13]. Therefore, elbow stability should be assessed in all lateral epicondylitis patients. Tenderness over the radiocapitellar joint may indicate elbow arthritis or a possible plica. The radial tunnel should also be palpated as tenderness in this area may indicate radial tunnel syndrome.

Radiographs reveal a lateral epicondyle spur in up to 20% of cases. As with medial epicondylitis, MRI adds little benefit to the diagnosis and treatment of lateral epicondylitis. Signal changes in the common extensor origin with or without partial or complete tears are often noted. Savnik et al. showed little correlation between ECRB signal changes on MRI and clinical symptoms [14].

Indications and Contraindications

Nonoperative measures have been shown to provide short-term improvement in symptoms, though the natural history of lateral epicondylitis has shown that nearly 90% of patients will be asymptomatic at 1 year regardless of treatment. Nonoperative measures for lateral epicondylitis include NSAIDS, activity modification, alteration of tennis equipment, physical therapy, bracing, and steroid injections.

Corticosteroid injections remain the mainstay of nonoperative treatment. Studies have shown excellent short-term improvement with corticosteroid injections but no long-term benefit. Smidt et al. performed a randomized study of 185 individuals, placing them into one of three groups: corticosteroid injections, physical therapy and a wait-and-see policy. At 6 weeks, the success rate for the corticosteroid group was 92%, as compared to 47% for physical therapy and 32% for the wait-and-see group. However, the 1-year follow-up success rates were clearly superior for the physical therapy group (91%) as compared to corticosteroids (69%) and wait-and-see group (83%) [15].

Several studies have shown promising results with autologous blood injection therapy. Edwards and Calandruccio noted complete relief of symptoms in 22 of 28 patients 3 weeks after autologous blood injection, even with strenuous activity [16]. Connell et al. also reported significant improvement in pain scores 6 months following ultrasound guided autologous blood injection in the 35 patients they evaluated [17]. Nevertheless, further controlled studies will be necessary to confirm the true effectiveness of autologous blood injection for lateral epicondylitis.

Extracorporeal shock wave therapy (ESWT) was initially a promising option in the treatment of lateral epicondylitis but studies have revealed its effectiveness to be limited [18].

Once nonoperative measures have been exhausted, surgery should be considered for refractory cases of lateral epicondylitis. Many techniques have been described for lateral epicondylitis; including percutaneous, arthroscopic and open common extensor origin release; and extensor origin debridement, with or without rotation of an anconeus muscle flap. Studies have not shown any clear superiority of any one of these methods and surgeons should perform the procedure with which he or she is most comfortable. Nevertheless, many, if not all, of these traditional surgical treatments center on debridement of the common extensor origin and consist of some variation of the classic Nirschl technique [1]. Nirschl noted that the lesion that was consistently identified at surgery was immature fibroblastic and vascular infiltration of the origin of the ECRB. A specific surgical technique was employed, including exposure of the ECRB, excision of the identified lesion, and repair.

As an alternative technique to the traditional lateral release, Dellon and Rose have proposed a lateral denervation procedure for treatment of lateral epicondylitis [19]. Partial joint denervation is the concept of preservation of joint function and relief of joint pain by interrupting the neural pathways that transmit the pain message from the joint to the brain. Dellon proposed the denervation procedure to multiple joints when traditional nonoperative musculoskeletal approaches fail [20]. Gardner first described the innervation of the elbow joint in 1947 [21]. Wilhelm noted that anatomical and clinical research had shown that the entire lateral epicondylar region is innervated only by radial nerve branches. Based on these investigations, he developed a surgical procedure for complete denervation that he recommended only in resistant cases of tennis elbow. He accomplished this blindly by disinsertion of certain muscles and reported 90% good to excellent results. Results of denervation did not improve by additional direct radial nerve release [8]. Dellon, in six fresh frozen cadaver dissections, found that a branch of the PCNFA innervated the lateral epicondyle in each case [20].

In an IRB-approved study, Dellon and Rose found that in 29 elbows in 26 patients, 86% of patients had good to excellent results when their lateral epicondylitis was primarily treated with partial lateral denervation [19]. Based on these findings, they proposed that partial lateral denervation is an acceptable surgical option in patients with lateral epicondylitis. Interestingly, two of the three failures in their study ultimately underwent surgery to decompress their radial tunnel resulting in complete relief of symptoms in both patients.

Operative Approach

Surgical management of lateral epicondylitis has traditionally been centered on release of the common extensor origin. This can be performed utilizing an open, arthroscopic or percutaneous technique. Clear identification of the pathologic tissue is essential for a successful surgical result.

The patient is placed in the supine position. The procedure is performed under tourniquet control. A 2- to 3-cm lateral incision is made centered over the lateral epicondyle (Fig. 20.8a). Dissection is carried through the subcutaneous tissue with care taken to identify and protect the superficial nerves. The interval between the extensor carpi radialis longus (ECRL) and EDC is identified by distinguishing the palpably softer, more muscular, more anterior ECRL from the more posterior EDC, which is covered by a relatively thicker aponeurosis (Fig. 20.8b). The ECRB is mostly covered by the ECRL, which must be elevated to identify the pathologic tissue in the ECRB origin. The cut in the ECRL should be only about 2-mm deep, as the ECRL is quite thin in this area. The ECRL is retracted anteriorly to bring the ECRB origin into view (Fig. 20.8c). All pathologic tissue is removed which usually requires excision of most, if not all, of the ECRB origin often to the level of the joint capsule (Fig. 20.8d). The pathologic tissue has a dull, grayish friable appearance as opposed to the normal firm, shiny, white appearance of healthy tendon. Typically, unhealthy diseased tissue can be scraped off with the broad portion of the surgical blade, whereas healthy tendinous tissue will remain in place with this scraping maneuver. Excision is performed in an elliptical fashion with care taken not to encroach into the lateral collateral ligament (LCL). The pathology often includes the anteromedial portion of the EDC and occasionally a small

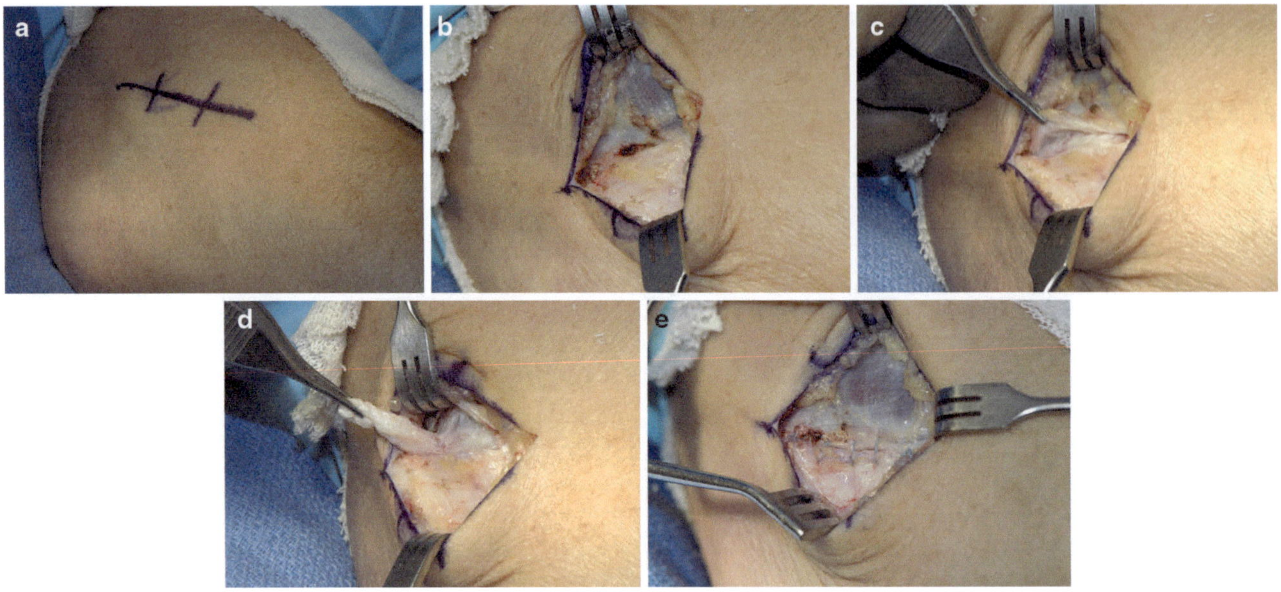

Fig. 20.8 (**a**) Longitudinal incision along the lateral epicondyle. (**b**) Identifying the interval between the ECRL and the EDC. (**c**) ECRL cut and elevated to bring the ECRB origin into view. (**d**) Excision of pathologic tissue from the ECRB. (**e**) Posterior edge of the ECRL sutured to the anterior edge of the EDC

portion of the undersurface of the ECRL. In 15–20% of patients, a calcific exostosis of the lateral epicondyle will be present and should be removed. Though intra-articular pathology is rare with lateral epicondylitis, a small arthrotomy can be made in the lateral capsule anterior to the LCL if intra-articular pathology is suspected preoperatively. One may opt at this point to drill one to two holes through cortical bone to cancellous depth in the triangular recess just distal and anteromedial to the epicondyle, stimulating hematoma formation and subsequent ingrowth of healthy healing tissue.

At this point the posterior edge of the ECRL is sutured to the anterior edge of the EDC to restore the normal anatomic extensor position (Fig. 20.8e). Care is taken to bury the suture knots. The skin is then closed in layers, preferably with an absorbable subcuticular suture.

Optimizing Outcomes

- Identify the interval between the ECRL and EDC by noting the softer, more muscular ECRL and the thicker aponeurosis covering the EDC.
- Incise the ECRL no more than 1- to 2-mm when elevating this structure to identify the underlying ECRB.
- Extending dissection posterior to a line midway bisecting the radial head may result in damage to the LCL with subsequent resulting posterolateral elbow instability.
- Use the “Scrape test” to differentiate between normal and abnormal tendinous tissue.
- Repair the extensor aponeurosis in a Watertight fashion.

Postoperative Care

The extremity is placed in a long arm splint with the elbow at 90° and the forearm neutral, leaving the hand free. Finger movement is encouraged immediately post-op. Active elbow exercises are started 2–3 days post-op and a removable splint is continued for 1 week post-op. The patient is allowed to resume normal activities of daily living during the first week after surgery. Wrist and forearm range of motion exercises without resistance are started 1 week after surgery. At 3 weeks, gradual resistance strengthening exercises including wrist resistance exercises with one pound weights are started. Patients wear a countertraction brace during these strengthening exercises for 2–3 months post-op while performing their activities of daily living. The countertraction strap is continued thereafter for sports and more strenuous work activities. Tennis players may resume easy strokes at 6 weeks post-op, while golfers may start chipping and putting 4 weeks post-op. Return to full strength and regular use in competitive athletes and manual laborers is allowed at 6 months after surgery. Patients may opt to continue prophylactic use of the countertraction strap thereafter.

Complications and Side Effects

Surgery success rates for lateral epicondylitis have been variably reported as 60–90% regardless of the specific technique used. Nevertheless, patients can experience some degree of lateral elbow pain for up to 1 year after surgery. The overall variability of success in operative procedures for lateral epicondylitis makes the need for reoperation uncommon but not infrequent either. One year of follow-up assessment is certainly appropriate to assess whether surgery has been successful. However, certain complications and postoperative problems may present within the first few months after surgery and surgical intervention may be indicated sooner.

Inadequate or Incomplete Procedure

Following lateral epicondylitis surgery, the most common reason for continued patient pain is inadequate removal of diseased tissue. This can be avoided by taking care at the primary operation to carefully identify and debride all diseased tendinous tissue.

Some patients may develop persistent elbow symptoms as a result of incomplete release or inadequate excision of pathologic tissue. In 35 secondary procedures for lateral epicondylitis, Nirschl found that pathologic tissue in the ECRB was not addressed at all in 27 and inadequately excised in seven [1]. With more extensive debridement of pathologic ECRB tissue, Nirschl noted that 83% experienced good or excellent results.

A local injection of 2 mL of lidocaine in the area of maximal tenderness is the first diagnostic maneuver. Complete relief of symptoms with this injection may indicate persistent pathology at the common extensor origin.

Unrecognized Radial Tunnel Syndrome

Unrecognized radial tunnel syndrome can be a source of persistent pain following standard lateral release. One study has shown posterior interosseous compression to be present in 5% of patients with lateral epicondylitis [22].

Synovial Fistula of the Radiocapitellar Joint

Wound problems may occur when an arthrotomy has been performed. In this scenario, some patients may form a subcutaneous synovial fluid collection or, more rarely, a draining cutaneous synovial tract. This can be avoided by repairing the synovium and capsule when possible. If the synovial fluid persists, this may indicate a persistent leakage of synovial fluid from the joint that on rare occasions may require reexploration and consideration of an anconeus rotational muscle flap to address the problem.

Lateral Collateral Ligament Damage

During aggressive debridement of the ECRB and EDC, iatrogenic injury to the LCL may occur, resulting in posterolateral elbow instability. Several authors have discussed this rare complication of lateral epicondylitis surgery [23]. Patients with this condition will typically develop mechanical elbow symptoms after surgery, often with subjective complaints of elbow instability.

Unrecognized Radial Tunnel Syndrome

Introduction

When patients have persistent lateral sided elbow symptoms following lateral release surgery, unrecognized radial tunnel syndrome should be considered as a possible etiology. Compression of the radial nerve in the forearm can result in radial tunnel syndrome, also known as posterior interosseous nerve (PIN) syndrome. Both lateral epicondylitis and radial tunnel syndrome can occur simultaneously. One study has shown posterior interosseous compression to be present in 5% of patients with lateral epicondylitis and unrecognized PIN entrapment was felt to be a cause for failure in 2 of 15 patients [22]. Patients with both conditions will often complain of pain or weakness after activities of forceful elbow extension or forearm rotation.

The radial nerve is one of two terminal branches of the posterior cord of the brachial plexus. After innervating the triceps in the arm, the radial nerve pierces the lateral intermuscular septum 10 cm proximal to the lateral epicondyle. It then sends branches to the brachialis muscle followed by the brachioradialis muscle. The anconeus is then innervated proximal to the joint line followed by the ECRL. The radial nerve enters the forearm anterior to the lateral epicondyle and splits into a superficial and deep branch PIN. The ECRB is innervated by either the superficial radial nerve or the PIN distal to the joint line. The PIN passes under the arcade of Frohse, a fibrous arch that originates on the lateral epicondyle that is often a source of PIN compression. Fibrous bands within the supinator may cause compression of the PIN in this area as well. The radial tunnel is approximately 4–5 cm in length. It is formed laterally by the ECRL, ECRB, and brachioradialis muscles, medially by the biceps tendon and brachialis and posteriorly by the radiocapitellar joint capsule.

The diagnosis of radial tunnel syndrome is based on clinical examination. Patients will typically have tenderness over the radial tunnel, specifically at the arcade of Frohse. Pain at the edge of the ECRB can be elicited with resistance of middle finger extension. Patients will also experience pain with resisted forearm supination. However, distinguishing between radial tunnel syndrome and lateral epicondylitis can be difficult for even the most astute clinician, as the two conditions often present with nearly identical symptoms and physical findings. The diagnosis of radial tunnel syndrome is strongly based on tenderness over the PIN in the interval between the brachioradialis and the ECRB muscles. It is imperative that the examiner also evaluates the contralateral asymptomatic extremity and assesses tenderness in the same areas.

A diagnostic injection of 2 mL of lidocaine may be considered. As mentioned above, a diagnostic injection into the common extensor origin will help discern whether or not the patient's persistent symptoms are a result from inadequate debridement of the common extensor origin at the original surgery. If the injection at the epicondyle is unsuccessful, and the physical exam indicates possible PIN entrapment, a second lidocaine injection may be considered in the region of the PIN as it enters the supinator muscle at the arcade of Frohse.

Electrodiagnostic studies are frequently negative in patients with radial tunnel syndrome and, therefore, not particularly useful in making the diagnosis.

Given the difficulty in distinguishing between lateral epicondylitis and radial tunnel syndrome and the fact that the two conditions can coexist in up to 10% of patients, it is not surprising that unrecognized or persistent radial tunnel syndrome can be an etiology for persistent pain following lateral epicondylitis surgery.

Indications and Contraindications

- Suspect PIN compression in all patients with persistent symptoms following lateral epicondylitis surgery.
- Patients will have localized tenderness over the PIN in the region of the arcade of Frohse.
- Pain with resisted middle finger extension and resisted forearm supination should raise clinical suspicion for PIN compression.
- Diagnostic lidocaine injection may be considered in the region of the PIN as it enters the supinator muscle at the arcade of Frohse.
- EMG studies are often normal and do not aid in the diagnosis.
- Consider decompression of the PIN in patients with persistent symptoms 6 months following lateral release surgery.

Preoperative History and Considerations

Patients who have persistent pain following lateral release surgery should be suspected of having posterior interosseous nerve compression. In these patients, postoperative symptoms are frequently similar to those that were present preoperatively. Findings include tenderness over the radial tunnel, pain at the edge of the ECRB with resistance of middle finger extension, and pain with resisted forearm supination. There are no sensory abnormalities in the hand. As mentioned above, examination of the contralateral asymptomatic extremity is imperative, particularly when assessing tenderness over the PIN. There is no specific nonoperative treatment for radial tunnel syndrome, though some suggest nerve gliding exercises may be helpful. Tennis elbow countertraction straps, while beneficial for lateral epicondylitis, can actually exacerbate the symptoms of radial tunnel syndrome because they place direct pressure on the PIN.

Preferred Operative Approach

The patient is placed in the supine position. The procedure is performed under tourniquet control. A 12-cm straight longitudinal skin incision is made along an imaginary line connecting the lateral epicondyle with Lister's tubercle. The incision is carried around the lateral epicondyle. The skin and subcutaneous tissues are elevated off the extensor fascia. The PCNFA is identified and protected throughout the procedure. Inspection of the common extensor origin with repeat debridement is recommended, as inadequate initial debridement of the common extensor origin can also be a source of persistent symptoms. Care is taken to ensure adequate debridement of the ECRB origin as covered above. The author has found that periosteal elevation of the distal portion of the ECRL and ECRB origin off the lateral epicondyle has been associated with a higher success rate when treating persistent or recurrent lateral epicondylitis.

The forearm fascia is incised in the interval between the EDC and the radial wrist extensors, noting that this interval is easier to distinguish distally. Proximally the ECRL and ECRB are elevated around the anterior edge of the humeral condyle, allowing identification of the underlying supinator muscle. The EDC muscle is partially detached from the lateral epicondyle to aid in exposure with care taken once again not to encroach into the LCL. Dissection is initiated distally and extended proximally to the lateral epicondyle.

Once the supinator is identified deep to the extensor muscles in the proximal third of the forearm, the PIN is identified at the proximal edge of the supinator. The fibrous leading edge of the ECRB and the tendinous edge of the supinator are released. The ECRB tendon and superficial head of the supinator must be adequately excised. The recurrent leash of Henry is also ligated. It is recommended that the supinator muscle be released to its distal border. The tourniquet is deflated and once meticulous hemostasis is obtained the fascia is loosely closed. The patient is placed in a long arm posterior splint extending to the fingertips, maintaining the wrist and fingers in the fully extended position.

Optimizing Outcomes

- Identify and protect the PCNFA.
- Preserve the nerve to the ECRB.

- The fibrous leading edge of the ECRB and the tendinous edge of the supinator must be adequately released.
- Ligate the recurrent leash of Henry vessels.
- Meticulous hemostasis is imperative.
- Splint the wrist and fingers in full extension and begin early ROM.

Complications and Side Effects

The PCNFA should be identified and protected throughout the procedure. It can be damaged during the initial dissection. Damage to this nerve will result in paresthesias along the dorsal aspect of the forearm and a painful neuroma. Should this occur and become evident in the postoperative period, excision of the painful neuroma with transposition is recommended.

Extensor lag in the digits can also result from extensive dissection of the EDC muscle and also from inadvertent injury to the small nerve branches innervating this muscle. Splinting of the wrist and fingers in extension can help prevent this complication, but should persistent extensor lag develop, it is best managed by buddy taping the involved digit to the adjacent digit.

Injury of the PIN is the most devastating potential complication of this procedure. This will result in a PIN palsy with extensor lags of all digits. A neuropraxia often will improve and resolve with benign neglect over a 3–4 month period. EMG/NCV studies can be beneficial in following the progression of nerve recovery. Reexploration of the PIN should be considered if the palsy persists beyond 4–6 months.

Postoperative Care

The patient is maintained in the long arm splint for 1 week post-op. The sutures are removed 10–14 days post-op. Range of motion exercises are initiated 1 week after surgery and the patient is protected with a removable long arm posterior splint extending to the fingertips between therapy sessions for 1 month post-op. Strengthening exercises are initiated 6 weeks after surgery. Two months post-op, the patient is allowed to return to regular activities.

Synovial Fistula of the Radiocapitellar Joint

Introduction

A very thin, elastic soft tissue envelope covers the elbow joint. As a result, this soft tissue envelope can be compromised after a failed lateral release procedure. A chronic synovial fistula of the radiocapitellar joint can develop, sometimes with open drainage of synovial fluid. Werner et al. found that synovial fistulas occurred as a complication in 4 of 149 percutaneous procedures [22]. Simple excision of the fistula and primary wound closure typically is not enough to resolve this rare but stubborn complication of lateral release surgery. Numerous soft tissue procedures have been described to cover the elbow ranging from random cutaneous flaps to pedicle muscle flaps.

The anconeous muscle provides excellent coverage of small to medium sized defects located on the posterior or lateral aspect of the elbow. The muscle is readily available on the lateral aspect of the elbow, and when it is used as a pedicled muscle flap, donor site morbidity is minimal. Schmidt et al. demonstrated that the anconeus has three arterial pedicles: the recurrent posterior interosseous artery (RPIA), the medial collateral artery (MCA), and the posterior branch of the radial collateral artery (PBRCA) [24]. Of the three, the RPIA was the main arterial pedicle to the anconeus while the MCA was the minor pedicle and anastomosed with the RPIA under the anconeus muscle. The MCA enters the anconeus proximally while the RPIA enters distally. They found that the anconeus on average covers an area of 7.3 cm over the elbow joint. The anconeus, based on the MCA, provides excellent coverage of small and medium sized defects on the lateral aspect of the elbow. The anconeus flap can also be raised off its distal pedicle, the RPIA, to cover more distal defects in the forearm. None of the 11 patients in the Schmidt's series demonstrated loss of elbow motion, stability, or extension strength and this has been the author's experience as well.

Indications and Contraindications

- Synovial fistula should be suspected when synovial drainage persists for weeks after elbow lateral release surgery.
- Wound cultures should be obtained and suspected infection managed appropriately.
- When a synovial fistula is present, damage to the LCL should be considered and posterolateral instability of the elbow should be assessed.
- Anconeus pedicle flap should be considered when drainage from a synovial fistula persists.

Preoperative History and Considerations

Patients who develop synovial fistulas may present with persistent drainage from their elbow wound. Other times, a fluctuant fluid collection will be evident over the lateral aspect of the elbow. When drainage is present, it will be thin and yellow in consistency and will have the appearance of joint fluid. If drainage persists for weeks or months following surgery, a synovial fistula should be suspected. Though synovial fistulas are typically noninfectious, cultures should be obtained and appropriate antibiotic coverage should be initiated.

Initially the synovial fistula can be managed nonoperatively with immobilization and activity modification in hopes that the fistula will seal itself off. When drainage persists beyond that expected for a typical surgical wound, a synovial fistula should be suspected and anconeus flap coverage should be considered. The presence of a synovial fistula should also raise the suspicion of damage to the LCL. Kalainov and Cohen noted three patients with posterolateral rotatory instability of the elbow in association with lateral epicondylitis and two of the three were noted to have synovial fistulas [13].

Preferred Operative Approach

The patient is placed in the supine position. The procedure is performed under tourniquet control. A longitudinal incision is made along the lateral aspect of the elbow with care taken to create an ellipse of skin around the fistula to ensure complete excision of the fistula with its tract. Skin flaps are elevated to expose the antebrachial fascia. The interval between the anconeus and the extensor carpi ulnaris (ECU) muscle is identified. For purposes of lateral radiocapitellar joint coverage, the proximal MCA pedicle is utilized. Therefore, the more distal RPIA is identified in the interval between the anconeus and the ECU and is carefully ligated to preserve the arterial pedicle on the deep surface of the anconeus muscle.

Dissection is carried down to the elbow joint where a capsular defect is identified. An arthrotomy is performed, preserving the joint capsule, and the articular surfaces are carefully inspected. The joint is copiously irrigated with antibiotic saline. The joint capsule is closed in a pants-over-vest fashion in an effort to seal off the original capsular defect.

The inferior border of the anconeus muscle is elevated subperiosteally off the ulna with care taken to preserve the elbow joint capsule as well as the arterial pedicle. It is safe to divide the posterior branch from the radial collateral artery as it enters the anconeus muscle from the lateral epicondyle. The anconeus can be completely elevated from both the olecranon and the lateral epicondyle and based on its proximal pedicle, the MCA (Fig. 20.9). The MCA can typically be identified when dissecting near the triceps muscle. It is essential that this pedicle be identified and preserved throughout the procedure. Ligation of the RPIA allows the anconeus to be raised on the MCA and rotated to cover the radiocapitellar joint capsule.

Once the anconeus is elevated off the olecranon and the lateral epicondyle, the tourniquet is deflated and meticulous hemostasis is obtained. The anconeus is inspected to ensure that the pedicle has been preserved and that the muscle is well perfused. The pedicled muscle flap is then rotated to cover the previous defect in the radiocapitellar capsule. The fascia accompanying and overlying the anconeus muscle can then be sewn to the adjacent extensor aponeurosis fascia. The skin is then closed in layers. A drain is optional but is not typically used by the author. The patient is placed in a long arm posterior splint with the elbow at 90° and forearm and wrist in neutral position.

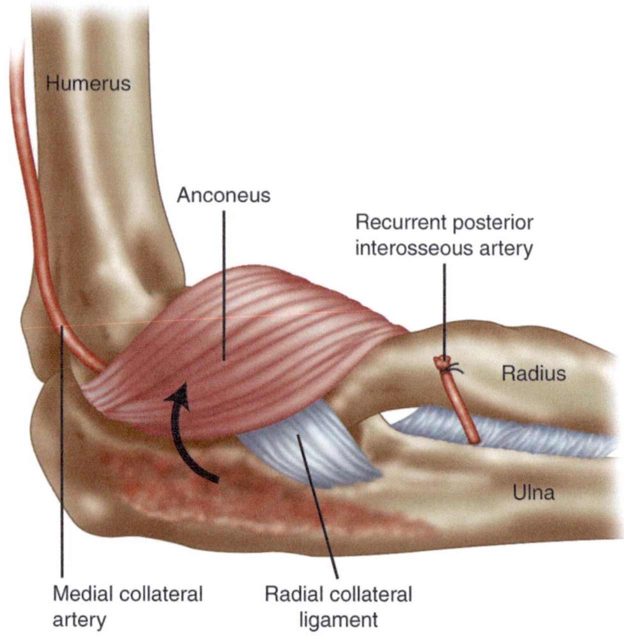

Fig. 20.9 The anconeus muscle is elevated subperiosteally off the ulna, raised on the MCA and rotated to cover the radiocapitellar joint

Optimizing Outcomes

- Make sure to excise the entire fistula within an ellipse of skin in skin incision.
- Identify the RPIA in the interval between the anconeus and the ECU and ligate this distal anconeus pedicle.
- For coverage of lateral elbow defects, the anconeus is raised on its proximal pedicle, the MCA, which can be identified at the triceps muscle.
- Elevate the anconeus from a distal/inferior to a proximal/superior direction.
- If possible, close the elbow capsule in a pants-over-vest type fashion to prevent synovial leakage.
- Ensure that the bulky muscular portion of the anconeus is placed over the prior defect in the radiocapitellar capsule.
- Preserve the fascia overlying the anconeus muscle so that this fascia can be used to attach the pedicle to the surrounding extensor aponeurosis fascia when insetting the muscle pedicle.

Complications and Side Effects

Patients can develop donor site morbidity as a result of anconeus muscle harvest but its clinical significance is uncertain. Electromyographical data have shown that the anconeus shows uniform activity in extension, pronation, and supination, implying a joint-stabilizing effect [25]. However, there have been no reports of elbow instability or loss of extension strength as a result of use of the anconeus muscle as a pedicle flap.

Cosmetically, the contour of the lateral aspect of the elbow may be altered following rotation of an anconeus flap and some patients will develop a concavity in the area previously occupied by the anconeus muscle. This is especially a concern in thin patients. All patients should be made aware of this potential cosmetic consequence.

Postoperative Care

The patient is maintained in a long arm posterior splint for 7–10 days after surgery. The splint is then removed and active and passive range of motion exercises are initiated. The patient is allowed to resume activities of daily living ten days after surgery but is instructed to avoid lifting and strenuous activities. A strengthening program is initiated at 6 weeks post-op. The patient is allowed to return to unrestricted activities 3 months after surgery.

Lateral Collateral Ligament Damage

Introduction

Lateral stability of the elbow is provided by the LCL and secondary soft tissue restraints. The LCL complex is comprised of three main components: the lateral ulnar collateral ligament, the annular ligament and the radial collateral ligament (Fig. 20.10). The etiology for posterolateral instability of the elbow is typically traumatic with a mechanism involving a combination of axial compression, external rotation, and valgus force such as when an individual falls on an outstretched hand. However, this pattern of instability can also be seen in patients following surgery for lateral epicondylitis and has been attributed to iatrogenic injury to the LCL [26]. Therefore, posterolateral instability should be considered in the differential diagnosis in patients with either persistent or recurrent lateral epicondylitis symptoms, particularly patients with mechanical symptoms and synovial fistulas.

Kalainov and Cohen described three patients with atraumatic lateral epicondylitis who also had clinical findings consistent with posterolateral rotatory instability of the elbow [13]. Two of the three patients were noted to have synovial fistulas evident on clinical examination and confirmed with

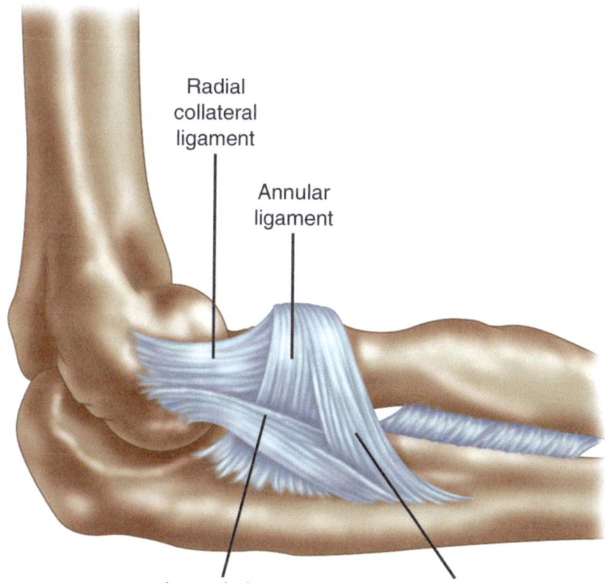

Fig. 20.10 Anatomy of the LCL complex

MRI scan. They postulated that degenerative changes in the extensor tendon origin may have also involved the underlying LCL but also felt that repeated corticosteroid injections into the tendon and ligament may have contributed to the weakening and ultimate failure of the common extensor origin and LCL.

Indications and Contraindications

- When a synovial fistula is present, damage to the LCL should be considered and posterolateral instability of the elbow should be assessed.
- Preoperatively, the clinical examiner should confirm the presence of an ipsilateral palmaris longus.
- MRI of the elbow may reveal a synovial fistula and can confirm insufficiency of the LCL.
- Lateral pivot-shift testing should be done to confirm the diagnosis.

Preoperative History and Considerations

Patients with posterolateral rotatory instability of the elbow often present with lateral sided elbow pain. They will often have mechanical symptoms, typically clicking with elbow extension, or the subjective feeling of elbow instability. They may complain of difficulty or inability to perform activities that require active elbow extension against resistance with forearm supination. Examples include the inability to open a heavy door or push themselves to stand from a seated position.

Often, skin depigmentation and subcutaneous atrophy may be noted as a result of multiple previous corticosteroid injections. The placement of prior skin incisions should be assessed, as incisions centered posterior to the mid-coronal plane raise the suspicion of inadvertent LCL damage. Cubitus varus should be screened as this can predispose a patient to tardy posterolateral rotatory instability. A fluctuant mass on the lateral aspect of the elbow should raise the suspicion of a synovial fistula. The posterolateral rotatory pivot-shift test can demonstrate posterolateral subluxation and relocation of the elbow joint. In this test, the examiner flexes and extends the elbow while applying a valgus force to the elbow and a supination force to the forearm. Posterolateral rotatory drawer test will demonstrate posterolateral subluxation of the proximal radius with forced supination. The chair sign is considered positive if the patient demonstrates reluctance to extend the elbow fully as they push themselves up from a chair using both upper extremities while keeping the forearms in supination and the arms abducted to greater than shoulder width [27].

Plain radiographs are typically normal. MRI findings will often include a disrupted common extensor origin, an insufficient LCL and a possible synovial fistula. Aspiration of the fluctuant synovial fistula typically reveals a noninflammatory synovial effusion with negative cultures.

Operative Approach

The patient is placed in the supine position. Examination under anesthesia should be performed to assess both posterolateral and varus stability. A lateral pivot shift test will often elicit a palpable clunk in the area of the radial head. The procedure is performed under tourniquet control. The common extensor origin and lateral epicondyle are exposed through a curvilinear incision on the lateral aspect of the elbow. Dissection is carried through the interval between the ECU and the anconeus muscle. A synovial fistula will occasionally be encountered and the common extensor origin may be found to have reruptured off the lateral epicondyle. The muscles are elevated off the lateral capsule and care is taken to preserve the capsule, if possible, as the graft is best placed extra-articular. The LCL is often found to be partially or completely disrupted and attenuated.

The humeral and ulnar tunnels are constructed next. The first ulnar tunnel is centered over the tubercle of the supinator crest. The second tunnel is placed proximally and posterior to the first leaving a 1–1.5-cm bone bridge between the two tunnels. The placement of the humeral tunnel is critical to ensure that the reconstruction will be isometric. The first humeral hole is placed at the geometric center of the capitellar articular surface. Proper tunnel placement is confirmed by running a nonabsorbable suture through the ulnar tunnel and selecting a point on the humeral epicondyle where the suture will maintain the same approximate tension through the entire arc of elbow motion. Once the point of isometry has been determined, the two proximal exit holes are created on the anterior and posterior aspect of the lateral humeral column.

The ipsilateral palmaris longus may be used as a graft. Alternatively, tendon allografts have been associated with the same outcomes and decrease the surgical time and morbidity associated with harvesting of the palmaris graft. The tendon graft is placed first through the ulnar tunnels and then docked into the anterior and posterior humeral tunnels, tying the sutures over the proximal aspect of the humeral condyle and the graft is appropriately tensioned. If possible, the remaining capsule is then sutured to seal the joint before the graft reconstruction is completed, ensuring that the graft is extra-articular. The graft is tensioned with the elbow reduced, the forearm in full pronation and the elbow in 45° of flexion. Additional tensioning of the graft may be achieved by suturing the two limbs of the graft to one another at one or more points.

Associated pathology should be addressed. If further degeneration of the common extensor origin is encountered, this should be appropriately debrided. Should the common extensor origin be completely detached from the lateral condyle, reattachment with anchors is appropriate and will help to augment stability provided by the ligament reconstruction. In cases where a synovial fistula is encountered, rotation of an anconeus muscle flap may be appropriate to provide adequate coverage.

Optimizing Outcomes

- Examination under anesthesia should be performed to assess both posterolateral and varus stability.
- Tendon allografts have been associated with the same outcomes and decrease the surgical time and morbidity associated with harvesting of the palmaris graft.
- Placement of the humeral tunnel is critical to ensure isometric tension of the reconstruction and can be confirmed by running a nonabsorbable suture through the ulnar tunnel and selecting a point on the humeral epicondyle where the suture will maintain the same approximate tension through the entire arm of elbow motion.
- The elbow capsule should be preserved in order to seal the joint before the graft reconstruction is completed, ensuring that the graft is extra-articular.
- Additional tensioning of the graft may be achieved by suturing the two limbs of the graft to one another at one or more points.

Complications and Side Effects

Persistent posterolateral instability can result when bone tunnels are not appropriately placed, resulting in the graft not being isometric. Sanchez-Sotelo et al. reported the Mayo Clinic experience in 44 cases, 12 who underwent ligament repair and 32 who underwent reconstruction. Stability was maintained in all but five cases [28].

Postoperative Care

Immediately following surgery, the upper extremity is immobilized with the elbow at 90° of flexion and the forearm in full pronation. One week post-op, early range of motion exercises are initiated in the confines of a hinged elbow brace that maintains the forearm in full pronation and also provides a 30° extension block. However, in cases with significant posterolateral instability, or in cases where patient compliance is questionable, cast immobilization may be continued for up to 4 weeks after surgery.

Because the lateral aspect of the elbow is facing upward during most activities of daily living such as keyboarding and writing, normal gravitational forces can place undue stress on the reconstructed LCL post-op. Therefore, patients will need to be educated about protecting the elbow from these forces for the first 3 months after surgery. Active overhead elbow flexion and extension exercises maintaining the forearm in pronation will protect the LCL reconstruction and avoid gravitational forces on the reconstructed ligament. Strengthening the extensor supinator group will also help to support the reconstruction. The patient is allowed to return to unrestricted activities 6 months after surgery.

Lateral Denervation

Indications and Contraindications

An alternative operative approach for lateral epicondylitis is partial lateral denervation. When joint pain persists, the differential diagnosis must consider that joint pain is of neural origin. As mentioned above, Dellon and Rose demonstrated 86% good to excellent results when partial lateral denervation was performed for lateral epicondyltis. Anatomic studies have shown that one or two small nerves have consistently been found to branch off the PCNFA and innervate the lateral epicondyle of the distal humerus (Fig. 20.11a, b). This nerve, or nerves, to the common extensor origin are purely afferent nerves. For joint denervation to be successful, one must be aware of joint innervation anatomy. Understanding that a nerve is the final pathway for pain, transection of this nerve(s) to the lateral epicondyle results in interruption of painful afferent nerve inputs from the common extensor origin. The noninjured joint afferents are preserved in partial denervation surgery.

In order to determine whether or not a patient is a good candidate for a partial lateral denervation procedure, patients undergo a diagnostic injection in the office. A 5-mL diagnostic lidocaine/marcaine injection is given 2 cm proximal to lateral epicondyle. Pre- and postinjection grip strength and tenderness are assessed. The patient is also asked to quantify his or her elbow pain pre- and postinjection using the visual analog scale (VAS). If anesthetic block of the nerve to the common extensor origin results in greater than or equal to a five-point reduction in visual analog scale score, 90% of the patients can expect good to excellent pain relief from partial joint denervation [19, 20].

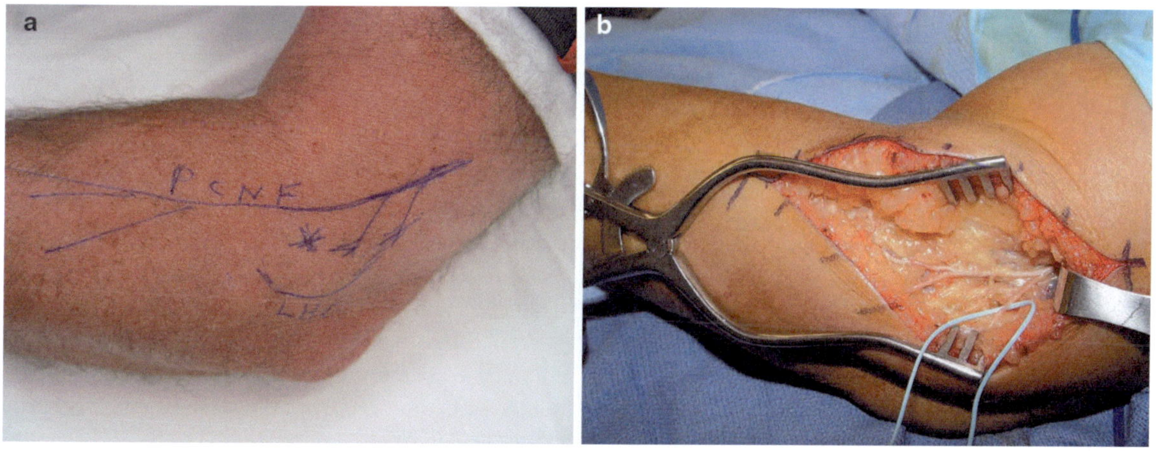

Fig. 20.11 (**a**) Skin drawing of the branches from the PCNFA innervating the lateral epicondyle. (**b**) Actual dissection of the branches from the PCNFA innervating the lateral epicondyle

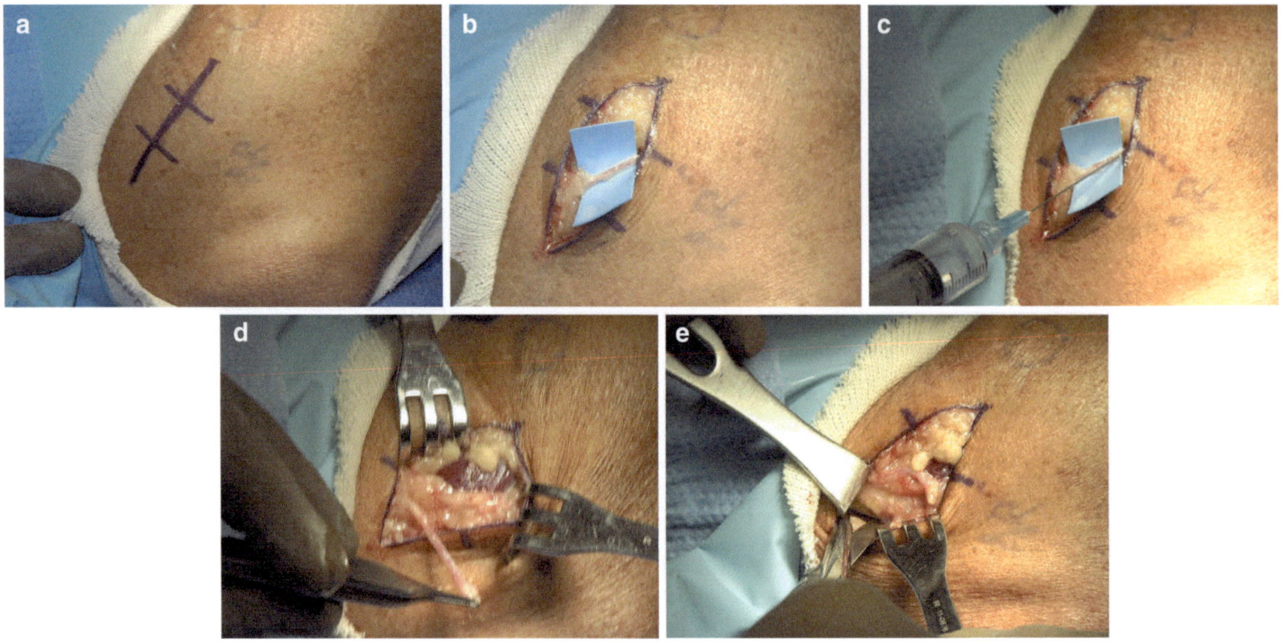

Fig. 20.12 (**a**) Ideal skin incision marked out two fingerbreadths proximal to the lateral epicondyle. (**b**) Identification of the nerves to the common extensor origin. (**c**) Nerve dissected as distally as possible and injected with 0.5% Marcaine. (**d**) Transection of the terminal nerve to the lateral epicondyle. (**e**) The nerve is buried within the triceps musculature posteriorly

Preoperative History and Considerations

For patients undergoing partial lateral denervation for lateral epicondylitis, the preoperative history and considerations are identical to those for patients undergoing a traditional lateral release procedure. Patients should have a minimum of 6 months of nonoperative management with symptoms that continue to affect their activities of daily living. In order to qualify as a good candidate for a partial elbow denervation procedure, the patient should experience significant subjective and objective improvement following the diagnostic lidocaine/marcaine injection. A 5 cc equal mixture of 1% lidocaine and 0.5% marcaine is placed in the subcutaneous tissues two fingerbreadths proximal to the lateral epicondyle. Following the diagnostic injection, the patient is asked to quantify the pain improvement based on the VAS scale and grip strength with the elbow in the flexed and extended position is measured and compared to preinjection values.

In Dellon and Rose's study, two of the three patients who failed to experience relief with lateral denervation surgery ultimately experienced complete relief of their symptoms with subsequent radial nerve decompression surgery. Therefore, patients should be screened for radial tunnel syndrome preoperatively with the realization that true distinction between radial tunnel syndrome and chronic lateral epicondylitis is very difficult clinically. Nevertheless, tenderness over the radial tunnel and forearm pain with resisted supination should be assessed and documented. Forearm and elbow pain with resisted middle finger extension should also be assessed. Patients undergoing lateral denervation surgery should also be informed that they may require a subsequent radial tunnel decompression should the lateral denervation procedure fail.

Lateral denervation for lateral epicondyltis can also be considered for patients with persistent symptoms following traditional lateral release surgery. Clinical trials are underway to examine this indication for the denervation procedure but early results have been promising.

Operative Approach

The patient is placed in the supine position. The upper extremity is prepped and draped in the usual sterile manner and placed on an arm board. A sterile tourniquet is optimal. A 3–4-cm incision is made two fingerbreadths proximal to the lateral epicondyle (Fig. 20.12a). Gentle superficial dissection is carried into the fat to identify the nerve or nerves to the common extensor origin (Fig. 20.12b). Care must be taken not to dissect too deeply in the subcutaneous fat because the nerves tend to be very superficial. The size and quantity of the nerve(s) to the lateral epicondyle can have tremendous variation. Once the nerve or nerves are found, great care must be taken to ensure that one has identified the nerve to the lateral epicondyle and not the more longitudinal posterior cutaneous nerve to the forearm (PCNFA). Often, gentle traction on the identified nerve will result in subtle skin puckering distally in the dermatome innervated by the nerve. This traction on the PCNFA will result in skin motion more distally in the forearm whereas gentle traction on the nerve to the lateral epicondyle will result in subtle movement of the skin over the lateral epicondyle. One can also inspect the orientation of the nerve, as the PCNFA has a more longitudinal path down the forearm while the nerve to the lateral epicondyle will be headed relatively more posteriorly towards the lateral epicondyle. Once appropriately identified, the nerve to the lateral epicondyle is dissected as distally as possible and injected with 0.5% Marcaine (Fig. 20.12c). The nerve is then transected (Fig. 20.12d) and buried within the triceps musculature posteriorly (Fig. 20.12e). The tourniquet is deflated and meticulous hemostasis is obtained. The wound is then closed with a running subcuticular stitch.

Optimizing Outcomes

- Patients who significantly improve with a preoperative diagnostic lidocaine/marcaine injection 2 cm proximal to the lateral epicondyle are good candidates for lateral denervation surgery.
- Avoid deep dissection in the subcutaneous fat as the nerves of interest tend to be relatively superficial in the subcutaneous fat.
- During surgery, confirm that one has found the nerve or nerves to the lateral epicondyle and not the PCNFA. This can be confirmed by examining the orientation of the nerve, ensuring it is headed to the lateral epicondyle, and also with gentle traction on the nerve, noting motion of the skin over the lateral epicondyle.
- Mobilize the nerve to the lateral epicondyle adequately to allow it to be transposed and buried within the triceps muscle.

Complications and Side Effects

A small proportion of patients who undergo lateral denervation of the elbow will experience hypoesthesias or dysesthesias in the posterolateral aspect of the proximal forearm. In the 29 elbows performed by Dellon and Rose, this was observed in three cases. In these three cases, the hypoesthesias or dysesthesias were not bothersome to the patient [19].

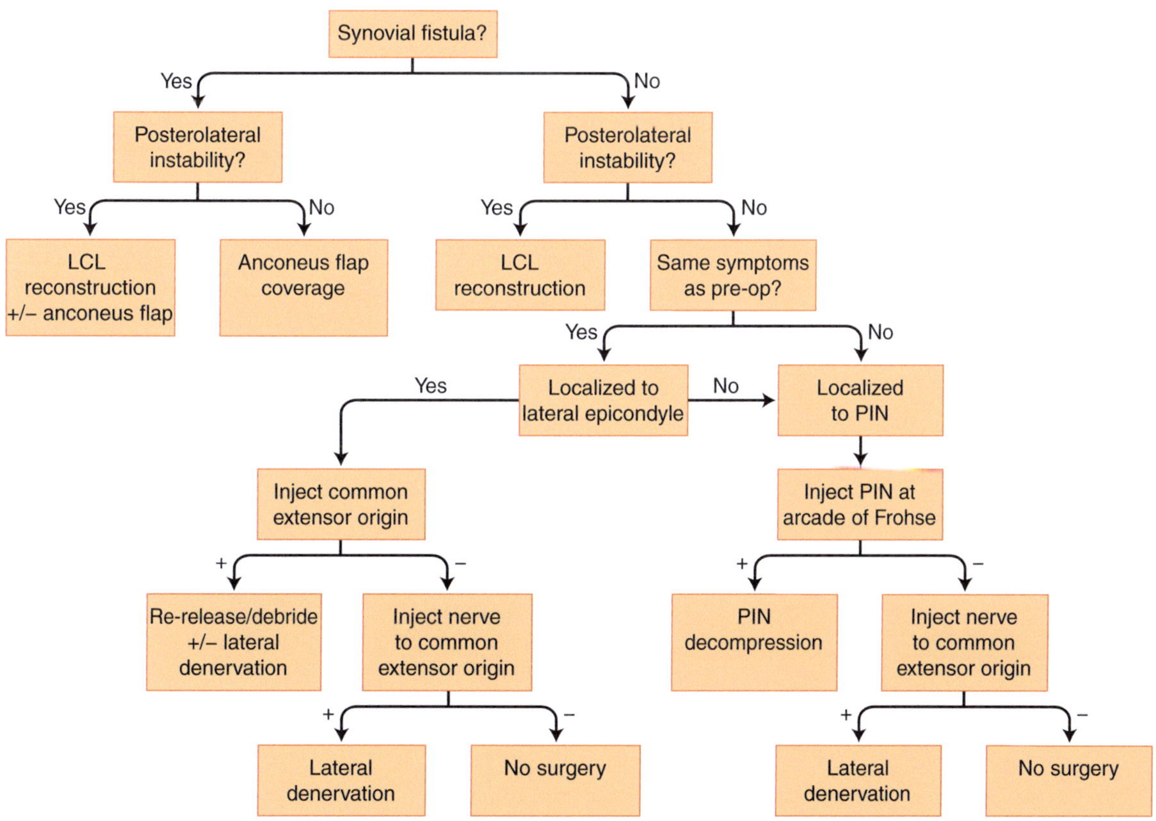

Fig. 20.13 Surgical algorithm for the management of patients who have failed surgical management of lateral epicondylitis

Though theoretically a painful neuroma could be encountered if the transposed nerve to the lateral epicondyle becomes displaced from its resting place in the triceps musculature, this was not observed by Dellon and Rose in their study [19].

Postoperative Care

Following denervation surgery, patients are placed in a soft dressing and a sling. They are encouraged to remove their sling several times a day and perform gentle elbow flexion and extension exercises. Patients are allowed to resume activities of daily living at 1 week post-op and are allowed to return to tennis or golf 4 weeks post-op.

Conclusion

Evaluating patients with incomplete relief of symptoms following lateral release surgery can be difficult. This is made even more difficult by the fact that many patients will experience some type of lateral elbow discomfort for up to 1 year following lateral release surgery. It is our hope that this chapter will allow the surgeon to follow a systematic approach for the evaluation and treatment of patients with persistent elbow symptoms following lateral release surgery. A surgical treatment algorithm showing the logical assessment and management of patients who have failed lateral release surgery is shown in (Fig. 20.13).

When a distinct etiology for persistent lateral sided elbow symptoms is identified (radial tunnel syndrome, posterolateral instability, synovial fistula) and symptoms persist despite nonoperative measures, surgery should be considered as outlined in the algorithm. Clinical acumen and diagnostic injections often play a critical role in differentiating between persistent lateral epicondylitis and radial tunnel syndrome. A diagnostic injection in the area of the nerve to the common extensor origin can also identify those patients who would potentially benefit from lateral denervation surgery. When the exact etiology of persistent lateral elbow pain is less clear, conservative management should be pursued. In the latter category of patients, lateral denervation surgery, with its low morbidity and relative quick recovery, can be considered when lateral elbow pain persists in spite of nonoperative measures.

References

1. Nirschl RP, Pettrone FA. Tennis elbow. The surgical treatment of lateral epicondylitis. J Bone Joint Surg Am. 1979;61(6):832–9.
2. Suresh SPS, Ali KE, Jones H, Connell DA. Medial epicondylitis: is ultrasound guided autologous blood injection an effective treatment? Br J Sports Med. 2006;40:935–9.
3. Hilburn JW. General principles and use of electrodiagnostic studies in carpal and cubital tunnel syndromes. Hand Clin. 1996;12:205–21.
4. Thompson WH, Jobe FW, Yocum LA, Pink MM. Ulnar collateral ligament reconstruction in athletes: muscle-splitting approach without transposition of the ulnar nerve. J Shoulder Elbow Surg. 2001;10(2):152–7.
5. Ahmad CS, Lee TQ, El Attrache NS. Biomechanical evaluation of a new ulnar collateral ligament reconstruction technique with interference screw fixation. Am J Sports Med. 2003;31(3):332–7.
6. Wilhelm A. ZurEntwicklungsgeschichte der gelenke der oberen extrmitat. Z Anatomieund Entwicklungsgesch. 1958;120:331–71.
7. Dellon AL, Ducic I, DeJesus RA. Innervation of the medial humeral epicondyle: implications for medial epicondylar pain. J Hand Surg Br. 2006;31(3):331–3.
8. Wilhelm A. Tennis elbow: treatment of resistant cases by denervation. J Hand Surg Br. 1996;21(4):523–33.
9. Rineer CA, Ruch DS. Elbow tendinopathy and tendon ruptures: epicondylitis, biceps and triceps ruptures. J Hand Surg Am. 2009;34(3):566–76.
10. Regan W, Wold LE, Coonrad R, Morrey BF. Microscopic histopathology of lateral epicondylitis. Am J Sports Med. 1992;20:746–9.
11. Nirschl RP, Ashman E. Elbow tendinopathy: tennis elbow. Clin Sports Med. 2003;22:813–36.
12. Dorf ER, Chhabra AB, Golish SR, McGinty JL, Pannunzio ME. Effect of elbow position on grip strength in the evaluation of lateral epicondylitis. J Hand Surg Am. 2007;32(6):882–6.
13. Kalainov DM, Cohen MS. Posterolateral rotatory instability of the elbow in association with lateral epicondylitis. A report of three cases. J Bone Joint Surg Am. 2005;87(5):1120–5.
14. Savnik A, Jensen B, Norregaard J, Egund N, Danneskiold-Samsoe B, Bliddal H. Magnetic resonance imaging in the evaluation of treatment response of lateral epicondylitis of the elbow. Eur Radiol. 2004;14:964–9.
15. Smidt N, van der Windt DAWM, Assendelft WJJ, Deville WLJM, Korthals-de Bos IBC, Bouter LM. Corticosteroid injections, physiotherapy, or a wait-and-see policy for lateral epicondylitis: a randomized controlled trial. Lancet. 2002;359:657–62.
16. Edwards SG, Calandruccio JH. Autologous blood injections for refractory lateral epicondylitis. J Hand Surg Am. 2003;28(2):272–8.
17. Connell DA, Ali KE, Ahmad M, Lambert S, Corbett S, Curtis M. Ultrasound-guided autologous blood injection for tennis elbow. Skeletal Radiol. 2006;35:371–7.
18. Staples MP, Forbes A, Ptasznik R, Gordon J, Buchbinder R. A randomized controlled study of extracorporeal shock wave therapy for lateral epicondylitis (tennis elbow). J Rheumatol. 2008;35:2038–46.
19. Rose NE. Partial lateral denervation for lateral epicondylitis. Presented at the American Society for Peripheral Nerve Conference. Boca Raton, FL; 2010
20. Dellon AL. Partial joint denervation I: wrist, shoulder and elbow. Plast Reconstr Surg. 2009;123(1):197–207.
21. Gardner E. The innervation of the elbow joint. Anat Rec. 1947;100:341–6.
22. Werner CO. Lateral elbow pain and posterior interosseous nerve entrapment. Acta Orthop Scand Suppl. 1979;174:1–62.
23. Nestor BJ, O'Driscoll SW, Morrey BF. Ligamentous reconstruction for posterolateral rotatory instability of the elbow. J Bone Joint Surg Am. 1992;74(8):1235–41.
24. Schmidt CC, Kohut GN, Greenberg JA, Kann SE, Idler RS, Kiefhaber TR. The anconeus muscle flap: its anatomy and clinical application. J Hand Surg Am. 1999;24A(2):359–69.
25. Basmajian JV, Griffin Jr WR. Function of anconeus muscle: an electromyographic study. J Bone Joint Surg Am. 1972;54(8):1712–4.
26. Morrey BF. Reoperation for failed surgical treatment of refractory lateral epicondylitis. J Shoulder Elbow Surg. 1992;1:47–55.
27. Regan W, Lapner PC. Prospective evaluation of two diagnostic apprehension signs for posterolateral instability of the elbow. J Shoulder Elbow Surg. 2006;15(3):344–6.
28. Sanchez-Sotelo J, Morrey BF, O'Driscoll SW. Ligamentous repair and reconstruction for posterolateral rotatory instability of the elbow. J Bone Joint Surg Br. 2005;87(1):54–61.

Secondary Reconstructive Options in Failed Fingertip and Nail Bed Injuries

21

Ryosuke Kakinoki

Abstract

Secondary reconstructive procedures for fingertip and nail bed injuries are frequently under appreciated by many surgeons. Complications from these injuries are not uncommon; however, many patients will just choose to live with their deformity. In other situations, the deformity with the fingertip injury leads to functional problems, and in these cases, the patient may seek out reconstructive options. These surgical efforts usually involve trying to make sure that the fingertip is covered with skin that has some sensation to it. It is also important that the skin be thick and durable to resist the significant forces placed upon it at the fingertip level. Just as important to the patient is the aesthetic and cosmetic appearance of the fingertip and nail; sometimes, this is even of greater concern to the patient than the functional deficits. This chapter discusses some of the reoperative options for dealing with failed fingertip and nail bed injuries.

Keywords

Medial • Lateral • Epicondylitis • Denervation • Revision

Fingertip Reconstruction

Sensation at the fingertips is important, as we use them to perceive the shape, surface nature, and temperature of items. Causalgia or abnormal sensations caused by complex regional pain syndrome, compression-related peripheral nerve neuropathy, or cervical radiculopathy drastically spoil manual function. Fingertips with poor sensation are susceptible to traumatic or heat injuries followed by ulceration or scar formation. The skin condition of the fingertips is also important. The skin and subcutaneous tissue of the finger pulp should be healthy and serve as a cushion against forces on the fingertip. This is a region where forces focus in pinching, gripping, and prehension. Injured or scarred skin at fingertips cannot resist the forces applied to the fingertips. Shortening of the fingertips because of trauma, surgery, or congenital conditions leads to weakness in these functions. In reconstruction, fingers should be kept as long as possible. In addition, the hand is the "second face" and often exposed to view. Thus, not only function but also the cosmetic appearance of fingertips is important. We must reconstruct fingertips keeping the following four essential points in mind:

1. The fingertip needs to be covered with skin providing good sensation.
2. The skin cover needs to be strong enough to resist shear or compression stress forces.
3. The digits must be long enough to enable grasping or pinching.
4. The reconstructed fingertip must have a good cosmetic appearance.

Anatomy of the Fingertip

Nail

The dorsum of the fingertip is covered by the nail plate. The proximal and lateral portions of this are covered by thin skin and are called the proximal (eponychium) and lateral

R. Kakinoki, MD, PhD (✉)
Department of Orthopedic Surgery, Kyoto University Hospital, 54 Shougoin Kawahara-cho, Sakyo-ku, Kyoto 606-8507, Japan
e-mail: kakinoki@kuhp.kyoto-u.ac.jp

S.F.M. Duncan (ed.), *Reoperative Hand Surgery*,
DOI 10.1007/978-1-4614-2373-7_21, © Springer Science+Business Media, LLC 2012

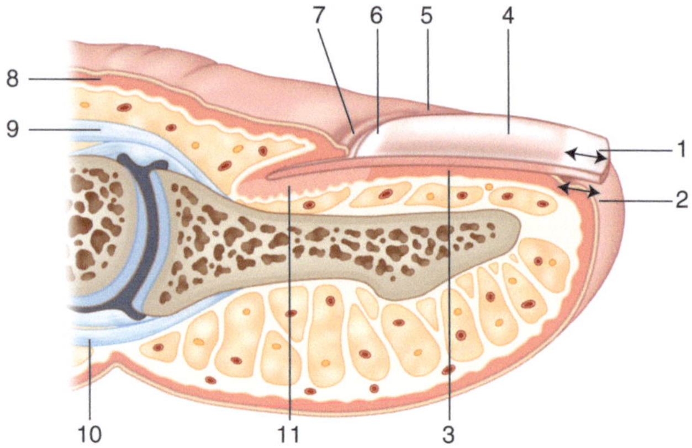

Fig. 21.1 Anatomy of the nail: *1* Terry zone, *2* hyponychium, *3* nail floor (nail bed), *4* nail plate, *5* paronychium, *6* nail lunate, *7* eponychium, *8* basement membrane, *9* extensor tendon, *10* flexor tendon (flexor digitorum profundus), *11* nail root or nail matrix

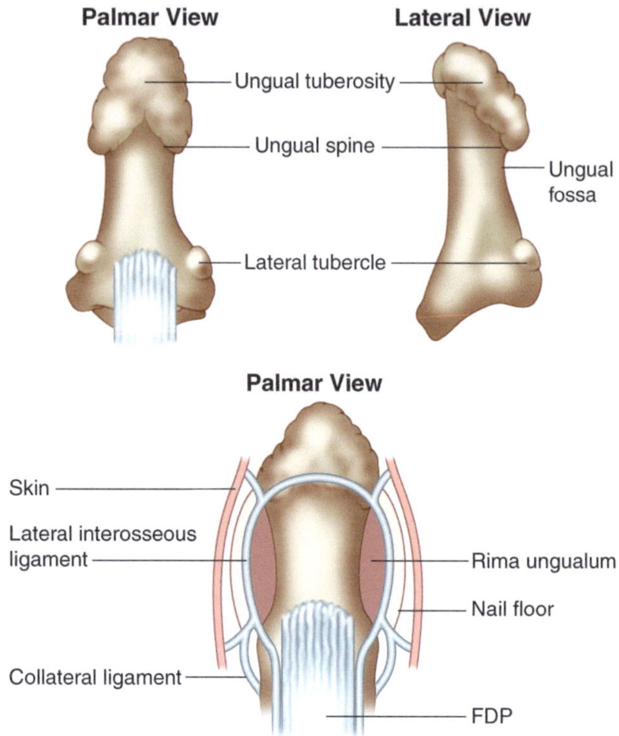

Fig. 21.2 Anatomy of the nail

(paronychium) nail folds, respectively. The proximal nail plate covered by the proximal nail fold is called the nail root or nail matrix. The nail plate demonstrates a pinkish color because of the blood flow to the underlying nail floor, except for the Terry zone, which is the most distal portion of the nail plate and is separated from the skin and the lunula. This has a whitish milky color just distal to the proximal nail fold. The skin where it separates from the nail plate in the Terry zone is called the hyponychium (Fig. 21.1). The nail floor and matrix are palmar to the nail plate and bind to the periosteum of the distal phalanx. Proximally, the nail matrix and bed bind strongly to the lateral tubercles of the distal phalanx to which the lateral interosseous ligaments attach and distally to the dorsal portion of the bilateral ungual spines that are on the nail tuberosities (Fig. 21.2). The other portion of the nail bed is attached to the distal phalanx loosely.

The nail bed covers the area from the distal margin of the lunula to the proximal margin of the Terry zone. The nail matrix is the area from the distal margin of the lunula to the attachment of the terminal tendon [1]. The nail bed is nourished by the terminal branches of the bilateral digital arteries. These pass through the space (*rima ungualum*) between the distal phalanx and the lateral interosseous ligaments and form two vascular arcades (nail matrix arcade and nail bed arcade) [2, 3]. The nail bed is innervated by the most dorsal branch of the palmar digital nerve that trifurcates just distal to the distal interphalangeal (DIP) joint [4].

Nail Regeneration

Lewis [1] performed histological studies on nail plate formation and found that there were three layers in the nail plate. According to this study, the superficial layer of the plate arises from the epithelium of the proximal nail fold. The intermediate layer is produced by cells in the lunula, and the ventral layer is formed by cells on the surface of the nail floor. When the nail plate is removed, the nail matrix starts to produce the nail plate, and the granular and cuticular layers are formed in the plate 1 month after removal. The newly formed nail plate regenerates distally in accordance with the distal extension of the granular and cuticle layers of the nail floor [5]. The nail matrix and nail floor are essential to create a new nail.

Finger Pulp

The finger pulp comprises adipose tissue and fibrous septa. The subcutaneous septa connect the palmar skin to the distal phalanx to prevent sliding of the skin when external shear forces are applied to the fingertip. A recent study has revealed that there is a dorsal septum in the dorsum of the DIP joint to confine hematoma to the distal phalanx after nail injuries and prevent proximal extension of ganglion cysts in the dorsal DIP joint [6].

The radial and ulnar palmar digital arteries connect with each other and form an arterial arch (the distal transverse palmar arch) just palmar to the distal phalanx at the level of the midpoint of the distal phalanx. Several branches (four or five) arise from the arch and extend distally just along the palmar cortex of the distal phalanx [7] (Fig. 21.3). Each of the radial and ulnar digital nerves trifurcates just distal to the DIP joint and innervates the fingertip [4]. The terminal tendon and bilateral oblique retinacular ligaments are attached to the dorsal base of the distal phalanx. The flexor digitorum longus tendon terminates in the proximal half of the palmar periosteum of the distal phalanx.

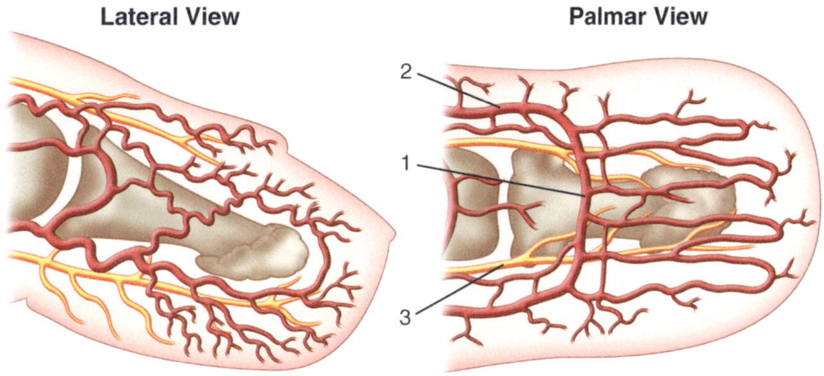

Fig. 21.3 Arterial anatomy of the fingertip: *1* distal transverse volar arch, *2* volar digital artery, *3* volar digital nerve

Classification of the Level of Fingertip Amputation

Tamai's and Ishikawa's classification schemes [8, 9] are popular tools to categorize the level of finger amputation (Fig. 21.4). The classification scheme by Ishikawa et al. is more specific to amputation in the distal phalanx. In Tamai's scheme, the finger distal to the DIP joint is divided into two zones. Zone 1 is the distal zone indicating from the fingertip to the base of the nail. Zone 2 is from the base of the nail to the DIP joint. In the scheme of Ishikawa et al., the finger distal to the DIP joint is divided into four parts. Zone 1 is the most distal part of the finger, from the tip of the finger to the level of the midpoint of the nail. Zone 2 is from the midpoint of the nail to the base of the nail (the proximal nail fold). The level of the base of the nail almost corresponds to the level of the distal transverse palmar arterial arch. The area from the base of the nail to the DIP joint is divided into two zones. Zone 3 is the distal half of the area, and zone 4 is the proximal half.

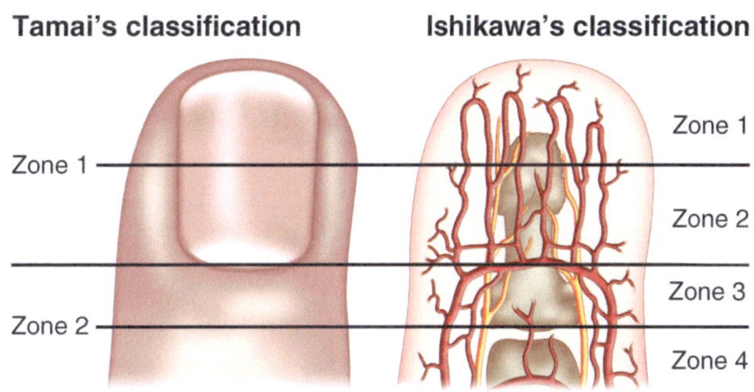

Fig. 21.4 Tamai's and Ishikawa's classification systems

Fingertip Replantation

Indication

According to Ishikawa et al. [8], the vessels are too small to perform vascular anastomosis in zone 1. However, because the mass of the amputated part of the finger is small in this zone, the amputated composite can survive without a vascular anastomosis. In zone 2, the amputated part might survive with only arterial anastomosis. If possible, adding venous anastomosis is preferable. In zones 3 and 4, venous as well as arterial anastomoses are necessary. In zones 2 and 3, if a venous anastomosis cannot be performed, drainage procedures such as fingertip incision or nail plate excision with or without heparin injection can be applied. In many cases with a zone 4 amputation, venous drainage procedures are not sufficient to vitalize the amputated part, and venous anastomosis is essential. Hattori et al. [10, 11] emphasized the importance of vascular anastomosis, especially venous anastomosis in patients with zone 1 and 2 amputations, because this can increase the success rate of replantations, decrease postoperative bleeding, and reduce the impact of postoperative tasks for doctors and nurses.

Presurgical Preparation

The amputated part should be washed well with sterilized water, wrapped in sterilized gauzes, and put in a plastic bag. The amputated finger in the plastic bag is then placed on pieces of ice and should be delivered as soon as possible to surgeons skilled in microsurgical techniques. Because the diameter of the vessels for anastomosis is around 0.3–0.5 mm in zone 2 injuries, the surgeons have to master "supermicrosurgery."

Anesthesia

Fingertip replantation can be performed using a digital nerve block. Patients who have the minimum compliance for immobilization such as children should have general anesthesia. The finger needs to be tied with a rubber band at the base.

Surgery

There are four or five arterial branches originating from the distal transverse arch of the palmar digital artery. Among them, one or two branches at the center of the distal phalanx are usually found to have the greatest diameter (central artery) and are the most suitable for anastomosis in zones 1 and 2 (Fig. 21.4). Stumps of the bilateral palmar digital arteries should be found in injuries to zones 3 and 4. The arterial and venous stumps should be searched for in the amputated part (distal segment) of the finger first using microscopy. Compression of the distal segment may facilitate blood oozing from the arterial or venous stumps, which help in locating vascular stumps. When a stump is found, it should be tagged temporarily with an 11–0 nylon suture. Vascular stumps should be located in the proximal segment of the injured finger in the same way as described for the distal segment. In zones 1 and 2, vein stumps are often found in the subcutaneous fat tissue just lateral to the nail fold or in the palmar pulp just beneath the skin. In zones 3 or 4, the dorsal terminal vein is the best candidate for vein anastomosis [11, 12] (Fig. 21.5).

One or two intramedullary K-wires (1.0- or 0.7-mm diameter) should be inserted into the bone of the distal segment retrogradely and pushed back to the proximal segment to fix the distal phalanx. The finger is then held with the palmar side up, and a small oblique skin incision is made in the palm across the amputated wound in both the proximal and distal segments. Each triangular palmar skin flap created in either segment is retracted laterally using 4–0 nylon sutures anchoring each flap. The redundant subcutaneous fat tissue should be removed to facilitate exposure of the marked arteries, attention being paid not to injure the marked venous stumps (Fig. 21.6). Nylon 11–0 or 12–0 sutures should be used for the arterial anastomosis. Four to five stitches are enough to get good blood inflow through the anastomosis sites. Three to four stitches are enough to for venous outflow. Single vein anastomosis is good enough for venous drainage [10]. When direct anastomoses of the arteries and veins are impossible, vein grafts harvested from the thenar eminence [12] or medial sole should be transplanted.

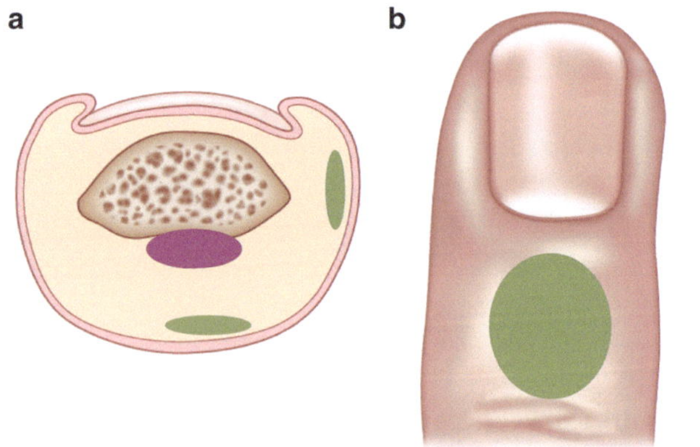

Fig. 21.5 Location of the central artery and veins for anastomosis. (**a**) A schematic diagram of a transverse section in zone 2. The central arteries are found just beneath the palmar cortex of the distal phalanx (*pink zone*), and vein stumps are often found out in the subcutaneous fat tissue just lateral to the nail fold or the palmar pulp just beneath the skin (*green zones*). (**b**) In zones 3 or 4, the dorsal terminal vein is the best candidate for vein anastomosis (*green zone*)

Venous Drainage and Postoperative Anticoagulation

If venous stumps cannot be found in the distal segment or vein-to-vein anastomosis is impossible, venous drainage procedures should be employed. Two types of venous drainage procedures have been described. One is to create a fistula using vein grafts between subcutaneous tissue in the distal segment and a vein stump in the proximal segment (venocutaneous fistula; [13]) or between a second arterial stump in the distal segment and a vein stump in the proximal segment (arteriovenous fistula) [14] for venous drainage. The other type of drainage is continuous external bleeding from the distal segment by creating a paraungual fishmouth incision [15] or by removing a partial nail plate to expose the nail floor [16, 17]. To maintain bleeding, a heparin–saline solution is dripped onto the fishmouth incision, and a gauze sponge soaked with the same solution is placed on the nail floor in the defect of the nail plate. These maneuvers are required for continuous bleeding for at least 4–5 days after surgery until the capillary connection is established between the distal and proximal segments of the finger. In a zone 4 amputation injury, continuous bleeding procedures using the fishmouth incision or nail plate removal with heparin immersion may not be enough to allow the amputated part to survive. Vein anastomosis is necessary in such cases. Koshima et al. [18]

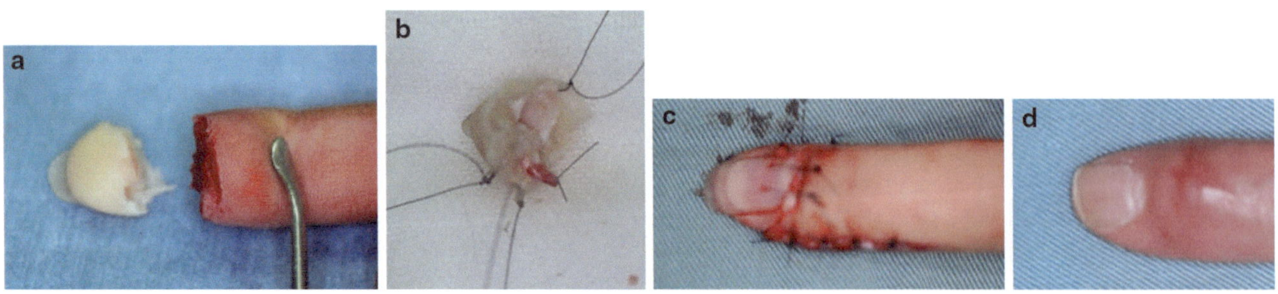

Fig. 21.6 Replantation of the fingertip in zone 3 injury. (**a**) Amputation in zone 3. (**b**) Vein graft was performed on the arterial stump of the distal segment. (**c**) Just after surgery. (**d**) Six months after the injury

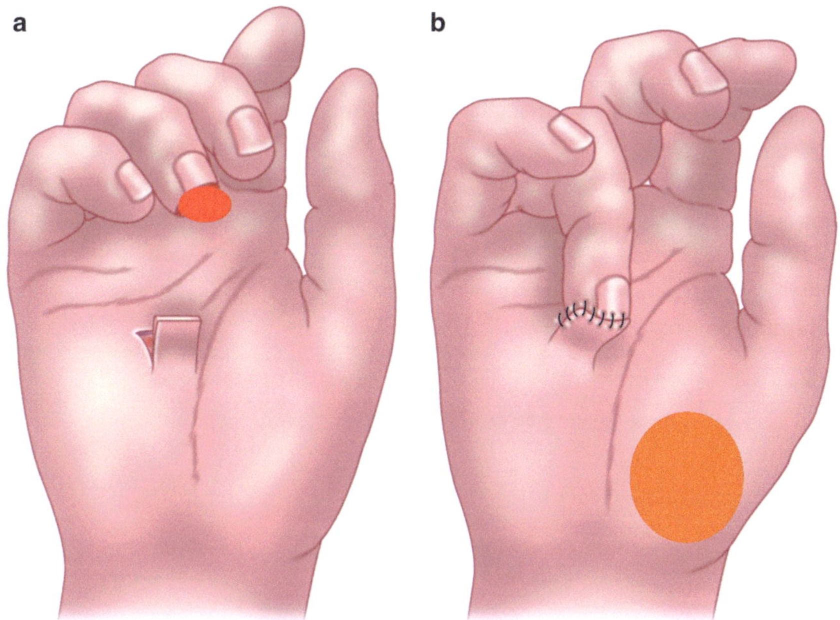

Fig. 21.7 (**a**) Thenar flap. This illustration is an example of a poorly crafted thenar flap. (**b**) The flap should be created in the thenar eminence allowing the injured fingertip more proximal interphalangeal (PIP) joint extension; this also allows the thumb to oppose the injured fingertip

recommended delaying a venous anastomosis in fingertip replantation when vein stumps cannot be found in amputated fingers on the day of the injury. Only the arterial anastomosis should be performed during the first surgery. On the next day, the second operation can be done for venous anastomosis. Dilated vein stumps caused by venous congestion in the distal segment make it easy to locate vein stumps and perform the anastomosis.

Fingertip Plasty

Brent's Procedure

Indication

This procedure is indicated for zone 2 amputation injuries according to Ishikawa's classification (see above). Although some authors have reported good results for zone 3 amputation injuries treated by this procedure, they are often followed by atrophy of the amputated segment or nonunion of the distal phalanx.

Advantage

Vascular anastomosis is unnecessary.

Disadvantage

Injuries in zones 3 and 4 are difficult to treat by this procedure.

Surgery

The procedure is simple. After the epidermis including the nail is denuded in the amputated segment, the amputated distal phalanx is fixed to the proximal part of the finger using an intramedullary K-wire. The distal stumps of the K-wire should be buried under the subcutaneous tissue in the fingertip. The denuded amputated segment with a K-wire fixation is inserted into a subcutaneous pocket created in the thenar eminence of the ipsilateral hand or the contralateral inguinal or chest area (Fig. 21.7a). The skin of the proximal segment is sutured to the skin around the skin pocket. Two weeks after the insertion, the sutures are removed and the amputated part is taken out. The denuded amputated part should have been vascularized by capillary invasion from the subcutaneous pocket and established a capillary connection with the proximal segment of the finger (Fig. 21.7b). The denuded amputated segment should undergo reepithelialization spontaneously within 2 weeks.

Aluminum Sheet Wrapping with Isodine Gel

Indication

This procedure can be indicated when the amputated tips are lost, not indicated or impossible for replantation.

Advantages

1. No vascular anastomosis is necessary.
2. Wound closure and creation of the finger stumps can be performed successfully without surgical intervention.

Disadvantages

1. Shortening of the finger might persist.
2. Severe nail deformity may occur in zones 2 and 3 injuries because of loss of the nail floor.

Treatment

The amputated wound is washed and sterilized with isodine sugar ointment. The amputated surface is wrapped with an aluminum foil sheet, which is replaced every other day. Any infectious signs of the finger stumps should be checked. The skin is created under the aluminum sheet within 2–3 weeks, and the amputated wound should undergo reepithelialization spontaneously.

Coverage of the Fingertip with Flaps

Random Pattern Flaps

Thenar Flap

Indication

This flap is used for treating fingertip injuries excluding the thumb tip.

Advantage

The operative procedure is easy and the flap is safe.

Disadvantages

1. The injured finger must be fixed to the thenar eminence for about 2 weeks.
2. During fixation, the injured hand must not be used.
3. The finger sometimes develops a flexion contracture at the proximal interphalangeal (PIP) joint, especially in elder patients.

Surgery

The amputated surface of the injured tip is cleaned. If the distal phalanx has protruded from the surrounding soft tissue, the bone must be osteotomized to level the amputated surface. A proximally based rectangular cutaneous flap is created at the radial border of the thenar muscles and elevated just above the fascia of the muscles. The ratio of the flap length to the width should be less than 1.5:1. The flap is sutured to the skin of the injured fingertip. The injured fingertip is kept attached to the flap for 2 weeks. During this time, the flap should have produced a new vascular connection with the injured fingertip. Two weeks after the surgery, the pedicle of the flap is transected at the thenar eminence. The skin defect created after harvesting the flap in the thenar eminence is usually closed primarily [19, 20].

Pitfalls

The flap should be created in the thenar eminence to which the injured fingertip can be approximated with maximum PIP joint extension, when the thumb is used to oppose the injured fingertip. In this position, the PIP joint of the injured finger is kept slightly flexed, and this can avoid the development of a flexion contracture.

Cross-Finger Flap

Indication

1. Fingertip injuries distal to the DIP joint.
2. In finger injuries proximal to the DIP joint, approximation of the amputated finger surface to the flap is difficult.

Advantages

1. The operative procedure is easy and safe.
2. The flap is available as a sensory flap.

Disadvantage

Like the thenar flap, the greatest demerit of this procedure is that the finger must be immobilized and kept flexed for 2 weeks.

Surgery

A rectangular flap is designed on the dorsum of the middle phalanx of a finger adjacent to the injured finger. The flap is elevated from the opposite side of the injured finger to the midlateral line facing the injured finger just above a paratenon of the extensor tendon. When the elevation reaches the midlateral line, the Cleland ligament should be transected. When a sensory flap is needed, the flap can be elevated containing the dorsal branches of the bilateral palmar digital nerves [21]. The branches should be exposed proximally to the bifurcation of the main trunk of the palmar digital nerves and transected. The skin defect created after elevation of the flap is covered by a full-thickness skin graft using a tie-over technique. The flap is trimmed to fit the injured skin defect and then sutured to the flap. The stumps of the bilateral dorsal branches of the palmar digital nerves should be approximated to the bilateral palmar digital nerve stumps of the injured finger under a microscope. A 1.2-mm K-wire is inserted from the distal phalanx of the injured finger to the middle phalanx of the donor finger to fix the injured finger to the flap. The flap is normally transected from the donor finger after fixation for 2 weeks (Fig. 21.8).

Pitfalls

When the flap is elevated from the donor finger, the Cleland ligament must be sectioned. The section provides mobility to the flap and prevents it from kinking, which may result in flap necrosis.

Axial Pattern Flap

Palmar V–Y Advancement Flap (Tranquilli-Leali 1935)

Vascularity

The flap is supplied by small arteries arising from the distal transverse palmar arch. The arteries are just palmar to the volar cortex of the distal phalanx. The flap must be mobilized while maintaining continuity of these arteries.

Indications

1. A finger pulp defect less than the distal one-third of the finger distal to the DIP joint
2. A distal dorsal oblique amputation of the finger pulp

Advantages

1. Flap elevation is very easy.
2. Postoperative fixation of the finger is unnecessary.

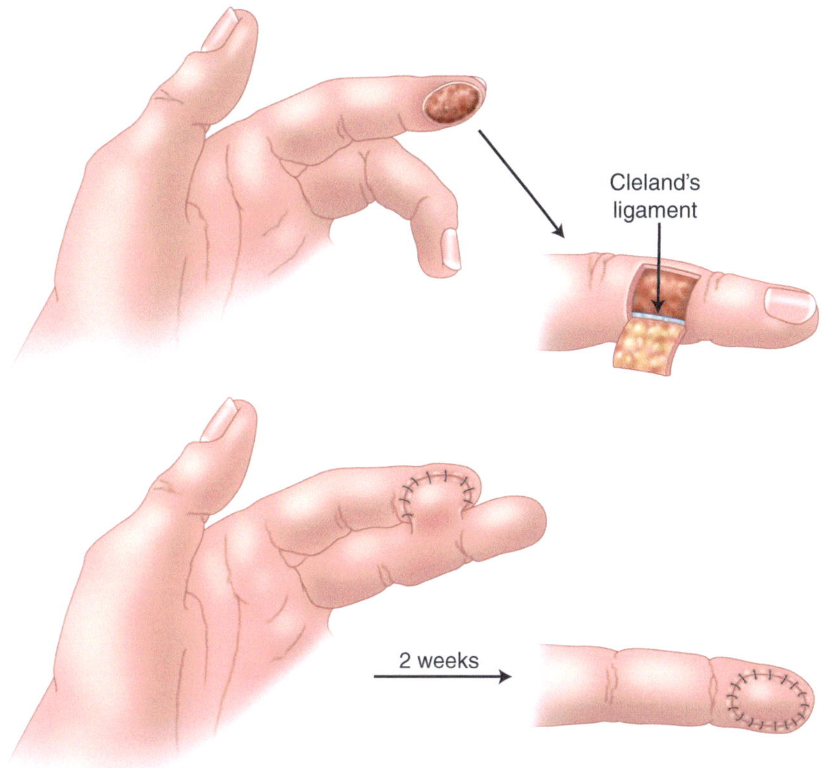

Fig. 21.8 Cross-finger flap

Disadvantages

1. Mobility of the flap is limited. Usually, the flap can advance within 5–7 mm.
2. The distal edge of the flap is prone to be avascular.

Surgery

After squeezing the finger, a finger tourniquet is applied around the base of the finger. A reverse triangular flap is designed at the finger stump. The base of the triangular flap is the amputated palmar skin edge. The bilateral oblique limbs extend proximally from either end of the base. The height of the triangular flap is 2–3 mm longer than that needed for flap advancement. The flap is elevated proximally in the subperiosteal layer from the tip of the finger. Because nutrient vessels are located just above the palmar cortex of the distal phalanx, the skin and subcutaneous fatty tissue should be incised, keeping the arteries intact. Because of the thick subcutaneous tissue in the tip of the finger, the flap can be mobilized for 5–7 mm distally. After the rubber band is released, blood circulation to the flap should be checked. At this time, the base of the triangular flap (the palmar skin edge of the amputation wound) is pulled distally and approximated to the nail and dorsal skin edge of the amputation wound. The skin defect created proximal to the flap is closed primarily in a Y-shaped fashion (Fig. 21.9).

Pitfall

The distal skin of the flap should be approximated to the nail and dorsal skin loosely to avoid ischemia of the distal edge of the flap.

Lateral V–Y Advancement Island Flap or Lateral Triangular Flap [22]

Indication

Skin defect following fingertip amputation.

Advantages

1. Vascularity of the flap is stable.
2. The flap is mobile for up to 1.5 cm distally by exposing the neurovascular bundle proximally.
3. Coverage of the amputated surface with a neurotized flap is possible.

Disadvantage

A skin defect of a finger supplied by a single palmar digital artery is a contraindication for this flap type.

Surgery

A distally based triangular flap is created in the hemilateral surface of the finger just proximal to the wound. The base of

Fig. 21.9 Palmar V–Y advancement flap

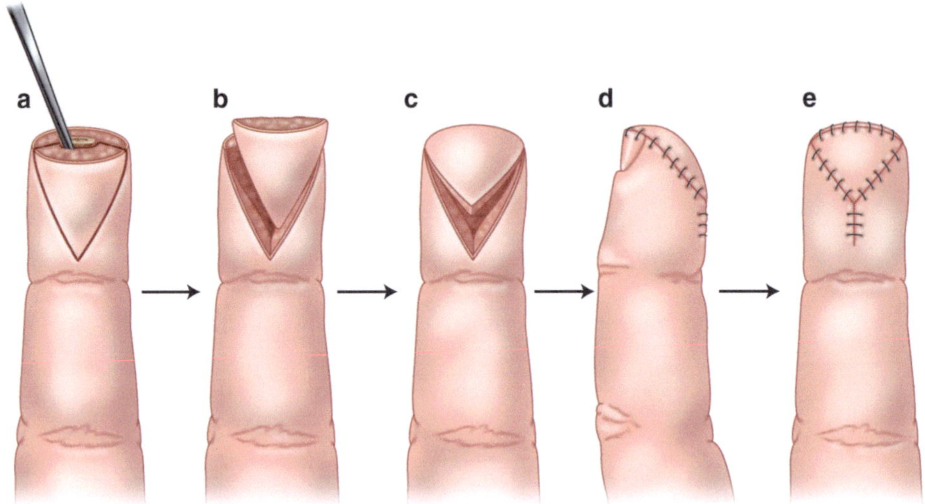

Fig. 21.10 Lateral V–Y advancement island flap or lateral triangular flap

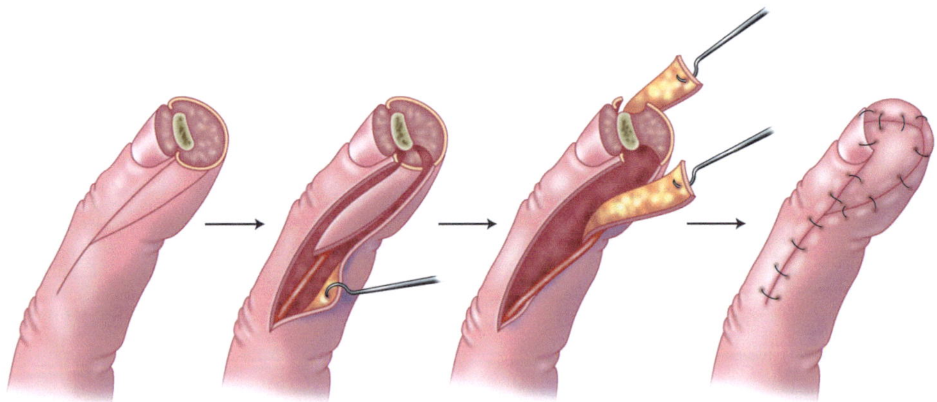

the triangular flap is the distal lateral edge of the amputation wound. The bilateral oblique limbs are extended proximally and connected to each other on the midlateral line of the finger. The size of the flap depends on the size of the skin defect, but the height and width of the triangular flap should be less than 1 cm. The skin incision is extended to the PIP level from the proximal tip of the triangular flap along the midlateral line. Through this incision, the neurovascular bundle is exposed after transection of the Cleland ligament. The flap is elevated proximally including the neurovascular bundle (Fig. 21.10). The flap should be mobile for about 1 cm. According to Kutler [22], the triangular flaps should be created on either side of the finger, and the two flaps are then moved distally to obliterate the skin defect in the fingertip. However, a skin defect at the fingertip can be covered by a hemilateral triangular flap including a neurovascular bundle elevated proximally [23]. The flap is then moved to the defect at the fingertip and sutured loosely. The finger should be fixed with a splint for 2 weeks with the PIP and DIP joints slightly flexed (Fig. 21.11).

Pitfall

Before starting the operation, the patency of the bilateral digital arteries of the injured finger should be examined.

Palmar Advancement Flap with V–Y Closure for Thumb Tip Injuries (Russell and Casas 1989; Bang et al. 1992)

Indication

A palmar pulp defect (about 1 cm long) of the thumb tip.

Advantage

The operative procedure is easy.

Disadvantage

The operative scar is conspicuous.

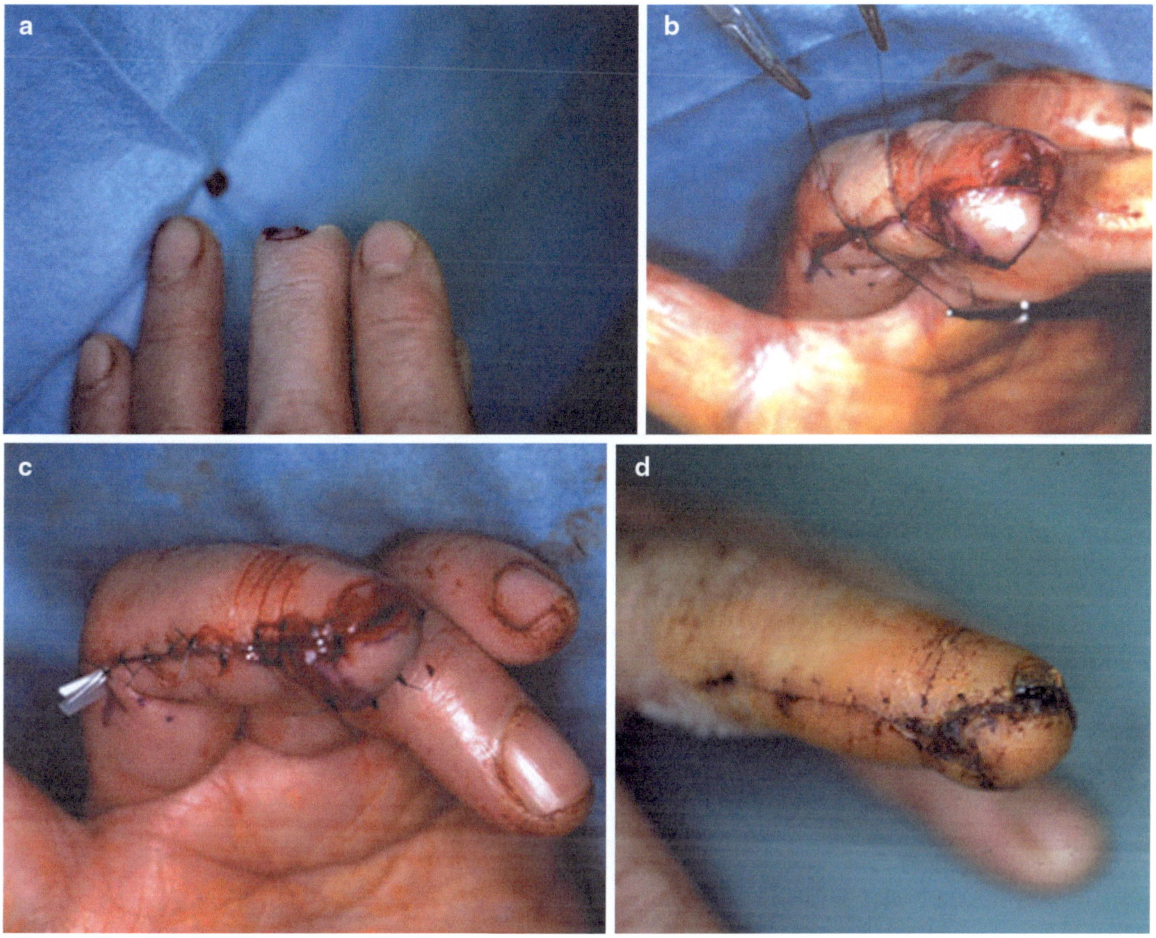

Fig. 21.11 Lateral V–Y advancement island flap or lateral triangular flap. (**a**) Amputation injury of the long finger. (**b**) Flap design and elevation. (**c**) Just after surgery. (**d**) Three weeks after surgery

Surgery

The incisions start from the wound along the bilateral midlateral line of the thumb. They turn palmar about 1 cm proximal to the proximal thumb crease and merge with each other at the palmar surface of the metacarpophalangeal (MP) joint. The palmar digital neurovascular bundle is included in the palmar flap, and the flexor tendon is excluded from the flap. In the proximal portion of the flap, the neurovascular bundles are exposed, and the skin and subcutaneous tissue of the palmar flap are separated. Thus, the palmar flap is completely elevated based on the bilateral neurovascular bundles. The flap is moved distally, and the distal margin of the flap is sutured to the nail and dorsal skin of the thumb tip (Fig. 21.12).

Skin Island Flaps

Reverse Vascular Pedicled Digital Island Flaps Based on the Palmar Digital Artery

Cutaneous island flaps supplied by a palmar digital artery can be harvested from the base of the finger. The skin island can be harvested from the distal palm (Fig. 21.13).

Vascularity

A hemilateral palmar digital artery nourishes this flap. When the flap is harvested from the dorsal surface of a finger, the flap is harvested including dorsal perforators originating from a palmar digital artery and extending to the dorsal skin of the finger. Because venous drainage is performed through venules in the adipose tissue around the palmar digital nerve and artery, the artery and the surrounding fatty tissue should be elevated.

Advantages

1. Mobility of the flap is good.
2. A sensitized flap can be harvested (Fig. 21.14).
3. Vascularity of the flap is stable, because the nutrient vessels are palmar digital arteries.
4. Harvesting a skin over the distal one-third of the palm is possible when a flap is raised including perforators originating from the palmar digital artery at the MP joint level (Fig. 21.15).

Disadvantages

1. To elevate the flap, one of the nutrient arteries of the finger must be sacrificed.

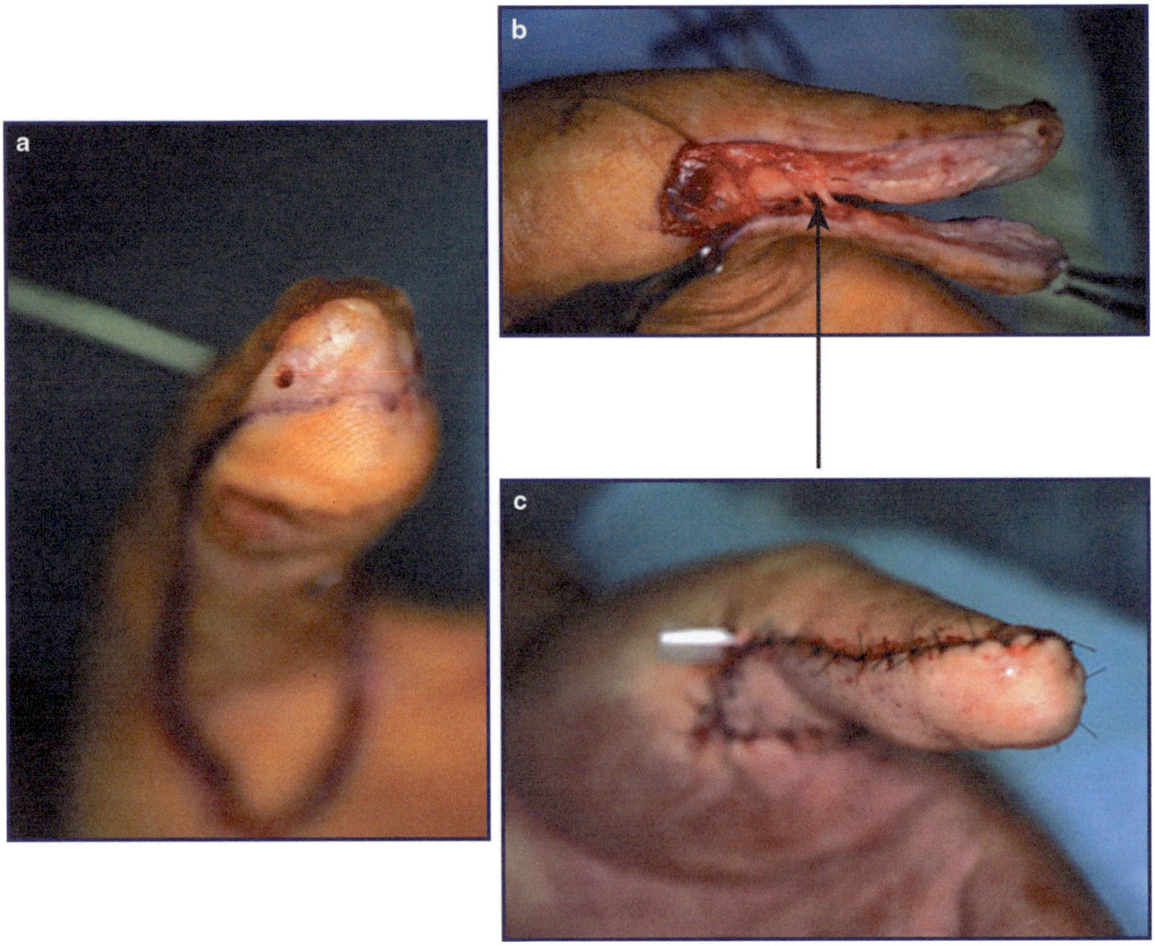

Fig. 21.12 Palmar advancement flap with V–Y closure for thumb tip injuries. (**a**) Thumb tip injury. (**b**) Elevation of the flap. *Arrow* perorating artery. (**c**) Just after surgery

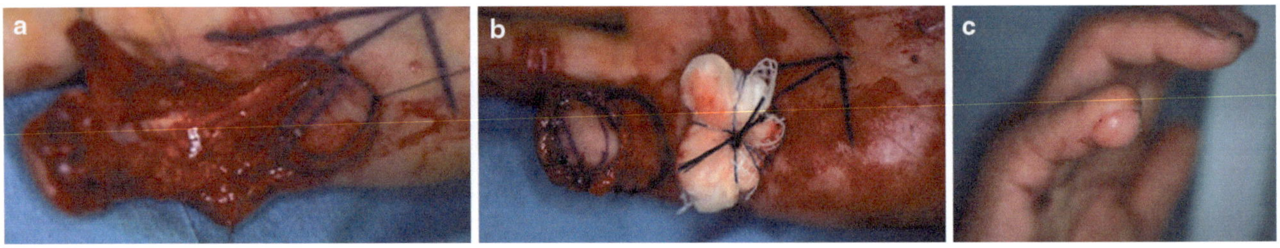

Fig. 21.13 (**a**) Flap elevation. (**b**) The donor site was closed using a full-thickness skin graft. (**c**) Two months after surgery

2. No vascular problems occur when a hemilateral palmar digital artery is sacrificed, provided the opposite palmar digital artery is intact.

Surgery

A skin island is designed on the lateral surface of the base of the finger distal to the interdigital web. When a sensitized flap is necessary, the flap should be created in the dorsolateral surface of the finger to include a dorsal digital nerve or a dorsal branch of a palmar digital nerve. The incision is made along the midlateral line of the finger connecting between the flap and the wound (Fig. 21.15a, b). After transecting the Cleland ligament, the neurovascular bundle is exposed distally to the midpoint between the wound in the fingertip and the distal margin of the flap. The digital nerve is separated from the neurovascular bundle, preserving the adipose tissue of the bundle attached to the palmar digital artery. After application of a vascular clip on the palmar digital artery proximal to the flap, the tourniquet is released to check vascularity of the entire finger and the flap. After good vascularity

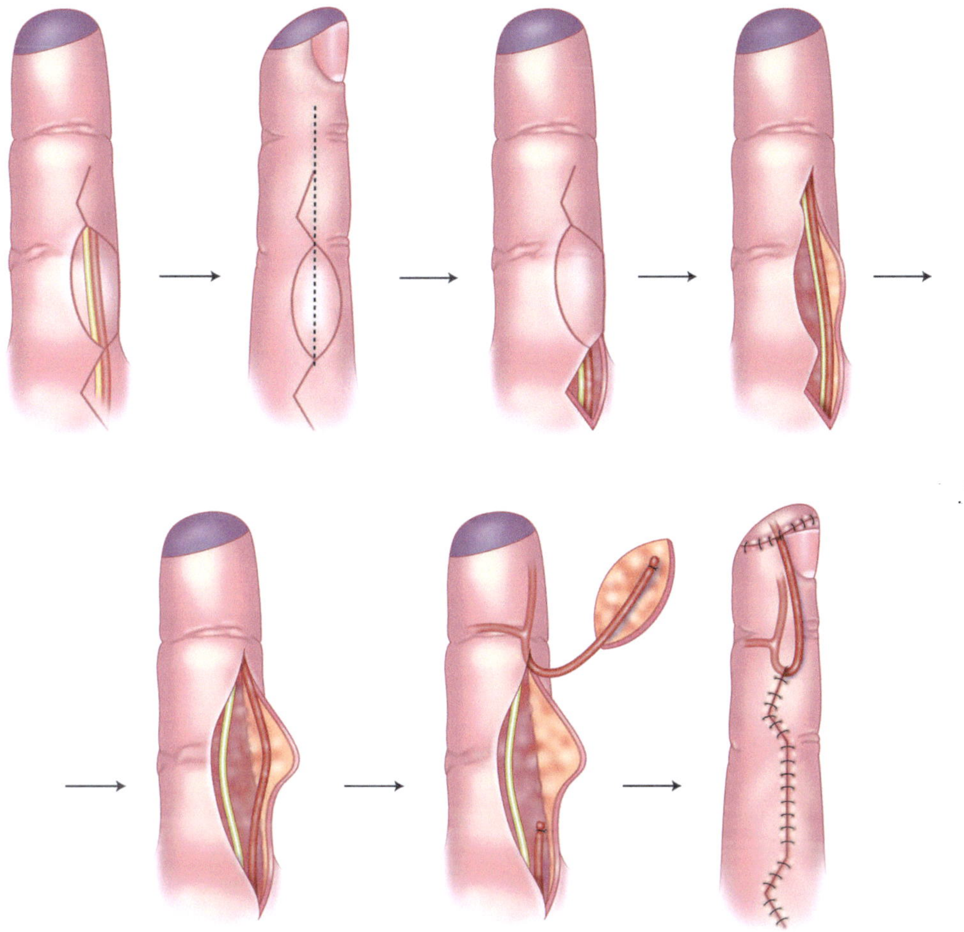

Fig. 21.14 Reverse vascular pedicle digital island flaps based on the palmar digital artery

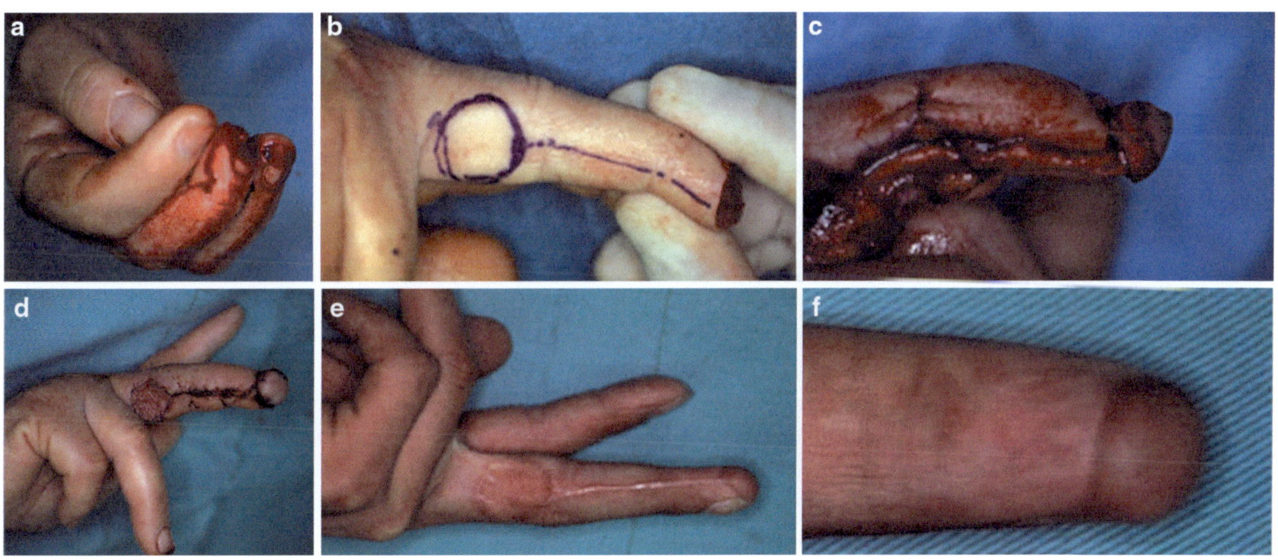

Fig. 21.15 Reverse vascular pedicle digital island flaps based on the palmar digital artery. (**a**) Injury of r-long fingertip. (**b**) Flap design. (**c**) The flap and vascular pedicle was turned distally. (**d**) Three weeks after surgery. (**e**, **f**) Two months after surgery

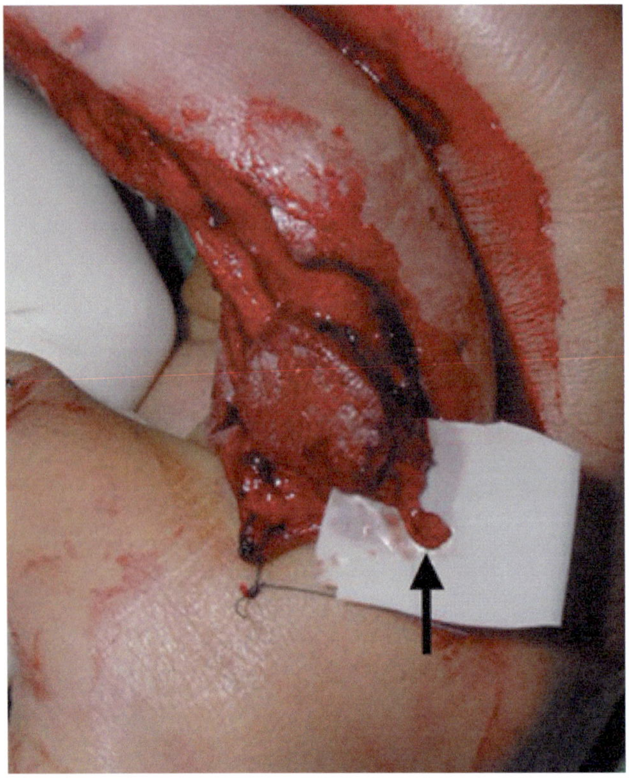

Fig. 21.16 Reverse vascular pedicle digital sensory island flaps based on the palmar digital artery. *Arrow* dorsal digital nerve

of the finger and the flap has been confirmed, the vascular bundle is ligated and transected where the vascular clip had been applied. The flap with the vascular bundle is turned distally and transplanted to the site of the wound without kinking or stretching of the vascular pedicle (Fig. 21.15c). The flap is loosely approximated to the skin around the amputated surface. A skin interval over the vascular pedicle is left open, turned distally. A fiber mesh sheet with antibiotic ointment should be placed over the vascular pedicle to avoid the adhesion of the gauze to the law surface over the vascular pedicle (Fig. 21.15d–f).

A flap including a dorsal digital nerve or a dorsal branch of a palmar digital nerve can be used as a sensory flap. To include a dorsal digital nerve, the flap is designed slightly dorsally. A dorsal digital nerve should be located in the subcutaneous tissue along a dorsal digital vein in the dorsoulnar or dorsoradial quadrant of each finger (Fig. 21.16). The nerve is pulled distally and cut as proximal as possible to leave a transected proximal nerve stump in the subcutaneous tissue in the dorsum of the hand. This is to prevent a neuroma forming on the transected stump. When a dorsal branch of the digital nerve is included in the flap, the flap should be harvested just proximal to the PIP joint. The dorsal branch is dissected proximally until the bifurcation from the palmar digital nerve and transected at the bifurcation. The dorsal branch distal to the flap should be pulled proximally and transected as distal as possible so that the transected stump is located just beneath a healthy subcutaneous fatty tissue in the dorsum of the finger. Any redundant nerve stump attached to the distal margin of the flap should be coagulated and removed. The proximal stump of the dorsal branch of the palmar digital nerve or the dorsal digital nerve included in the flap should be approximated to the distal stump of a contralateral palmar digital nerve stump using 10–0 nylon sutures [24].

Pitfalls

1. When a flap is harvested from the dorsolateral surface of the finger, the flap is connected to the palmar digital artery with a tissue containing perforators arising from the artery.
2. Adipose tissue should be preserved around the palmar digital artery when the vascular pedicle is being elevated. Special care should be taken not to separate the fatty tissue from the artery when the digital nerve is separated from the neurovascular bundle.
3. Kinking or stretching of the vascular pedicle must be avoided.
4. The skin over the vascular pedicle turned distally should be left open and covered by a fiber mesh with fradiomycin sulfate (Sofra-Tulle).

Skin Island Flaps Based on the Dorsal Digital Arterial Network

An arterial structure should be located in the subcutaneous layer on either radial or ulnar side of the dorsal aspect of the finger, for example, a palmar digital artery that is on either radial or ulnar side of the palmar aspect of the finger. Unlike a palmar digital artery, the arterial structure in the dorsum of a finger is not an established independent artery but is composed of longitudinal connections of several small perforating arteries arising from a palmar digital artery in the dorsum of a finger and hand. Thus, it should be called the dorsal digital arterial network (DDAN) rather than dorsal digital arteries. Distal to the PIP joint, the DDAN is concomitant with a dorsal branch of the palmar digital nerve and is called a dorsal branch of the palmar digital artery. It consists of several perforator connections with the palmar digital artery [25] (Fig. 21.17). Because the DDAN has a lower blood pressure than the palmar digital artery, its blood flow is easily compromised by kinking or stretching of the vessel. Flaps with orthograde or retrograde blood flow can be harvested based on the DDAN and dorsal metacarpal arteries in any region of the dorsum of the digits and hand.

Vascularity

Although the DDAN is accompanied by venules, subcutaneous veins should be included in the vascular pedicle composed of DDAN to facilitate venous drainage of the flap.

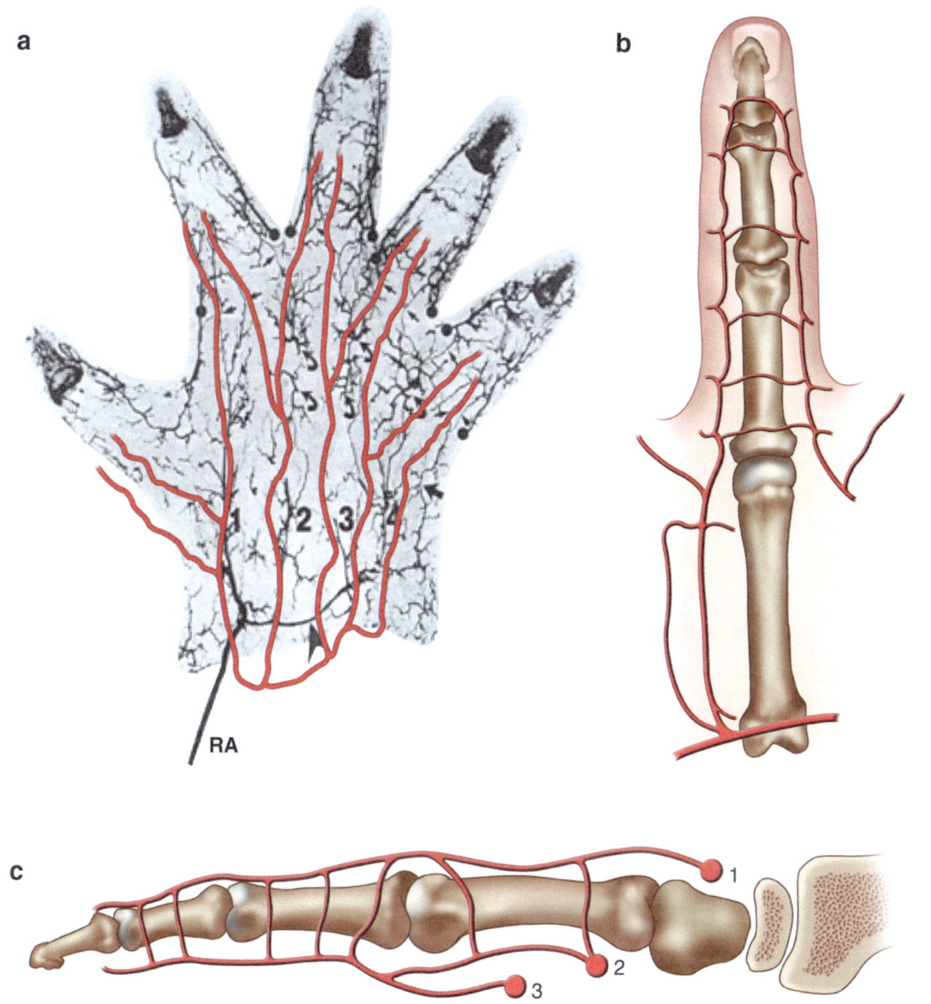

Fig. 21.17 (**a**, **b**) Dorsal digital arterial network (DDAN). (**c**) Connection between the palmar digital artery and the dorsal digital arterial network

Advantages

1. Skin islands can be harvested anywhere on the dorsum of the hand and digits.
2. A flap can be harvested orthogradely or retrogradely based on the DDAN and dorsal metacarpal arteries.

Disadvantages

1. Because of their unstable vascularity, flaps based on DDAN easily develop congestion or necrosis [25, 26].
2. The length of the vascular pedicle and the size of the flap should be restricted because of the unstable vascularity of the DDAN.

Surgery

A skin island should be designed over either the ulnar or radial dorsal quadrant of a finger. The width of the flap should not exceed that of the dorsal quadrant of the finger. A straight skin incision is made along a midline of the ulnodorsal or radiodorsal quadrant of the finger. The skin incision should stay in the dermis and extend laterally in the subdermal layer to expose the subcutaneous fatty layer including subcutaneous veins. The vascular pedicle is the subcutaneous adipose tissue of the ulnar or radial dorsal quadrant of the finger. The flap (including the subcutaneous vascular pedicle) is elevated distally toward the skin defect just above the paratenon of the extensor tendons until the flap is turned distally to reach the skin defect. The flap is loosely approximated to the wound. A skin interval over the turned subcutaneous pedicle should be left open (Fig. 21.18). A split-thickness skin graft may be indicated on the skin interval over the flap pedicle. However, in most cases, the interval will epithelialize spontaneously. Like the palmar digital artery, the dorsal digital flaps can acquire sensation if a dorsal digital nerve or a dorsal branch of the palmar digital nerve is included in the flap.

Pitfalls

As the vascularity of a flap based on the DDAN is unstable and the blood pressure in the DDAN is also weak, harvesting

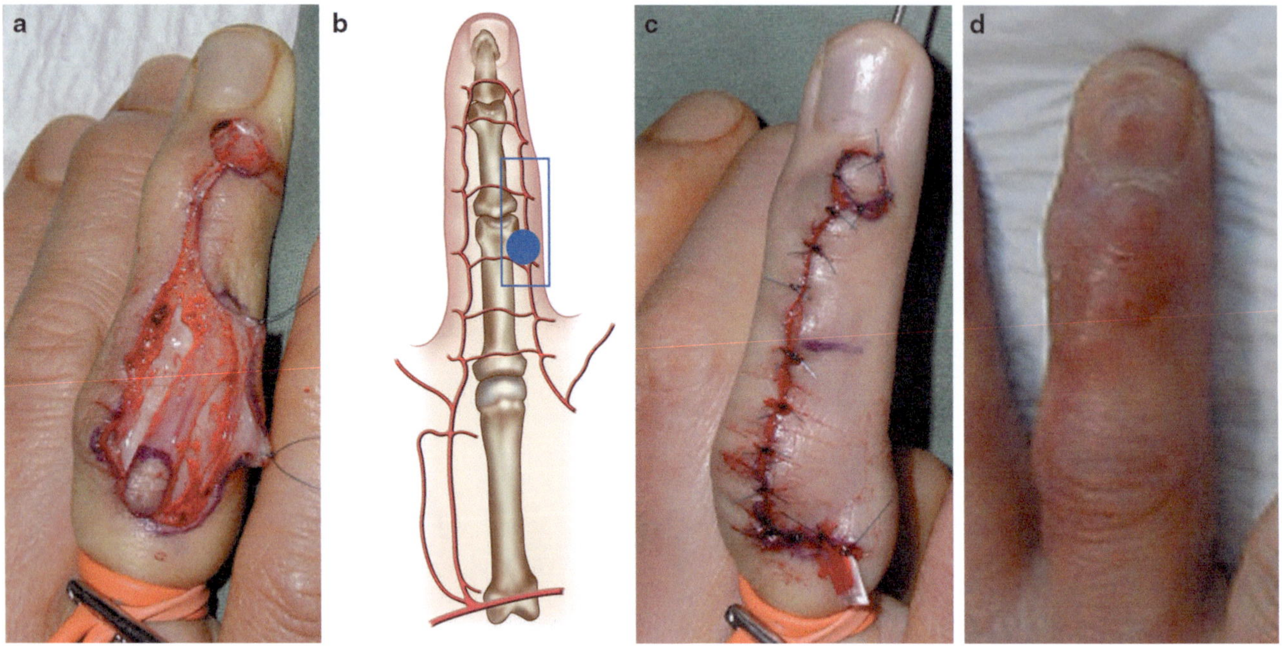

Fig. 21.18 (**a**, **b**) A mucous cyst in the distal interphalangeal (DIP) joint. A skin island based on the DDAN was harvested. (**c**) Just after surgery. (**d**) Three months after surgery

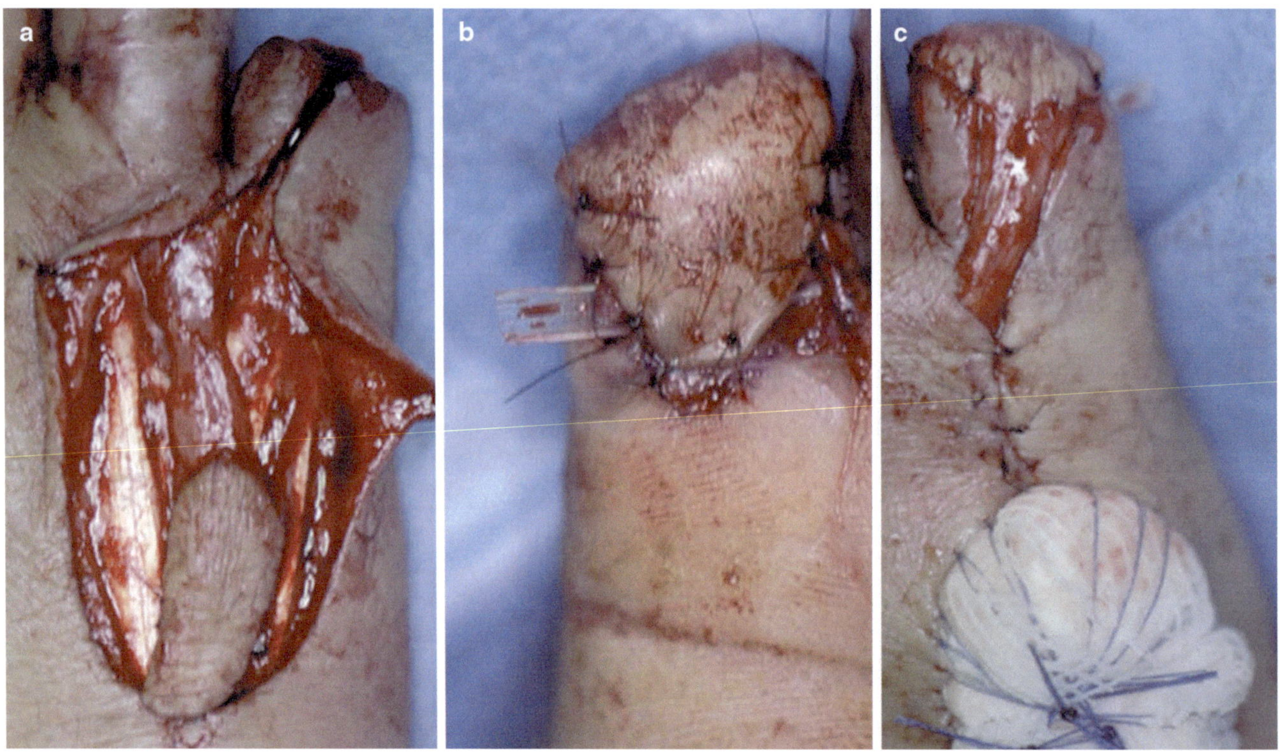

Fig. 21.19 Finger amputation covered by a skin island nourished by a dorsal metacarpal artery. (**a**) Flap elevation. (**b**) Coverage of the amputated finger with the dorsal metacarpal flap. (**c**) The donor site was covered by a full-thickness skin graft

huge flaps based on DDAN should be avoided. Flaps with a long subcutaneous pedicle risk necrosis. From the author's experience, the flap should be harvested from the radial or ulnar quadrant of the dorsum of the finger. When the flap is taken from a finger, the length of the vascular pedicle should be less than one-third of that of the finger (from the web to the fingertip). In the thumb, the pedicle length should be the whole length of the thumb (Fig. 21.19).

Modification of the Skin Island Based on the Dorsal Digital Arterial Network

Kite Flap (Foucher and Braun 1979)

A line connecting the midpoint between the common extensor tendon and the radial midlateral line at the MP joint level to the point where the pulsation of the radial artery is palpable at the base of the first web corresponds to the course of the second dorsal metacarpal artery. It is advisable to confirm the existence of the second metacarpal artery along this radial index finger line in the first web space using Doppler sonography before surgery. A flap should be designed on the radial quadrant in the dorsum of the index finger in the proximal phalanx level and elevated subcutaneously just above the paratenon of the extensor tendon. The skin incision of the flap should be connected proximally to the incision along the radial index finger line. Only skin and dermis should be incised along the line in the first web space and separated from the underlying subcutaneous fatty tissue. Subcutaneous fatty tissue with a 1-cm width including the second dorsal metacarpal artery, subcutaneous veins, and fascia over the adductor pollicis muscle and first dorsal interosseous muscle should be elevated because the second dorsal metacarpal artery is located just above the fascia. The incision is extended along a new line connecting the point of the radial artery pulsation to a skin defect in the thumb tip along the thumb–ulnar midlateral line. The subcutaneous tissue is dissected, and a subcutaneous space is created along this incision to accommodate the vascular pedicle within it. After the vascular pedicle has been shifted to the incision, the flap is sutured to the skin defect in the thumb tip. The radial index finger incision is closed primarily, and the skin defect created after harvesting the flap in the index finger is covered using a full-thickness skin graft taken from the forearm. The ulnar–thumb incision should not be closed primarily to avoid compromising the vascularity of the vascular pedicle of the flap. Spontaneous reepithelialization can be found in a skin interval over the vascular pedicle along the ulnar–thumb incision (Fig. 21.20).

To avoid compression of the subcutaneous vascular pedicle and facilitate skin closure over the transferred pedicle, the vascular pedicle (including an overlying skin strip about 0.5 cm wide) can be harvested along the radial index finger incision and shifted to the ulnar–thumb incision as described by Holevich [27] (Figs. 21.21 and 21.22).

Flaps Based on the Ulnodorsal Digital Artery of the Thumb (Brunelli et al. 1999)

This flap type is categorized among those based on the DDAN. However, unlike the DDAN of fingers, that of the thumb is well developed and recognized as an established artery. Blood flow in the DDAN of the thumb is quite stable. A longitudinal incision starts from a skin defect at the thumb tip, passes along the center of the ulnodorsal quadrant of the thumb, and ends in the first web space. An ulnodorsal digital artery and concomitant nerve should be identified deep to subcutaneous veins. A flap is then created in the first web space over the ulnodorsal digital artery (Fig. 21.23a, b). The ulnodorsal artery, nerve, and subcutaneous vein are found proximal to the flap. The ulnodorsal digital nerve, which is a branch of the superficial branch of the radial nerve, is pulled distally and transected as proximal as possible, so that the transected stump is located in healthy subcutaneous tissue in the first web space. When the nerve branch is large, the stump can be buried in the muscle belly of the adductor pollicis muscle or inserted into the lumen of a subcutaneous vein to prevent neuroma formation. The ulnodorsal digital artery and subcutaneous veins should be ligated or coagulated proximal to the flap. The flap is elevated distally to the interphalangeal (IP) joint level including the ulnodorsal digital artery, nerve, subcutaneous veins, and the surrounding adipose tissue. The flap is then turned distally along the skin incision (Fig. 21.23c, d). The ulnodorsal nerve stump of the flap is approximated to the palmar digital nerve stump to restore sensation to the flap. The skin defect created after removal of the flap is usually closed primarily.

Free Flaps

The wraparound flap method is sometimes used for fingertip reconstruction; however, it is more likely to be used for thumb reconstruction. The second toe is often used to reconstruct fingertip injuries. Even with thumb amputation, the second toe is preferred to the great toe for reconstruction. Regarding thumb amputation, a thumb reconstructed by using the wraparound flap is cosmetically much better than that created using toe transfer. If the MP joint function of the amputated thumb is to be preserved, the wraparound flap is recommended. However, if the amputation level is proximal to the MP joint level, a toe transfer can provide the MP joint with function in combination with tendon reconstruction.

Wraparound Flap [28]

Indications

1. Fingernail reconstruction
2. Thumb amputation distal to the MP joint
3. Finger amputation distal to the PIP joint level

Advantage

It is possible to restore the fingertip or thumb tip with excellent cosmetic appearance.

Disadvantages

1. Deformity of the great toe or delaying healing of the donor site may occur.
2. This flap cannot be used in growing children.

Fig. 21.20 Kite flap

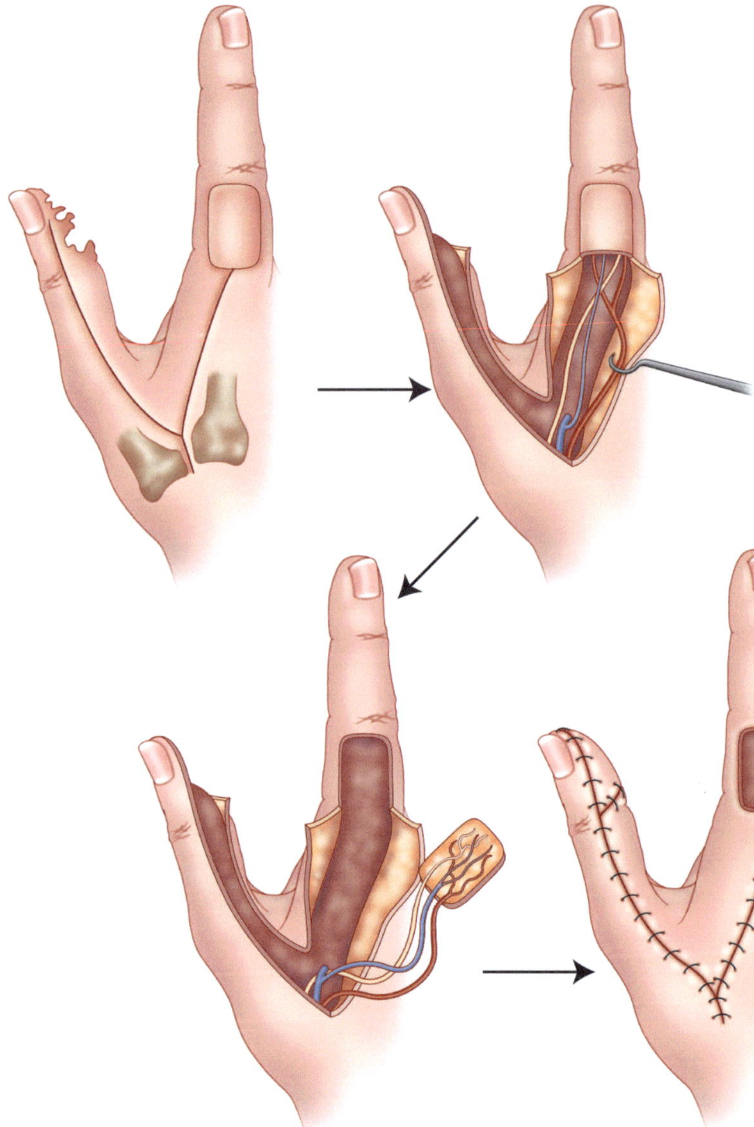

Surgery

Flaps with a Short Vascular Pedicle (Often Used for Nail Reconstruction)

Before surgery, the circumference, length, width, and nail size of the opposite normal thumb are measured. A template is made for marking the flap on the donor big toe. A zigzag incision is made in the first web space. The incision is extended distally to the dorsum of the IP joint of the big toe. The subcutaneous veins originating from the dorsum of the big toe are exposed proximally. Because the big toe nail is wider than the thumb nail, a proximal and lateral nail, nail matrix, and the underlying distal phalanx of the great toe are harvested to match the size of the nail of the opposite thumb. The flexor and extensor tendons are divided, and the toe IP joint is disarticulated. The nail, the underlying distal phalangeal bone, and skin tissue large enough to create the missing thumb are harvested from the distal lateral portion of the big toe, including the lateral plantar neurovascular bundle and the dorsal digital veins. The medial plantar neurovascular bundle is preserved to nourish the remaining medial part of the big toe. The lateral plantar digital neurovascular bundle is exposed proximally and transected in the first web space (Figs. 21.25 and 21.26).

The skin, nail, and distal phalanx including the lateral plantar digital artery (LPDA) and nerve (LPDN) and dorsal subcutaneous veins are transferred to the thumb. The LPDA and LPDN are approximated to the radial or ulnar digital artery and nerve of the thumb, respectively. The subcutaneous veins of the big toe are sutured to the subcutaneous veins in the dorsum of the hand (Fig. 21.24a, b).

Fig. 21.21 Holvitch's method

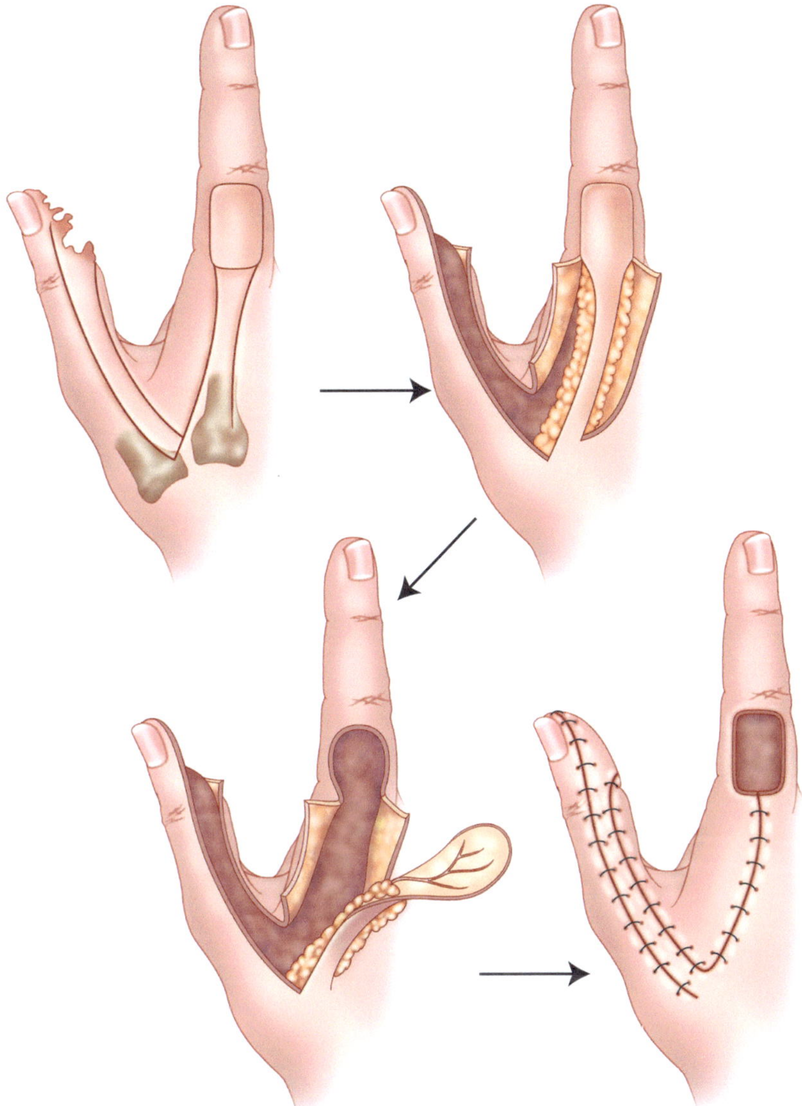

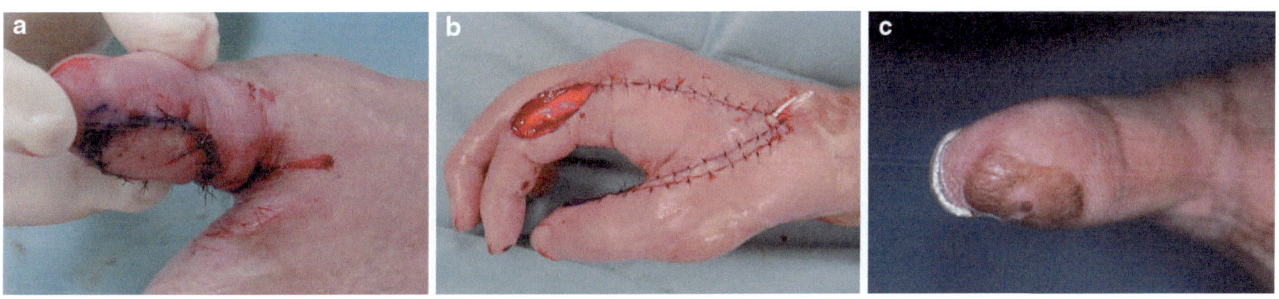

Fig. 21.22 Holvitch's method. (**a**, **b**) During surgery. The donor site was covered by a full-thickness skin graft later. (**c**) One year after surgery

Flaps with a Long Vascular Pedicle

A zigzag incision is made from the first web space to the base of the first and second metatarsal bones. Subcutaneous veins originating from the dorsum of the big toe are exposed proximally to the great saphenous vein. The LPDA and LPDN of the big toe (LPDABT and LPDNBT) are identified, and the LPDABT is exposed proximally in the first web space. The branching portion of the LPDABT, the medial plantar digital artery (MPDA) of the second toe (MPDAST), the first dorsal metatarsal artery (FDMA), the first plantar metatarsal artery

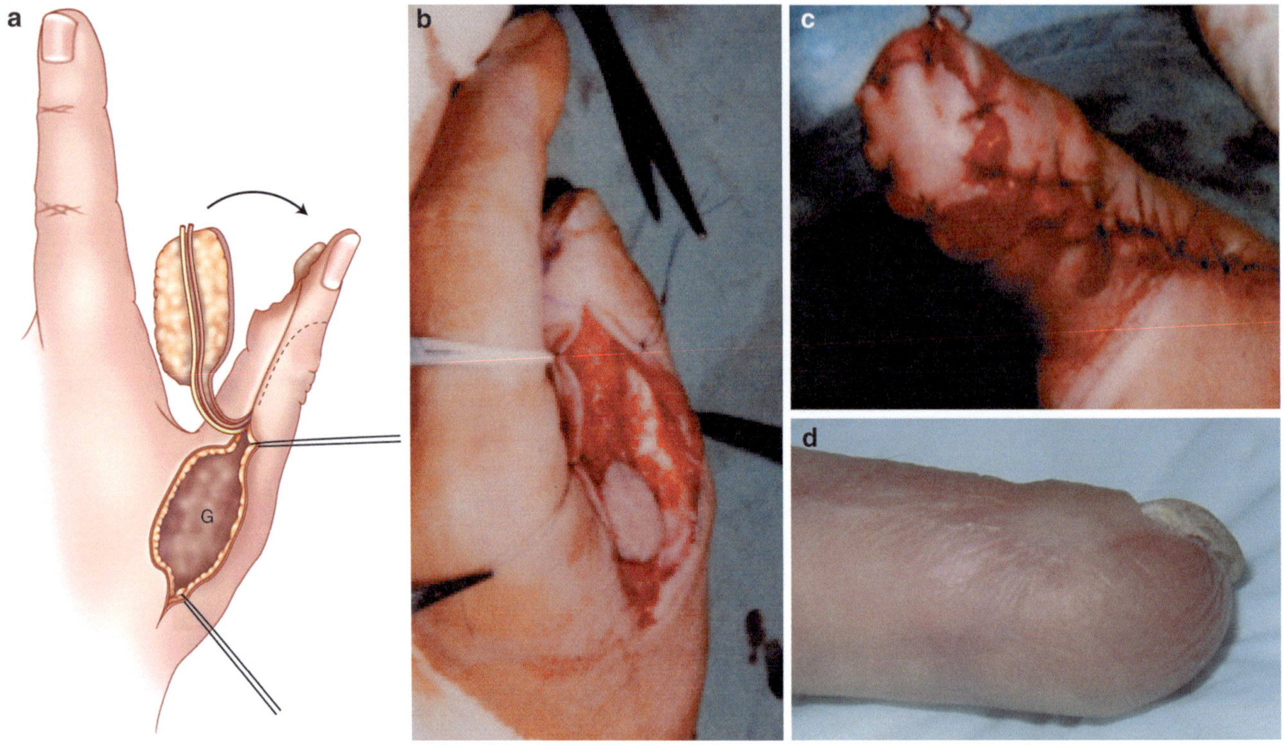

Fig. 21.23 Flaps based on the ulnodorsal digital artery of the thumb. (**a**, **b**) Flap elevation. (**c**) Coverage of the thumb tip. (**d**) One year after surgery

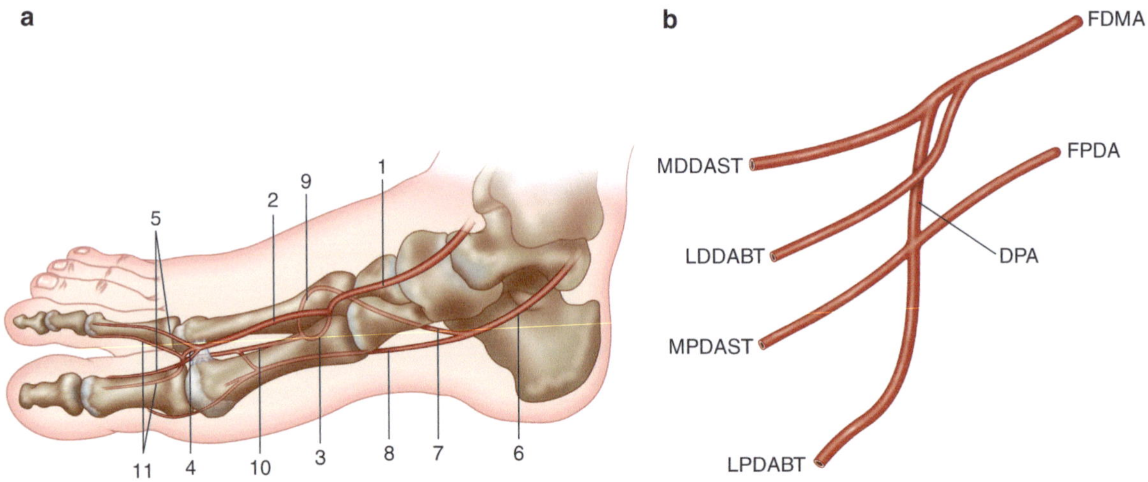

Fig. 21.24 (**a**) Arterial anatomy of the foot: *1* dorsalis pedis artery, *2* first dorsal metatarsal artery, *3* deep plantar artery, *4* distal connecting artery, *5* dorsal digital arteries, *6* posterior tibial artery, *7* lateral plantar artery, *8* medial plantar artery, *9* plantar arch, *10* first plantar metatarsal artery, *11* plantar digital arteries. (**b**) Arterial anatomy of the first web space: *FDMA* first dorsal metatarsal artery, *FPMA* first plantar metatarsal artery, *MDDAST* medial dorsal digital artery of the second toe, *LDDABT* lateral dorsal digital artery of the big toe, *MPDAST* medial plantar digital artery of the second toe, *LPDABT* lateral plantar digital artery of the big toe, *DPA* distal perforating artery

(FPMA), and the communicating artery between the FDMA and FPMA are exposed carefully. Because the FDMA is usually larger than the FPMA, the latter is exposed proximally to the dorsalis pedis artery after ligating the MPDAST or the FPMA. When the FDMA is not suitable for a nutrient artery, the FPMA should be exposed proximally through a palmar incision between the first and second metatarsal bones (Fig. 21.24a, b). The nail, nail matrix, the distal phalanx, and skin are harvested as described previously.

The FDMA or dorsalis pedis artery is transected to harvest an arterial pedicle that is long enough to reach the radial artery in the snuffbox. The deep peroneal nerve that is

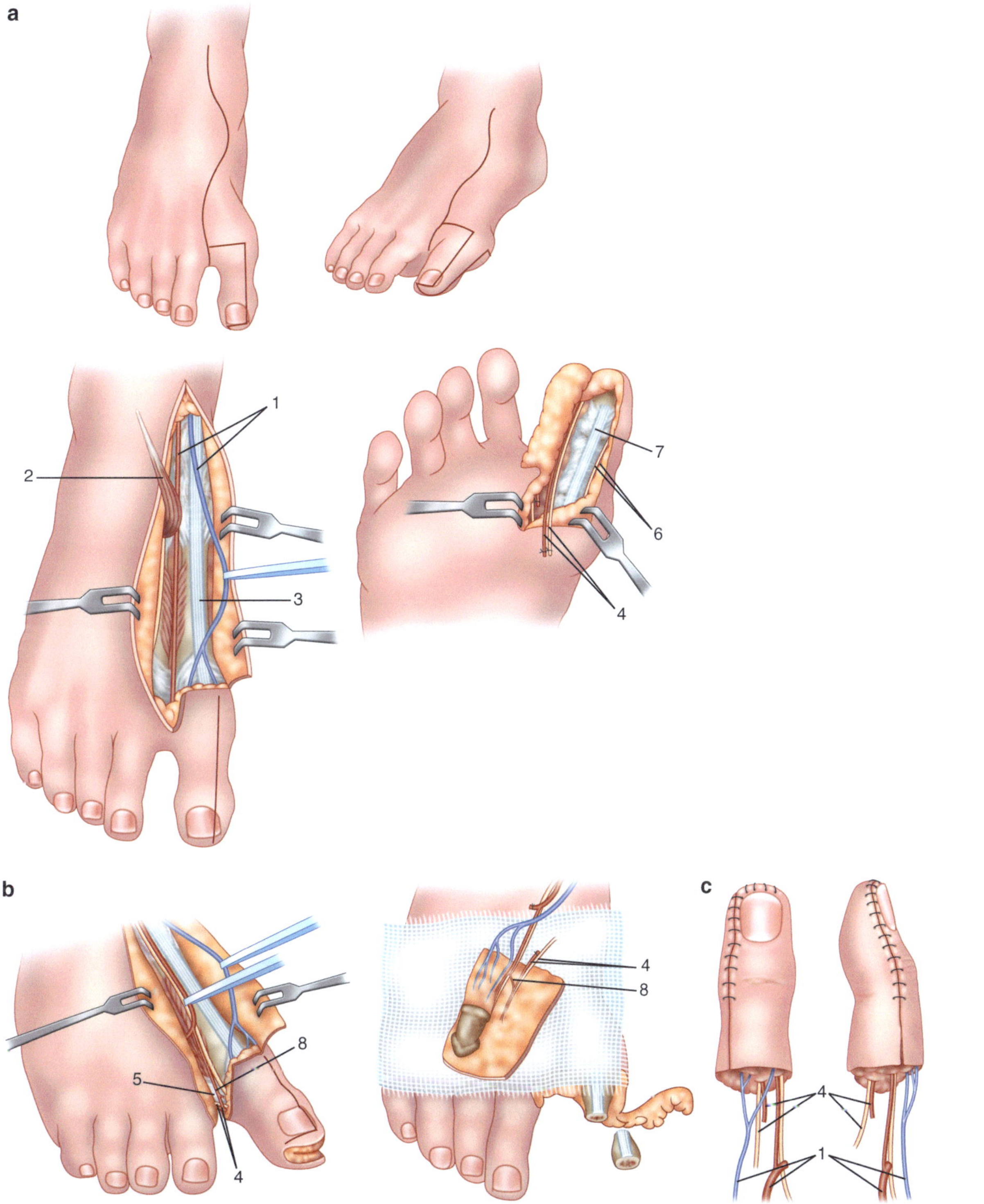

Fig. 21.25 Wraparound flap: *1* dorsalis pedis artery and great saphenous vein, *2* extensor hallucis brevis muscle, *3* extensor hallucis longus tendon, *4* lateral plantar digital artery and nerve, *5* deep transverse metatarsal ligament, *6* medial plantar digital artery and nerve, *7* long flexor hallucis muscle tendon, *8* distal perforating artery

concomitant with the FDMA and dorsalis pedis artery is also transected at the same level as the artery. The LPDNBT is also transected proximally through a plantar incision in the first web space. Thus, the skin, nail, distal phalanx, and subcutaneous veins based on the FDMA or dorsalis pedis artery are transferred to the thumb (Figs. 21.25–21.27). An iliac bone graft should be interposed between the distal phalanx of the big toe and the thumb phalanx to adjust the length of

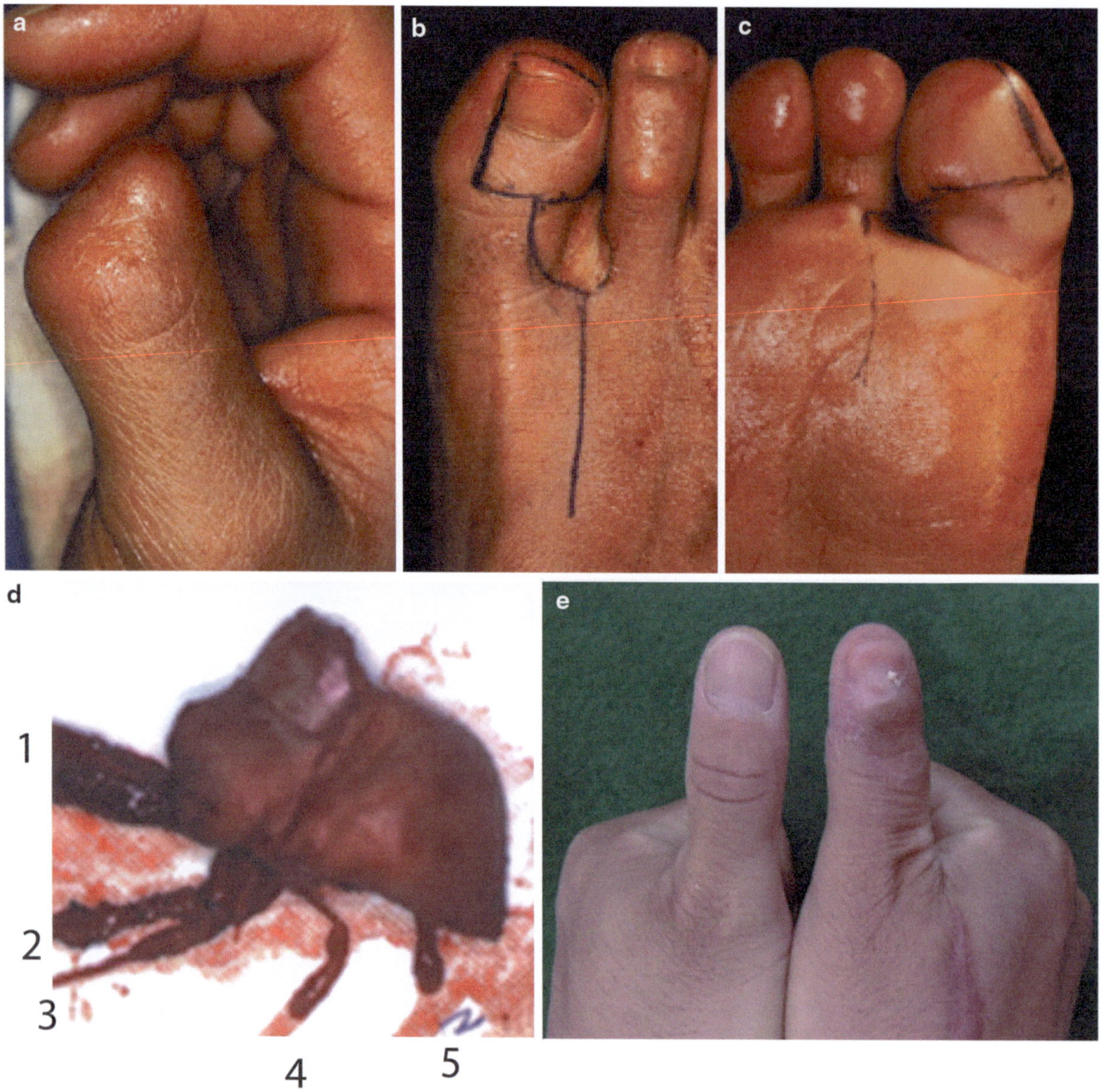

Fig. 21.26 Wraparound flap for thumb nail reconstruction. (**a**) Amputation of thumb tip. (**b**, **c**) Flap design. (**d**) Harvested nail and skin. *1* Subcutaneous vein, *2* lateral plantar digital artery, *3* deep peroneal nerve, *4* lateral plantar digital nerve, *5* medial plantar digital nerve. In this case, the medial plantar digital nerve was included in the flap, (**e**) Post-operative appearance

the thumb [29]. After the iliac bone graft, the FDMA or dorsalis pedis artery is approximated to the radial artery at the snuffbox. The LPDNBT and deep peroneal nerve are approximated to the radial and ulnar digital nerves of the thumb, respectively. The great saphenous vein is sutured to a subcutaneous vein of the hand. The remaining portion of the big toe after harvesting the flap can be obliterated by a free vascularized cutaneous flap or bone shortening.

Toe-to-Finger Transfer

Second Toe Transfer (Yoshimura 1980; Lister et al. 1983; Leung 1985)

Indications

1. Thumb amputation proximal to the MP joint level
2. Toe or finger reconstruction in growing children
3. Finger amputation proximal to the proximal nail fold in the ulnar fingers
4. Fingernail reconstruction

Advantage

It is possible to reconstruct a cosmetically acceptable fingertip.

Disadvantage

Because the second digit and nail are short compared with the normal fingernail, the second toe transfer is better, cosmetically, when used for reconstruction of the ulnar fingers than when used for thumb or radial finger reconstruction.

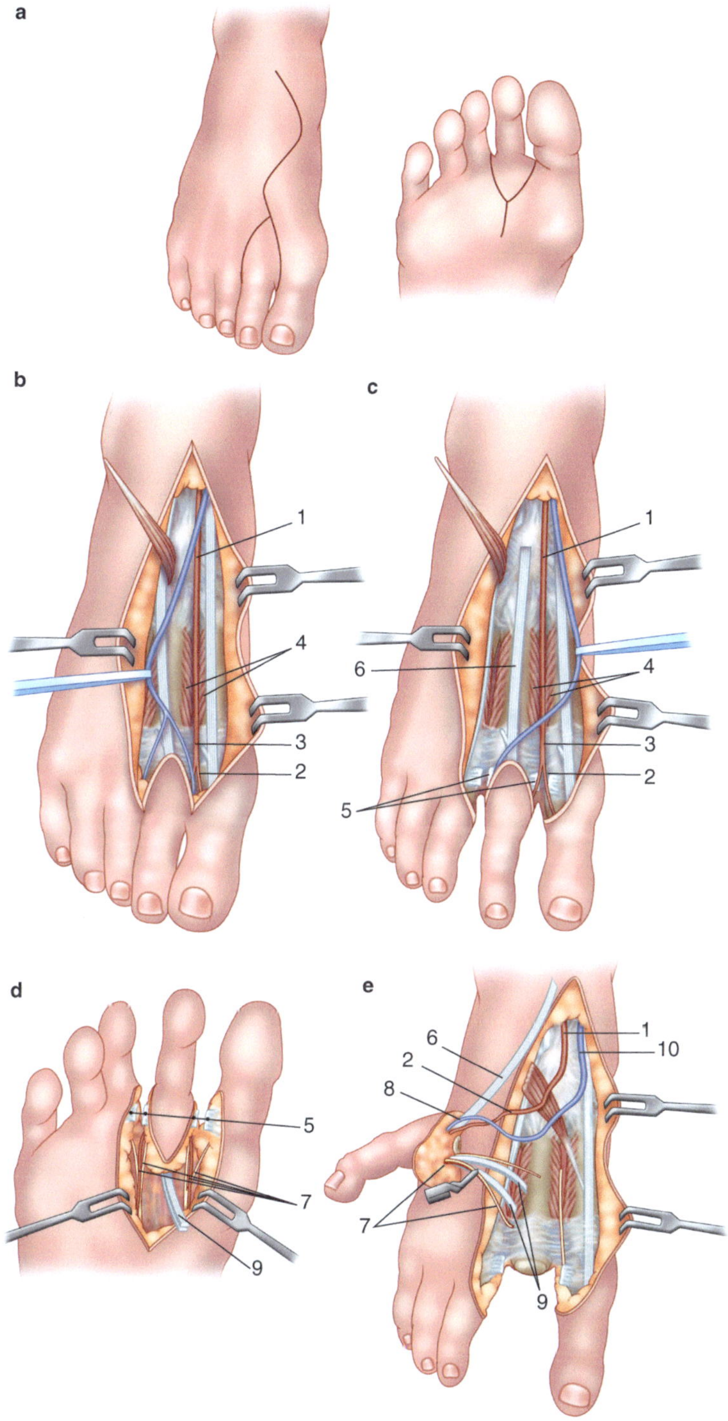

Fig. 21.27 Second toe transfer: *1* dorsalis pedis artery, *2* first dorsal metatarsal artery, *3* deep plantar artery, *4* interosseous muscle, *5* deep transverse metatarsal ligament, *6* extensor tendon, *7* plantar digital nerve and artery, *8* dorsal metatarsal vein, *9* flexor tendons, *10* great saphenous vein

Surgery

Dorsal subcutaneous veins should be exposed in the dorsum of the MP joint of the second toe and elevated distally toward the PIP joint of the second toe. At the first and second web space, the medial and lateral plantar digital arteries and concomitant nerves of the second toe are then identified. The medial and lateral plantar digital arteries and nerves should be divided in the first and second webs, respectively. The digit is osteotomized depending on the length required for reconstruction of the finger. The long extensor and deep flexor tendons are exposed proximally through a dorsal and plantar incision extended proximally, respectively, and transected as long as they are needed. In the fingertip, the bilateral palmar digital arteries, nerves, extensor and flexor

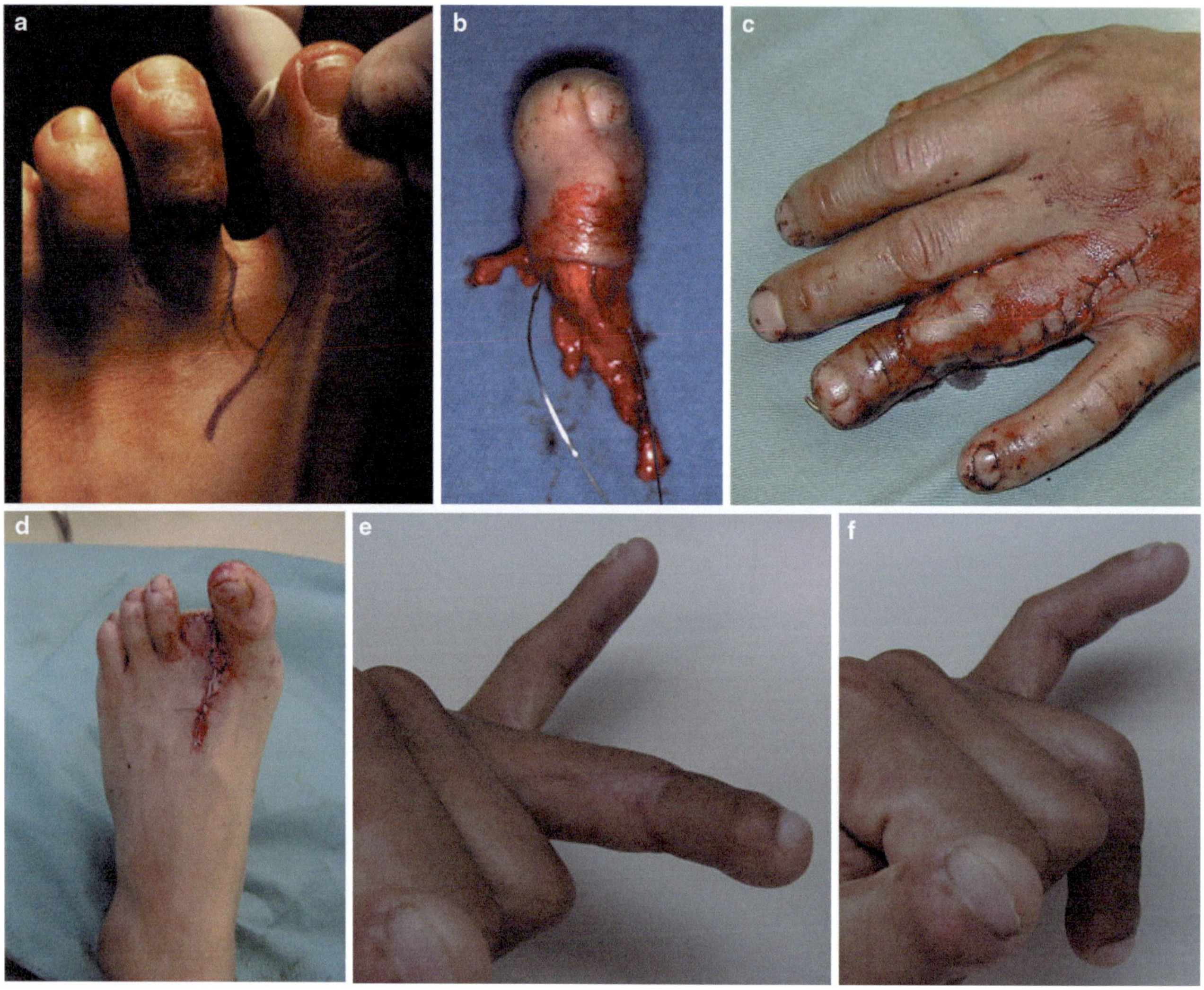

Fig. 21.28 (a) Flap design. (b) Harvested second toe. (c) Fingertip reconstruction using a second toe flap. The proximal phalanx of the second toe was joined to the proximal phalanx of the ring finger. Tenodesis was performed on the DIP joint. (d) Wound closure. (e) Six months after surgery. Active extension of the PIP joint. (f) Six months after surgery. Active flexion of the PIP joint

tendons, and subcutaneous veins should be exposed. The toe phalanx is fixed with the finger phalanx using crisscrossed K-wires and/or tension-band wiring. The bilateral palmar digital nerves and arteries of the toe are approximated with those of the finger. The toe veins are also sutured to the dorsal subcutaneous veins of the finger. The deep flexor tendon of the toe is sutured to the deep flexor tendons of the finger in the palm using interlacing. The long extensor tendon of the toe is sutured to the extensor digitorum communis tendon of the hand. Arthrodesis of the toe DIP joint is necessary (Fig. 21.28).

When a long vascular pedicle is necessary, the second toe should be elevated on the LPDABT and the FDMA or FPMA, as described for the wraparound flap. When a second toe with a long metatarsus is needed, branches of the FDMA or FPMA supplying the second metatarsal bone should be preserved during the vascular pedicle elevation (Fig. 21.29).

Hemipulp Flap [30–33]

Indication

The ideal indication of this procedure is loss of the finger pulp, although the nail and the underlying distal phalanx should remain intact.

Advantage

The flap is strong for shear or compression loads.

Disadvantages

Deformity of the big toe or delayed healing of the donor site might occur.

Surgery

In the first web space, the LPDA and LPDN of the big toe should be identified and exposed distally. The cutaneous flap is designed on the distal lateral plantar pulp of the big toe

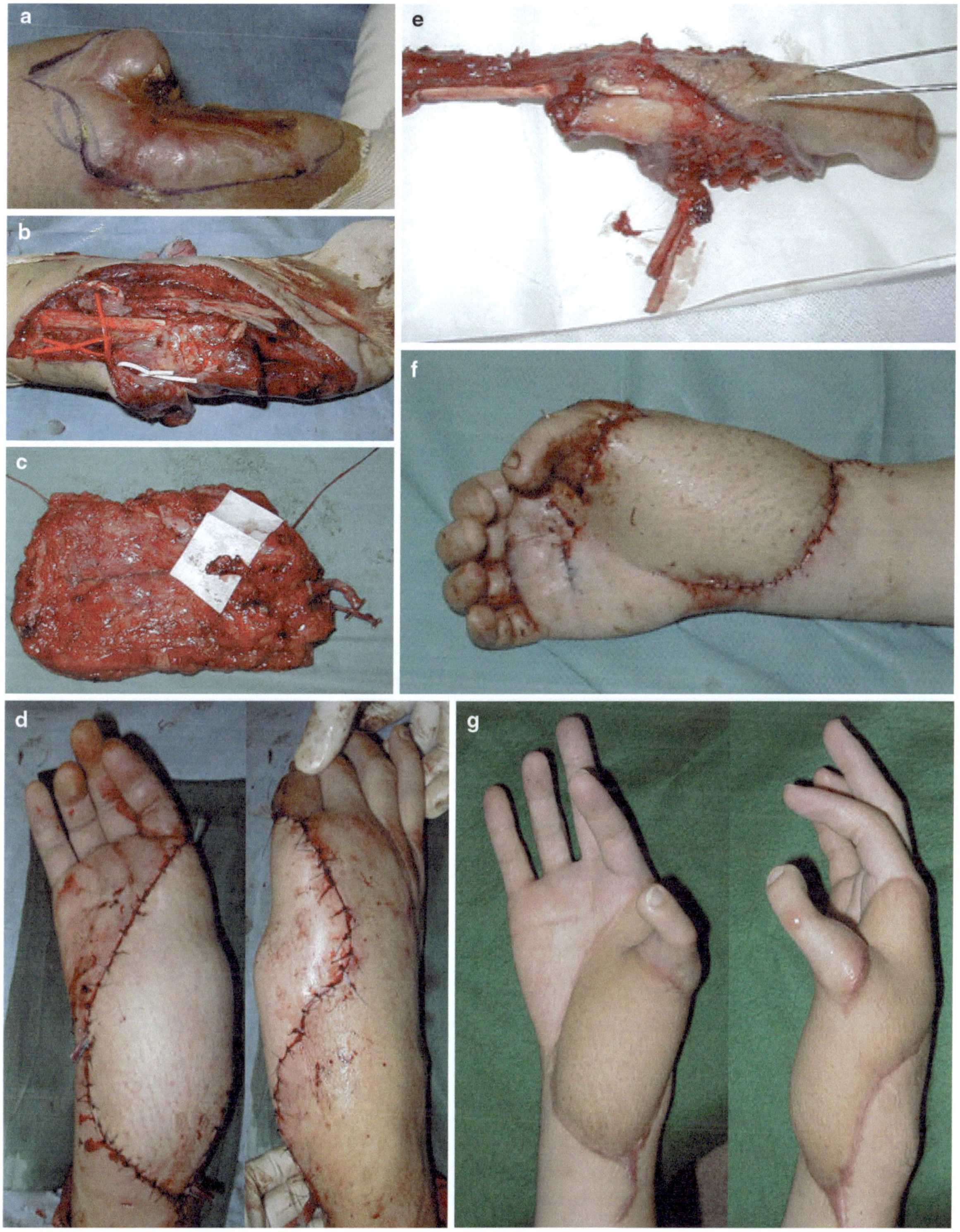

Fig. 21.29 (**a**) Thumb amputation. (**b**) Digital nerve reconstruction (sural nerve graft) and debridement. (**c**) Groin flap. (**d**) Transplantation of the groin flap. (**e**, **f**) Second toe transfer at the metatarsal level. Arthrodesis was performed on the DIP and PIP joints. (**g**) Six months after surgery

including the LPDA and LPDN. In the proximal dorsal portion of the flap, a subcutaneous vein is identified and exposed proximally. The flap is elevated including the LPDA, the LPDN, and the subcutaneous vein. The skin defect created after removal of the flap is covered using a full-thickness skin graft (Fig. 21.30).

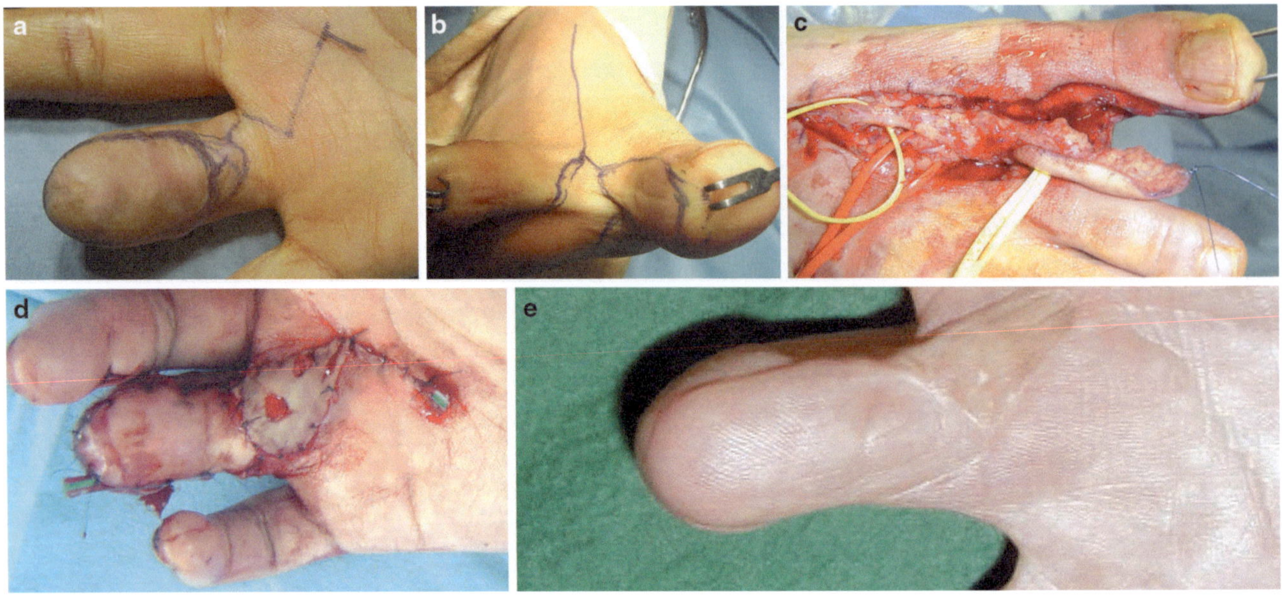

Fig. 21.30 Hemipulp flap. (a) The palmar aspect of the ring finger was covered by a skin graft in the previous operation. (b) A hemipulp flap was designed. (c) Elevation of the flap based on the FDMA. (d) The FDMA was approximated to a common digital artery in the palm and the great saphenous vein was sutured to the dorsal subcutaneous vein of the hand. Note skin graft on the vascular pedicle. (e) One year after surgery

Fingertip Reconstruction Using an Arterialized Venous Skin Graft

Indications

1. Skin coverage of fingertip injuries with a phalangeal bone exposure
2. Guillotine amputation of fingers
3. Fingertip injuries occurring on people who do not wish for a toe transfer

Advantage

Harvesting donor skin is quick and easy.

Disadvantages

1. The skin might be weak against mechanical forces applied to the fingertip.
2. Unpredictable skin necrosis can occur, even though vascularity within the flap is good.

Surgery

The loss of the phalanx is reconstructed by transplantation from the iliac bone. Skin including subcutaneous fatty tissue, a subcutaneous vein, and the medial forearm cutaneous nerve should be harvested from the medial aspect of the medial anterior forearm. The flap width is slightly greater than a half of the circumference of the amputated surface of the finger. The flap length should be determined from the length of the iliac bone graft and thickness of the subcutaneous tissue of the flap. The proximal portion of the iliac bone graft is inserted into the medullary cavity of the phalanx and fixed with a K-wire. The proximal stump of the subcutaneous vein is approximated to the palmar digital artery stump, and the distal one is sutured to a dorsal subcutaneous vein of the finger. The forearm cutaneous antebrachial nerve is sutured to either the radial or the ulnar digital nerve stump (Fig. 21.31).

Pitfalls

1. For arterialized venous flaps, the subcutaneous vein of the flap is included in the center of the flap.
2. The flaps should not be harvested from a portion where a thick subcutaneous fat layer is between the subcutaneous veins and the dermis.
3. The flap size should be small.
4. The vascularity of the flaps should be flow-through pattern.
5. The vein of the flap should be interposed between an artery and a vein or between arteries [34].

Nail Reconstruction

Principle of Nail Reconstruction

Nail growth is determined by three factors: the nail matrix, nail floor, and underlying bone. The nail matrix produces nail tissue. Once the nail matrix is injured and lost, it should be transplanted from a toenail as a vascularized composite. The nail bed and underlying bone are necessary to extend the nail tissue distally. Even if the nail matrix and nail floor are intact, the nail will be deformed if the distal phalanx is deformed or lost. Deformity of the distal phalanx can be

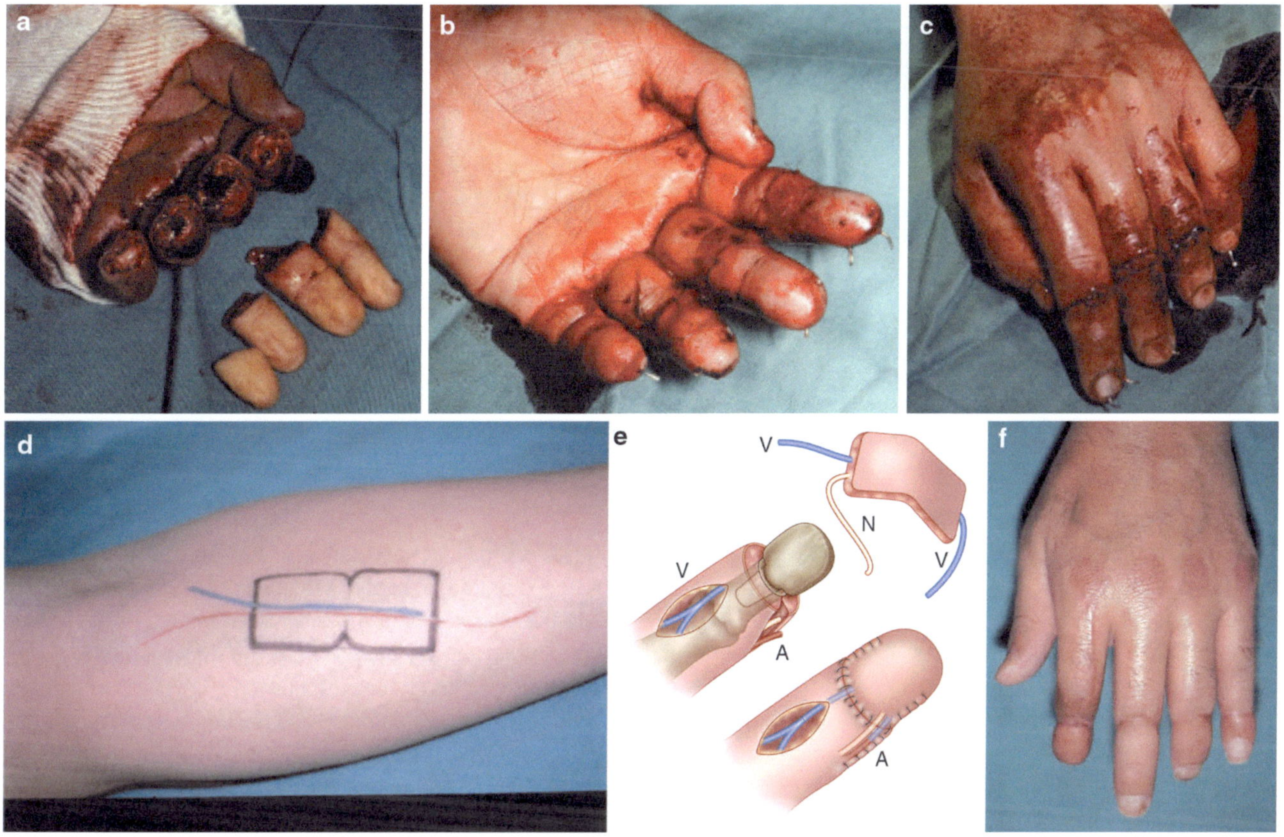

Fig. 21.31 (a) Four finger amputation. (b, c) Replantation. The index finger stump got necrosis a week after surgery. (d) A skin island including a subcutaneous vein and the forearm cutaneous nerve was harvested from the ipsilateral forearm. (e) An iliac bone graft was performed at the proximal phalanx. The proximal stump of the subcutaneous vein was sutured to the digital artery, and the other end of the vein was approximated to the dorsal subcutaneous vein of the finger. (f) One year after surgery

repaired by osteotomy. When the nail floor is injured or lost, the nail deformity occurs even if the nail matrix and distal phalanx are intact. If the defect of the nail floor is partial and limited, a split-thickness nail bed taken from the toenail can survive on the finger phalanx as a composite that can be vascularized by capillary invasion from the underlying bone and surrounding remaining nail floor [35, 36].

Nail Deformity

Hook Nail Deformity

A hook nail deformity of the fingernail is a palmar curling of the nail caused by a defect of the tip of the distal phalanx. When the defect is limited to the distal one-fifth of the distal phalanx, the nail floor elevation can be elevated by soft tissue transplantation where the distal phalanx is deficient. If the bone defect of the distal phalanx is more than the distal one-fifth and the nail matrix does not have bony support, bone transplantation is necessary. However, if nonvascularized bone is transplanted, the tip of the transplanted bone is often reabsorbed. Thus, when the bone defect of the distal phalanx is extensive even though the nail and nail floor remain, vascularized toe transplantation or nail transplantation is indicated. Atasoy et al. [37] noted that a hook nail deformity was caused by palmar bending of the nail floor caused by loss of the subungual skin and treated it by transplantation of a cutaneous flap to a skin defect created after elevating the nail floor including the subungual skin.

Surgery

The deformed nail is removed from the nail floor. A transverse incision is made in the finger palm where the nail floor bends palmar. The skin underlying the nail floor is elevated dorsally to straighten it. Two or three thin K-wires are inserted from the fingertip to keep the nail floor straight. The palmar skin defect created after elevating the nail floor is covered by a reverse digital skin island taken from the base of the finger or a cross-finger flap [37]. The curled nail is straightened by placing several small lateral incisions at either end of the bending portion of the nail and fixed on the straightened nail floor. A sculptured nail can be an alternative to the original nail. The straightened or sculptured nail is fixed until the new nail has formed beneath it and replaced it. The K-wires are removed 3 weeks after the surgery (Fig. 21.32).

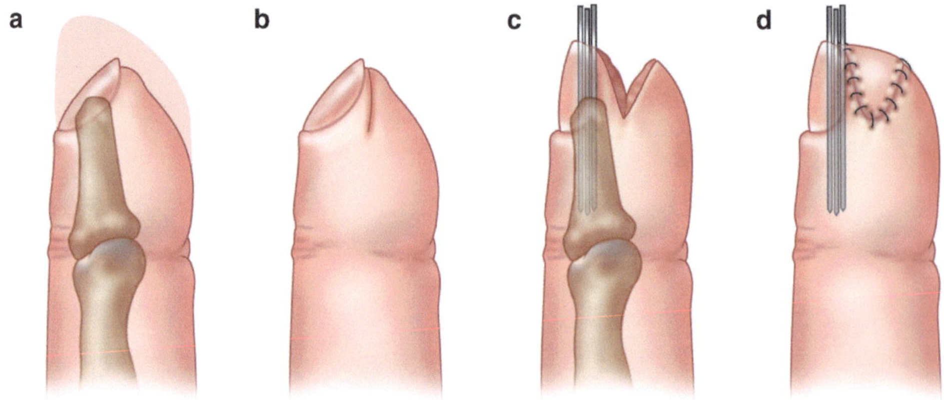

Fig. 21.32 (**a**) Hook nail deformity. (**b**) The deformed nail floor was elevated. (**c**) The nail floor was fixed with several K-wires. (**d**) The skin defect created after elevation of the nail floor was covered by a skin flap

Partial Defect of the Nail Floor

A defect of the nail floor often causes an ugly deformity of the nail. After removal of the nail, scar tissue is removed from the nail floor. A split-thickness nail floor is taken from the second toe using a scalpel, transplanted to the defect of the fingernail floor, and sutured using 5–0 absorbable sutures. The transplanted nail floor is fixed and compressed to the dorsal cortex of the distal phalanx by fixing a sculpture nail or the original nail after correction of the deformity on the repaired nail floor. The original toenail was returned to the toenail floor after harvesting the nail floor [35, 36].

Vascularized Toenail Transfer (Osteo-onychocutaneous Flap)

Vascularized Second Toe Nail Transfer

Indication

Dorsal fingertip loss including the nail and distal phalanx, even though the skin of the finger pulp remains.

Advantage

The reconstructed nail is acceptable cosmetically.

Disadvantage

The nail may be small, when it is used for reconstruction of the radial fingernails.

Surgery

A straight skin incision is made from the dorsum of the MP joint to the DIP joint in the second toe. The skin incision is extended laterally and medially just over the DIP joint to avoid injury to the toenail matrix. The lateral and medial incisions are turned distally along the midlateral line of the toe. Both incisions extend around the toe tip (about 2–3 mm plantar to the lateral and distal nail folds) and merge with each other at the tip of the toe. In the dorsal subcutaneous tissue proximal to the flap, one or two subcutaneous veins should be found and elevated proximally to the MP joint level. In the first web space, the medial plantar neurovascular bundle of the second toe is exposed and elevated distally. Through the bilateral midlateral incisions and the distal incision around the toe tip, the distal phalanx is osteotomized and divided into the dorsal and plantar segments. The dorsal segment of the distal phalanx including that overlying the nail, nail matrix, and a surrounding 2–3-mm-wide region of skin nourished by the MPDA and dorsal subcutaneous veins is separated from the plantar toe segment. The lateral neurovascular bundle is attached to the plantar toe and nourishes it. The subcutaneous veins are transected around the MP joint level, and the medial plantar neurovascular bundle is separated in the first web space. The scar in the dorsal distal phalanx of the finger including the remnant of the nail matrix is removed completely. The dorsal portion of the distal phalanx of the finger is osteotomized to accommodate the dorsal segment of the toe phalanx, securing the attachment of the terminal extensor tendon and flexor digitorum profundus. The toe distal phalanx is then fixed to the distal phalanx of the finger using a small K-wire. The nail with its surrounding skin is sutured to the palmar finger pulp. The MPDA is approximated to a palmar digital artery of the finger. The subcutaneous veins attached to the nail are joined to the dorsal subcutaneous veins of the finger (Fig. 21.33).

Vascularized Big Toenail Transfer

This is a modification of the "wraparound flap" approach [14, 38–40].

Indication

A vertical amputation of the distal and middle phalanges.

Advantages

1. The reconstructed nail is cosmetically excellent.
2. The nail size can be adjusted depending on the finger or thumb to be reconstructed.

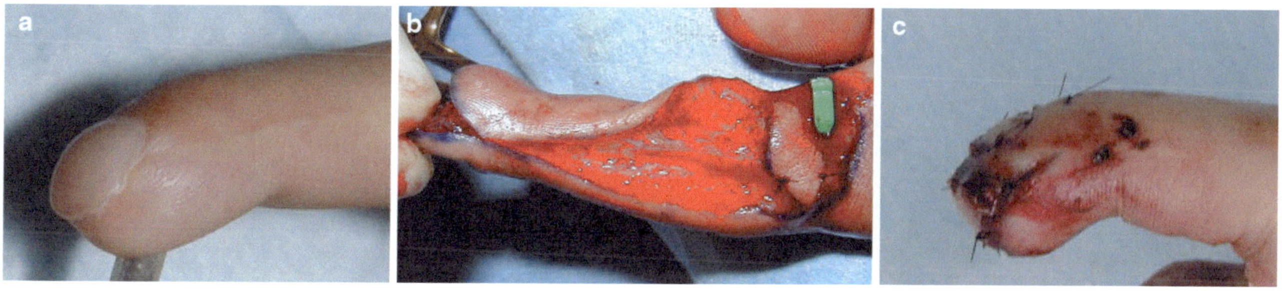

Fig. 21.33 (**a**) Hook nail deformity. (**b**) A reverse digital skin island flap was taken from the base of the finger. (**c**) The skin island flap was transplanted to a skin defect created after elevation of the nail floor

Disadvantages
To close the skin defect after harvesting a flap from the big toe, flaps or shortening of the big toe is necessary.

Surgery
See section "Wraparound Flap," flaps with a short vascular pedicle (often used for nail reconstruction).

Arterialized Venous Nail Graft
Indication
Nail and nail matrix have been lost; however, the distal phalanx and the palmar pulp of the finger have been preserved.

Advantages
1. The cosmetic appearance of the reconstructed nail is acceptable.
2. The operative procedures are easy.

Disadvantages
1. The nail may be too small, when used for reconstruction of the radial fingernails.
2. Unpredictable partial or superficial necrosis can occur. The flap sometimes demonstrates congestion resulting in an atrophic nail.

Surgery
The skin incision is the same as that for a vascularized second toe nail graft. The nail, nail matrix, and the surrounding 2-mm-wide region of skin are elevated, including a thin dorsal cortex of the distal phalanx. Two subcutaneous veins connected to the nail composite are found proximal to the nail in the dorsum of the finger. The nail composite is transferred to a fingernail defect where the dorsal cortex of the distal phalanx is removed. The bone included in the flap is not needed to fix the palmar distal phalanx. The marginal skin of the nail composite is sutured to the palmar pulp of the finger. One of the subcutaneous veins is approximated to a digital palmar artery, and the other is joined to the dorsal subcutaneous vein of the finger. However, the nail composite with arterialized venous flow tends to show congestion. Some part of the composite may turn necrotic, followed by atrophy of the transplanted nail (Fig. 21.34). A vascularized toenail graft is recommended rather than the arterialized venous nail graft for reconstruction of the nail [41].

Treatment of Traumatic Painful Neuromas

Fingertip neuromas are troublesome for the patient. They often generate severe pain or uncomfortable sensations called causalgia. Simple resection of neuromas is not effective for relieving pain, and new neuromas are easily formed at the site of the resection. Treatment of painful cutaneous neuromas is a challenge for surgeons. There have been several procedures reported to treat painful cutaneous neuromas: simple resection and wrapping of the nerve stump in its epineurium, coagulation or freezing of the nerve stumps, use of chemical agents to inhibit axonal regeneration, or the use of silicone to cap the nerve endings. However, none is successful uniformly. Here, three different procedures for treating painful cutaneous neuromas are described.

Resection of a Neuroma and Insertion of the Nerve Stump into a Pedicled Subcutaneous Vein

Lundborg [42] reported that a peripheral nerve stump joined to an end of a silicone tube, with the other end left free, terminated without forming a neuroma, and suggested the possibility of treating neuromas this way. Herbert and Filan [43] treated painful cutaneous neuromas by inserting the proximal nerve stump into the lumen of a pedicled subcutaneous vein instead of a silicone tube and reported good or excellent results in 10 of 13 patients. Kakinoki et al. [44] reported events occurring at the end of the nerve stump inserted into a pedicled vein using a rat femoral nerve model. When the femoral nerve stump remaining after removal of a neuroma

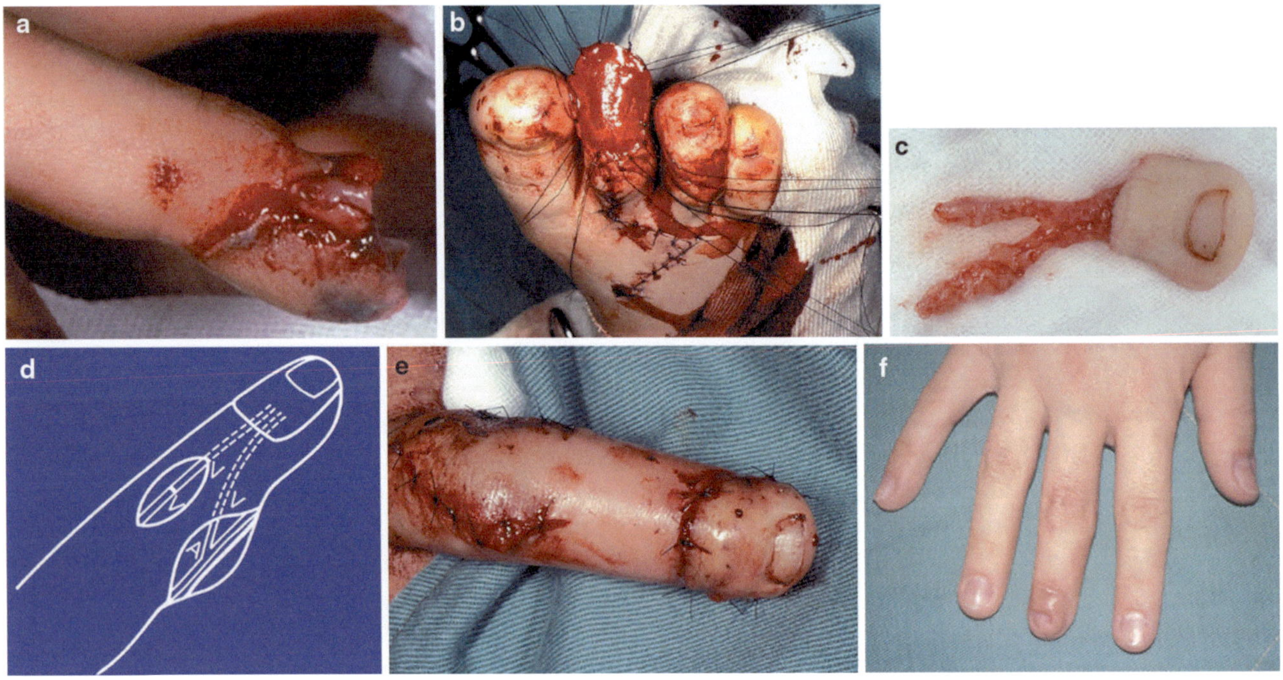

Fig. 21.34 (**a**) Dorsal fingertip injury. (**b**, **c**) A nail including two subcutaneous veins was harvested from the second toe. (**d**) One of the veins was approximated to the palmar digital artery, and the other was joined to a subcutaneous vein of the finger. (**e**) Just after surgery. (**f**) The nail is atrophic 2 years after surgery

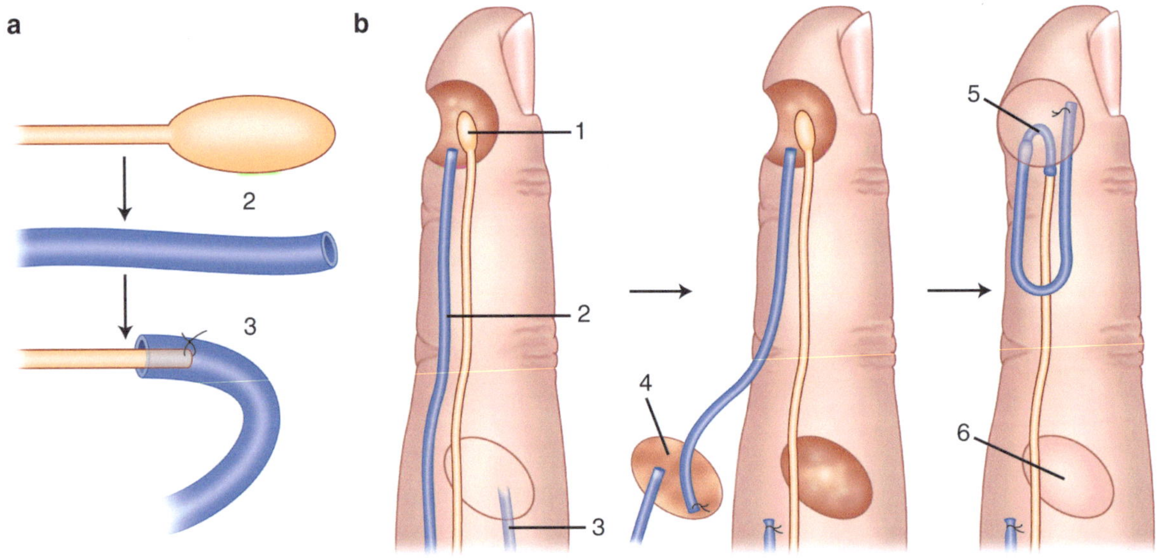

Fig. 21.35 Treatment of painful neuromas at the fingertip. (**a**) Resection of a neuroma and insertion of the nerve stump into a pedicled subcutaneous vein. (**b**) After resection of a neuroma, the nerve stump is sutured to a nerve of a neurovascular island flap

was inserted into the proximal stump of the femoral vein, nerve fibers extended from the stump along the inner surface of the vein wall. However, they started to show retraction 6 weeks after implantation. Finally, the proximal nerve stump did not form a neuroma but a hemispherical nerve ending that was covered by a layer of endothelial cells at 12 weeks after the surgery (Fig. 21.35a).

Resection of a Neuroma and Insertion of the Transected Nerve Stump into a Muscle Belly or the Medullary Cavity of Finger Phalangeal Bones

A nerve stump after removal of a neuroma is exposed proximally and inserted into the muscle belly after transection of the fascia. The nerve stump is sutured to the fascia over the muscle with a small suture to prevent protrusion of the stump [45]. This method is hardly indicated for treatment of neuromas in the fingertip. The stump must be exposed proximally for a long distance to reach the intrinsic muscle. The alternative method is insertion of the transected nerve stump into a medullary cavity of finger phalangeal bones instead of a muscle belly.

After Resection of a Neuroma, the Nerve Stump Is Sutured to a Nerve of a Neurovascular Island Flap

This operation is indicated for a neuroma formed at the fingertip. Most are caused by trauma, and the skin over the neuromas is also injured. Mackinnon et al. [45] reported that injured skin could be a target organ of small diameter nerve fibers and that they would regenerate from the neuroma toward the overlying skin, which can cause allodynia or painful or uncomfortable sensation. In this procedure, the injured skin over a neuroma is replaced by a neurovascular skin island including a subcutaneous nerve that is connected to the transected digital nerve stump after removal of the neuroma. The neurovascular skin islands nourished by a palmar digital artery or a dorsal digital arterial network are usually harvested from the base of the finger or thumb. Nerve fibers regenerated from the digital nerve stump are introduced to the skin island and contribute to sensitizing the flap. The site of the neurorrhaphy is covered by a healthy subcutaneous tissue of the skin island, and nerve fibers with small diameters extending from the transected nerve stump at the site of the neurorrhaphy lose the target tissue for extension. In addition, the subcutaneous adipose tissue of the skin island might cover the neurorrhaphy site and acts as a cushion for the site [46] (Fig. 21.35b).

References

1. Lewis BL. Microscopic studies of fetal and mature nail and surrounding soft tissues. AMA Arch Derm Syphilol. 1954;70:732–47.
2. Brunelli F, Brunelli G. Vascular anatomy of the distal phalanx. The hand and upper limb 7. In: Foucher G, editor. Fingertip and nail bed injuries, vol. 17. Edinburgh: Churchill Livingstone; 1991. p. 1–9.
3. Flint MH. Some observation on the vascular supply of the nail bed and terminal segments of the finger. Br J Plast Surg. 1956;8:186–95.
4. Zook EG, van Beek AL, Russel RC, et al. Anatomy and physiology of the perionychium: a review of the literature and anatomic study. J Hand Surg. 1980;5:528–36.
5. Zaias N, Alvarez J. The formation of the primate nail plate: an autoradiographic study in squirrel monkey. J Invest Dermatol. 1968; 51:120–36.
6. Slattery D, Aland R, Durbridge G, Cowin G. Dorsal digital septum of the distal interphalangeal joint. J Hand Surg. 2009;34A:467–73.
7. Strauch B, Moura W. Arterial system of the fingers. J Hand Surg. 1990;15A:148–54.
8. Ishikawa K, Ogawa Y, Soeda H, Yoshida Y. A new classification of the amputation level for the distal part of the finger. J Jpn Soc Reconstr Microsurg. 1990;3:54–62.
9. Tamai S. Twenty years' experience of limb replantation—review of 293 upper extremity replants. J Hand Surg. 1982;7:549–56.
10. Hattori Y, Doi K, Ikeda K, Abe Y, Dhawan V. Significance of venous anastomosis in fingertip replantation. Plast Reconstr Surg. 2003;111: 1151–8.
11. Hattori Y, Doi K, Sakamoto S, Yamasaki H, Wahegaonkar A, Addosooki A. Fingertip replantation. J Hand Surg. 2007;32A: 548–55.
12. Hattori Y, Doi K, Ejiri S, Baliarsing AS. Replantation of very distal thumb amputations with pre-osteosynthesis interpositional vein graft. J Hand Surg. 2001;26B:105–7.
13. Kamei K, Shinokawa Y, Kishibe M. The venocutaneous fistula: a new technique for reducing venous congestion in replanted fingertips. Plast Reconstr Surg. 1997;99:1771–4.
14. Koshima I, Moriguchi T, Soeda S, et al. Free thin osteo-onycocutaneous flaps from the big toe for reconstruction of the distal phalanx of the fingers. Br J Plast Surg. 1992;45:1–5.
15. Han SK, Lee BI, Kim WK. Topical and systemic anticoagulation in the treatment of absent or compromised venous outflow in replanted fingertips. J Hand Surg. 2000;25A:659–67.
16. Gordon L, Leitner DW, Buncke HJ, Alpert BS. Partial nail removal after digital replantation as an alternative method of venous drainage. J Hand Surg. 1985;10A:360–4.
17. Hirase Y. Salvage of fingertip amputated at nail level: new surgical principles and treatments. Ann Plast Surg. 1997;38:151–7.
18. Koshima I, Yamashita S, Sugiyama N, Ushino S, Tsutsui T, Nanba Y. Successful delayed venous drainage in 16 consecutive distal phalangeal replantation. Plast Reconstr Surg. 2005;115:149–54.
19. Gatewood MD. Plastic repair of finger defects without hospitalization. J Am Med Assoc. 1926;87:1479.
20. Crikelair GF, Crowley RT, Miller H. Management of severe trauma to distal digital extremities. Am J Surg. 1953;85:322–6.
21. Bralliar F, Horner RL. Sensory cross-finger pedicle graft. J Bone Joint Surg. 1969;51A:1264–8.
22. Kutler W. A method for repair of finger amputation. Ohio State Med J. 1944;40:126.
23. Segmüller G. Modifikation des Kutler-Lappens: neuro-vaskuläse stielung. Handchirurgie. 1976;8:75–6.
24. Del Ben M, et al. Reverse dorsal digital island flap. Plast Reconstr Surg. 1994;93:552–7.
25. Maruyama Y. The reverse dorsal metacarpal flap. Br J Plast Surg. 1990;43:24–7.
26. Quaba AA, Davison PM. The distally-based dorsal hand flap. Br J Plast Surg. 1990;43:28–39.
27. Holevich J. A new method of restoring sensibility to the thumb. J Bone Joint Surg. 1963;45B:596–602.
28. Morrison WA, O'Brien BM, MacLeod AM. Thumb reconstruction with a free neurovascular wrap-around flap from the big toe. J Hand Surg. 1980;5A:575–83.
29. Doi K, Kuwata N, Kanai S. Reconstruction of the thumb with a free wrap-around flap from the big toe and an iliac crest graft. J Bone Joint Surg. 1985;67A:439–45.
30. May JW, Chait LA, Cohen BE, O'Brien BM. Free neurovascular flap from the first web of the foot in hand reconstruction. J Hand Surg. 1977;2A:387–93.
31. Morrison WA, O'Brien BM, Macleod AM, Gilbert A. Neurovascular free flaps from the foot for innervation of the hand. J Hand Surg. 1978;3A:235–42.
32. Bunkey Jr HJ, Rose EH. Free toe-to-finger tip neurovascular flaps. Plast Reconstr Surg. 1979;63:607–12.

33. Foucher G, Merle M, Maneaud M, Michon J. Microsurgical free partial toe transfer in hand reconstruction: a report of 12 cases. Plast Reconstr Surg. 1980;65:616–27.
34. Kakinoki R, Ikeguchi R, Atiyya AN, et al. Treatment of posttraumatic painful neuromas at the digit tip using neurovascular island flaps. J Hand Surg. 2008;33A:348–52.
35. Shepard GH. Treatment of nail bed avulsions with split-thickness nail bed grafts. J Hand Surg. 1983;8:49–54.
36. Shepard GH. Management of acute nail bed avulsions. Hand Clin. 1990;6:39–56.
37. Atasoy E, Godfrey A, Kalisman M. The "antenna" procedure for the "hook-nail" deformity. J Hand Surg. 1983;8:55–8.
38. Koshima I, Soed S, Takase T, et al. Free vascularized nail grafts. J Hand Surg. 1988;13A:29–32.
39. Koshima I, Moriguchi T, Soeda S, et al. Free second toe transfer for reconstruction of the distal phalanx of the fingers. Br J Plast Surg. 1991;44:456–8.
40. Koshima I, Moriguchi T, Umeda N, et al. Trimmed second toe tip transfer for reconstruction of claw nail deformity of the fingers. Br J Plast Surg. 1992;45:591–4.
41. Nakayama Y, Iino T, Uchid A, et al. Vascularized free nail raft nourished by arterialized inflow from the venous system. Plast Reconstr Surg. 1990;85:239–45.
42. Lundborg G. Tubular repair of nerves. In: Staffar P, Amadio PC, Foucher G, editors. Current practice in hand surgery. London: Martin Dunitz; 1997. p. 161–9.
43. Herbert TJ, Filan SL. Vein implantation for treatment of painful cutaneous neuromas. J Hand Surg. 1997;23B:220–4.
44. Kakinoki R, Ikeguchi R, Matsumoto T, et al. Treatment of painful peripheral neuromas by vein implantation. Int Orthop. 2003;27:60–4.
45. Mackinnon SE, Dellon AL, Hudson AR, Hunter DA. Alteration of neuroma formation by manipulation of its microenvironment. Plast Reconstr Surg. 1985;76:345–53.
46. Kakinoki R, Ikeguchi R, Nankaku M, Nakamura T. Factor affecting the success of arterialized venous flaps in the hand. Injury. 2008;39 Suppl 4:18–24.

Additional References

Bang H, Kojima T, Hayashi H. Palmar advancement flap with V-Y closure for thumb tip injuries. J Hand Surg. 1992;17A:933–4.

Brunelli F, Vigasio A, Valenti P, Brunelli GR. Arterial anatomy and clinical application of the dorsoulnar flap of the thumb. J Hand Surg. 1999;24A:803–11.

Foucher G, Braun JB. A new island flap transfer from the dorsum of the index to the thumb. Plast Reconstr Surg. 1979;63:344–9.

Foucher G, Merle M, Maneaud M. Microsurgical vascularized compound toe transfer for traumatic dorsal loss of the thumb. Plast Reconstr Surg. 1991;87:310–4.

Han SK, Chung HS, Kim WK. The timing of neovascularization in fingertip replantation by external bleeding. Plast Reconstr Surg. 2002;110:1042–6.

Koshima I, Soeda S, Moriguchi T, Higaki H, Miyakawa S, Yamasaki M. The use of arteriovenous anastomosis for replantation of the distal phalanx of the fingers. Plast Reconstr Surg. 1992;89: 710–4.

Leung PC. Thumb reconstruction using second-toe transfer. Hand Clin. 1985;1:285–95.

Lister GD, Kalisman M, Tsai TM. Reconstruction of the hand with free microvascular toe-to-hand transfer: experience with 54 toe transfers. Plast Reconstr Surg. 1983;71:372–86.

Russell RC, Casas LA. Management of finger tip injuries. Clin Plast Surg. 1989;6:405–25.

Tranquilli-Leali E. Riconstruzione dell'apice falangi; ungueall mediante autoplastica volare peduncolata per scorrimento. Infort Traumatol Lav. 1935;1:186–93.

Yamano Y. Replantation of the amputated distal part of the fingers. J Hand Surg. 1985;10A:211–8.

Yang D, Morris SF. Vascular basis of dorsal digital and metacarpal skin flaps. J Hand Surg. 2001;26:142–6.

Yoshimura M. Toe-to-hand transfer. Plast Reconstr Surg. 1980;66: 74–84.

Reoperative Options in Failed Proximal Interphalangeal and Metacarpophalangeal Joint Arthrodesis and Replacement

22

Marco Rizzo

Abstract

Revising previous arthroplasties done in either the metacarpophalangeal joint or the proximal interphalangeal joint can be technically very difficult. Frequently, the bone stock has been either resorbed or eroded, making potential reimplantation of new joint replacements quite challenging. Furthermore, the soft-tissue envelope is usually severely scarred, and there can be issues with tendon imbalance as well as ligamentous laxity. This combination of bone and soft-tissue factors sometimes precludes the ability to perform revision implant surgery. In these circumstances, arthrodesis can be of benefit; however, care needs to be taken to try and not unduly shorten the digit, which could lead to tendon imbalance. Ultimately, in some cases where there is such significant structural loss of the finger or where the finger has no functional usage, amputation can be considered. Ultimately, the patient needs to understand that the revision surgery is unlikely to yield improved motion but is done in order to try and help preserve hand function while reducing any pain or other symptoms that the patient may be having.

Keywords

Revision • Metacarpophalangeal • Proximal • Interphalangeal • Joint • Arthroplasty

Metacarpophalangeal Joint

Key Points

- Treatment options for failed MP joint arthroplasty mainly include revision arthroplasty and arthrodesis.
- Bone stock will be a major factor in determining the feasibility of revision arthroplasty.
- Soft-tissue stability plays a major role in determining the choice of implant for revision arthroplasty.
- Limit the amount of bone resection when performing the revision cuts in preparing the revision implants.
- Upsizing of the implant is usually necessary for successful revision.
- Impaction bone grafting can be utilized in cases of significant osteolysis and limited intramedullary bone stock.
- Tagging and securing the collateral ligaments will help with stability of the revision arthroplasty.

(continued)

M. Rizzo, MD (✉)
Department of Orthopedic Surgery, Mayo Clinic College of Medicine, 200 1st Street SW, Rochester, MN, 55905, USA
e-mail: Rizzo.marco@mayo.edu

S.F.M. Duncan (ed.), *Reoperative Hand Surgery*,
DOI 10.1007/978-1-4614-2373-7_22,

- Rehabilitation following surgery will be determined by the stability of the joint at the time of surgery.
- Arthrodesis is reserved for cases of inadequate bone stock for arthroplasty and soft-tissue incompetence.
- Success of fusion can be enhanced with bone graft and rigid fixation.
- Stabilization of the collateral ligaments may be afforded with ligament reinforcement, reconstruction, or suture stabilization.
- Sagittal band insufficiency and ulnar drift may be corrected with radial placation of the extensor mechanism, ulnar intrinsic release, and/or sagittal band reconstruction.

Introduction

Metacarpophalangeal (MP) joint arthroplasty has been utilized in the treatment of arthritis for nearly 50 years. Early designs were hinged and made of silicone. These implants continue to be utilized and are indicated for patients with soft-tissue incompetence and joint subluxation or dislocation, as commonly seen in patients with rheumatoid arthritis. Newer-generation MP joint replacements utilize metal and plastic or pyrolytic carbon materials. These designs are unconstrained and have the advantage of less strain on the implant. However, they require that the joint has more inherent stability afforded from the soft tissues. The wear characteristics of the new designs are favorable compared to silicone, and they avoid the risk of silicone particulate-related synovitis and osteolysis.

Silicone is the preferred implant for patients with significant deformities of the joints and/or soft-tissue incompetence, as is seen in rheumatoid arthritis (RA). Failure of these joint replacements is typically secondary to wear and cyclic loading. Silicone has been known to fracture over time and result in recurrent deformity and accelerated rates of silicone synovitis [1, 2]. While more recent evaluation of the clinical ramifications of silicone implant failure suggests worse clinical outcome, the literature remains conflicted on this issue [3, 4].

The pyrocarbon and metal/plastic designs offer an excellent option in patients with osteoarthritis or early nondeforming RA [5]. Wear characteristics are favorable when compared to silicone implants (although fracture has been known to occur) [6]. Comparable long-term survivorship data to the silicone prostheses will become available over time.

Indications and Contraindications

The indications for revision arthroplasty of the MP joint are dependent primarily on the cause of primary joint failure, the amount of residual bone stock, and the competence of the associated soft tissues. Failures secondary to infection pose significant challenges and necessitate eradication of the infectious process prior to proceeding with any surgical reconstruction. This typically requires long-term intravenous antibiotics and a period of time with placement of an interposing antibiotic impregnated polymethylmethacrylate spacer. Upon successful treatment of the infection, reconstruction options can be weighed. Unfortunately, the infectious process associated with repetitive surgeries challenges the success of revision arthroplasty, and many of these patients are best treated with arthrodesis.

Lack of bone stock and the quality of remaining bone will be a significant determinant of the surgical options following failed primary MP arthroplasty. The ligament competence and soft-tissue integrity will also be an important determining factor. Patients who have undergone primary joint replacement with the use of cement will generally have limited residual bone due to increased bone loss during cement removal. However, cement can be utilized as an adjunct in revision surgery, with the understanding that future surgery will carry the same challenges, if necessary. My preference is to upsize the implants whenever possible and avoid the use of cement altogether.

Soft-tissue augmentation and reconstruction is sometimes feasible to enhance joint support. In cases of instability of the primary implant with good osseous integration, I prefer to keep the original implant and supplement the soft tissues with augmentation or reconstruction. The revision to hinged implants (in previously unconstrained joints) will afford more inherent stability to the joint and may be a viable option in the treatment of failures due to soft-tissue incompetence.

Silicone synovitis and osteolysis may lead to pain, loss of bone stock, and even fracture of the metacarpal or phalanges. I find that these patients can be treated with two options following the removal of the inflamed synovitis: bone grafting of the osteolytic bone with or without revision implant arthroplasty.

Revision Arthroplasty

Technique (Fig. 22.1)

A dorsal approach to the joint is utilized, typically through the previous incision. Extension of the incision and dissection is necessary to provide appropriate exposure and reveal the joint appropriately. I prefer to incise along the radial border of the common extensor tendon. This will allow for plication of this layer to help correct recurrent ulnar drift of the digits when closing the wound. If possible, approaching the joint through layers is advised. Deep to the tendon and sagittal band layer lies the capsule. It can be divided in the midline, and the joint will then be exposed. The collateral ligaments can be removed from their metacarpal origins and tagged with a 3-0 FiberWire suture for reattachment following revision arthroplasty. Drill holes can be made with a 0.45 or 0.54 K-wire at their insertion site following implant removal, and the sutures can be pulled through the drill holes prior to placement of the revision implant. Removal of the implants can then be performed. This can be best performed with the joint in flexion. Silicone implants will generally be pulled out. In addition, the pyrocarbon prostheses can be removed with relative ease as they tend to have less osseous ingrowth when compared to the metal designs. The titanium implants are usually the most difficult to remove. If the implant is well positioned and well seated, I prefer to leave it whenever possible and address other causes for failure. In cases where cement removal is necessary, I prefer to use curved osteotomes between the bone-cement intervals to extract the cement. This can be very challenging as it commonly results in some bone loss. Following implant removal, the metacarpal and proximal phalanx are cleared of any additional debris and osteolysis in preparation for revision. Impaction grafting can be a suitable supplement for limited bone stock, and I prefer to utilize distal radius bone graft with or without demineralized bone matrix. Upsizing of the implants will also help afford added stability and fill larger cavities. My preference is to avoid the use of cement.

Implant selection is based on the amount of remaining bone stock, deformity of the joint, and the competence of the surrounding soft tissues. Practically speaking, a nonconstrained design is frequently not possible. It is important to have plans A, B, C, etc. based on the intraoperative findings. I think the silicone replacements are usually the most feasible in revision situations. This is consistent with previously published reports [6]. Upon choosing the optimal implant, recutting the bone ends can be performed. Whenever necessary, bone grafting can be placed at this time. I prefer to utilize distal radius bone cancellous bone graft mixed (on occasion) with demineralized bone graft. This allows for an impaction grafting effect when broaching. Rebroaching is then performed, followed by placement of the trial implant. It is important to assess stability at this time through the range of motion of the MP joint. The intrinsics can be released if tight and affecting the reduction and stability of the joint. Fluoroscopy can be helpful in confirming the alignment and position of the joint. The medullary canals are prepared and cleared of all loose debris or bone graft, and the real implant is then placed.

Following revision joint insertion, the collateral ligament reattachment can be completed by securing the 3-0 FiberWire to the bone while holding the joint reduced. The capsule is closed with an absorbable interrupted suture (3-0 Vicryl). The tendon can then be secured with a 2-0 Dexon or 3-0 FiberWire suture and plicated if necessary. Plication can be performed by utilizing a pants-over-vest technique of interrupted sutures. The tourniquet is then deflated, and all bleeding is controlled with bipolar cautery and pressure hemostasis. The skin can be closed over a Silastic drain with an interrupted 4-0 Prolene or nylon suture. I then apply a bulky dressing and splint, holding the MP joints at zero degrees and extending to the interphalangeal (IP) joints.

Optimizing Outcomes

- The presence of competent collateral ligaments will significantly help in ensuring the success of revision arthroplasty.
- Take time to be meticulous when removing cement to minimize bone loss.
- Be prepared for a fallback plan depending on the intraoperative findings.
- Minimize bone cuts at the time of revision.
- Upsizing the implant will help with fitting the components in the canals of the metacarpal and phalanx.

Complications and Side Effects

Complications following revision arthroplasty of the MP joint may include instability, implant loosening, limited range of motion, recurrent deformity, pain, and neurovascular compromise. Instability and recurrent deformity are the most common concerns in my opinion. This is most commonly associated with "pushing" the envelope in attempting arthroplasty with insufficient bone stock and/or surrounding soft-tissue stabilizers. Instability may be preventable with prolonged immobilization following surgery. In addition, protected rehabilitation in patients where instability is a concern may be helpful. Appropriately fashioned splints with attachments such as derotational slings are also helpful. When instability occurs, repeat surgery is likely necessary. In cases of nonconstrained revision, I would consider graduation to either a constrained implant or a fusion of the MP joint. In cases of instability with a constrained revision, I would recommend graduation to an arthrodesis.

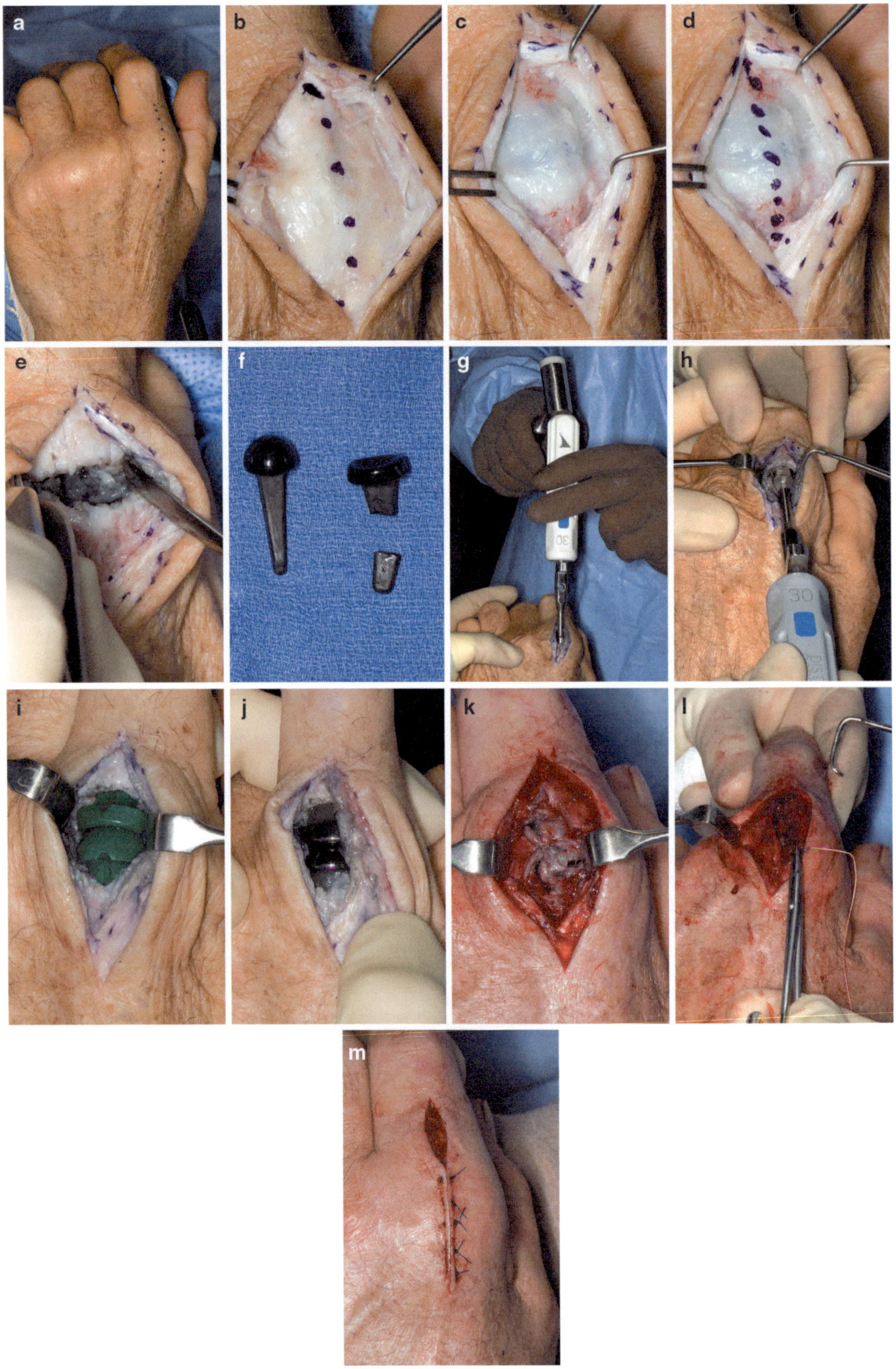

Fig. 22.1 Illustrative case of a 66-year-old male patient with osteoarthritis who underwent revision MP arthroplasty. (**a**, **b**) A dorsal approach to the MP joint. (**c**, **d**) The extensor tendon is sharply released from the midline (frequently from the radial side in patients with RA). (**e**) The capsule is revealed and can be divided longitudinally. In this specific case, metallosis is noted secondary to the fractured distal component. (**f**) The implants are removed. When necessary (usually in patients with RA), drill holes in the metacarpal can be used to allow for reattachment of the ligaments following revision. (**g**, **h**) The canals are prepared and rebroached. (**i**) The revision implant is trialed, and the joint is run through range of motion and stability assessed. (**j**) The final implant is inserted. (**k**, **l**) The capsule is closed, and the extensor tendon layer is reattached and plicated to centralize the tendons. (**m**) The skin is closed

Postoperative Care

Postoperative care following surgery includes removal of the Silastic (when utilized) implant on day 1. When concerned, the incision can be inspected at that time. I typically will immobilize the MP joints in extension while allowing IP joint motion for approximately 2 weeks. I prefer to err on the side of stiffing the joint in revision cases. In patients who take disease-modifying anti-inflammatory drugs, it is preferable to wait at least 2 weeks prior to removing the sutures. Further immobilization of the MP joint following suture removal is often warranted, especially in patients with RA and/or cases where joint stability is a concern. Following immobilization, structured therapy can be initiated. In patients with RA, dynamic daytime splinting, holding the MP joints extended and allowing active flexion, can be utilized in conjunction with static nighttime splinting. Four to six weeks following the initiation of therapy, strengthening can be initiated. It is important to individualize the postoperative regimen based on the intraoperative findings and the patient's medical condition.

Arthrodesis

Technique (Fig. 22.2)

A dorsal approach that incorporates the previous incision is utilized. The dissection is carried out in a similar fashion as revision arthroplasty. I want to stress that arthrodesis may not be the primary option hoped for at the time of revision and the decision to proceed with this option may occur at the time of surgery. Thus, it is important to methodically expose, even though the soft tissues will become less important in cases of fusion. The joint is removed, and the bone ends are prepared for arthrodesis. My preference is to fuse the MP joint in a position of 40° of flexion, but it is important to discuss arthrodesis in detail with the patients so that they understand what to expect and any special needs or circumstances are reviewed and addressed. Cancellous bone graft from the distal radius or iliac crest is helpful in facilitating successful fusion. It can be packed into the intramedullary canals of the metacarpal and phalanx. In cases of significant

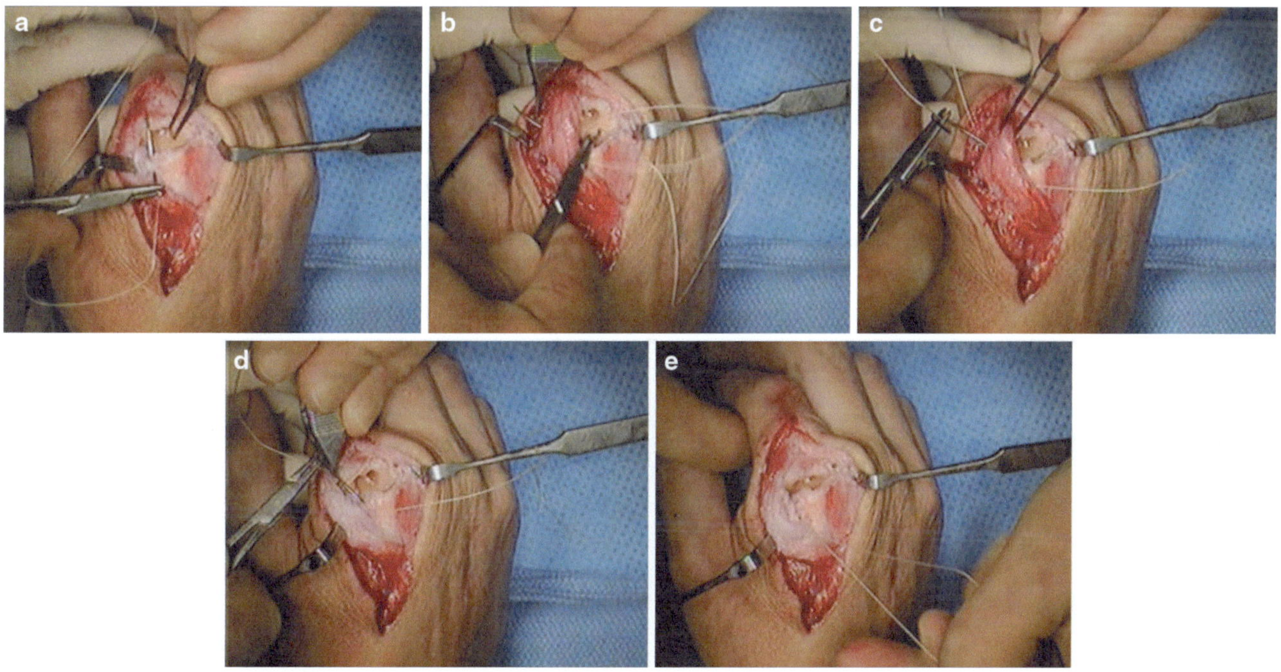

Fig. 22.2 Video technique of collateral ligament-stabilizing suture for MP revision. An O-Vicryl or Dexon suture with a large-diameter needle is used to capture the collateral ligament at its insertion in the base of the proximal phalanx. The ability to pull the proximal phalanx up with the suture confirms that the suture will effectively reinforce the ligament and stabilize the MP joint

bone loss, structural bone graft (preferably from the iliac crest) can be harvested and fashioned to prevent excessive shortening of the digit.

My preference for securing the arthrodesis is K-wires and tension band. I like to utilize two 0.45 K-wires in parallel from the dorsal cortex of the metacarpal into the medullary canal of the phalanx. A 25-gauge wire folded on itself is utilized as a tension band. It is passed through an ulnar-to-radial drill hole (created with a 0.54 K-wire) in the midportion of the proximal phalanx. The wire is fashioned into a figure-of-8 form and pulled beneath the K-wires at the metacarpal. Tensioning is performed through tightening of the tension band. Care should be taken not to overtighten, especially in patients with poor bone quality. Upon completion of the tensioning, the K-wires are gently pulled out, bent back on themselves to create a crook, and cut. It is then rotated so that the crook secures the tension band and the wire is pushed back into place. Fluoroscopy is helpful in all phases of the procedure to confirm appropriate position of fusion, hardware placement, appropriate compression, and overall final alignment.

Following hardware placement, the wound is closed in layers. The capsule can be closed with interrupted 3-0 Vicryl sutures. The extensor tendon layer is closed with interrupted 2-0 Dexon or 3-0 FiberWire. The tourniquet is then deflated, and bleeding is controlled with pressure hemostasis and bipolar cautery. The wound can be closed over a Silastic drain with 4-0 Prolene or nylon sutures. A bulky dressing and splint is then applied, holding the MP immobilized to protect the fusion.

Optimizing Outcomes

- It is important to appropriately prepare the medullary canals and bone ends including removal of all inflammatory tissues and debris.
- The liberal use of bone grafting is helpful in facilitating successful fusion.
- Creation of a strong hardware construct will help ensure stability during the healing process.
- Understanding the patients' needs and catering the position of fusion to help meet them will help ensure that preoperative expectations will be met.
- Refrain from hardware removal until complete healing has occurred.
- Fusion of multiple digits will pose challenges due to the loss of abduction and adduction of the fingers. In these cases, it is important to allow enough room in the web spaces for appropriate hygiene.

Complications and Side Effects

Nonunion and delayed union are common concerns and complications following attempted arthrodesis. In addition, prominent hardware can occur in thin patients or patients with less subcutaneous tissue. Additional complications include limited finger range of motion, malpositioning of the digit, loss of function, and neurovascular injury. Successful fusion can be ensured with appropriate technique and the use of bone grafting. It is important that patients who use tobacco be urged to cease their habit prior to surgery. The use of bone stimulators can be a helpful adjunct. My preference is the ultrasound stimulators. They typically require approximately 30 min daily, and the device is very portable, helping with patient compliance.

Postoperative Care

The immediate postoperative regimen following fusion requires immobilization of the MP joint. The decision of when to allow IP joint motion will depend on the stability and fixation of the MP arthrodesis site. In cases where the fixation is good, I will allow some degree of IP motion within the first few days following surgery. If not, I will choose to immobilize the IP joints for approximately 2 weeks (until suture removal). Overall, the MP fusion site is protected for approximately 6 weeks. Radiographs will help confirm healing. At 6–8 weeks following surgery, the patient will likely progress toward strengthening and light use of the hand.

Miscellaneous Issues

The Unstable MP Joint with Well-Fixed Prosthesis

If the joint is unstable, angulated, or frankly dislocated and the arthroplasty is well fixed, the surgeon may direct his/her attention on the soft-tissue stabilizers. Achieving stability in these cases can be difficult and challenging. If the collateral ligaments are incompetent, reconstruction may be an option with either auto- or allograft tendon. An alternative option includes materials such as AlloDerm to reinforce the ligaments. Securing the tendon can be difficult because placing drill holes in the bone (for suture anchors) is frequently impossible with a well-fixed implant in the medullary canal. A deep collateral ligament-stabilizing suture technique has been described to help provide stability (Fig. 22.3). It typically involves the use of an O-Vicryl or Dexon suture with a large-diameter needle. The suture

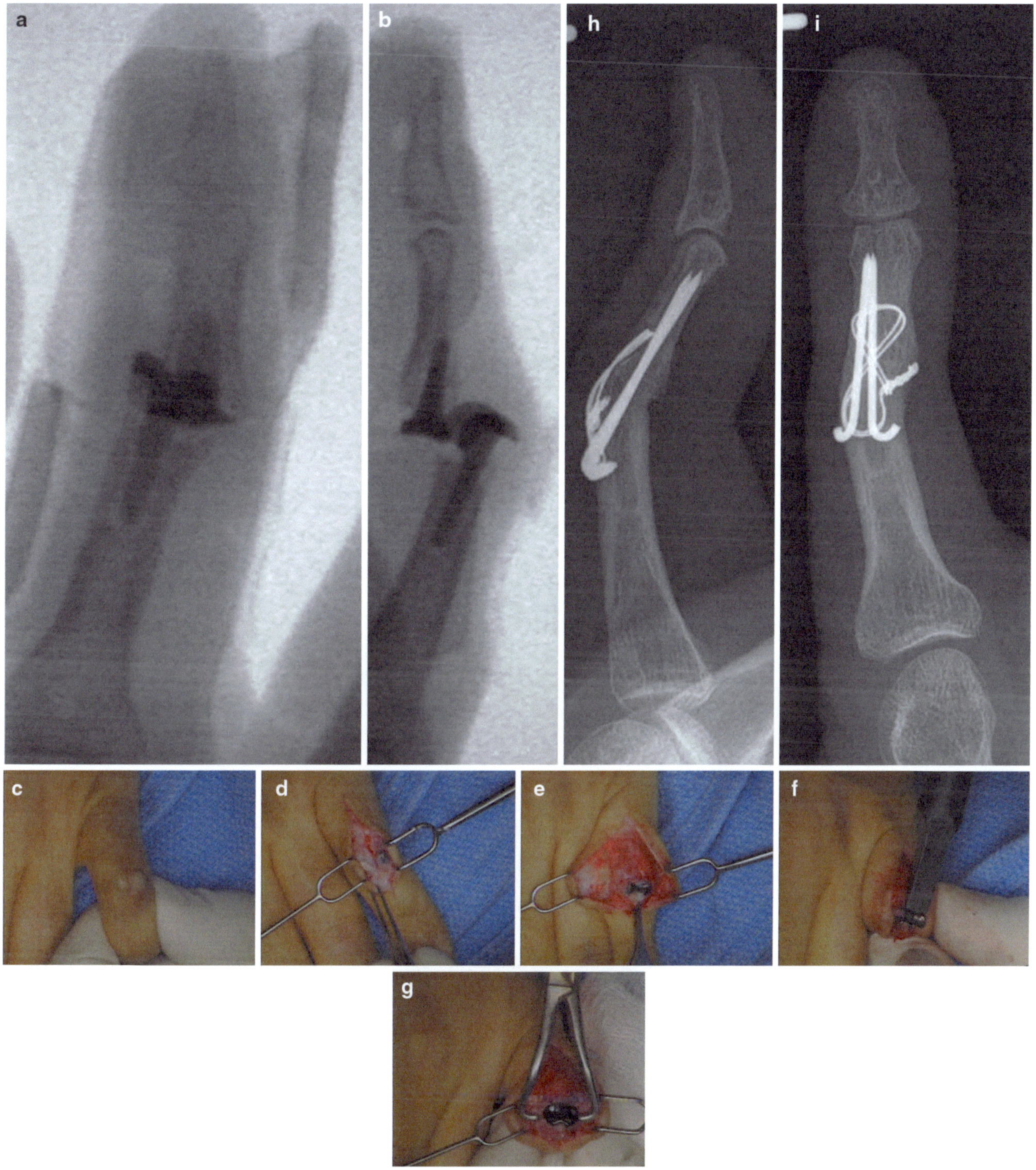

Fig. 22.3 PIP arthrodesis. (**a**, **b**) Images show AP and lateral X-rays of a patient with chronic dislocation following PIP arthroplasty. (**c**) The previous incision is utilized. (**d**, **e**) The extensor tendon may be split to reveal the joint. In the case shown, the extensor tendon was incompetent, and the joint was revealed following incision. (**f**, **g**) The joint is removed, and the bone ends are prepared for arthrodesis. Bone graft from the distal radius can be packed into the medullary canals of the proximal and middle phalanges. (**h**, **i**) X-rays at 1 year postsurgery show successful fusion with K-wires and tension band construct

passes through the collateral ligament at the insertion of the ligament in the proximal phalanx. It can then be secured and anchored to the dorsal soft-tissues. A pull on the suture that affects a dorsal pull on the proximal phalanx confirms that the suture will achieve its desired effect. This suture can also be utilized in revision arthroplasty cases to afford additional stability.

Sagittal Band Insufficiency and Recurrent Ulnar Drift of the Fingers

Patients with rheumatoid arthritis may develop recurrent ulnar drift of the digits. Typically (but not always), this occurs in association with implant failure. Stabilizing and reinforcing the sagittal band can be a challenge in some of these patients. Approaching the joint from the radial aspect of the tendon can be helpful in centralizing the tendon via placation at the time of closure. Release of tight ulnar intrinsics can also help centralize the extensor tendons and prevent tendency toward ulnar drifting. If the sagittal band remains incompetent and the fingers continue to drift ulnarward, the radial one-third of the extensor tendon may be released from the remaining tendon distal to the sagittal band while leaving it attached proximally. The segment of tendon may then be passed beneath the radial intermetacarpal ligament and reattached to the remaining extensor tendon through a Pulvertaft weave-type of repair. This will allow for anchoring of the tendon. Unfortunately, it does require a period of MP joint immobilization for approximately 1 month.

Conclusion

Revision surgery following failed MP arthroplasty can be challenging. The primary treatment options include revision arthroplasty and arthrodesis. Many factors will help determine the best option for each patient. The amount of residual bone stock and competency of the stabilizing soft tissues are primary factors. I think it is important for the surgeon to have a variety of plans prior to surgery and proceed appropriately depending on the intraoperative findings. Postoperative regimen will be largely determined by the intraoperative stability of the MP joint. Arthrodesis is a fallback option in cases where arthroplasty is not feasible. Collateral ligament reconstruction and reinforcement and ligament-stabilizing sutures are reasonable options for instability in patients with well-fixed implants. Intrinsic release, extensor tendon plication, and sagittal band reconstruction are surgical options and techniques useful for patients with sagittal band incompetence and ulnar drift.

Proximal Interphalangeal Joint Arthroplasty

Key Points

- The amount of residual bone stock is an important factor in considering the optimal surgical treatment option.
- Soft-tissue stability plays a major role in determining the choice of implant for revision arthroplasty.
- Limit the amount of bone resection when performing the revision cuts in preparing the revision implants.
- Impaction bone grafting can be utilized in cases of significant osteolysis and limited intramedullary bone stock.
- Tagging and securing the collateral ligaments will help with stability of the revision arthroplasty.
- Rehabilitation following surgery will be determined by the stability of the joint at the time of surgery.
- Arthrodesis is reserved for cases of inadequate bone stock for arthroplasty and soft-tissue incompetence.
- Success of fusion can be enhanced with bone graft and rigid fixation.
- Well-fixed implants with instability can be treated by reinforcement of the collateral ligaments.
- Fixed swan-neck deformities can be managed with a V-Y lengthening of the extensor tendons and flexor digitorum superficialis hemitenodesis and preservation of the implants.

Introduction

Like MP joint arthroplasty, arthroplasty of the proximal interphalangeal (PIP) joint has been utilized for many years in the management of arthritis. Silicone was introduced over 40 years ago for the damaged PIP joint [7]. These hinged implants continue to be utilized in patients with significant soft-tissue laxity and significant deformity. Metal and plastic designs, as well as pyrocarbon implants, have also been introduced and utilized [8, 9]. These implants are unhinged and are more dependent on the bone stock and soft tissues for helping afford stability.

The limitations and shortcomings of the silicone implants are similar to those of the MP joints. Failure secondary to fracture and recurrent deformity are established complications with these implants [10]. The metal/plastic and pyrocarbon designs are made of more durable material that is less likely to fracture or subside. Earlier designs were cemented, although many surgeons currently avoid the use of cement secondary to difficulties with extraction at revision surgery in cases of prior methyl methacrylate use. However, more recent reports suggest that the use of cement minimizes failure secondary to loosening [11]. Outcomes with pyrocarbon have demonstrated excellent pain relief and improved grip strength. However, range of motion was not significantly improved, and the reoperation rates have been nearly 30% at an average 4-year follow-up [9]. Longer-term data will help better define the roles of these newer implants.

Indications and Contraindications

Like MP joint reoperations following failed arthroplasty, the indications for revision arthroplasty in the PIP joint rely heavily on the reason for primary failure, amount and quality of residual bone stock, and the competence of the associated soft-tissues. In addition, failures due to infection pose the added burden of thorough eradication of the infection prior to implant placement and are generally considered a relative contraindication to revision arthroplasty. In my opinion, this is more poignant in the PIP joint when compared to MP infections, as the amount of residual bone stock is less to start with. Extraction of the implant followed by placement of an antibiotic polymethylmethacrylate spacer for usually 6 weeks is usually required prior to attempting revision surgery. Oftentimes, the best option in these patients is to undergo arthrodesis.

The quality and quantity of residual bone stock will help determine the feasibility of revision PIP arthroplasty. Like MP reoperations, the use of cement is controversial. Patients who have undergone prior implant with the use of cement will have challenges related to cement removal and additional loss of bone stock. However, cement can be utilized to help implant fixation, with the understanding that subsequent surgery will be complicated by cement removal.

In cases of joint instability, upsizing the prosthesis or conversion to hinged implants may help afford stability. Due to the challenges associated with bone stock, well-fixed implants with deformities and instability are best managed by avoiding removal of the prosthesis. Soft-tissue augmentation, releases, and reconstruction can be utilized in these cases.

Patients with silicone synovitis and/or osteolysis can be treated with excision of the offending implant, synovectomy, and bone grafting. Depending on the joint stability and residual bone stock, revision arthroplasty or arthrodesis can be performed.

Revision Arthroplasty

Technique

I prefer to utilize the same approach that was utilized for the primary surgery unless there were unique concerns that require a dorsal approach. For example, an incompetent extensor mechanism or dorsal dislocation of the joint will likely benefit from a dorsal approach regardless of which technique was previously utilized. While not reported on for revision cases, the lateral approach affords the preservation of the extensor mechanism. The joint can be exposed with either a Chamay [12] or extensor tendon-splitting approach. Every attempt should be made to preserve the collateral ligaments. If the joint is stable and the implant can be removed without having to take them down, I prefer to leave them attached to their origin. Otherwise, they can be sharply removed from the proximal phalanx and tagged. Following implant removal, drill holes with 0.45 or 0.35 K-wires can be created at the insertional footprint, and the ligament can be reattached following reimplantation. I prefer to use a 3-0 FiberWire or Surgilon suture. The sutures can be passed prior to final implant placement, and the ligament can be tightened down following definitive joint placement. When necessary, tensioning of the ligament can be done through this method as well. Appropriate tensioning can be gauged at the time of trialing of the prosthesis.

Implant removal can be challenging. My experience with the pyrocarbon and silicone implants is that they are generally readily removable, whereas previously cemented or titanium implants are more difficult. Like the MP joint cases, whenever possible, I try and leave a well-fixed implant and address the specific cause of the failure. Cylindrical curved and straight osteotomes are helpful in extracting cement from the cement-bone interface. Meticulous technique will help minimize the amount of bone loss, which is critical in determining options following extraction. Following implant and cement removal, the medullary canals are cleared of additional debris and prepared for broaching, trailing, and reimplantation. Complete removal of residual metallosis and silicone-related osteolysis and synovitis should be performed prior to broaching. Minimal cuts of the middle and proximal phalangeal bone ends are usually done (if at all). I usually cut only if the bone ends are not parallel and contribute to a deformity. Impaction grafting can be utilized to help provide additional structural support to the bone. However, in the PIP joint, I have found it to be less useful when compared to the MP joints. Upsizing of the implants can help fill the medullary canals and is likely the best way to fill the bone canals and afford a stable joint. A benefit of some of the implant systems in the PIP joint is that (unlike the MP joints) size mismatches are allowable to some degree. This allows more options for optimizing the arthroplasty stability. Like the MP joints, I prefer to avoid the use of cement.

The implant choices include hinged and unconstrained designs. The optimal choice is dependent on the amount of residual bone stock and the competence of the surrounding stabilizing soft tissues. Like the MP joint revision cases, it is important to have alternate plans depending on the intraoperative findings. Whenever feasible, following a failed unconstrained implant, I prefer to aim for revising to a nonconstrained device. They share the load better and are less likely to fail secondary to fracture. The hinged implants afford more stability and are a reasonable fallback if the unconstrained implant is not feasible. Arthrodesis can be utilized whenever the hinged implant is not a workable option. Upon trialing, the joint is assessed for stability and alignment throughout its range of motion. The use of fluoroscopy is essential in helping with implant alignment and canal fill through all steps of the revision procedure.

Following reimplantation, the ligaments are secured to the bone (if detached from their insertion), and the capsule can be closed with a 3-0 Vicryl suture. The extensor mechanism can be secured with 3-0 FiberWire, 3-0 Surgilon, or 2-0 Dexon interrupted sutures. When closing a tendon-splitting approach, the distal interphalangeal (DIP) joint should be held in flexion during the closure to avoid overtightening of the interval, which can result in hyperextension of the PIP joint. The tourniquet can then be deflated and bleeding be controlled. Skin can be closed with 4-0 Prolene or nylon interrupted sutures over a Silastic drain. A bulky finger dressing and splint holding the PIP joint in extension is applied.

Optimizing Outcomes

- Preserving the bone stock is critical in allowing for successful revision surgery. Meticulous technique to preserve bone is time well spent.
- Preservation of the collateral ligaments and soft-tissue stabilizers will also help maximize stability of the revision joint.
- Preoperative planning and discussions with the patient are critical in realizing expectations and planning for contingencies.
- Upsizing the implant will help fill the bone canal and improve stability.
- Hinged implants can be utilized when unconstrained implants are not feasible.
- Arthrodesis is a reasonable contingency for persistent failure of either constrained or nonconstrained joint replacements.

Complications and Side Effects

Complications following revision arthroplasty of the PIP joint can be numerous and include instability, limited motion, implant failure/loosening, recurrent deformity, pain, and neurovascular compromise. Practically, the primary concerns are instability, recurrent deformity, and implant survivorship. Like MP joint revision arthroplasty, these problems are usually the result of "pushing" the envelope and indications for arthroplasty. Prolonged immobilization may be helpful in allowing scar tissue to develop and afford ligament healing in hopes of providing a more stable joint. However, the PIP joint is generally less forgiving than the MP joint with respect to range of motion. In addition, limited motion at the PIP joint is more noticeable and functionally limiting to the patient than MP stiffness. Splints can be helpful in providing added external stability for the finger. In addition, derotational slings are useful in correcting rotational deformities. Prolonged immobilization may also lead to tendon adhesions. Additional surgery may be necessary for recalcitrant cases that fail conservative measures.

Postoperative Care

Postsurgical care includes removal of the Silastic drain (if utilized) on day 1. If concerned about the incision, the wound may be inspected at that time. Further immobilization is generally warranted. I prefer to immobilize in 0–15° of extension. However, care must be taken not to hyperextend the PIP joint. Like the MP joint, many of these fingers will necessitate a longer period of immobilization when compared to the primary joint replacement rehabilitation protocol. In addition, patients on disease-modifying anti-rheumatoid medications will take longer to both heal the wound and form scar tissue. Following a period of immobilization, therapy can be initiated. I prefer dynamic splinting with care taken again not to hyperextend the PIP and allowing for active flexion with passive extension. This will minimize stress at the extensor mechanism while initiating joint motion. Flexion is protected—initially starting to 30° and increased every 1–2 in intervals of 10–15°. A nighttime resting splint is also utilized. Once the patient approaches 90° of flexion and the joint is clinically and radiographically stable, gentle strengthening may be initiated. Individualization of the postoperative regimen is important as the findings at the time of surgery and the patient's early postoperative course will significantly determine the optimal course for therapy. I also prefer to get long-term radiographic and clinical analysis yearly, or at 2-year intervals.

Arthrodesis

Technique (Fig. 22.3)

It is not uncommon for arthrodesis to be a first option for reoperation. I prefer a dorsal approach for arthrodesis of the PIP joint following failed arthroplasty. It allows for excellent visualization of the joint and appropriate fixation and hardware placement. The approach is similar to that for revision arthroplasty. However, in these cases, I prefer a tendon-splitting technique to expose the joint. In addition, less emphasis is placed on preservation of the collateral ligaments and supporting soft-tissues. The implant is removed, and the bone ends are prepared. Again, minimal bone resection is preferred. This will minimize the already significant shortening effect of the arthrodesis. I prefer to liberally use distal radius bone graft. Alternatives include the proximal ulna and iliac crest. Typically, the distal radius will provide enough to fill the medullary canals across the anticipated fusion site. If the finger has substantial bone deficit, a structural graft can be utilized with cancellous bone. Allograft can also be used. The position of fusion is usually 45–60° depending on the digit. The natural resting cascade of the hand incrementally increases the PIP joint flexion from the index finger to the small finger. Thus, 45° at the index finger with increasing 5° intervals to 60° for the small finger is typically appropriate. However, it is important to discuss the position of fusion with the patient in detail so as to accommodate for expectations and address special needs.

Arthrodesis can be fixed with plates, screws, wires, and/or tension band. My preference is to utilize K-wires and tension band construct to secure fixation. While technically somewhat more challenging than plates, I find that excellent compression can be achieved with low-profile hardware. This can be done with two 0.35 or 0.45 K-wires placed across the fusion site in line with the shaft of the middle phalanx. I then utilize a 25-gauge wire and pass it through a radial-to-ulnar drill hole (usually with a 0.45 K-wire) in the middle phalanx. It is crossed over the dorsum of the finger and passed beneath the prominent K-wires in the proximal phalanx. It can be folded on itself to enhance the strength of the construct and allow for easier passage through the middle phalanx (which can be sometimes difficult due to the wire bending). Tensioning is performed with a large needle driver. Care should be taken not to overtighten the band as it could cut out the soft bone. I find the tension to be appropriate if the construct moves as a unit and allows no gapping with flexion of the finger. The K-wires are each then pulled back slightly from the proximal phalanx, bent back to create shepherd's crook, and then cut. It is then rotated so that the crook lies over and secures the tension band at the distal aspect of the proximal phalanx. The liberal use of fluoroscopy is helpful in determining the appropriate position of fusion, the degree of compression, and hardware placement.

Upon completion of the construct, the wound is closed in layers. The extensor interval is closed with 3-0 FiberWire, 3-0 Surgilon, or 2-0 Dexon interrupted sutures. Care should be taken to not close the extensor mechanism too tightly as it may result in hyperextension of the DIP joint. Occasionally, this results anyway and can be remedied by either intrinsic release or tenotomy of the extensor mechanism at the distal phalanx. The tourniquet can then be deflated, and bleeding be controlled with pressure hemostasis and bipolar cautery. The skin is closed with 4-0 Prolene or nylon interrupted sutures over a Silastic drain. A bulky dressing and splint follows, maintaining the finger at the position of fusion.

Optimizing Outcomes

- It is important to meticulously prepare the bone canals and remove any inflammatory tissue and debris.
- The liberal use of bone grafting is helpful.
- Many of these fingers have a prolonged time to fusion. It is important to have a durable and strong hardware construct to help facilitate fusion.
- Refrain from hardware removal, if possible, until successful fusion has been achieved.
- The optimal position of fusion depends on the finger and any specific needs of the patient.
- The use of ultrasound or electrical stimulation may be useful in cases of delayed or nonunion.
- Due to the position of fusion and the fact that many of these patients have bone loss, arthrodesis will result in shortening of the finger.

Complications and Side Effects

The primary complications associated with arthrodesis of the PIP joint following failed arthroplasty are delayed union and nonunion and their sequelae. Prominent and painful hardware is another common problem associated with these procedures. Additional complications include limited function, limited motion of the MP and DIP joints, malpositioning of the digit, pain, infection, and neurovascular compromise. Successful fusion can be ensured with appropriate technique, stable fixation, and the use of bone graft. Patients who consume products with nicotine should be counseled to quit

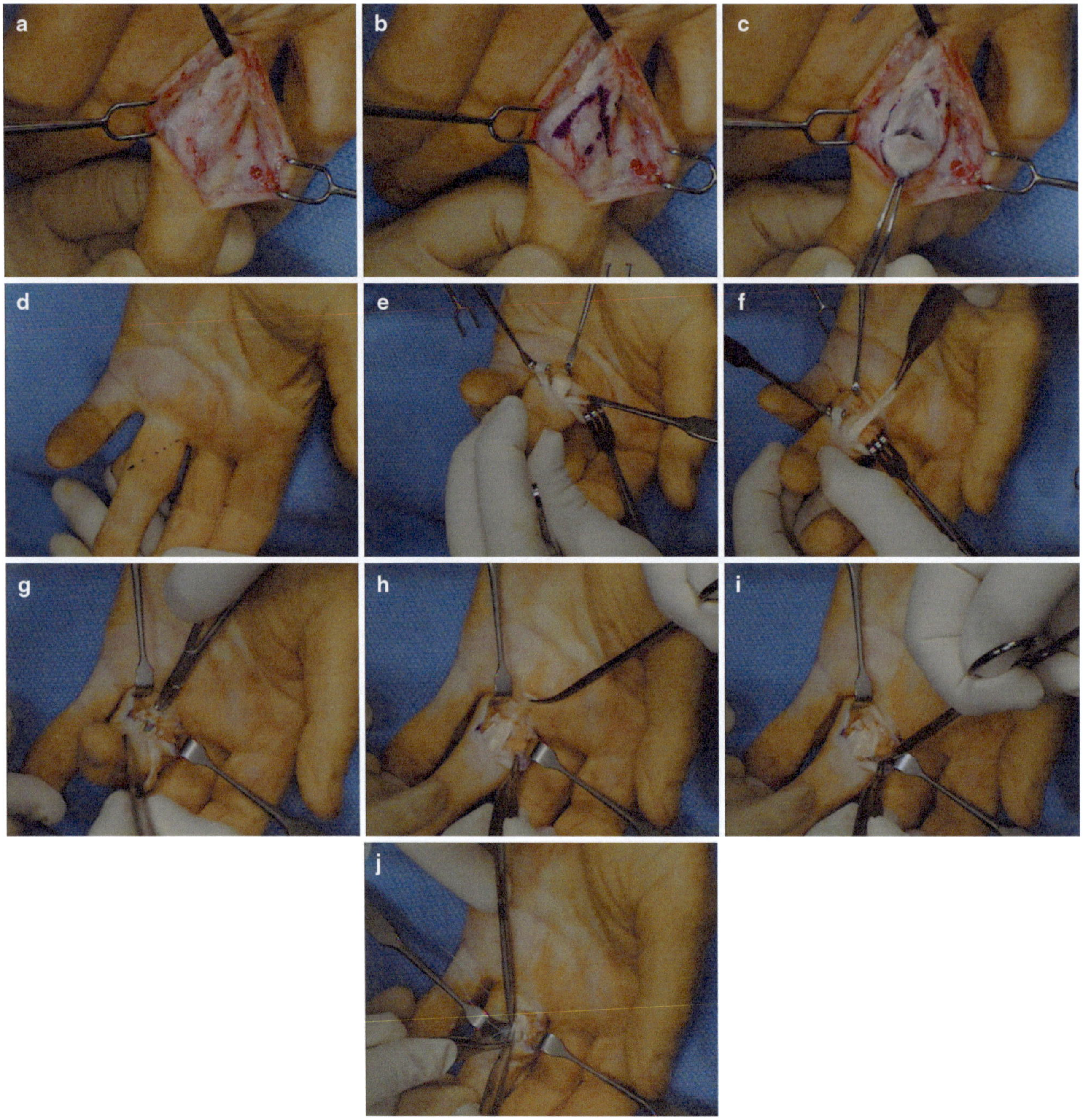

Fig. 22.4 (**a**) The previous dorsal incision to the PIP joint is utilized. (**b**, **c**) A "V"-shaped cut is utilized in the extensor mechanism, and the flap is raised. (**d**) A volar Bruner-type incision can be made to expose the flexor tendon sheath. (**e**) Picture demonstrates the two slips of FDS and underlying FDP. (**f**) In this example, the radial slip is released proximal to the A-2 pulley while leaving it attached at its insertion on the middle phalanx. (**g**–**j**) The slip is then pulled beneath the pulley and sutured back to itself (using a 2-0 nonabsorbable suture) with the finger in approximately 30–45° of flexion. The dorsal extensor mechanism is closed in a V-Y fashion prior to wound closure

prior to performing arthrodesis. Bone stimulators (electrical or ultrasound types) can be utilized as an adjunct to facilitate fusion. Like the MP joints, my preference is the ultrasound-type devices due to their ease of use and portability. I find that this helps with patient compliance.

Postoperative Care

The postoperative regimen following PIP fusion is simpler than that following arthroplasty. I prefer to immobilize the entire finger for a full 2 weeks or until the wound is healed and sutures removed. Thereafter, depending on the stability of fixation, I will graduate the patient to a splint that immobilizes the PIP joint and allows for MP and DIP motion. The splint can be liberally used until fusion has been achieved. Strengthening (without the use of a splint) can be initiated when the patient has demonstrated good radiographic consolidation and is pain-free at the fusion site. Typically, this is at least 6 weeks and can be up to several months.

Miscellaneous Conditions

PIP Instability with Well-Fixed Implants

Collateral ligament reinforcement and reconstruction options can be similar to those of the MP joints. Like the MP joint, my preference is to perform a collateral ligament-stabilizing suture.

Fixed Swan-Neck Deformity with Well-Fixed Implants (Fig. 22.4)

Fixed swan-neck deformity can result following PIP arthroplasty. While most of these patients are pain-free and have well-fixed implants, this can be disabling. This may be remedied with a soft-tissue procedure to reposition the PIP joint in a more flexed posture. A V-Y lengthening of the dorsal extensor mechanism can be performed in conjunction with a volar flexor digitorum superficialis hemitenodesis. The finger is then splinted and immobilized in a similar fashion as a PIP arthrodesis. The net effect of the procedure is not to improve motion; rather, it is to afford a "soft-tissue" fusion.

Conclusion

Reoperation for failed PIP arthroplasty can be difficult and challenging. The primary surgical options include revision arthroplasty and arthrodesis. Factors that affect the success of reoperation include the amount of residual bone stock, the quality of remaining bone, and the competency of the adjacent soft tissues. The decision regarding the best treatment will largely be dependent on the intraoperative findings. It is important for the surgeon and patient to outline contingencies based on these situations and findings. The postoperative regimen should be customized to the patient based on the intraoperative stability of the PIP joint. Arthrodesis may be considered a first option or may be a fallback in cases where arthroplasty is not feasible.

References

1. Goldfarb CA, Stern PJ. Metacarpophalangeal joint arthroplasty in rheumatoid arthritis. A long-term assessment. J Bone Joint Surg Am. 2003;85-A(10):1869–78.
2. Burgess SD, Kono M, Stern PJ. Results of revision metacarpophalangeal joint surgery in rheumatoid patients following previous silicone arthroplasty. J Hand Surg Am. 2007;32(10):1506–12.
3. Wilson YG, Sykes PJ, Niranjan NS. Long-term follow-up of Swanson's silastic arthroplasty of the metacarpophalangeal joints in rheumatoid arthritis. J Hand Surg Br. 1993;18(1):81–91.
4. Parkkila T, et al. Osteolysis after Sutter metacarpophalangeal arthroplasty: a prospective study of 282 implants followed up for 5.7 years. Scand J Plast Reconstr Surg Hand Surg. 2006;40(5):297–301.
5. Parker W, et al. Nonrheumatoid metacarpophalangeal joint arthritis. Unconstrained pyrolytic carbon implants: indications, technique, and outcomes. Hand Clin. 2006;22(2):183–93.
6. Cook SD, et al. Long-term follow-up of pyrolytic carbon metacarpophalangeal implants. J Bone Joint Surg Am. 1999;81(5):635–48.
7. Swanson AB. Silicone rubber implants for replacement of arthritis or destroyed joints in the hand. Surg Clin North Am. 1968;48(5):1113–27.
8. Linscheid RL, et al. Development of a surface replacement arthroplasty for proximal interphalangeal joints. J Hand Surg Am. 1997;22:286–98.
9. Bravo CJ, et al. Pyrolytic carbon proximal interphalangeal joint arthroplasty: results with minimum two-year follow-up evaluation. J Hand Surg Am. 2007;32(1):1–11.
10. Takigawa S, et al. Long-term assessment of Swanson implant arthroplasty in the proximal interphalangeal joint of the hand. J Hand Surg Am. 2004;29(5):785–95.
11. Jennings CD, Livingstone DP. Surface replacement arthroplasty of the proximal interphalangeal joint using the PIP-SRA implant: results, complications, and revisions. J Hand Surg Am. 2008;33(9):1565 e1–11.
12. Chamay A. A distally based dorsal and triangular tendinous flap for direct access to the proximal interphalangeal joint. Ann Chir Main. 1988;7(2):179–83.

Reoperative Surgery in Failed Wrist Arthroplasty

23

Kevin J. Renfree

Abstract

Despite wrist arthritis and other degenerative conditions of the wrist being quite common, total wrist arthroplasty is a relatively uncommon procedure, especially when compared to arthroplasty about the hip, knee, and shoulder. Newer implants require minimal bone resection; however, not only are there still numerous older implants still in patients, but these newer implants can still have complications. Revising a wrist arthroplasty to another implant is believed to have a rather high complication and failure rate, although no large studies are available. In most cases of wrist arthroplasty revision, wrist arthrodesis will be considered the procedure of choice. Given bone loss, there is usually the need for a significant amount of structural bone grafting that can either be in the form of autograft or allograft. Plate fusion is most commonly utilized, but newer intramedullary fusion implants do offer some unique possibilities. In some circumstances, the wrist may be fused as a temporary measure to establish more bone stock, and then the wrist fusion taken down and a new arthroplasty implant placed. The patients suffering with these conditions frequently may have loss in finger range of motion secondary to scarring of the extensor and flexor tendons. The challenges of implant revisions should be thoroughly reviewed with the patient as there is the possibility of significant complications

Keywords

Revision • Total • Wrist • Arthroplasty • Fusion

Key Points

- The wrist is the most frequently involved joint in patients with rheumatoid arthritis.
- Published outcomes for total wrist arthroplasty (TWA) are based on multiple implants, many of which are no longer in use.
- Currently available fourth-generation implants require minimal bone resection. Also, they don't require cement fixation, so they are easier to revise to fusion in the event of failure. This may lower the threshold for their use in primary reconstruction.
- There are no good outcome studies available for revision wrist arthroplasty using current-generation implants.
- Revision wrist arthroplasty has a high complication and failure rate.
- Wrist arthrodesis should be the first choice in most cases of revising failed wrist implants, unless one can identify a clear source of pain (i.e., malrotation) which is easily addressed.

(continued)

K.J. Renfree, MD (✉)
Department of Orthopedic Surgery, Mayo Clinic Hospital, 5777 East Mayo Boulevard, Phoenix, AZ 85054, USA
e-mail: Renfree.Kevin@mayo.edu

S.F.M. Duncan (ed.), *Reoperative Hand Surgery*,
DOI 10.1007/978-1-4614-2373-7_23, © Springer Science+Business Media, LLC 2012

- Structural bone grafting is often needed when revising failed wrist implants to restore carpal height.
- Plate fixation is the preferred method of fixation to allow compression and provide stable fixation.
- Case reports have shown that wrist fusions can be "taken down" and converted to wrist arthroplasty. Making fusions a rare option for increasing bone mass as a preliminary step before revision wrist arthroplasty.

Introduction

The wrist is the upper extremity joint most frequently involved in patients with rheumatoid arthritis [1]. Although the initial presentation of rheumatoid arthritis involves the wrists in 3% of the cases, the wrist frequently becomes involved and may demonstrate bilateral involvement in 95% of the cases as the disease progresses [2]. Despite the fact that evolutionary changes in design and technique have taken place since Swanson introduced his silicone wrist spacer in the late 1960s, primary TWA is a procedure that should still only be considered in a small subset of patients. Current indications would include patients over 65 who are very low demand (don't require use of the affected arm for ambulatory aids or frequent transfers) and perhaps patients who have a fused wrist on the opposite side. The latter is a relative contraindication, since bilateral wrist fusions have been reported with acceptable functional results and patient satisfaction [3]. Patients must also have adequate bone stock to support the implant, especially the distal component. Although published outcomes for TWA are based on multiple prostheses, most of which are no longer in use, reports have shown that long-term failure is frequent with rates of up to 52% at 6 years; with bony resorption seen in more than 75% of the patients [4, 5]. Three fourth-generation implants approved by the FDA (ReMotion Total Wrist, Small Bone Innovations, Inc., Morrisville, PA; Maestro Wrist Reconstruction System, Biomet, Inc., Warsaw, IN; and the Universal 2 Total Wrist Implantation System, Integra Life Sciences Holding Corporation, Plainsboro, NJ) are currently in use in the United States. The most significant design characteristic that these implants share is that they require minimal bone resection and allow implantation of both proximal and distal components without cement. As a result, the threshold for their use in even elderly patients with osteoarthritis may be lowered, since theoretically it should be easier to achieve a fusion in cases of failure. Unfortunately, at the time this chapter is written, there are very few reports available on the intermediate and long-term outcome of these implants, and no reports on their use in revision cases. Distal component loosening was probably the most common cause of prosthetic failure in older generation implants. My personal experience with the newer generation implants have suggested that this problem may not have been eliminated with the current designs, which do not have single- or multiple-stemmed implants placed into the metacarpals (see Fig. 23.1).

The current surgical options for patients with failed primary TWA include resection arthroplasty, silastic interposition arthroplasty, revision wrist arthroplasty, or arthrodesis. Resection, or soft-tissue arthroplasty, should rarely be considered as an option, and only if revision or arthrodesis is contraindicated due to sepsis or unmanageable soft-tissue defects. Beckenbaugh has noted that this procedure will occasionally lead to a painless wrist, but they usually become unstable over time, drifting into ulnar deviation and flexed positions, with poor resulting function [6]. Talwalker reported good results in a small group of patients who had excisional arthroplasties for salvage of failed biaxial wrist arthroplasties. Using the three parameters of pain relief, range of movement, and function, he found that the excision arthroplasties had an excellent result and were better than the wrist fusions or revision TWA patients [7]. Excision arthroplasty may be a consideration as a salvage procedure in cases

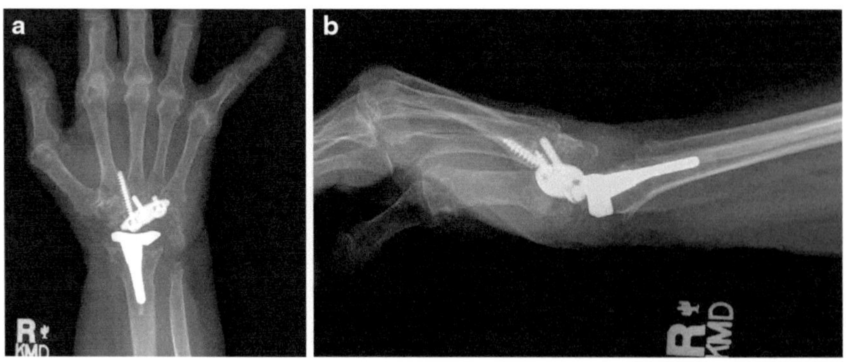

Fig. 23.1 (**a**, **b**) Radiographs (AP and lateral) of a failed distal component secondary to aseptic loosening with volar displacement. Patient presented with wrist pain and clinically apparent rupture of flexor digitorum profundus tendons to ring and small fingers, and carpal tunnel syndrome

with inadequate bone stock, and where the patient is a poor candidate for a large structural bone (i.e., vascularized fibula) graft. Postoperative management can be prolonged and difficult.

The Swanson II Wrist implant (Wright Medical Technology, Inc., Arlington, TN) is still available commercially and has been modified with a shorter distal stem and titanium grommets to lessen the risk of cutting or abrasion of the flexible implant from contact with resected bone. As in resection arthroplasty, in order to consider this option, patients must have an adequate soft-tissue envelope, but also functioning tendons and adequate bone stock to support the implant. Results reported for flexible implant radiocarpal wrist arthroplasties done with protective grommets offer significant improvement over those reported without [8]. One must balance the desire for a limited arc of motion (40–50°) against the risks of early implant failure and silicone wear-induced osteolysis and more extensive bone loss.

Other authors agree that indications for revision TWA are rare and that arthrodesis should be considered as the "gold standard" for salvage of failed TWA, since this will predictably lead to a stable, painless wrist in most cases [4, 9]. Cobb has pointed out that a major advantage of arthrodesis is that it offers patients a single procedure that effectively resolves their problem permanently [9]. Palmer showed that total wrist fusion provided more reliable relief than even a primary TWA in rheumatoid patients [10]. When comparing arthrodesis to arthroplasty (first generation Universal), Cavaliere noted that even just primary wrist arthroplasties done in a similar group of patients (all with rheumatoid arthritis) had a significantly higher rate of major and total complications, and a lower rate of patient satisfaction compared to an arthrodesis group.

When revising a failed TWA to an arthrodesis, structural bone graft and internal fixation is recommended. Significant bone loss results from the carpal resection during the original implant insertion, as well as osteolysis-induced bone loss which results from implant loosening and metallosis. Arthrodesis, however, has a high success rate with union rates above 90% reported [11, 12].

Rettig reported on 13 failed total wrist arthroplasties managed with revision TWA and reported a 38% failure rate of their "re-visions," with failures typically not becoming apparent for at least 2 years [13]. Despite the addition of long-stemmed and multistemmed distal carpal implants seated in the metacarpals with cement fixation, Beckenbaugh noted that results tended to deteriorate with time [6]. There are no good outcome studies available for revision wrist arthroplasty using current-generation implants.

Indications

In my opinion, there are few indications for revision arthroplasty, unless one is able to identify a specific problem, such as component malrotation. Other indications might include clearly identifiable problems such as isolated small perforations of the proximal metacarpal or distal radius that can be bypassed easily by a long stem component [14]. Other frequent causes for prosthetic revision or replacement include: instability, which can be revised in some cases with changing to a thicker elliptical polyethylene bearing; soft-tissue deformity; or contracture. They might be addressed by soft-tissue balancing procedures such as tendon transfer. Loosening of the prosthesis can occasionally be addressed by cementation if the implant had been previously implanted in an uncemented fashion (see Fig. 23.2a–d). This technique may complicate any future revision with an arthrodesis, because of increased bone loss from the cement, particularly if a long stem component(s) is used.

Contraindications

Contraindications are many, and similar to those for primary wrist arthroplasty, although the threshold for the latter has been lowered because of the minimal amount of bony resection required and the potential for easier revision to fusion if a failure occurs.

The more common contraindications are listed below:

- Posttraumatic or degenerative joint disease.
- Loss of innervation (neurologically impaired wrist).
- Poor active motion (less than 40° arc).
- Sepsis (local or remote).
- Poor bone stock (particularly loss of carpal bones).
- Need to use extremity for weight-bearing activities (frequent transfers, ambulatory aids).
- Soft-tissue insufficiency (loss of wrist extensors, poor skin coverage).
- Severe deformity or instability.
- Severe systemic disease requiring systemic steroids or tumor necrosis factor (TNF) inhibitors which may raise the risk of wound-healing problems or infection.

Preoperative History and Considerations

Jolley has identified multiple theoretic reasons for implant failure including: active disease with progression, poor rebalancing at the time of operation, advanced preoperative deformity, poor component design, poor component materials,

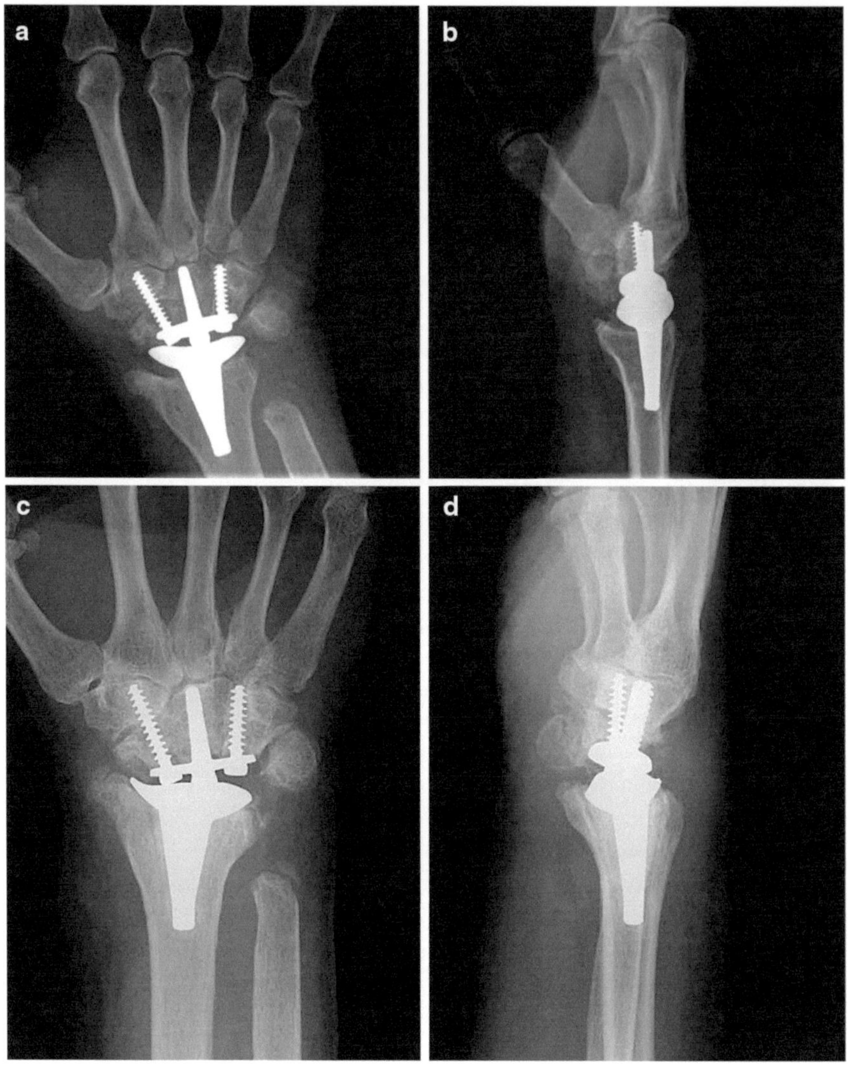

Fig. 23.2 (**a**, **b**) AP and lateral views of an uncemented wrist arthroplasty with pain and loosening. (**c**, **d**) AP and lateral views of the same wrist after revision to a cemented implant

and excessive patient demands (use of ambulatory aids) [5]. Prosthetic fracture is associated with increasing wrist pain, instability, and deformity with decreasing strength and function. In patients who present with failed silicone implants, usually from fracture, excessive motion is seen and the wrist often develops progressive ulnar deviation and flexion deformity (see Fig. 23.3). In evaluating a patient with a painful wrist arthroplasty, it is important to look for other sources of pain, such as distal radio-ulnar joint arthritis, which may be addressed with a distal ulnar resection. Clicking or catching may indicate wrist subluxation or impingement. These findings are often absent during passive movement of the wrist observed by the examining surgeon. Such symptoms may be evident only with active use such as grasping or while performing certain motions [15]. In cases of distal component loosening and migration, the flexor tendons should be evaluated to make sure that they are intact or without impending rupture (crepitus, and/or pain against resistance). Carpal tunnel syndrome should also be ruled out, because of potential compromise of the carpal tunnel space. Laboratory studies should include a CBC, sedimentation rate (ESR), and C-reactive protein (CRP), as a screening tool for infection. If a revision arthroplasty is expected, a urinalysis to rule out a urinary tract infection should be done. If positive, treatment can be instituted promptly to avoid seeding of any postoperative hematoma.

Radiographic studies should include plain radiographs, which can be evaluated for loosening, migration of components, prosthetic and cement fracture, cortical bone resorption/fracture, and radiolucency [9]. Radiographs may also be examined for lucent lines around the implants (particularly if >2 mm in width or progressive on serial radiographs), implant subsidence and shift, and/or erosion of the tip of the implant through the cortex. Cobb has pointed out that subsidence of the proximal implant was estimated in a similar fashion by using the distal ulna as a reference point, and that 3-mm

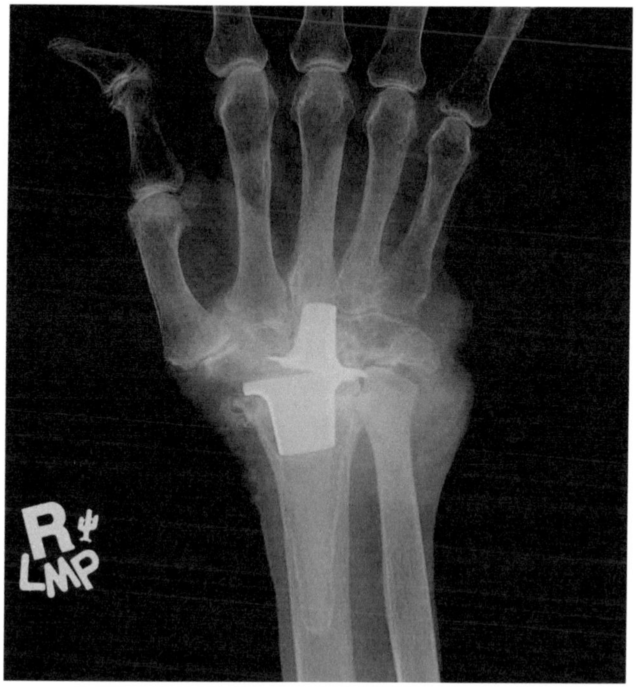

Fig. 23.3 Classic radiographic presentation of a patient with a failed wrist silicone implant

subsidence was significantly associated with failure of the implant [9]. Subsidence of the distal component may be determined by loss of carpal height on serial radiographs. Compression or distraction roentgenograms, or motion views with loading (during grip), may demonstrate a change in the position of the prosthetic stems, dorsal or volar subluxation of the prosthesis, or bone impingement [15]. Silicone or wear-induced osteolysis will often show cystic changes and bony resorption, in addition to some of the changes in prosthetic position mentioned above. Although prosthetic fracture is a common cause of failure in silicone implants, fractures of metallic stems or base plates can also lead to failure. Computed tomography can occasionally be helpful in looking for component malposition, or impingement. Nuclear studies can be helpful to confirm prosthetic loosening or infection.

Operative Approach

The surgical approach to the wrist for revision arthroplasty or arthrodesis is through a dorsal, longitudinal, midline incision. An attempt to incorporate previous surgical scars should be made. I prefer to incise the extensor retinaculum in a stepwise fashion, so that it can be lengthened at the time of closure. Alternatively, if necessary, one slip can be placed deep to the extensor tendons to act as a protective soft-tissue barrier above the dorsal lip of the radial component, or a bony edge. Care should be taken to evaluate the extensor tendons for rupture or attenuation. If the posterior and/or interosseous nerves are intact, a 1-cm segment should be excised 3–5 cm proximal to the wrist, with the hope that nerve entrapment in scar is avoided and postoperative pain is reduced.

When a revision arthroplasty is planned, a distally based, U-shaped capsular flap should be raised, leaving a cuff of tissue on the dorsal lip of the radius for repair. Synovial tissue should be harvested and sent for frozen section intraoperatively to rule out the possibility of infection before reimplantation of another implant. Removal of the implant can be facilitated by wrist hyperflexion over a bump, which will improve access to both proximal and distal components. Bone tamps, vice grips with a slap hammer attachment, flexible osteotomes, can be helpful in removing the implants. In the event of a cemented implant, cement removal instruments should also be available. An osteotome will usually suffice in separating the polyethylene from the base plate. An attempt to limit bone loss should be made during implant removal.

If infection is encountered or highly suspected, a resection arthroplasty is performed. This may be the definitive procedure planned if the conditions mentioned earlier in this chapter preclude revision arthroplasty or arthrodesis. In this case, the dorsal flap can be folded down and sewn into the volar capsule and tensioned to promote soft-tissue stability as well as acting as a soft-tissue "spacer". Prolonged immobilization (10–12 weeks) in a cast or external fixator (if soft tissue/wound care is required) is necessary. Long-term supportive wrist bracing may be needed. If the resection arthroplasty is temporary (infection), and a staged arthrodesis or arthroplasty is anticipated, an antibiotic-impregnated cement spacer or beads are placed in the defect. The patient is placed on susceptibility-based intraveneous antibiotics for 6 weeks before the definitive procedure.

When an arthrodesis is performed, a structural bone graft is necessary to replace missing bone and restore length. Options include a tricortical iliac crest autogenous graft, in which case the cortical portion of the graft should be placed longitudinally in line with the radial shaft and third metacarpal (see Fig. 23.4). Other options include the ipsilateral distal ulna which can be measured for length, cut proximally and "rolled" into the defect (Fig. 23.5). Soft-tissue stripping of the distal ulna should be minimized (especially in the region of the interosseous membrane) in order to preserve its blood supply. Fresh-frozen allograft femoral heads fashioned to fit the defect have also been shown to yield good results [11]. Beckenbaugh, however, has reported nearly a 50% nonunion rate with allograft, but admits that it is very appealing in the elderly population with low demand and at a higher risk for complications of the larger iliac crest surgery [6]. If the bony defect is very large (>6–8 cm), a vascularized fibular graft could be considered in the appropriate patient. Buried Steinman pins are an option for fixation, particularly if the patient has poor quality soft-tissue on the dorsum of the wrist

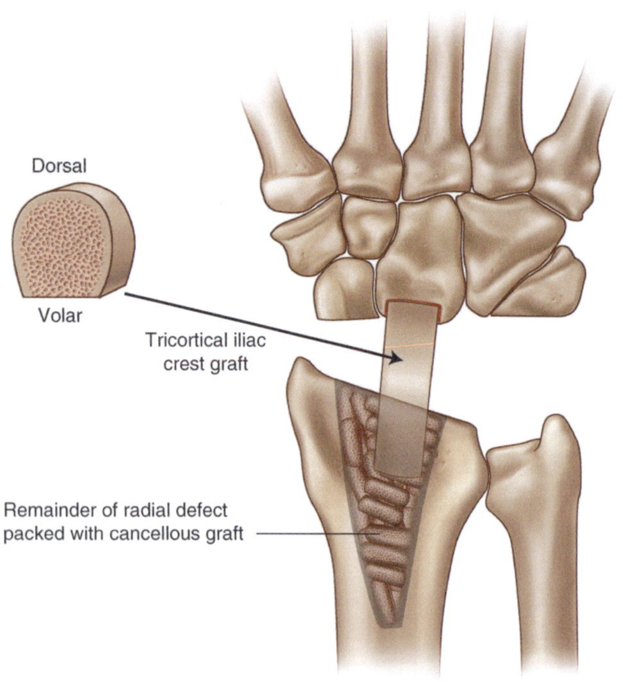

Fig. 23.4 Tricortical iliac crest autogenous bone graft utilized to replace missing bone and restore length

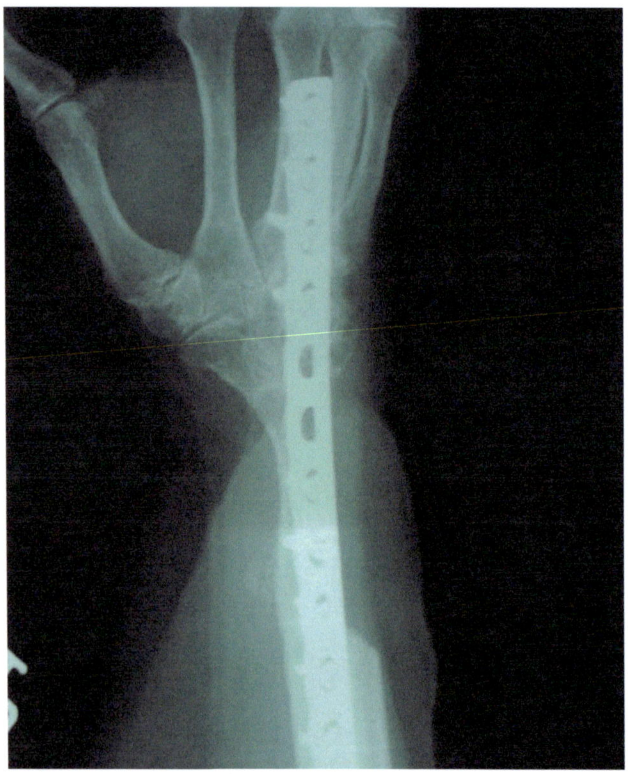

Fig. 23.5 Ipsilateral distal ulna rolled into the bone defect and held together with plate fixation

and is at risk for wound breakdown or dehiscence. If soft-tissue quality is good, my preference is to use a locking wrist fusion plate (Synthes USA, West Chester, PA) or a 3.5 DCP locking plate. It is often necessary to position the wrist in neutral or in just a slight amount of flexion or extension (<5–10°) so that the graft does not fracture. The carpometacarpal joints should be prepared and included in the arthrodesis, and in cases of bilateral involvement, the nondominant hand may be placed in 5–10° of flexion to better assist in such activities as perineal care [3].

When a revision arthroplasty is performed, three main goals must be achieved: (1) the prosthesis must be properly centered, (2) adequate prosthetic fixation is essential, and (3) the soft tissues must be balanced [15]. Since most deformities are in ulnar deviation and flexion, tendon transfers such as the extensor carpi ulnaris to the extensor carpi radialis longus or the flexor carpi ulnaris to the extensor carpi radialis brevis can be performed [15]. To my knowledge, custom modification of currently available implants is necessary if long stem components are needed. One may not be able to place longer screws perfectly up the metacarpal shafts through the fixed angles on the holes of the carpal base plate. If an adequate press-fit of the implant is not possible, cementation can be considered. Impaction bone grafting for patients with poor bone stock, using fresh frozen allograft from the femoral head, might also be a consideration [16, 17]. Mutimer has described a case where a revision arthroplasty was staged via a wrist fusion [17]. There is very little clinical experience with this procedure, however, and assurance must be made that wrist extensor function can be restored and joint-capsule ligament restraints restored.

Postoperative Care

Much of the postoperative care was outlined in Sect. Postoperative Care. Additional specific recommendations for revision TWA would include the following:

- Wound suction drain to prevent hematoma.
- Prophylactic antibiotics until intraoperative cultures return negative.
- Immobilization with wrist in neutral for 3–4 weeks to allow healing of capsular repair.
- Immediate active range of motion of digits to prevent adhesions and stiffness.
- Resting splint with wrist in neutral for an additional 4 weeks (until 8 weeks post-op). Patient is to remove for active range of motion exercises several times a day. The limits of flexion and extension should be noted intraoperatively at the time of the procedure, and the therapist notified not to try and exceed these limits in therapy. A 60° arc of motion is a very satisfactory goal.

- Patient may also begin light grip/pinch and wrist flexion and extension exercises with a 1–2 lb dumbbell at 8 weeks.
- Patients are discouraged from using the wrist for any transfer activities (i.e., pushing/pulling oneself up from a chair) for 12 weeks postoperatively.
- Remind patients that wrist arthroplasty is a very low-demand implant!

Optimizing Outcomes

Arthrodesis for a failed TWA.

- The plate can be applied to the index or ring finger metacarpal if the long finger metacarpal is inadequate.
- Bone graft substitutes (demineralized bone matrix, rh-BMP, etc.) may improve union rates.
- Supplemental external immobilization (casting) should be used for at least 6 weeks if bone quality is poor.
- Consider prophylactic simultaneous carpal tunnel release.
- Initiate immediate active range of motion exercises of the digits postoperatively.
- If patients use an ambulatory aid, consider a platform walker or wheelchair until bony union of the arthrodesis is confirmed radiographically.
- Discuss temporary discontinuance of medications that might impair bone or wound healing (i.e., TNF inhibitors, methotrexate) with rheumatologist prior to surgery.
- Always complete due diligence to rule out infection both preoperatively and intraoperatively before committing to bone grafting and hardware placement. Stage if unsure.
- Perform distal ulnar resection if distal radial ulnar joint ("DRUJ") arthritis present or ulnacarpal abutment is identified intraoperatively (clinically and radiographically).
- Use a wound suction drain to prevent a postoperative hematoma.

Complications

Even in primary wrist arthroplasty, complications are common and can be very problematic to treat. Acute prosthetic instability can often be prevented by careful evaluation intraoperatively. The smallest polyethelene ellipsoid spacer should be used that provides for a stable arc of motion. A larger (thicker) spacer will usually increase stability, but at the expense of decreased motion. To my knowledge, there are no constrained implants currently available. Soft-tissue balance should also be confirmed. In a patient with severe ulnar deviation deformity, a tendon transfer (ECU to ECRL) should be considered. Good medical control of their rheumatoid disease should be in place to prevent deterioration of the soft-tissue support structures postoperatively. Late instability is often due to component subsidence.

Distal component loosening is, in my experience, still probably the most common cause of implant failure. Metallosis, tendon rupture (usually flexor), and/or carpal tunnel syndrome may all occur as a result of component migration. Periprosthetic fractures of the radius can also occur. In Dawson's series, all fractures required prolonged cast immobilization. Three patients developed either delayed union or union with deformity. Significant interference with hand function resulted in those three; two required revision arthroplasty to salvage a satisfactory result [18].

Complications specific for arthrodesis include: nonunion, deep infection, ulnocarpal impaction, hardware failure, hematoma, and wound dehiscence. Finger stiffness from extensor tendon adhesions can result if postoperative hand therapy is not used or is inadequate.

Conclusion

There is a high failure rate reported for older generation primary wrist arthroplasty designs. There is scant outcome data for current-generation implants currently available on the market, and it is very short-term [4]. There is no outcome data on use of these available implants for revision arthroplasty, and their use for this purpose would need to be done on a custom basis. Takwale has pointed out that fewer than half of primary arthroplasties achieve a range of movement which is defined as functional [16]. In Talwalker's series, even though revision wrist replacements and excision arthroplasties had insufficient extension, adequate flexion was usually achieved [7]. Clayton and Ferlic believe that flexion is more important in rheumatoid arthritis than extension above neutral [19]. Therefore, maintaining wrist motion should always be a goal, if reasonable and appropriate for that patient.

There is very good clinical evidence that wrist fusions are well tolerated in the rheumatoid population. Arthrodesis achieves the goals of pain relief and stability, at the expense of grasp and the more sophisticated hand movements, such as buttoning clothes [16]. Personally, I prefer wrist arthrodesis as the primary means of revising a failed wrist arthroplasty. Through stability and pain relief, hand function is optimized.

References

1. Ferlic DC, Jolly SN, Clayton ML. Salvage for failed implant arthroplasty of the wrist. J Hand Surg Am. 1992;17(5):917–23.
2. Davis RF, Weiland AJ, Dowling SV. Swanson implant arthroplasty of the wrist in rheumatoid arthritis. Clin Orthop Relat Res. 1982;166:132–7.

3. Rayan GM, Brentlinger A, Purnell D, Garcia-Moral CA. Functional assessment of bilateral wrist arthrodeses. J Hand Surg Am. 1987;12(6):1020–4.
4. Cavaliere C, Chung KC. A systematic review of total wrist arthroplasty compared with total wrist arthrodesis for rheumatoid arthritis. Plast Reconstr Surg. 2008;122:813–25.
5. Jolly SL, Ferlic DC, Clayton ML, Dennis DA, Stringer EA. Swanson silicone arthroplasty of the wrist in rheumatoid arthritis: a long-term follow-up. J Hand Surg Am. 1992;17(1):142–9.
6. Beckenbaugh RD. Commentary: APH total wrist arthroplasty. J Hand Surg Am. 2003;28A:795–6.
7. Talwalker SC, Hayton MJ, Trail IA, Stanley JK. Management of the failed biaxial wrist replacement. J Hand Surg Br. 2005;30(3):248–51.
8. Capone RA. The titanium grommet in flexible implant arthroplasty of the radiocarpal joint: a long-term review of 44 cases. Plast Reconstr Surg. 1995;96(3):667–72.
9. Cobb TK, Beckenbaugh RD. Biaxial long-stemmed multipronged distal components for revision/bone deficit in total-wrist arthroplasty. J Hand Surg Am. 1996;21(5):764–70.
10. Palmer AK, Werner FW, Murphy D, Glisson R. Functional wrist motion: a biomechanical study. J Hand Surg Am. 1985;10:39.
11. Carlson JR, Simmons BP. Wrist arthrodesis after failed wrist implant. J Hand Surg Am. 1998;23:893–8.
12. Radmer S, Andresen R, Sparmann M. Total wrist arthroplasty in patients with rheumatoid arthritis. J Hand Surg Am. 2003;28A:789–94.
13. Rettig ME, Beckenbaugh RD. Revision total wrist arthroplasty. J Hand Surg Am. 1993;18(5):798–804.
14. Lorei MP, Figgie MP, Ranawat CS, Inglis AE. Failed total wrist arthroplasty. Clin Orthop Relat Res. 1997;342:84–93.
15. Cooney WP, Beckenbaugh RD, Linscheid RL. Total wrist arthroplasty. Problems with implant failures. Clin Orthop Relat Res. 1984;87:121–8.
16. Takwale VJ, Nuttall D, Trail IA, Stanley JK. Biaxial total wrist replacement in patients with rheumatoid arthritis. J Bone Joint Surg Br. 2002;84-B:692–9.
17. Mutimer JN, Giddins GEB. Maintaining wrist function in severe rheumatoid arthritis: a case study of revision Swanson wrist arthroplasty staged via a wrist fusion in rheumatoid arthritis. Hand Surg. 2002;7(2):183–5.
18. Dawson WJ. Radius fracture after total wrist arthroplasty. J Hand Surg Am. 1989;14(4):630–4.
19. Clayton M, Ferlic D. Silicone arthroplasty of the wrist in rheumatoid arthritis. (Letters to the Editor). J Hand Surg Am. 1993;18(1):166.
20. Sollerman C, et al. One year result from an ongoing multicenter study of the Avanta wrist implant. Abstract presented at: Meeting of the International Federation of Societies for Surgery of the Hand, March 2007, Sydney, Australia.
21. Rettig ME, Beckenbaugh RD. Revision total wrist arthroplasty. J Hand Surg Am. 1993;18A:798–804.

Secondary Surgery Following Failed Forearm Reconstruction

24

Shushan Jacob, Tsu-Min Tsai, and A. Lee Osterman

Abstract

It is not uncommon for longitudinal forearm instability to be recognized quite late after the injury. Frequently, this injury is not appreciated until there have already been changes at both the wrist (ulnar carpal abutment) and the elbow (radiocapitellar abutment). These late cases frequently require an ulnar shortening osteotomy, as well as radial head prosthesis and/or reconstruction of the interosseous ligament. If continued problems result and there are degenerative changes or chronic pain at the radial capitellar joint, a radiocapitellar prosthesis can be considered. The final treatment for some patients may require creation of a one-bone forearm. This prevents any further longitudinal instability of the forearm; however, it obviously results in loss of forearm rotation. These injuries are best treated early and aggressively, as later reconstructive options will usually result in decreased function of the extremity. This chapter goes through the different reconstructive options that are available to the reoperative surgeon.

Keywords

Forearm • Interosseous • Ligament • Reconstruction • Dissociation

Key Points

- Forearm instability can result from trauma, bone loss secondary to infection, or tumor resection and congenital malformation.
- The three main stabilizers of the forearm are the radial head, the interosseous ligament (IOL), and the triangular fibrocartilage complex (TFCC). In order for traumatic longitudinal dissociation of the radius and ulna to occur, there must be an axial loading force that disrupts all three of them.
- Early diagnosis is essential, as treatment of acute injuries with reestablishment of the radiocapitellar articulation results in satisfactory outcomes 80% of the time (Clin Orthop Relat Res 234:61–69, 1988; J Bone Joint Surg Am 74(10):1486–1497, 1992), while treatment of missed injuries is difficult and results in a significant failure rate (J Bone

(continued)

S. Jacob, MD
Department of Orthopedic Surgery, Division of Hand and Microsurgery, UT Southwestern Medical Center, Dallas, TX, USA

T.-M. Tsai, MD
Department of Hand and Microsurgery, Christine M. Kleinert Institute of Hand and Microsurgery, University of Louisville School of Medicine, Louisville, KY, USA

A.L. Osterman, MD (✉)
Department of Orthopedic Surgery, Philadelphia Hand Center, Thomas Jefferson University, King of Prussia, PA, USA
e-mail: loster51@verizon.net

S.F.M. Duncan (ed.), *Reoperative Hand Surgery*,
DOI 10.1007/978-1-4614-2373-7_24, © Springer Science+Business Media, LLC 2012

Joint Surg Am 87(8):1828–1833, 2005; Clin Orthop Relat Res 234:61–69, 1988; J Bone Joint Surg Am 74(10): 1486–1497, 1992).

- Chronic longitudinal radioulnar dissociation (longitudinal radioulnar dissociation) resulting in ulnocarpal abutment can be addressed with an ulnar shortening osteotomy. This procedure corrects only the ulnar impaction and does not address the forearm instability. Therefore, reestablishment of longitudinal stability with either a radial head prosthesis or a reconstructed IOL is essential to prevent recurrent symptoms at the wrist.
- If axial instability persists even after adequate reestablishment of the radiocapitellar articulation, the continued increased load transmission can result in radiocapitellar joint arthritis. This is a concern for a metallic radial head prosthesis wearing against capitellar cartilage. In this scenario, reconstruction of the IOL and stabilization of the TFCC in addition to the radial head prosthesis may be prudent (Hand Clin 23:195–208, 2007).
- If significant radiocapitellar arthritis is present with axial instability, the use of a hemielbow arthroplasty may be considered.

Introduction

A forearm instability injury pattern was first documented by Brockman in 1931 [1] and Curr and Coe in 1946 [2]. However, it was Essex-Lopresti in 1951 [3], who made many of the observations and conclusions regarding longitudinal radioulnar dissociation (longitudinal radioulnar dissociation). He described the triad of radial head fracture, tear of the interosseous membrane (IOM), and acute distal radioulnar joint (DRUJ) dislocation resulting from a traumatic axial load transmitted from wrist to elbow [3]. Essex-Lopresti recognized that wrist pain and forearm swelling may not be present despite injury to wrist and forearm soft tissue structures. Following his contributions, considerable advancements in understanding the anatomy and biomechanics of the forearm have been made. MRI and ultrasound imaging have improved ability to visualize the IOM. Early recognition and treatment of this injury pattern are essential. Eighty percent success rate has been reported when longitudinal radioulnar dissociation is diagnosed and treated acutely, whereas delayed treatment despite attempts to stabilize the forearm axis can result in a failure rate of up to 80% [4–6].

The three main stabilizers of the forearm are the radial head, the central band of the IOM, and the TFCC of the DRUJ. In order for longitudinal dissociation of the radius and ulna to occur, there must be an axial loading force that disrupts all three of them. Cadaver studies suggest that such axial injury occurs with a forceful fall on the pronated forearm [7]. With continued loading and absence of support from the fractured radius at the radiocapitellar joint, the radius is forced proximally. If there is enough force, the secondary structures preventing this migration are injured, namely, the IOM and the TFCC. The proximal migration of the radius leads to a positive ulnar variance with DRUJ dysfunction or impingement of the remaining proximal radius on the capitellum. As the TFCC is the primary stabilizer of the DRUJ, an unstable DRUJ indicates the presence of a TFCC injury. Acute injuries may not necessarily present with wrist pain after trauma to the radial head [3]. Chronic cases present 12 weeks or longer after the injury and are typically unrecognized injuries to the IOM that were treated with a radial head resection. In both cases, the compromised forearm stability causes pain, instability, and decreased motion at the elbow and wrist.

Galeazzi fractures (radial shaft fracture with associated DRUJ dislocation) and Monteggia fractures (ulna shaft fracture with associated radial head dislocation) can also lead to forearm instability. These fracture patterns are usually easily diagnosed and treated early.

Anatomy and Biomechanics of the Forearm

The forearm unit consists of the radius and ulna bound together distally at the DRUJ, proximally by the proximal radioulnar joint and centrally by the IOM.

The IOM is the fibrous tissue that extends from the interosseous crest of the radius to that of the ulna. It behaves more like a ligament, and therefore, a more descriptive term for this structure is the IOL complex [8–10].

The central band is composed mostly of collagen organized in parallel arrangement with very little elastin and has the mechanical properties of a ligament.

The components that comprise the IOL complex include the central band, proximal band, accessory bands, and distal oblique band [8]. Figure 24.1 illustrates the gross anatomy of the IOL complex. The most important component of the IOL complex is the central band, also called the IOL

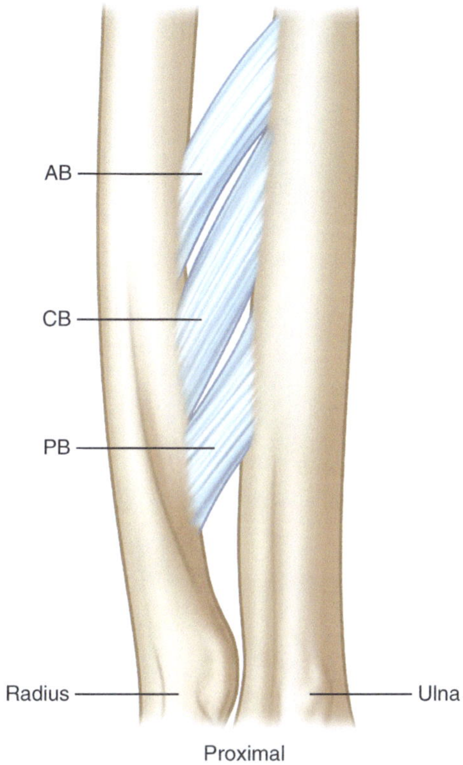

Fig. 24.1 Anatomy of the interosseous ligament complex (ILC). The proximal band (PB) is oriented perpendicular to the central band (CB). The accessory bands (AB) are distal to the central band

[11, 12]. It is a wide, flat, trapezoidal structure found consistently in the forearm [11, 13]. The material properties of the central band are similar to those of the patellar tendon [9, 11]. There are two bundles within the central band that have different stress and strain relationships [8, 12]. The proximal bundle of the central band experiences the most strain across it in neutral rotation with an intact radial head, suggesting that this is the position a graft should be tensioned [10, 11]. The central band has a thickness of 1–2 mm and a width of 1 cm [10, 11, 14] (Fig. 24.2c). The length of the intact central band measures about 40 mm, but the minimum graft length necessary for reconstruction is 112 mm [15]. The origin begins at an average of 7.7 cm from the radial head, angles at 21° to the longitudinal axis of the radius, and inserts approximately 13.7 cm from the tip of olecranon (Fig. 24.2b, c). For the purpose of reconstruction, it is more useful to note, as in Fig. 24.2a, that the center of the origin is approximately 60% of the radial length from the radial styloid and inserts one third of the ulnar length from the ulnar styloid, which is about 3.2 cm [10, 11, 15]. The average length of the ulnar insertion is longer, measuring about 4.2 cm, than the radial origin, which measures around 3.4 cm [10, 15]. A second ligament of the IOL complex, named the proximal band (also called oblique cord), originates from the same area as the central band but is oriented perpendicularly and courses proximally (Fig. 24.1). This proximal band has been reported to be present in 85% of forearms [10, 16], is located on the dorsal surface of the forearm, and angles at 28° to the longitudinal axis of the ulna. It inserts approximately 9.7 cm from the distal tip of the olecranon and is 4 mm in width [9].

The proximal oblique cord has been studied by several investigators [8, 17–20]. These investigators have concluded that the proximal oblique cord has little function in humans.

Accessory bands vary in quantity from one to five [9, 10]. They are located distally to the central band and run in the same orientation (Fig. 24.1). They are consistently found in the forearm like the central band, but accessory bands are less substantial, and their role in forearm stability is minor [9]. The distal oblique band is important in DRUJ stability, but not as much in axial stability [8, 21, 22].

The forearm functions as a unit to provide forearm rotation, stability, and load transfer from the wrist to the elbow. The IOL complex acts to stabilize the forearm and serves as an attachment for the deep flexors in the forearm in addition to transferring load from the radius to the ulna. The radius is important for rotation around the ulna and in load transfer to the capitellum. The radial head is the primary restraint to proximal migration of the radius; however when the radial head is fractured or resected, this primary restraint is lost. The secondary restraints, which are the IOL complex and the TFCC, then become important in preventing proximal migration of the radius [11, 23] and must transfer entire load of radius to the ulna. If the primary and secondary restraints are injured, there is a dissociation between the radius and ulna that allows unabated motion of the radius, thus creating longitudinal radioulnar dissociation.

With an ulnar neutral wrist in zero forearm rotation, the force at the wrist is transmitted through the radius and diminishes at the proximal radius across the radiocapitellar joint [24–26]. Conversely, the ulnar load increases from the wrist to the proximal ulna, suggesting that there is force transferred from distal radius to proximal ulna.

The IOL complex is a soft tissue structure that has been shown to be important for load transfer from the distal radius to the proximal ulna with the most crucial component being the IOL. In the same study that demonstrated transference of load from radius to ulna, data collected after transecting the IOL revealed that the load in the distal radius was equal to that of the proximal radius [25]. Therefore, the IOL becomes

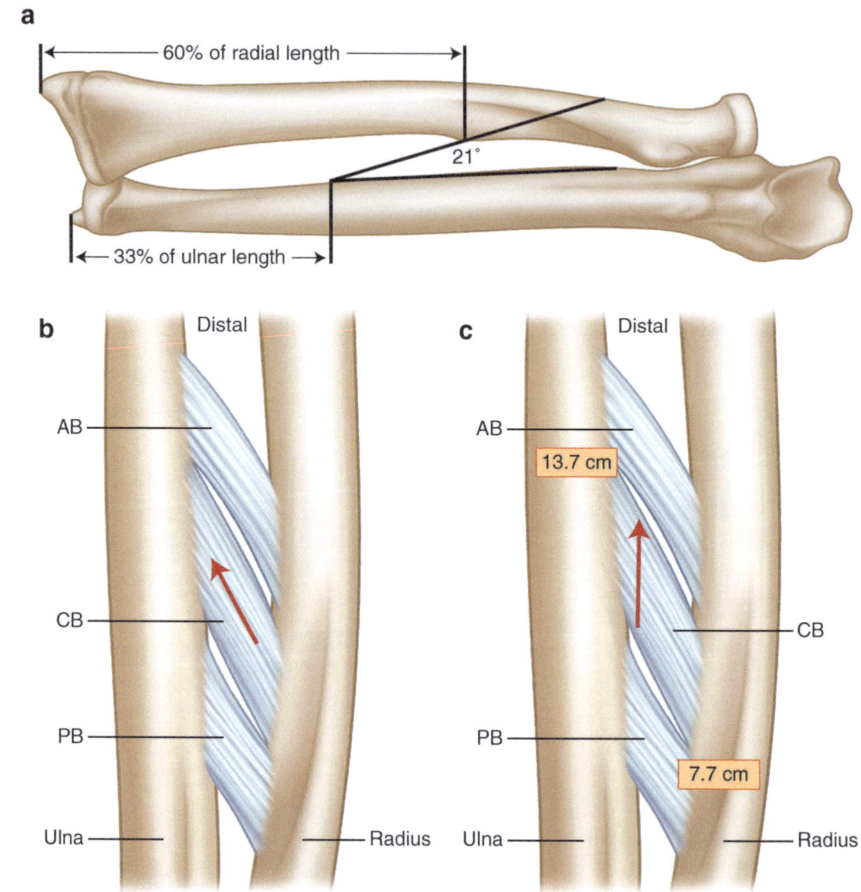

Fig. 24.2 (**a**) Ulnar origin of the interosseous ligament begins one third of the length of the ulna from the ulnar styloid. The insertion is 60% of the length of the radius from the radial styloid. The angle of the ligament from ulna to radius is 21°. These landmarks and values are important to remember when attempting reconstruction. (**b**) The fibers of the central band at a 21° angle as shown by the arrow. (**c**) The origin of the central band from the radius is approximately 7.7 cm from the radial head, and its insertion onto the ulna is 13.7 cm from the olecranon tip. Its width (*arrow*) is 1.1 cm

increasingly important for load transfer in the event that the radiocapitellar articulation is lost.

The increased demand placed on the IOL complex in the absence of an intact radiocapitellar joint may stretch the ligament and account for the various reports of 1–2 mm of asymptomatic proximal migration seen years after radial head resection, seen especially in those who put a greater strain across the IOL complex, such as laborers who use their forearms for strenuous activities [27–32].

In the absence of a radial head, the central band bears 71% of the longitudinal stiffness, while the TFCC is responsible for 8% of the stiffness (Fig. 24.3) [11]. When both of these secondary stabilizers are injured, more than 7 mm of migration can be detected clinically [12]. In addition to transferring load from the radius to ulna, the IOL complex also keeps the forearm bones from separating or bowing through a transverse component [33].

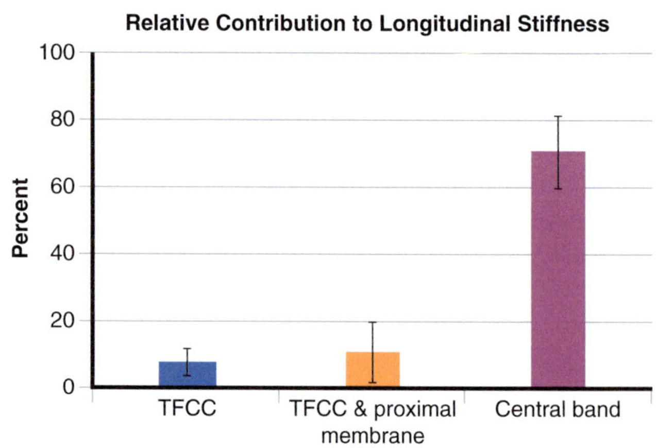

Fig. 24.3 Contribution of each anatomic structure to longitudinal stability. The central band contributes approximately 71% to longitudinal forearm stiffness [11]

Preoperative History and Considerations

History

Patients with longitudinal radioulnar dissociation typically have a history of a forceful axial load to the pronated forearm. Pain in the wrist and forearm in addition to an elbow injury should alert the examiner to the possibility of this diagnosis.

Physical Exam

These patients commonly may have a dorsal prominence of the ulna, decreased extension and ulnar deviation of the wrist, and decreased supination of the forearm. Grip strength will be decreased, and the provocative maneuvers of pronation and power grip will increase wrist pain and reveal increased ulnar variance on radiographs. In acute cases, central band forearm tenderness may be present. These findings must always be compared with the opposite extremity. Stability of the DRUJ in neutral, supination, and pronation should be assessed. Aspiration with intra-articular injection of lidocaine into the elbow can aid with anesthesia for a proper exam and possible reduction. Supination and pronation should be evaluated for the presence of a bony restriction.

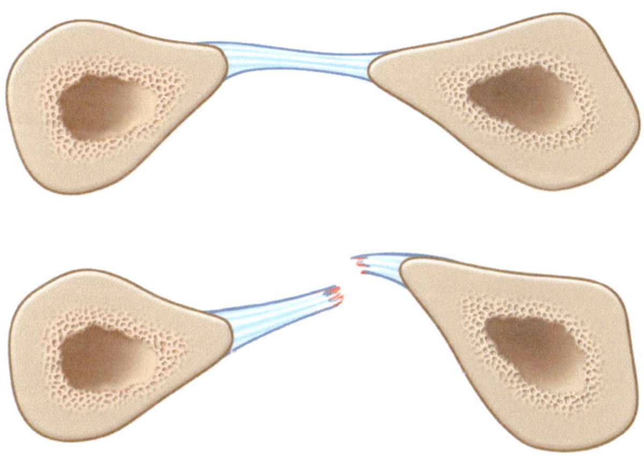

Fig. 24.4 Illustration of a T2-weighted image demonstrating normal IOL and disruption of the IOL on MRI

Diagnostic Modalities

Posteroanterior (PA) and lateral radiographs of the elbow and wrist are standard. Grip views can be helpful in detecting dynamic radial shortening, which is very important in patients with failed radial head resection and wrist pain [34]. An MRI can be used to evaluate the integrity of the IOL complex. On T1-weighted images, the central band appears as a dark line with "crisp detail" [35]. It is best viewed on axial cuts of fat-suppressed T2-weighted images, where an acute injury to the IOL complex can be seen as increased signal intensity around the ligament representing edema and hemorrhage. The linear low-intensity signal in the middle one third of the forearm between the radius and ulna represents the IOL and will be discontinuous with injury (Fig. 24.4) [35]. On ultrasound [36], the IOL complex is a hyperechoic structure that is at least 2 cm in length in the central one third of the forearm and appears as a thick continuous line distinguishable from the muscles (Fig. 24.5). An injured IOL complex appears as a wavy, bowed, and discontinuous band [14, 35]. Both MRI and ultrasound are equivalent in their capacity to diagnose IOL complex pathology. US can be done much quicker and is less expensive than MRI. In addition, it can be used in patients with ferromagnetic implants and in those with

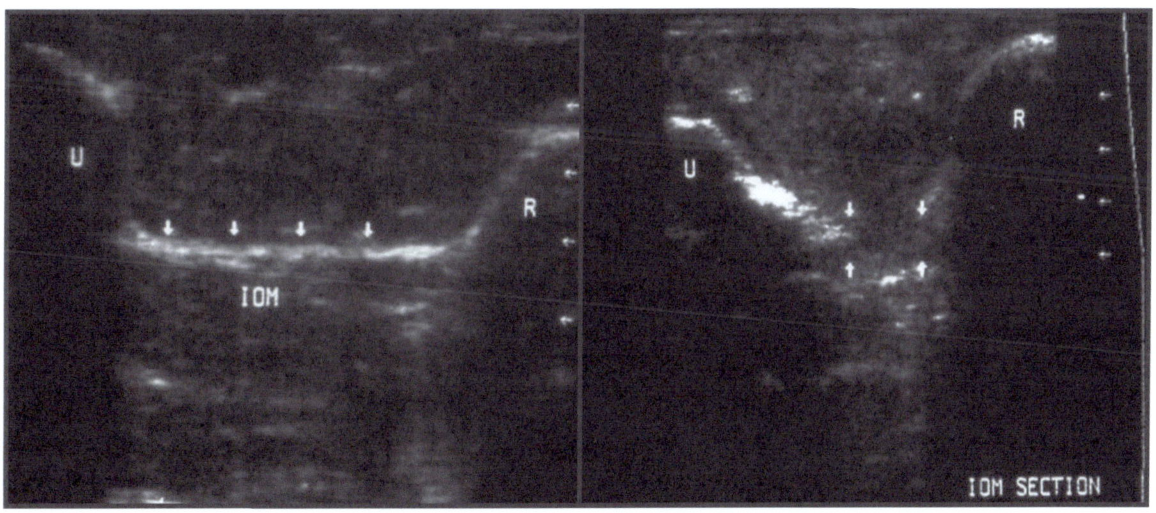

Fig. 24.5 Illustration of a normal IOL as viewed by ultrasound. The second image showing disruption of the IOL

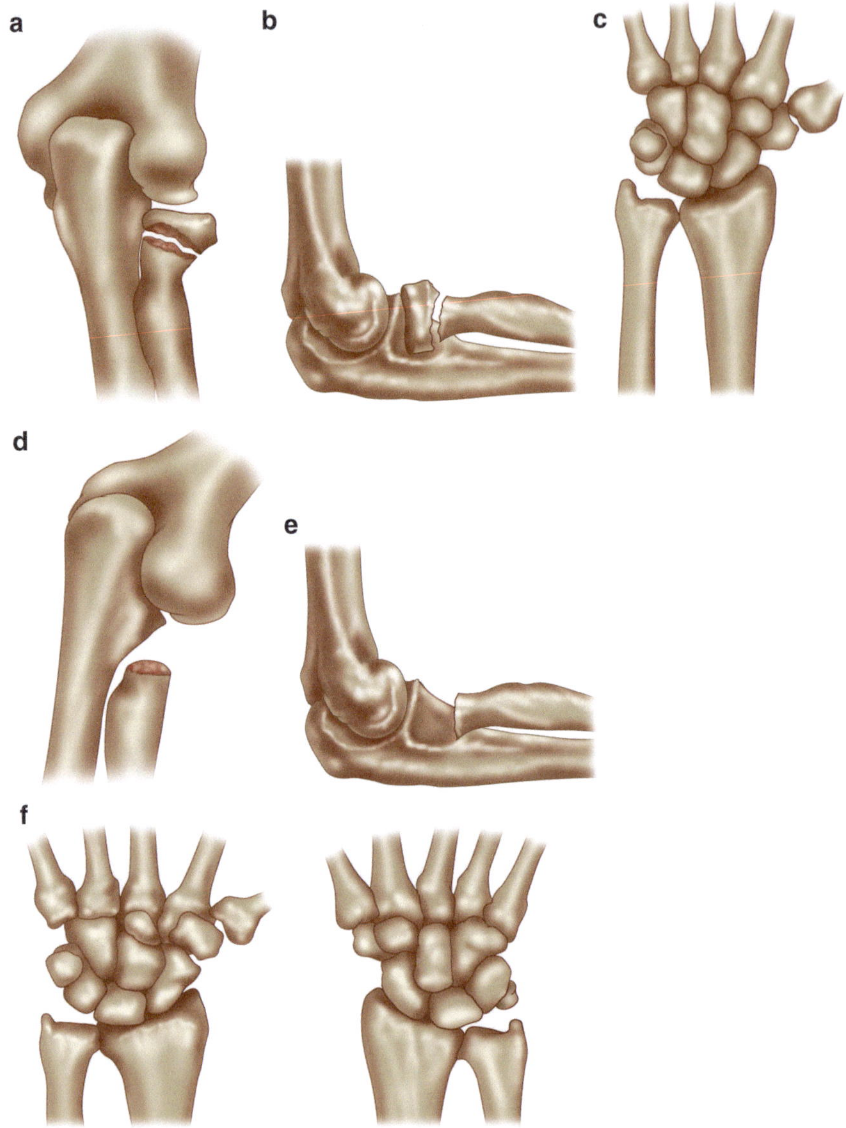

Fig. 24.6 Axial load injury results in a radial head fracture (**a**, **b**). Ulnar positive variance of 2 mm is seen at the initial evaluation (**c**). Radial head resection was performed to treat the fracture (**d**, **e**). However, this has now resulted in worsening of the ulnar positive variance and subsequent wrist pain (**f**)

claustrophobia. Clinically, however, MRI may be more convenient to assess the TFCC at the same time for associated pathology. While they are excellent at visualizing the central band in cadaver studies, they have yet to prove clinically useful in most cases. In acute cases, the diagnosis of longitudinal radioulnar dissociation is confirmed by significant proximal migration of the radius, obvious injury to the DRUJ, or an intraoperative push/pull test. In chronic cases, the diagnosis of proximal radial migration is usually straightforward.

The radius pull test is a useful intraoperative aid [37]. After radial head removal, load is applied with a bone reduction tenaculum to the proximal radius. With the patient's shoulder positioned in 90° of abduction and 90° of internal rotation and the wrist in neutral, imaging is used at the wrist to determine ulnar variance. If 3 mm or more of proximal radial migration is noted, the IOL complex is likely disrupted. A migration of 6 mm or more occurs when both IOL complex and TFCC are incompetent.

Classification

Edwards and Jupiter [5] classified longitudinal radioulnar dissociation into three types. Type I fractures have large displaced radial head fragments that can be fixed with ORIF. Type II fractures are too comminuted for ORIF and require excision and replacement. Type III fractures involve old injuries with irreducible proximal migration of the radius that could be managed with ulnar shortening and radial head prosthetic replacement [5]. Another surgical option for Type III injuries includes reconstruction of the IOL. Longitudinal radioulnar dissociation is distinct from the proximal migration of the radius that occurs slowly over years after radial head excision [27]. Lack of osseous support at the elbow from radial head excision can result in stretch and strain of the IOL complex, resulting in gradual proximal migration of the radius (Fig. 24.6). If this migration becomes symptomatic, the patient can be managed similar to having a Type III injury.

Treatment

Indications and Contraindications

- To avoid proximal migration after excision of radial head in all radial head fractures, the radiocapitellar articulation should be reestablished with either ORIF or prosthetic replacement if IOL injury is suspected.
- Radial head excision only may be appropriate in the setting of axial and valgus stability.
- Currently, metallic implants are recommended for radial head arthroplasty. No study has proven the effectiveness of unipolar over bipolar constructs. There is some concern over the long-term effects of metal on the articular cartilage surface of the capitellum.
- In chronic longitudinal radioulnar dissociation resulting in symptomatic positive ulnar variance, treatment at the wrist is centered on achieving a level joint, most commonly accomplished through an ulnar shortening osteotomy (ulnar shortening osteotomy).
- Ulnar shortening osteotomy should not be used alone as it does not address the forearm instability and there is a tendency for further migration of the radius.
- Reestablishment of longitudinal stability with central band reconstruction and/or prosthetic radial head replacement is often essential to prevent recurrence of symptomatic proximal migration.

Treatment

Acute Longitudinal Radioulnar Dissociation

In an acute longitudinal radioulnar dissociation, each of the three components of the injury should be addressed. If the DRUJ is unstable, arthroscopic or open repair with reattachment of the TFCC is indicated. The radiocapitellar articulation should be reestablished with either ORIF or replacement [38, 39].

Options to address the central band injury include primary repair, transient internal fixation, or reconstruction. While repair is possible by exposing the central band in line with the fifth extensor compartment, we have not found such repairs to be very satisfying. The disrupted ligament is difficult to approximate because of the bowing of the forearm bones and the interposition of muscle. In our acute series, 70% were central disruptions which were repaired with 2–0 PDS suture; the others were bony avulsions repaired with anchors. Without such an approximating repair, there is a real question as to whether the IOM can heal. Transient stabilization by cross pins or a radioulnar screw without such a repair is not predictable. IOM reconstruction has been studied in cadaveric models and performed in patients for the treatment of longitudinal radioulnar dissociation [40–43]. Currently, we favor augmentation of the central band using a pronator teres rerouting graft as described by Ruch and Kuzma [44].

Chronic Longitudinal Radioulnar Dissociation

Treatment of chronic longitudinal radioulnar dissociation at the wrist involves management of ulnocarpal abutment and lesions of the TFCC. Ulnar variance needs to be determined, and if it is symptomatic, treatment at the wrist is centered on achieving a level joint, most commonly accomplished through an ulnar shortening osteotomy (ulnar shortening osteotomy). In the presence of radiocapitellar arthritis secondary to chronic axial instability, a hemielbow arthroplasty may be considered.

Wrist arthroscopy is often done concurrently to assess and debride, if necessary, the TFCC and lunotriquetral ligament. Ulnar shortening does not reestablish longitudinal stability, and thus, a reconstructed IOL and/or a radial head prosthesis is usually required to prevent recurrent symptoms at the wrist. Various tendon grafts have been used in the reconstruction of the IOL. Use of palmaris longus or half of the flexor carpi radialis (FCR) tendon does not provide adequate strength [45]. A single weave of the FCR tendon has been shown to be successful in preventing complete migration of the radius on to the capitellum, but is not capable of restoring longitudinal stability of the forearm [45, 46]. Using Achilles tendon allograft restores approximately 50% of the transferring force of the native IOL [47]. A double FCR weave, however, is an improved approach that provides mechanics across the distal and proximal radius equal to the intact IOL complex [46]. The use of nylon rope to perform a flexible IOL reconstruction by Sellman et al. restored stiffness, but only when the radiocapitellar articulation was restored [48]. Ruch and Kuzma reported the use of the pronator teres transfer to reconstruct the central band in chronic longitudinal radioulnar dissociation. At an average follow-up of 22.75 months, all patients demonstrated clinical improvement and were satisfied with the outcome [44].

We have treated patients for chronic longitudinal radioulnar dissociation injuries with ulnar shortening osteotomy and bone-ligament-bone reconstruction using a patellar tendon graft. This bone-ligament-bone construct most closely simulates the mechanical qualities of the deficient central band [40]. Sixteen patients were treated with this procedure in the initial prospective series [16]. Concomitant procedures included radial head excision (1), removal of radial head prosthesis (2), wrist arthroscopy (3), DRUJ resection (1), Suave-Kapandji (1), and carpal tunnel release (1).

The initial diagnoses were radial head fracture (7), radial head fracture with posterior dislocation (2), Monteggia fracture (3), radial head fracture with distal radius fracture (1), and Essex-Lopresti fracture (2). IOL instability was identified an average of 10 months after radial head excision (range of 2 months to 12 years), with 75% of patients presenting within 2 years. The average ulnar variance was 3 mm (range of 2–5 mm) on standard PA radiographs [16].

At 78 months postoperatively, 15 of 16 patients had improved wrist pain. No patient was worse in terms of pain or function than before surgery. None had radiocapitellar impingement, and none needed secondary surgery for forearm instability. Grip strength improved from 59% to 86% of the unaffected limb. Ten of the 14 patients who were previously employed returned to their regular work duties, while 3 of the 14 required job modification. Initial postoperative ulnar variance was −2 mm (range of −4 mm to +1 mm) and on follow-up averaged −1.5 mm (range −3 mm to +1 mm). Complications included one ulnar nonunion, one ulnar delayed union, one patient with extensor tendon adhesions, and four patients with knee aches. To avoid the complication of knee pain, we have begun to use bone-patellar tendon-bone allograft [16].

Tejwani et al. [40] measured the abilities of 3 graft tissues (palmaris longus tendon, FCR tendon, and a 1-cm bone-patellar tendon-bone allograft) to limit proximal radial displacement compared with the native IOM in a radial head-deficient cadaver model. The bone-patellar tendon-bone allograft allowed the least proximal radial displacement and displayed the least permanent elongation after 10 cycles of mechanical loading of the wrist.

One-Bone Forearm

The final salvage procedure to prevent the proximal migration of the distal radius is to create a radioulnar arthrodesis. Hey-Groves initially described this procedure in 1921 as the construction of an osseous bridge between the ulna and radius to provide functional stability to the forearm [49]. Radioulnar arthrodesis can be accomplished by creation of a one-bone forearm or radioulnar synostosis [50]. The creation of a one-bone forearm is defined by the end-to-end fusion of the distal radius to the proximal ulna. A radioulnar synostosis procedure is defined by side-to-side juxtaposition of the distal radius shaft and proximal ulna shaft stabilized by internal fixation across the proposed fusion site. Both methods essentially create a single-bone forearm [50]. The forearm is fused in a neutral or slightly pronated position and provides a stable lever to facilitate hand function, but at the expense of forearm rotation [50–52]. In failed radioulnar synostosis procedures, the combination of plate osteosynthesis and bone grafting together has established union [50].

Vascularized Fibula Bone Graft

Segmental defects of the forearm bones can result from tumor resection, following trauma or debridement of osteomyelitis/infected nonunions, previous failed attempts at bone healing by other means, and nonunions from radiation necrosis [53–55]. Taylor reported the first successful free vascularized fibular transfer in 1975, when he used a fibular segment from the opposite lower extremity to reconstruct a large tibial defect [56]. Autogenous nonvascularized bone grafts for reconstruction of large skeletal extremity defects have obvious limitations including prolonged time for bone union or failure to achieve union. The advantages of vascularized bone grafts over nonvascularized grafts for large segmental bony defects of the extremity have been well described [57–62] in the literature. When autologous bone is harvested using conventional means, only the surface osteocytes survive the transfer [53]. The remaining bone becomes necrotic within a week, and diffuse marrow fibrosis can be anticipated [60]. Viable bone eventually surrounds and replaces the necrotic bone, called "creeping substitution" [61]. The replacement of nonvascularized necrotic bone is incomplete, with a net decrease in overall transferred osseous volume [53, 62]. Graft hypertrophy is a phenomenon seen only in vascularized bone transfers. It is not seen following conventional bone grafting [53].

The actual length of the bony defect requiring free vascularized bone transfer continues to be debated. Long bone defects exceeding 6 cm have been considered an indication for free vascularized bone transfer [53, 63–65]. Alternatively, Enneking has shown that in defects as large as 10 cm, healing with conventional bone grafting techniques can be anticipated if an adequate soft tissue envelope exists [53, 66]. Similarly large defects have been reconstructed with allograft bone [67]. In most situations, a long bone defect between 6 and 10 cm is justification for a free vascularized bone graft procedure [53]. Vascularized fibular segments 24 cm or greater can be harvested with a peroneal artery pedicle up to 8 cm. Weiland and several other authors [59, 63, 64, 68–70] have described the use of vascularized bone grafts in the treatment of a variety of extremity conditions, including tumor resection, posttraumatic bone defects, and congenital pseudoarthrosis. Specific indications for the use of vascularized bone grafts in upper extremity disorders have been outlined [71–74].

The presence of peripheral vascular disease is a contraindication to harvest the fibula from the diseased extremity. Other contraindications described in the literature include patients with multiple cardiac risk factors, current substantial smoking history, and previous lower extremity vascular trauma [53].

The proximal fibula has been used for vascularized hemiarthroplasty at the distal radius [75–78], in order to preserve wrist motion. However, in our practice, we have found this procedure to be associated with instability and pain at the wrist secondary to distal radioulnar incongruity and articular malalignment, as reported in other studies as well [71]. Arthrodesis with a vascularized bone graft after long-segment distal radius resection offers a more stable, pain-free grasp with the preservation of pronation and supination.

Cases 24.1–24.3 are individual cases of forearm reconstruction with vascularized free fibula.

Operative Approach: Authors' Preferred Technique

Ulnar Shortening Osteotomy and Bone-Ligament-Bone Reconstruction of Interosseous Membrane with Allograft in Chronic Longitudinal Radioulnar Dissociation (Fig. 24.7)

The wrist must be examined under anesthesia and ulnar variance confirmed under fluoroscopy. The prepped hand and arm is placed in a wrist traction tower, and a diagnostic and therapeutic wrist arthroscopy is performed to evaluate and document the ulnar impaction which is commonly present in this scenario. A fibrillated lunotriquetral ligament and the central TFCC tear are debrided.

A skin incision is made along the subcutaneous border of the ulna, extending longitudinally for about 14 cm. The fascia is incised between the ECU and the FCU. The dorsoulnar sensory nerve and ulnar vascular bundle are identified and protected. The ulna is exposed extraperiosteally. A 3.5-mm dynamic compression plate or one of the ulnar shortening osteotomy specific plates is applied over the ulna's dorsal surface, with its distal edge about 1 cm proximal to the sigmoid notch. Care is taken not to disrupt the sheath of the extensor carpi ulnaris. If a standard compression plate is chosen, the two most distal screws are inserted neutrally. The osteotomy site must be marked on the ulna either with the oscillating saw or electrocautery. A longitudinal mark is made to ensure proper rotational alignment after the osteotomy. The plate can be swung away from the ulna after the most distal screw is loosened and the other screw removed. An oblique cut is made at the marked osteotomy site with a second cut made parallel to it. The width of the osteotomy is predetermined to achieve an ulnar negative variance of 2 mm. If the ulnar positive variance is greater than 4 or 5 mm, then an external compression device is helpful in achieving the desired shortening. The plate is swung back in place, and the distal screws are replaced and tightened. One or two proximal screws are inserted eccentrically in the dynamic compression mode. An interfragmentary compression screw is inserted across the oblique osteotomy. Bone graft from the osteotomy site is morselized and placed at the osteotomy site. Fluoroscopy is used to confirm adequate position of the screws as well as to confirm the ulnar negative variance of 2 mm at the radioulnar joint.

An autograft or allograft bone-ligament-bone using the patellar ligament is then fashioned to round wafers of bone. Starting ulnarly at the midportion of the ulnar shaft, a Kelly clamp is used to start dissecting beneath the extensors in the plane of the IOMs, toward the radius. Care is taken to protect the anterior and posterior interosseous nerves. Staying in this plane, the dissecting Kelly clamp is brought over the dorsal radius. A counter incision is made over the Kelly clamp on the proximal radius. The dorsal radial sensory nerve is avoided. The wrist extensors and brachioradialis are identified. The radius shaft is exposed in the plane between the brachioradialis and the radial wrist extensors.

The bone-ligament-bone (bone-ligament-bone) graft is then levered into place. It is attached distally first by creating a trough in the ulna at the level of midplate, just proximal to the osteotomy site. The bone wafer of the bone-ligament-bone graft is then laid in this trough and fixed in place with an AO screw. The tension is set with the forearm in neutral to midsupination, and the bone-ligament-bone graft is directed proximally at an angle of 20° toward the radius. At the point on the radius, where the bone-ligament-bone graft meets it, a trough is made with a burr. The proximal bone wafer of the bone-ligament-bone graft is placed in this trough and fixed with an AO screw. Fluoroscopy is used to confirm the placement of the bone-ligament-bone allograft. The forearm motion is tested for full pronation and supination, and stability at the DRUJ is also assessed.

Optimizing Outcomes

Applying autogenous bone graft at the ulnar shortening osteotomy site in addition to compression provided by the plate encourages healing of the osteotomy.

Establishing ulnar variance at 2 mm negative allows for some subsidence over time.

The bone-ligament-bone graft used to reconstruct the IOM must be fixed distally before it is fixed proximally. It is essential to ensure that the tension in the graft is set with the forearm in neutral to midsupination and the graft directed proximally at an angle of 20° toward the radius, before it is fixed proximally at the radius.

The anterior and posterior interosseous nerves as well as the dorsal ulnar and radial sensory nerves must be identified and protected.

Complications

Complications include ulnar nonunion or delayed union, joint stiffness more at the wrist than the elbow, nerve injury especially to the posterior interosseous or the dorsal radial sensory nerve, and extensor tendon adhesions.

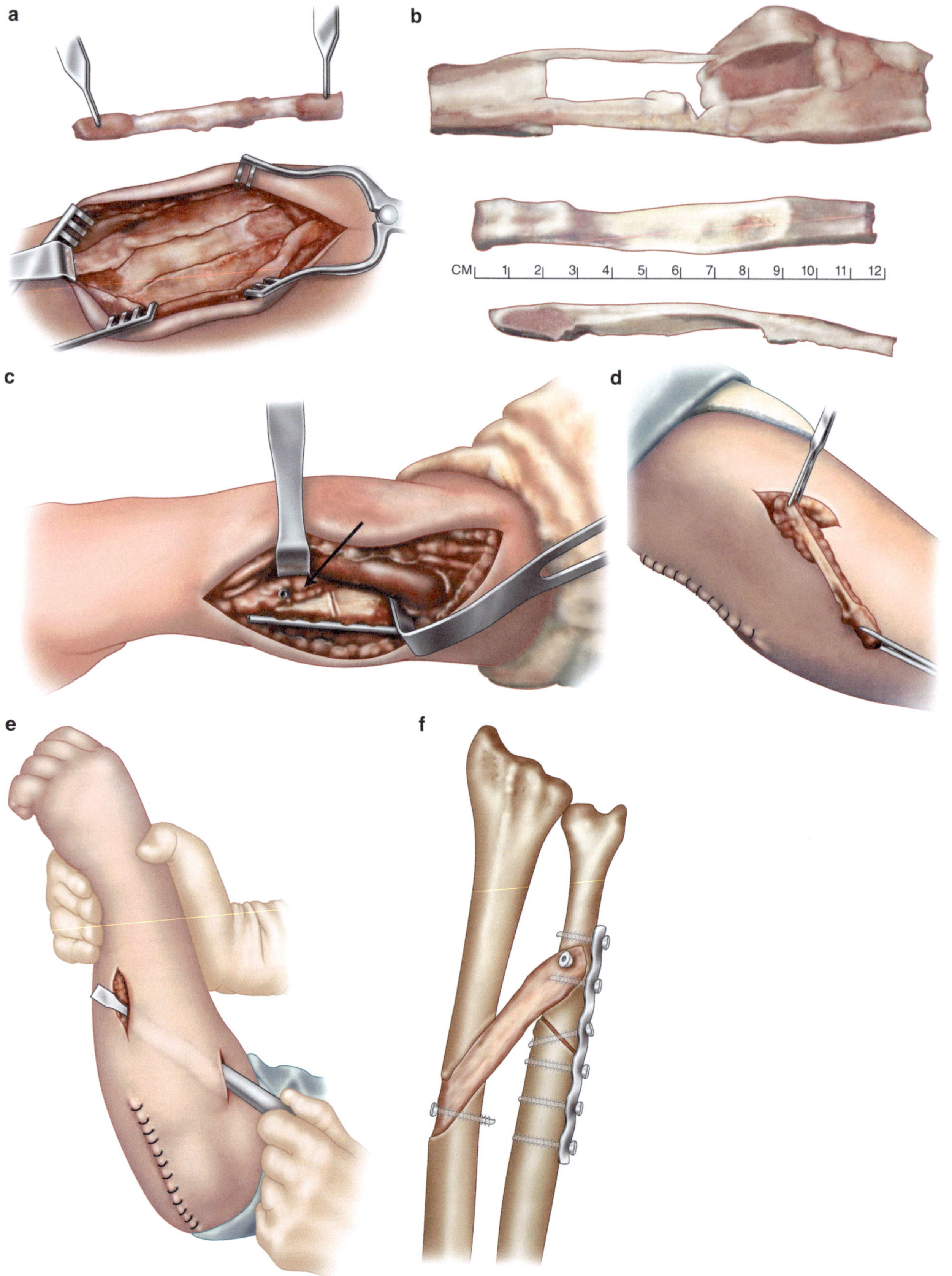

Fig. 24.7 (**a**) Illustration of patellar tendon graft used for bone-ligament-bone reconstruction of the IOM. (**b**) To avoid the complication of knee pain, we have begun to use bone-patellar tendon-bone allograft. (**c**) After completion of the ulnar shortening osteotomy, the graft is attached distally at the osteotomy site (*note arrow*). (**d**, **e**) The graft is then directed at an acute angle to the radius so that it can be attached to the radius proximally. The tension is set with the forearm in neutral to midsupination. The plane of dissection is beneath the extensors. (**f**) The bone wafers of the BLB graft are laid in troughs burred into the ulna and radius and fixed with AO screws

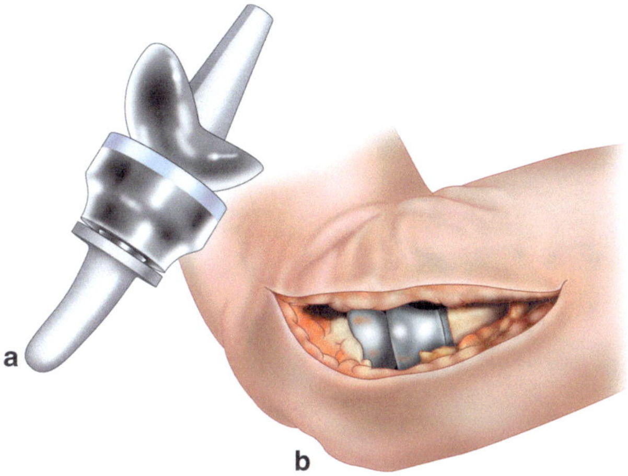

Fig. 24.8 (**a**) Radiocapitellum replacement system (Small Bone Innovations, Inc.). (**b**) Radiocapitellar prosthesis in place

Postoperative Care

Postoperatively, a long arm splint at 90° of elbow flexion and neutral forearm rotation is used. After 1–2 weeks, a thermoplastic splint with the same specifications is used by the patient for 4–6 weeks, removing only for range-of-motion activities. On day 10, wrist and elbow active range of motion (AROM) is begun with neutral forearm rotation. At week 6, AROM of the forearm is also begun, followed by assisted AROM at week 8. Passive ROM is not allowed at this time point. At week 10, strengthening and passive ROM is begun, avoiding rotational stress.

Hemielbow Arthroplasty (Fig. 24.8)

If there is radiocapitellar arthritis with longitudinal radioulnar dissociation, we prefer use of the UNI-Elbow™, a radio capitellum replacement system (*Small Bone Innovations, Inc.*) over radial head prosthetic replacement. In our opinion, this articulating prosthesis will tolerate axial load better than a metal radial head on capitellar cartilage.

The elbow is examined under anesthesia to assess lateral collateral complex stability. A classic Kocher skin incision is made, identifying the interval between the anconeus and the extensor carpi ulnaris. The dissection is carried down to the joint capsule. The extensor carpi ulnaris may be split longitudinally in line with its fibers staying anterior to the attachment of the lateral collateral ligament. The lateral capsule is divided slightly anterior to the collateral ligament, and the annular ligament and capsule are reflected anteriorly and posteriorly, respectively, to expose the radiohumeral joint.

The axis of rotation locator clamp and capitellum template are assembled. Using image intensification, a drill guide is placed against the lateral epicondyle and aligned. A 0.062 K-wire is placed through the drill guide and advanced into the capitellum. The K-wire should be advanced to the midline of the distal humerus when viewed on the posteroanterior plane. Care should be taken not to extend the K-wire through the medial epicondyle. Leaving the K-wire in place, remove the axis of rotation locator clamp and template. The resection guide is placed and cut for the appropriately sized prosthesis. Care is taken not to disrupt the trochlea. Sizing is performed and the appropriate capitellar trial is placed. Next, the radial head is prepared. A resection guide and appropriate broaches are used. Sizing is performed and the appropriate radial head trial is placed. With the capitellar and radial head trials in place, the elbow is carried through flexion, extension, supination, and pronation with image intensification confirming trial tracking and alignment. The capitellum is also broached, and the definitive capitellar and radial head implants are placed. The wound is closed by simple reapproximation of the Kocher interval. Final fluoroscopy images of the elbow are taken, confirming stability and alignment of the prosthesis. A pivot shift test must also be performed, confirming preservation of the collateral ligament complex. If unstable, the ligament must be reconstructed.

Optimizing Outcomes

Care must be taken to preserve the lateral collateral ligament complex and avoid injury to the trochlea.

Complications

Infection of the prosthesis is a dreaded complication of any joint replacement, and meticulous soft tissue handling and antibiotic prophylaxis are important.

Inadvertent injury to the lateral collateral ligament complex is a possibility. This must be recognized intraoperatively and repaired.

The radial nerve must be protected.

Postoperative Care

Postoperatively, the extremity is placed in a long arm splint in 90° of flexion and 30° of pronation. On day 10, AROM of the elbow is begun. At week 3, assisted AROM is begun, avoiding combined elbow extension and supination. PROM is begun at 4 weeks, followed by strengthening at 6–8 weeks.

Vascularized Free Fibula Flap (Cases 24.1–24.3)

The patient is positioned supine with the entire leg draped free. The fibula is measured, and its middle third is identified. In a cadaveric study [79], we have shown that the most reliably found skin branch was located within 2 cm of the fibula midpoint. Skin branches from the distal two thirds of the peroneal artery were usually affixed to the posterior crural septum. Our cadaveric study [79] reinforced the fact that a large skin island supplied by branches of the peroneal artery can be

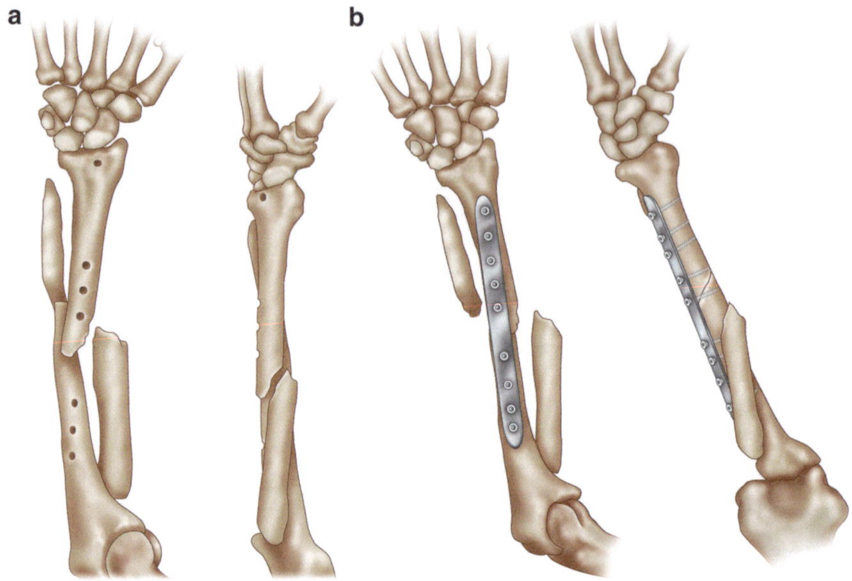

Fig. 24.9 (**a**) Illustration of a forearm after multiple procedures including a radial head resection and distal ulna resection presenting with a floating forearm, unstable distal ulna stump, and severe pain at the wrist and elbow.(**b**) Illustration of a one-bone forearm in treating the aforementioned problem. A seven-hole locking plate is applied to bridge the distal radius stump transferred onto the proximal ulna stump. This procedure can result in a stable forearm with resolution of pain and improvement in grip strength

harvested with the fibula flap, and that the most reliable cutaneous vessels are found in the lower two thirds of the leg, running posterior to the fibula in the posterior crural septum.

After inflation of the tourniquet, an incision is made directly along the fibular longitudinal axis laterally and taken down through skin and subcutaneous tissue. The anterior border of the skin flap is incised, and the interval between the peroneus longus muscle and the soleus is identified. This interval is developed with blunt dissection, beginning in the middle third of the bone. The cutaneous vascular perforators supplying the skin may be visualized passing through the posterior crural septum or through the adjacent soleus. Dissection is continued progressively proximally, elevating the soleus from the fibula. Next, the lateral compartment muscles are elevated from the fibula protecting the peroneal nerve at all times. The anterior compartment is elevated next, and the anterior tibial artery as well as the IOM is identified. The bone is divided proximally and distally with a Gigli saw, protecting neurovascular structures. Although the entire proximal fibula may be harvested if the articular surface or physis is required, 7–8 cm of distal fibula should be preserved to prevent valgus instability of the ankle.

The IOM is divided and the peroneal artery is identified at the distal osteotomy and ligated. The vessels are tagged to facilitate proximal dissection of the vessel. Dissection then proceeds from distal to proximal. The tibialis posterior and flexor hallucis muscles are divided to expose the peroneal vessels. Multiple perforators to these muscles must be identified and ligated while protecting the underlying peroneal vessels.

The vessels are dissected as far proximally as possible to their origin from the posterior tibial artery. After separation of the artery and venae comitantes, the venae comitantes may be dissected more proximally past the bifurcation of the peroneal and posterior tibial vessels, depending on the length of vein required. Planning to harvest this additional length of venae comitantes may help avoid harvesting saphenous vein graft in situations where additional vein length is required.

At this point, the sole remaining attachment of the fibula is its peroneal vessel pedicle. The tourniquet is then released, and the osteocutaneous fibula flap is allowed to perfuse while careful hemostasis is obtained in the leg. We recommend perfusion for at least 30 min prior to dividing the pedicle, to allow drainage of oxygen-derived free radicals formed during reperfusion of the limb. Following this, the artery and veins in the pedicle are occluded with microvascular clamps, ligated proximally, and divided to detach the flap.

Optimizing Outcomes

The skin paddle included in the osteocutaneous free fibula flap should ideally be in the middle third of the fibula, as the most reliably found skin branch is located within 2 cm of the fibula midpoint.

While the peroneal artery has to be divided at the point of bifurcation of the posterior tibial artery proximally, the venae comitantes accompanying the peroneal artery may be dissected for a longer distance proximally to obtain additional length of vein when required and thus avoid harvesting saphenous vein to be used as vein graft.

The osteocutaneous fibula flap must be allowed to perfuse for at least 30 min prior to division of the pedicle, to allow for drainage of oxygen-derived free radicals that are produced during reperfusion.

Performing a careful preoperative evaluation of donor leg suitability is essential as the presence of peripheral vascular disease would preclude the use of that extremity as the donor leg for fibula harvest.

Complications

Reported recipient site complications include nonunion, malunion, infection, stress fracture, nerve injury, compartment syndrome, free graft microvascular failure, and flexor/extensor tendon dysfunction [65, 68, 69, 80–82]. Donor site complications include hammertoe formation, paresthesias, weakness, pain, ankle instability, subjective discomfort, slower gait, and loss of ankle or knee motion [53, 83–87].

Postoperative Care

Immediately postoperatively, the forearm is placed in a long arm splint with a window to monitor the flap. Two weeks postoperatively, the long arm splint is changed to a long arm cast. Range-of-motion exercises are begun when radiographic union is seen.

One-Bone Forearm (Fig. 24.9)

Our preferred technique is a direct radius to ulnar transfer rather than a syndesmotic technique. A 16-cm dorsal incision is started at the distal third of the radius and continued proximally toward the ulna. A forearm fasciotomy is done from the proximal extensor retinaculum to the proximal third of the forearm. The radius is exposed from the ulnar side, elevating the second extensor compartment.

The ulna is exposed subperiosteally beneath the extensors. The radius and ulna are mobilized leaving the pronator segment intact on the proximal radial fragment. The anterior and posterior interosseous nerves are identified and protected. The radius and ulna are obliquely cut at their midshaft levels, maintaining rotational alignment and length. The very proximal portion of the distal ulna stump as well as some of the radius is excised to be used as bone graft. With the arm in 60° of pronation, a direct transfer of the distal radius stump onto the proximal ulna stump is performed, noting rotational alignment. This alignment is locked into position with provisional pins and confirmed under fluoroscopy. A seven-hole locking plate is then applied to bridge the distal radius stump now transferred onto the proximal ulna stump. Ideally 6 (and minimum 4) cortices must be engaged proximal and distal to the union. An interfragmentary screw is applied at the site of union, where morselized bone graft is placed after completion of plate application. Fluoroscopy is used to confirm adequate plate placement and the wrist and elbow are evaluated as well, to confirm the absence of ulnar or radial translation at these joints.

The tourniquet is taken down and hemostasis is achieved. Wounds are closed in layers over a Hemovac drain. Sterile dressings are applied. Final X-rays of the elbow, forearm, and wrist in posteroanterior, lateral, and oblique views are obtained, and a long arm splint is applied.

Optimizing Outcomes

Use of autogenous bone graft with a locking plate encourages union. Pronation as the position of fusion was preferable to our patients as it allows for keyboard use.

Complications

Nonunion is the most common complication. This is treated by revision procedures as described below.

Postoperative Care

Postoperatively, the arm is placed in a long arm splint for 1–2 weeks with elbow in 90° of flexion and forearm in 60° of pronation. Following removal of sutures at first follow-up visit, the arm is placed in an orthoplast splint with the same specifications for a total of 6–8 weeks postoperatively. At week 6, AROM of wrist and elbow is begun. At week 8, after confirmation of adequate bony healing, assisted AROM of wrist and elbow is allowed avoiding rotational stress. Strengthening is begun at week 10.

Revision of the Ununited Radioulnar Arthrodesis [50]

Prior incisions are used when possible. The surgical approach is dorsal and similar to the one-bone forearm procedure (as described above) in all our cases [50]. The position of arthrodesis is 10–25° of pronation in each patient. We used the following three methods.

Plating of Distal Radius Shaft to Proximal Ulna in End-to-End Fashion (Revision of the One-Bone Forearm) (Fig. 24.10)

These patients underwent takedown of their nonunion site with subsequent fixation of the distal radius stump end-on to the proximal ulna with a dynamic compression plate (Fig. 24.10). The remaining proximal stump was not incorporated into the arthrodesis and was merely left free. Autogenous bone graft obtained from the iliac crest was added to the arthrodesis site. Demineralized bone matrix was used instead of iliac crest graft in the morbidly obese.

Side-to-Side Arthrodesis of the Radius and Ulna Using an S-Plate (Radioulnar Synostosis) (Fig. 24.11)

These patients underwent takedown of the nonunion site and subsequent fixation with a 3.5-mm reconstruction plate contoured in an S-fashion to incorporate the previous synostosis site into the dorsal plate fixation of the distal radius shaft to the proximal ulna segment. Additional transverse compression screws spanning the previous synostosis site were also used to augment the fixation, and autogenous cancellous bone graft from the iliac crest was added to the site of arthrodesis.

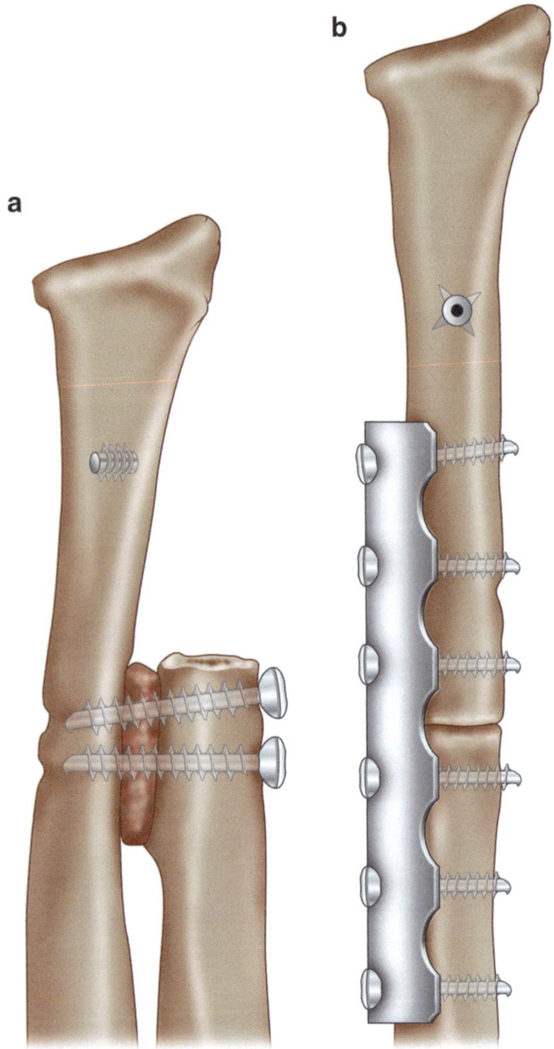

Fig. 24.10 (**a**, **b**) Image depicting a failed radioulnar synostosis procedure (**a**). Revision of the ununited synostosis one-bone forearm to a traditional distal radius to proximal ulna one-bone forearm

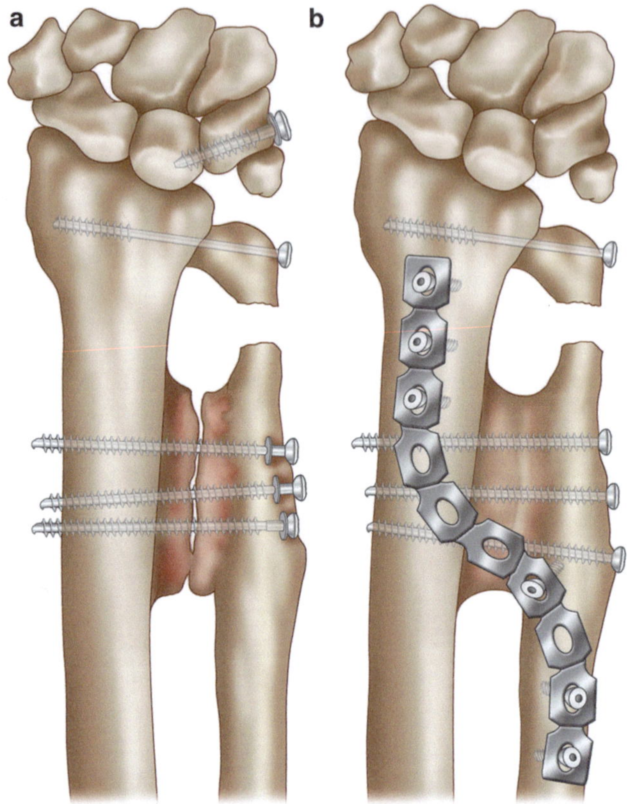

Fig. 24.11 (**a**, **b**) Image showing a failed radioulnar synostosis with a healed Suave-Kapandji procedure (**a**). Revision imaging showing a dorsal plate contoured in an "S"-type fashion to bridge the synostosis nonunion and well as aggressive bone grafting

Side-to-Side Arthrodesis of the Radius and Ulna with Screw/Pins (Radioulnar Synostosis)

This involved takedown of the pseudoarthrosis with replacement of the transverse screws, followed by local bone grafting from the proximal ulna or autogenous iliac crest repeat bone grafting with retention of the majority of the traversing large Steinmann pins. An additional radial counterincision is used in the latter case.

Optimizing Outcomes

Rigid fixation between the radius and ulna is essential for successfully establishing union. Use of a rigid compression plate facilitates the healing process by primary bone healing as the fracture gap is reduced, enabling capillary and Haversian extension across the fusion site [88].

Bone morphogenetic proteins (BMPs) are being used for their osteoinductive properties to promote bone union. The recombinant human BMPs extensively studied are rh-OP-1 (osteogenic protein 1), rh-BMP-2 (Genetics Institute, Cambridge, MA), and rh-BMP-7 (Creative Biomolecules, Hopkinton, MA) [89]. The osteogenic activity of OP-1 has been proven in a validated critically sized fibular defect in human subjects [90]. INFUSE (Medtronic Sofamor Danek, Minneapolis, MN) is a new investigational material containing genetically engineered recombinant human BMP-2 with a collagen sponge carrier. A prospective randomized controlled human clinical pilot trial had shown definite evidence of osteoinduction with the use of rh-BMP-2 in interbody fusion cages for single-level lumbar degenerative disk disease [91].

OP-1 and INFUSE can be applied at the site of arthrodesis to induce differentiation of undifferentiated stem cells to osteogenic cells or induce stem cells to proliferate and thus promote bony union.

Complications

Of the two patients in our series [50] who underwent revision without plate fixation, one progressed to union and the other had persistent symptomatic nonunion despite two revision attempts. Based on our series [50] and peer-reviewed literature, we advocate use of plate fixation with aggressive bone grafting for revision of failed radioulnar synostosis.

Postoperative Care

All patients are placed in a long arm cast in 10–25° of pronation and 90° of elbow flexion for 4–6 weeks, followed by a clam shell orthoplast splint and initiation of occupational therapy.

Conclusion

Forearm instability can result from trauma, infection with bone loss, tumor resection, or congenital malformation.

In traumatic longitudinal radioulnar dissociation (Essex-Lopresti), proximal migration of the radius may result if the stability of the forearm is not reestablished. To prevent this migration, the fractured radial head as the primary stabilizer must be fixed or replaced. Attention must also be directed to the secondary stabilizers, the central band of the IOM and the TFCC. In the acute injury, a pronator teres augmentation is used in conjunction with repair. In the chronic longitudinal radioulnar dissociation, we prefer a patellar bone-ligament-bone allograft in association with ulnar shortening osteotomy to neutralize the variance.

If radiocapitellar impingement arthritis is present, then lateral compartment arthroplasty using either an anconeus technique [92] or more recently a UNI-Elbow™ replacement may be considered.

Forearm instability in the setting of structural bone defects presents a difficult reconstructive challenge. Treatment of these angular, axial, and rotational deformities with their associated bone loss is problematic. Nonoperative management includes functional bracing or activity modification [51]. The surgical management of the incompetent forearm can include several options: structural or nonstructural bone grafting with rigid internal fixation, vascularized bone transfer or osteogenic bone transport. When these procedures fail, radioulnar arthrodesis can be performed as a salvage procedure. In select cases, radioulnar arthrodesis may be preferred as a primary option [50].

Case 24.1

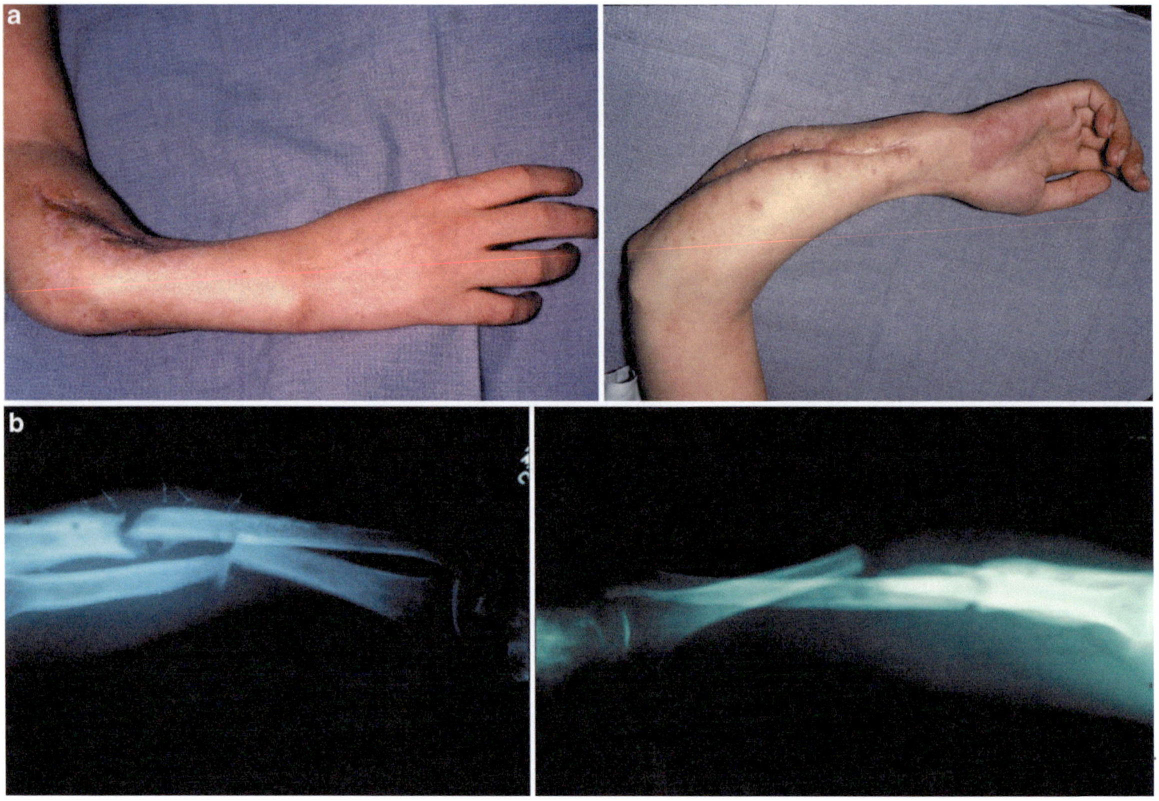

(**a** and **b**) Initial presentation—28-year-old male with flail right arm due to infected nonunion of compound fractures of both radius and ulna (s/p multiple operations including sequestrectomies of the infected nonunions).

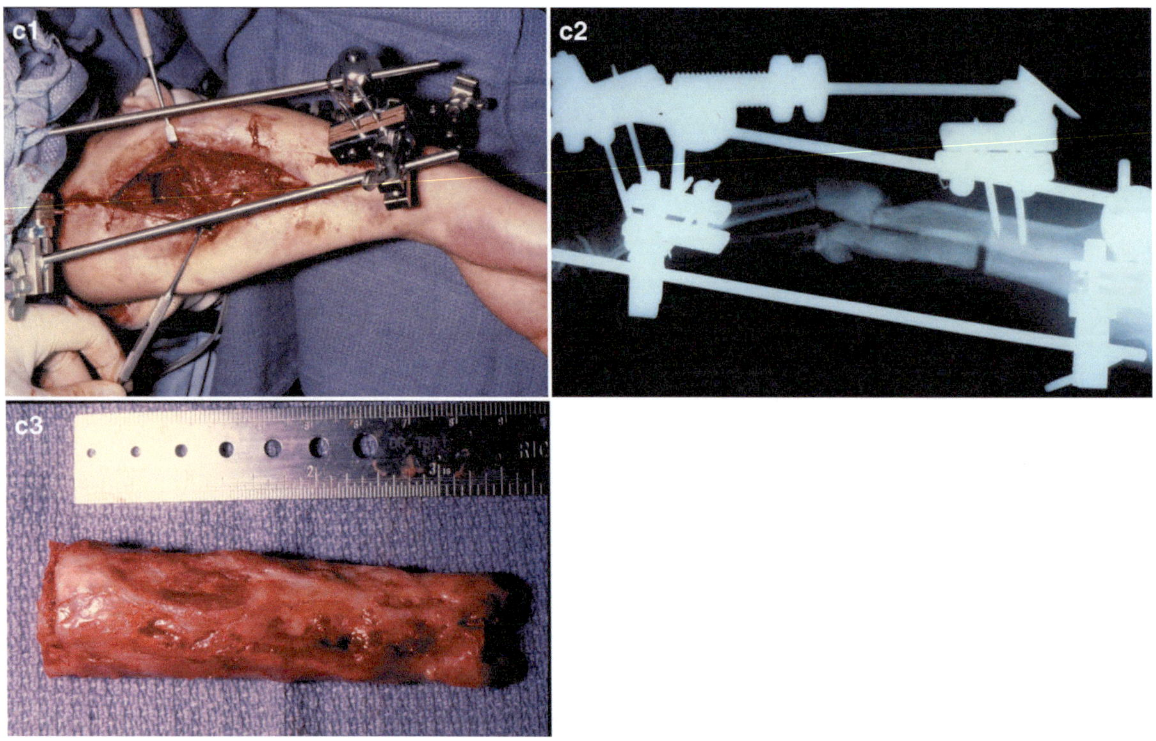

(**c**) Initially underwent segmental bone resection (2.5 cm of radius and 7.5 cm of ulna) and interposition of antibiotic-impregnated bone cement.

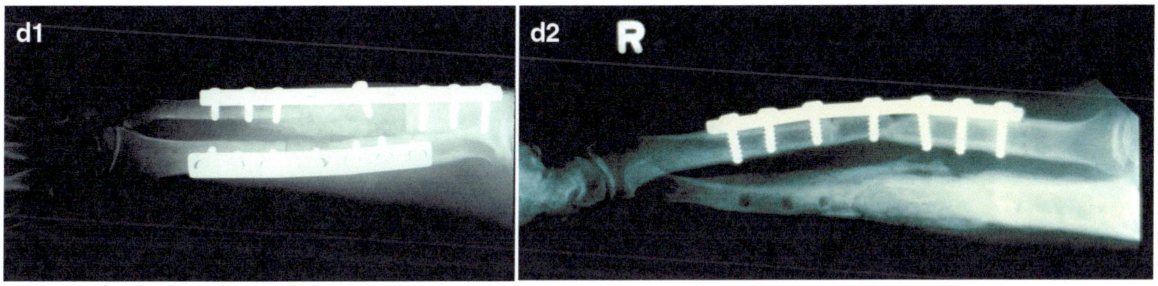

(**d**) Four weeks later, removal of external fixator and open reduction and internal fixation (ORIF) of long bones with iliac crest bone graft (ICBG). Four weeks after ORIF, presented with draining osteomyelitis of ulna and excision of ICBG to ulna, removal of plate, insertion of tobramycin cement, and replating of the large ulnar defect. One week later, bone cement was trimmed leaving a cylinder the same diameter as the ulna plus a bridge of cancellous bone graft from the iliac crest. Two months later, presented again with purulent drainage from ulna. Therefore underwent removal of ulnar plate and second cancellous bone grafting (from iliac crest) to ulna, held in place by the periosteal envelope. The radius was healing.

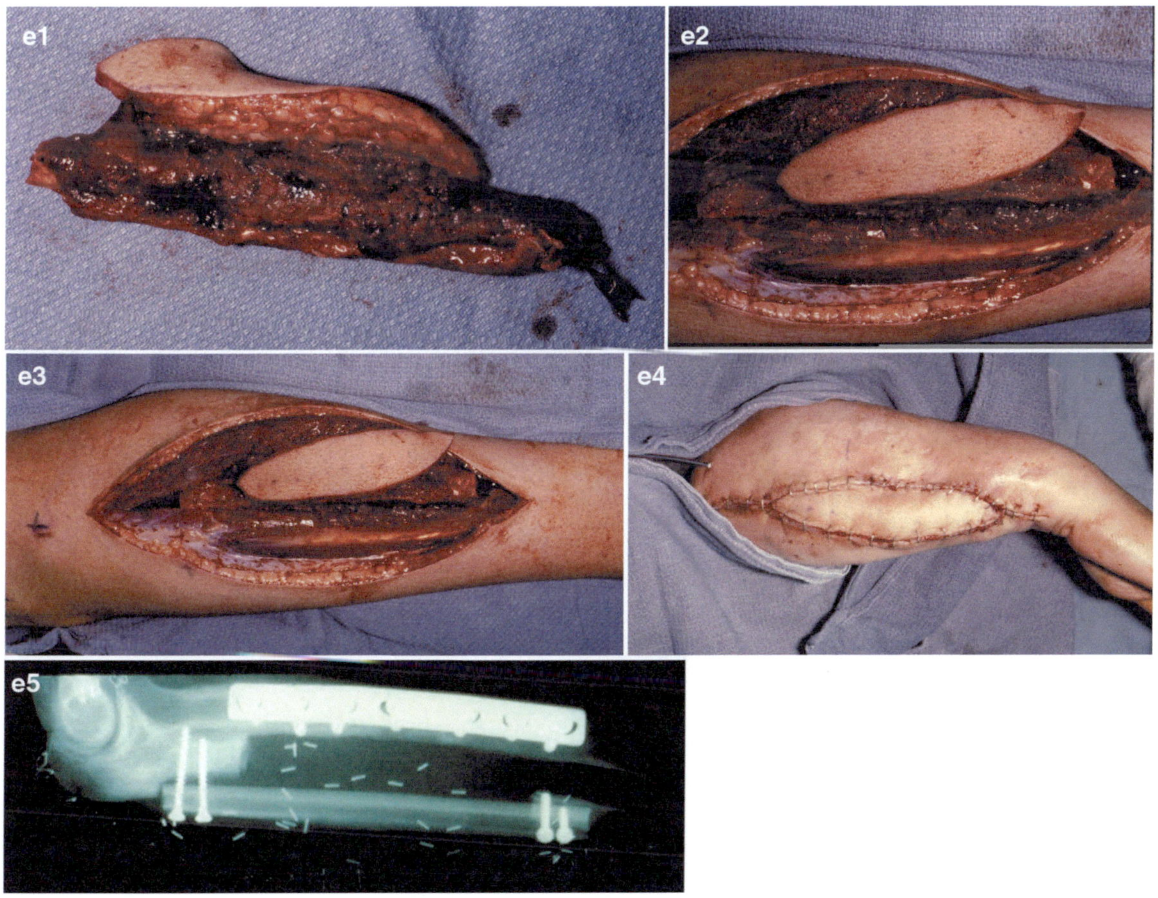

(**e**) Despite multiple debridements, antibiotics, and bone grafting, chronic symptomatic osteomyelitis of ulna persisted. Therefore, partial excision of ulna and free vascularized osteocutaneous fibular graft to the ulna was performed.

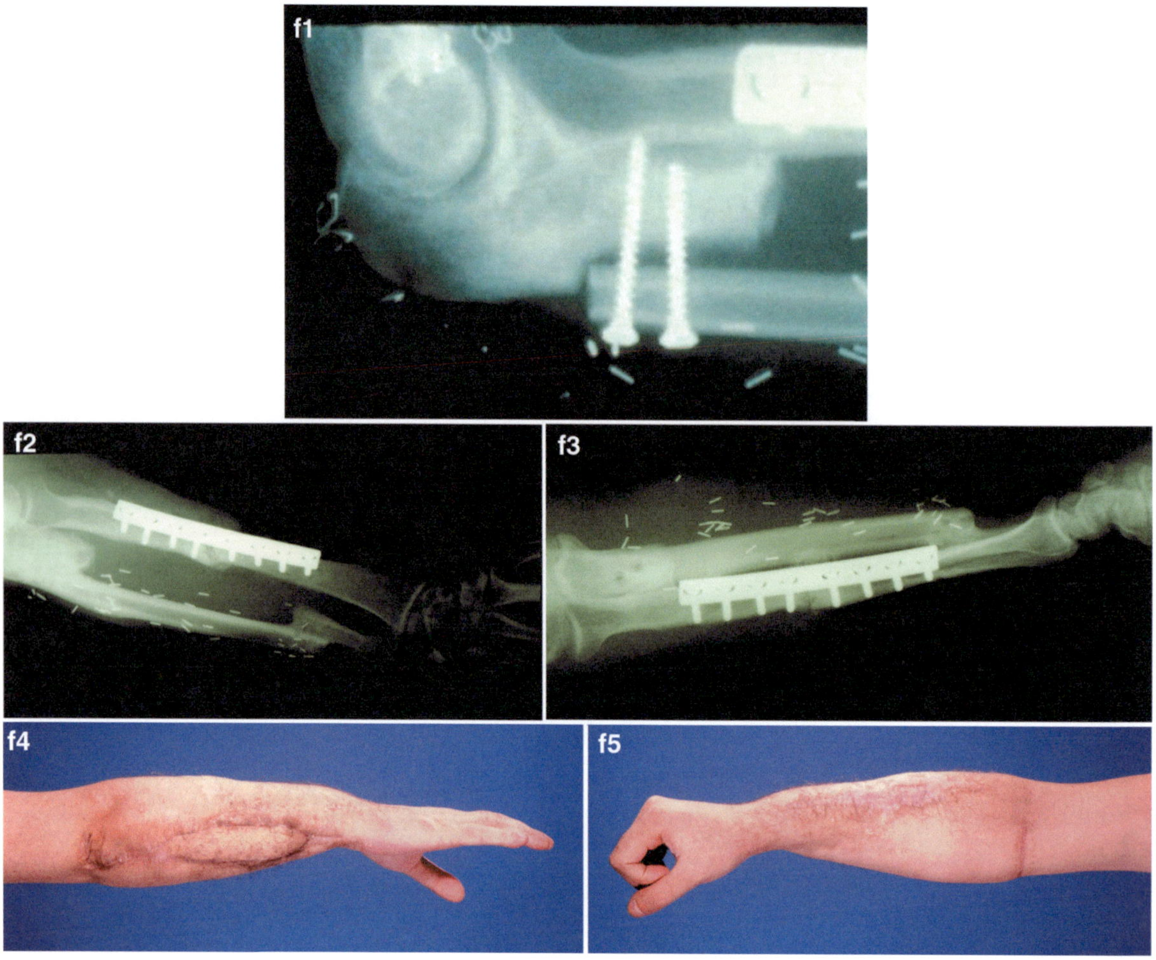

(**f**) The cortices of the overlapping ulnar stump and fibular graft are taken down to promote union. However, as good apposition of these surfaces was not achieved with screw fixation, as seen in this radiograph, fibrous nonunion persisted. Subsequently, this fibrous nonunion was excised with placement of ICBG and AO plating. Five months later, satisfactory union was achieved, as seen in the radiographs below.

Case 24.2

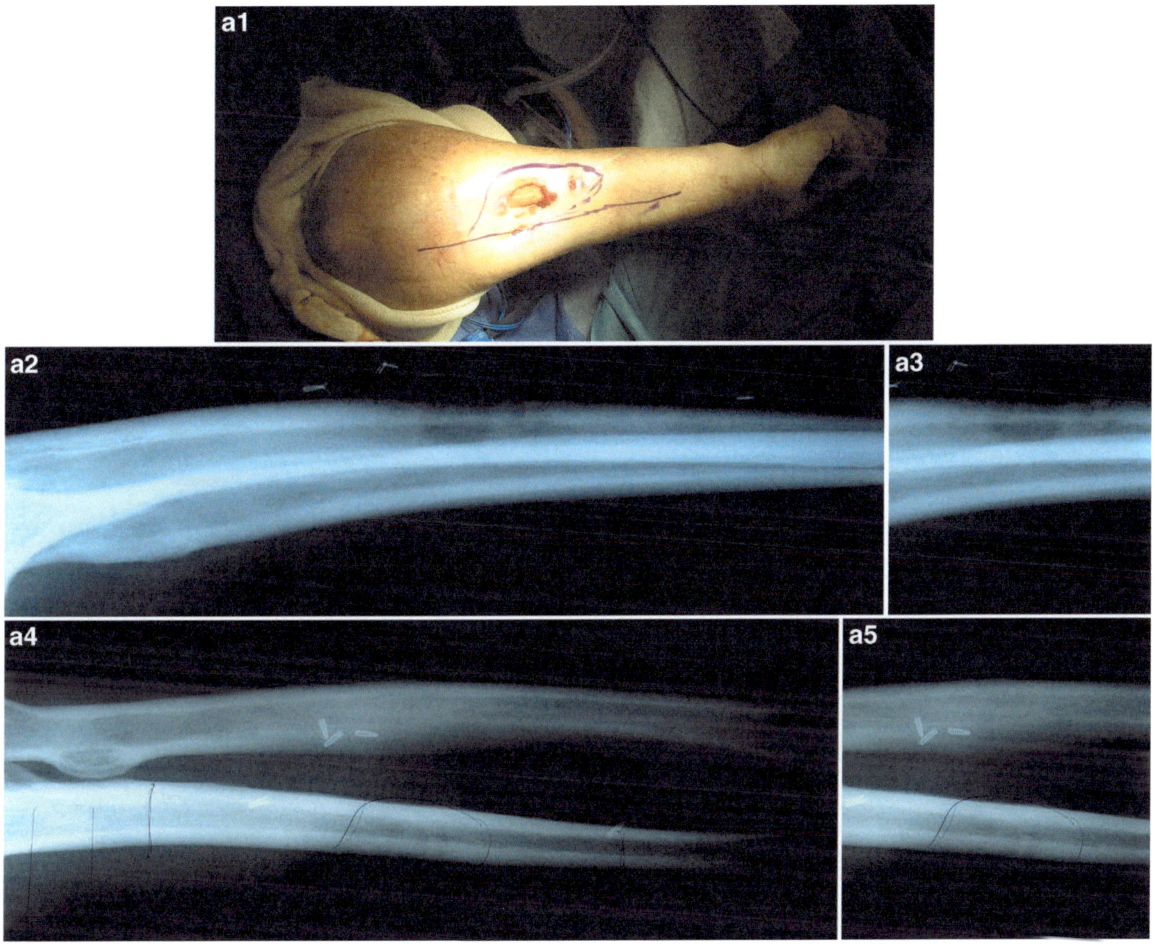

(**a**) Initial presentation—68-year-old male presenting with wound over ulna in proximal forearm (h/o soft tissue sarcoma in same region resected, followed by resection of recurrences × 2 and intraoperative radiation). Radiographs (X-ray and MRI) showed osteonecrosis and chronic osteomyelitis.

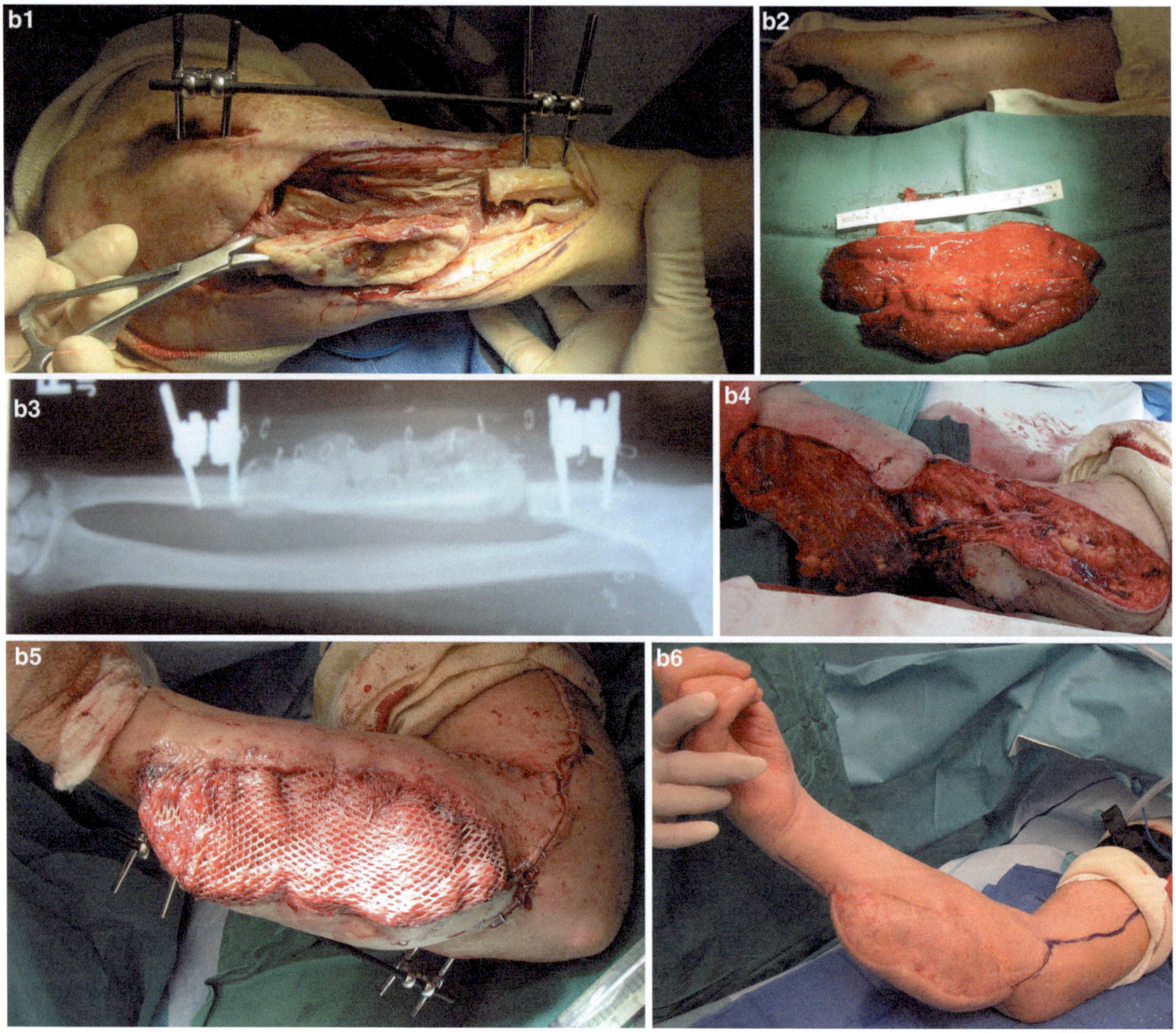

(**b**) Initial operation—excision of ulceration and 12 cm of infected ulnar bone. Placement of antibiotic-impregnated bone cement and external fixator followed by gracilis myocutaneous flap and split thickness skin graft.

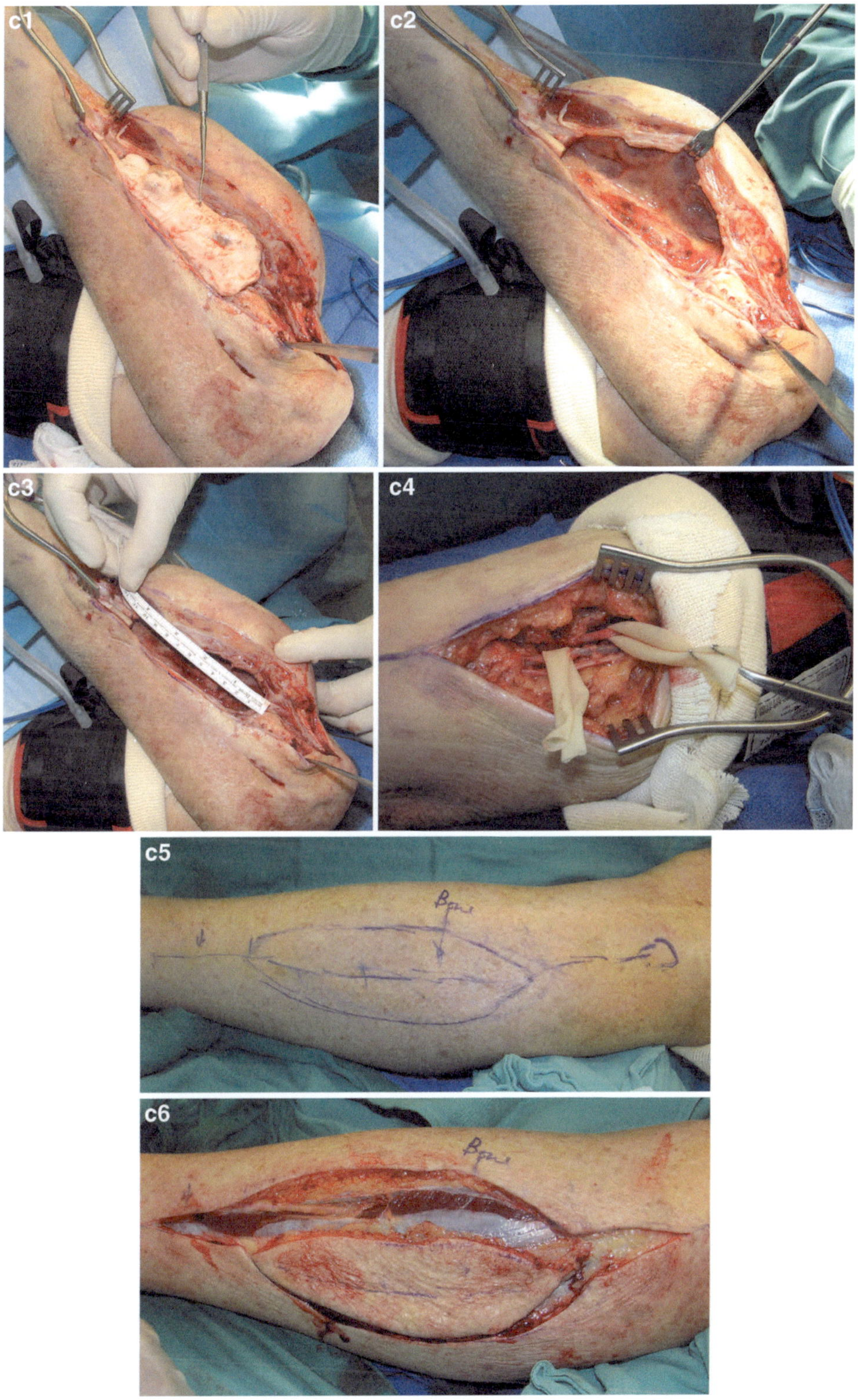

(**c**) Two months later, external fixator and bone cement were removed. Vascularized osteocutaneous free fibula flap was performed. Because of recent irradiation to forearm, brachial artery and basilic vein outside field of irradiation were chosen as recipient vessels. The fibula is measured and its middle third is identified. Fasciocutaneous perforators from the peroneal artery supply the skin at intervals, especially along middle third of the fibula.

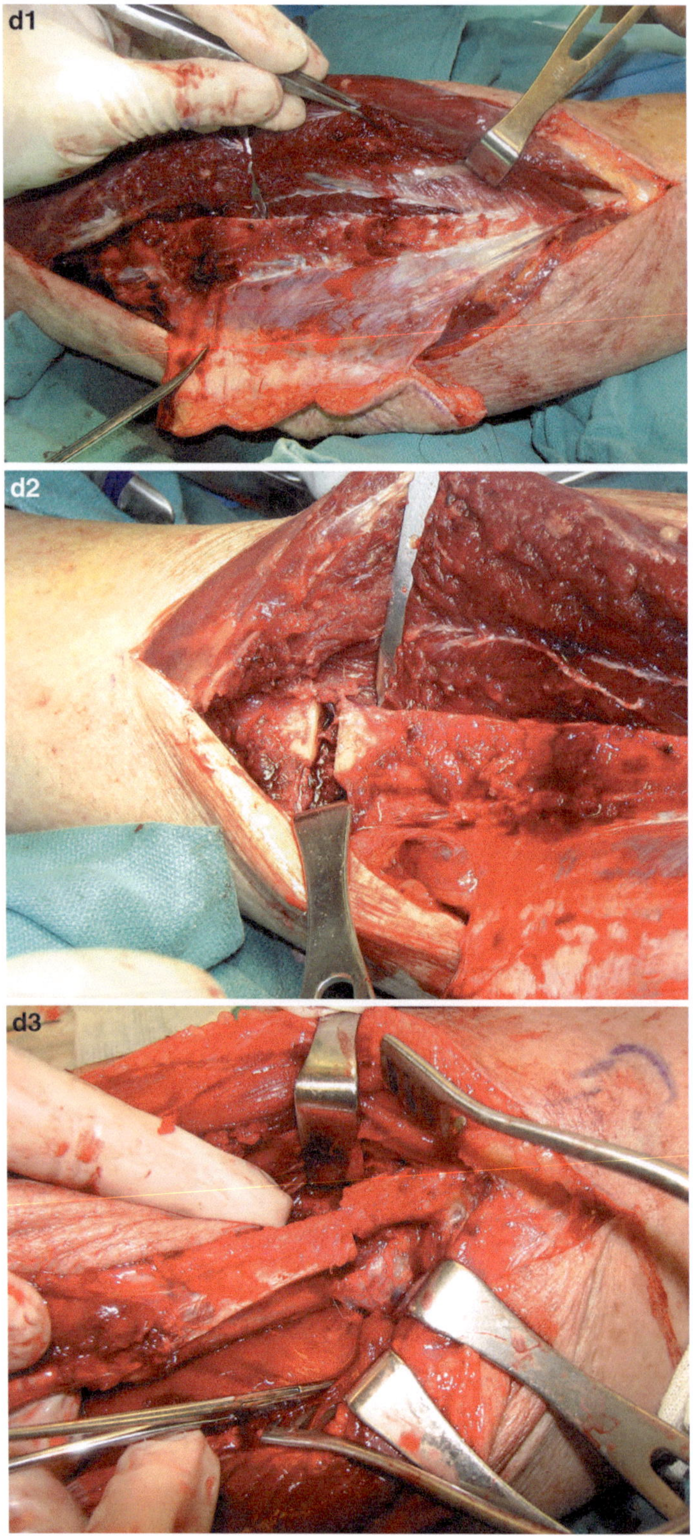

(**d**) Lateral and anterior compartment muscles are freed from fibula, protecting both deep and superficial branches of peroneal nerve. The interosseous membrane is exposed and divided. The distal fibula is exposed and cut 7–8 cm above the lateral malleolus. The proximal fibular cut is also made, protecting the peroneal nerve and vessels.

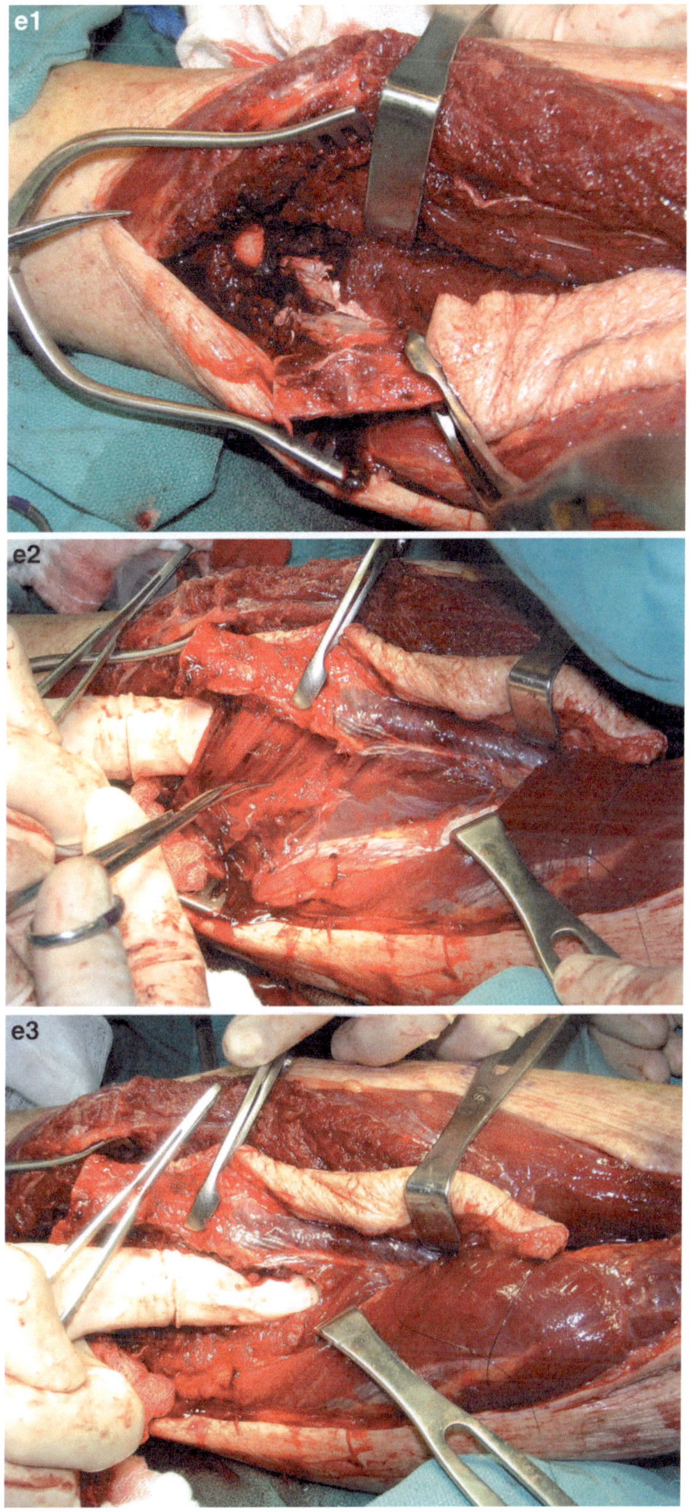

(**e**) The peroneal vessels are visualized and ligated distally. The flexor hallucis longus (FHL) muscle is separated from the fibula. Next, the tibialis posterior (TP) muscle is separated from the fibula. A cuff of FHL and TP muscle may be left around the vessels, to protect them.

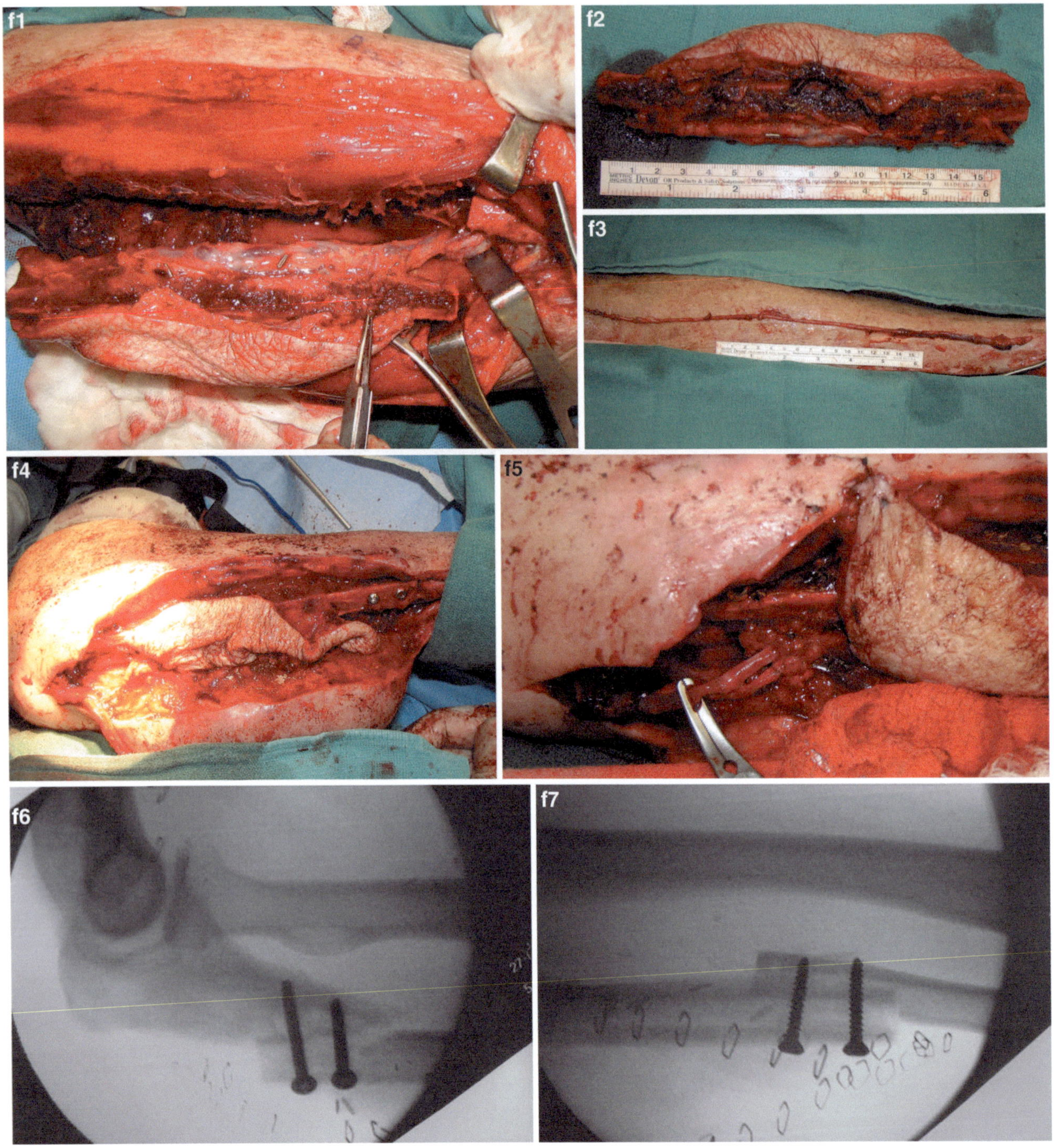

(**f**) The osteocutaneous fibula flap is left attached by the proximal peroneal vessels, while the tourniquet is let down and the flap is allowed to perfuse for 30 min prior to harvest. Below—the free osteocutaneous fibular flap. Saphenous vein is harvested to be used as vein graft connecting the peroneal artery and vein to the brachial artery and vein, respectively. Below—completed anastomosis. Osteocutaneous fibular graft in place. The fibular graft overlaps the proximal and distal ulnar stumps (see radiographs below). The overlapping apposing cortices are taken down and fixed rigidly with two AO screws each, to promote union.

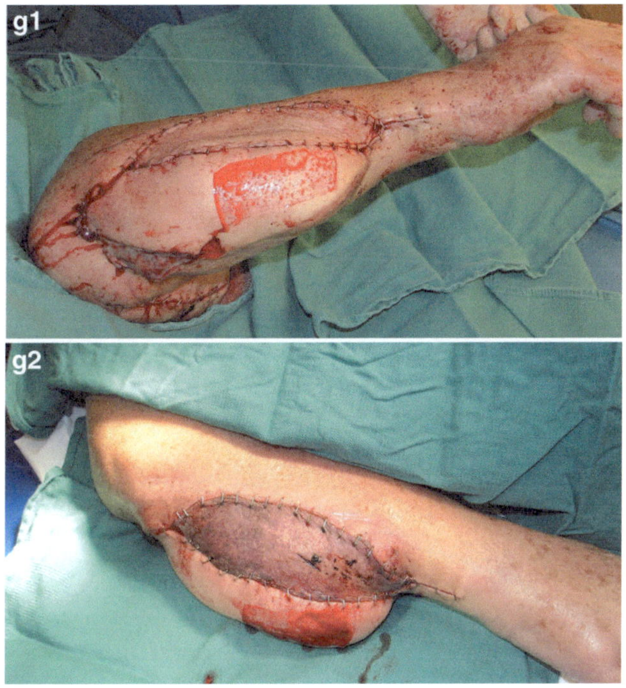

(**g**) Immediately postoperative—osteocutaneous fibular flap in place with well-perfused skin paddle. Postoperative day 2—venous congestion and hematoma under the skin paddle was noted. Patient was taken back to operating room, hematoma was evacuated, and a thrombosed venous anastomosis was taken down and repaired. The arterial anastomosis was intact. Postoperative day 3—patient suffered hypotension, was transferred to ICU, and was diagnosed with pneumonia. The flap died.

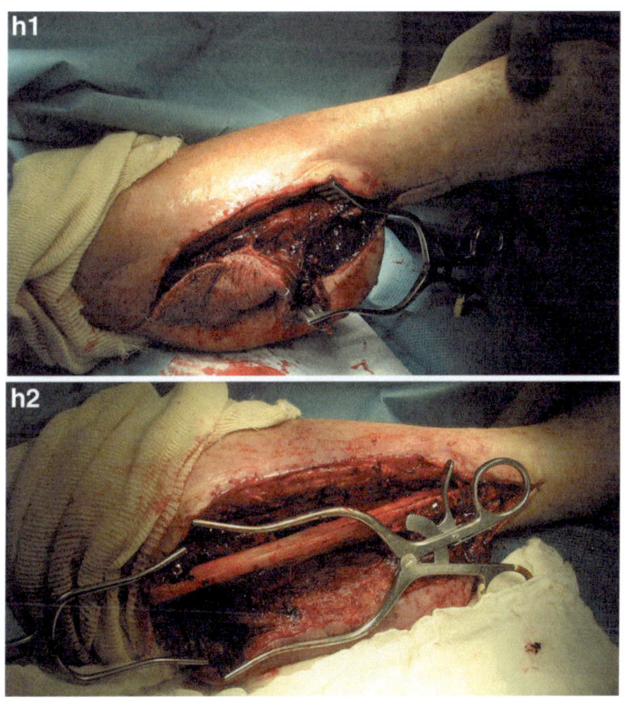

(**h**) Postoperative day 4—patient was stabilized and taken to OR. Soft tissue and periosteum beneath the skin paddle were found to be devoid of blood supply. The peroneal vessels were found to be thrombosed and were ligated. All soft tissue was stripped off the fibular graft which was left in situ to be incorporated as a nonvascularized bone graft. The proximal two AO screws were found to be broken. These were removed and interosseous wire times three was used to hold the fibular graft proximally. The skin was easily apposed, even after excision of the skin paddle.

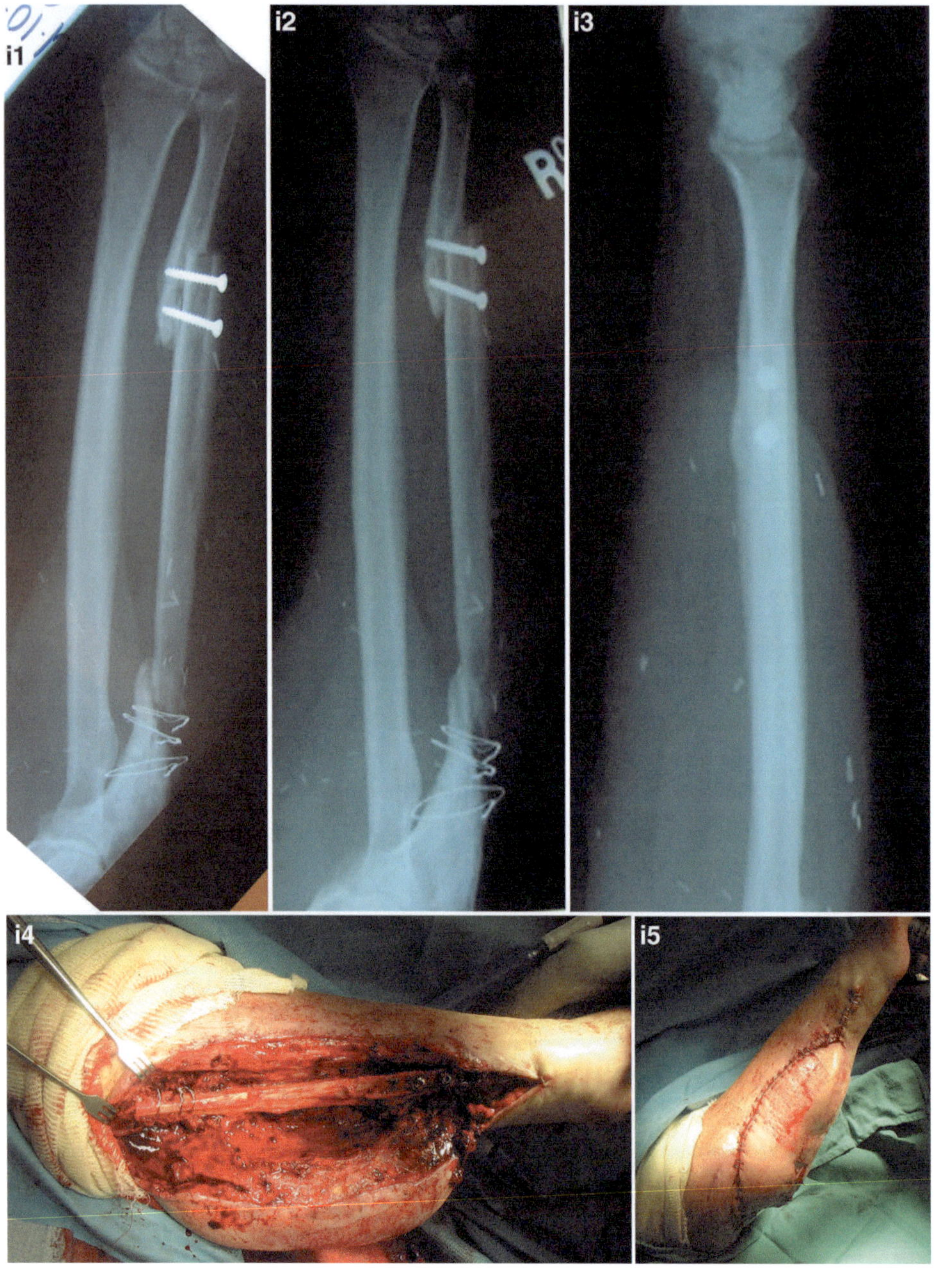

(**i**) Eight months postoperatively, union has not been achieved. One year postoperatively, radiographs reveal proximal and distal union of the fibular graft.

Case 24.3

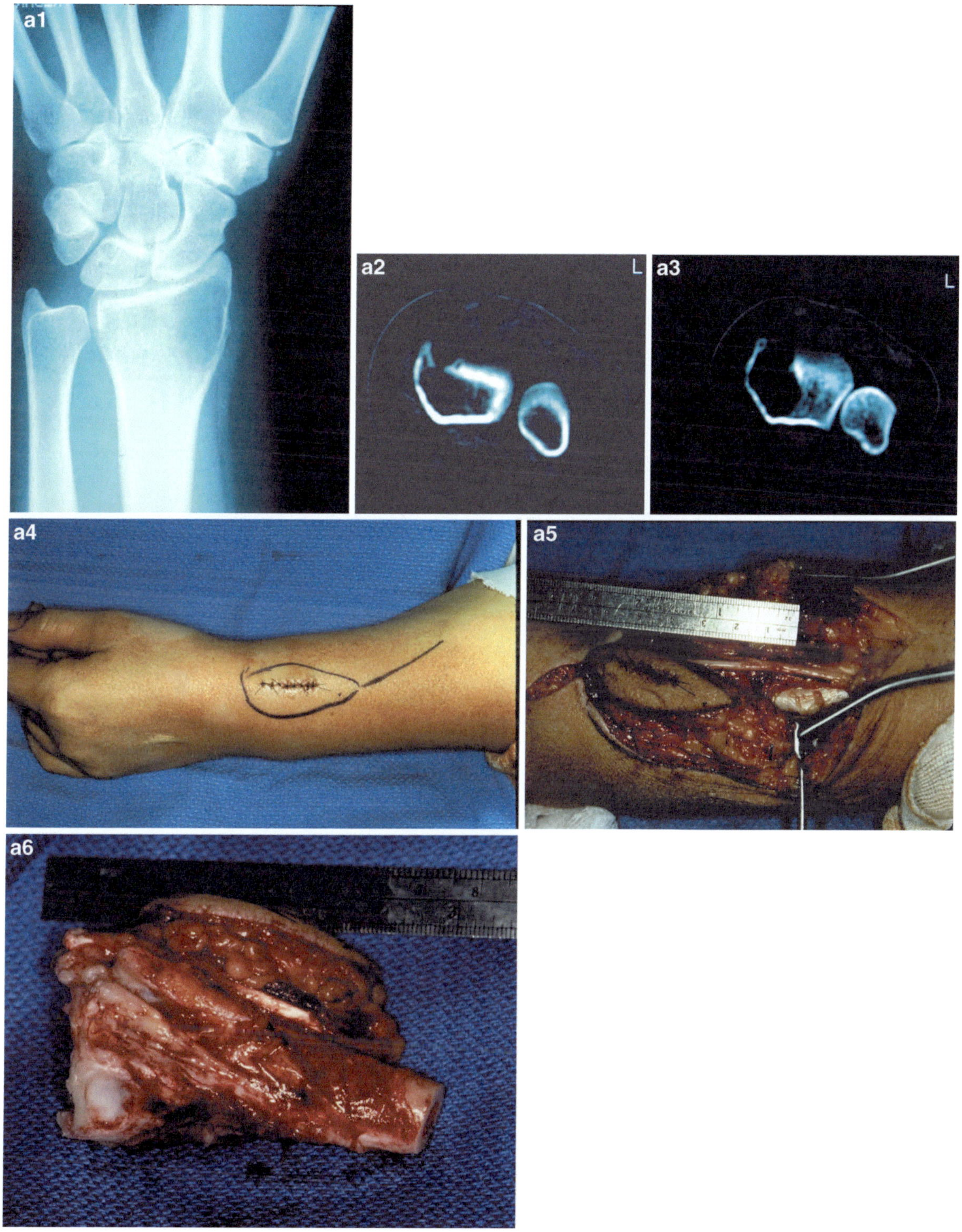

(**a**) Initial presentation—43-year-old female with 1 year of wrist pain. Radiograph—lytic lesion in distal radius. CT—erosion of dorsal cortex of radius by tumor. Biopsy revealed giant cell tumor.

Resection of giant cell tumor of distal radius included:

- Ellipse of skin enclosing biopsy site tract
- Contents of first extensor compartment
- Half of second extensor compartment
- Distal brachioradialis
- 6 cm of distal radiusIntraoperative frozen section of soft tissue margins was negative for tumor. The fibula is measured and its middle third is identified.

Note—radical excision of giant cell tumors as performed above is controversial. Some authors advise less radical operations, such as enucleation of the tumor and cancellous bone grafting.

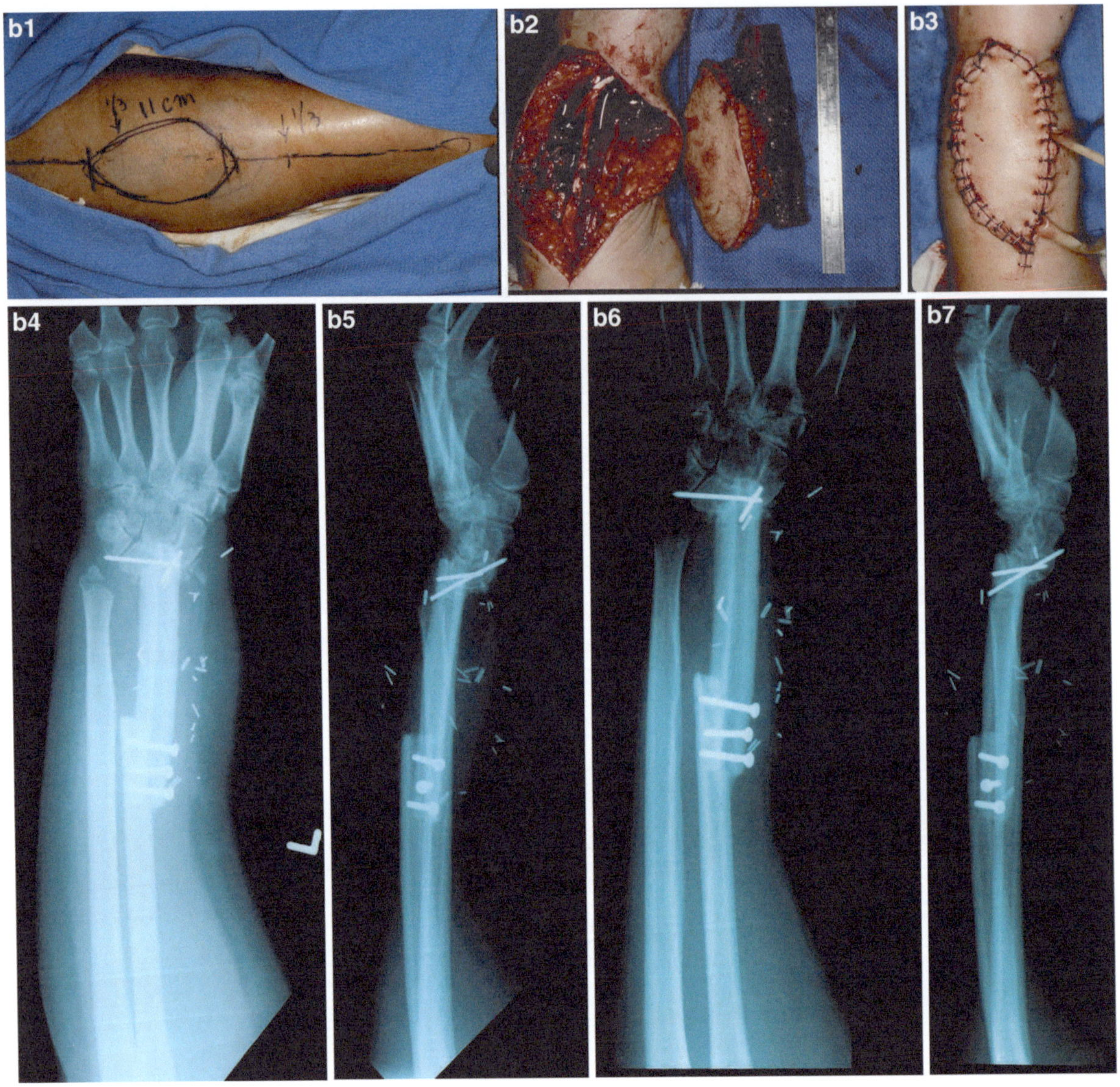

(**b**) An osteocutaneous vascularized fibula flap is harvested with peroneal artery and its venae comitantes. Two long toe extensors are harvested to reconstruct the first and second extensor compartments in the wrist. A step cut was made in the proximal radius to accept to accept the fibular bone graft. The dorsal cortices of the scaphoid and lunate were removed in a block fashion to accept the fibula. The ends of the fibula were cut to match the osteotomies of the radius proximally and scaphoid and lunate distally. Proximal fixation was with three 2.7-mm AO screws. Distal fixation was with two 0.062-in. Kirschner wires passed across the fibula into the carpal bones. Postoperative X-rays revealed union in 3 months. However, the ulna was subluxed dorsally and was of positive variance. Patient presented with instability of her distal ulna with pain and laxity. Subsequently, a modified Darrach with ECU stabilization was performed, as seen in radiographs below.

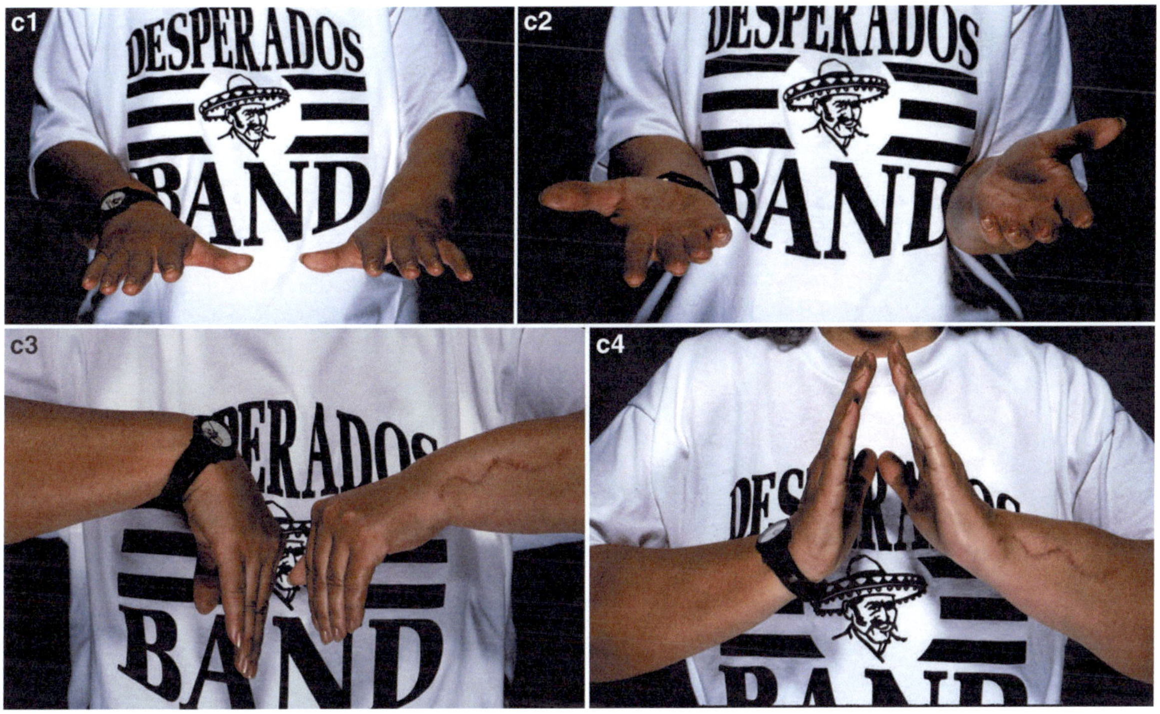

(c) Wrist motion at 1 year postoperatively.

References

1. Brockman EP. Two cases of disability at the wrist joint following excision of the head of the radius. Proc R Soc Med. 1931;24:904–5.
2. Curr JF, Coe WA. Dislocation of the inferior radioulnar joint. Br J Surg. 1946;34:74–7.
3. Essex-Lopresti P. Fractures of the radial head with distal radio-ulnar dissociation; report of two cases. J Bone Joint Surg Br. 1951;33(2):244–7.
4. Karlstad R, Morrey BF, Cooney WP. Failure of fresh-frozen radial head allografts in the treatment of Essex-Lopresti injury. A report of four cases. J Bone Joint Surg Am. 2005;87(8):1828–33.
5. Edwards Jr GS, Jupiter JB. Radial head fractures with acute distal radioulnar dislocation. Essex-Lopresti revisited. Clin Orthop Relat Res. 1988;234:61–9.
6. Trousdale RT, Amadio PC, Cooney WP, et al. Radioulnar dissociation. A review of twenty cases. J Bone Joint Surg Am. 1992;74(10):1486–97.
7. McGinley JC, Hopgood BC, Gaughan JP, et al. Forearm and elbow injury: the influence of rotational position. J Bone Joint Surg Am. 2003;85:2403–9.
8. Noda K, Goto A, Murase T, et al. Interosseous membrane of the forearm: an anatomical study of ligament attachment locations. J Hand Surg Am. 2009;34A:415–22.
9. Skahen 3rd JR, Palmer AK, Werner FW, et al. The interosseous membrane of the forearm: anatomy and function. J Hand Surg Am. 1997;22(6):981–5.
10. McGinley JC, Kozin SH. Interosseous membrane anatomy and functional mechanics. Clin Orthop Relat Res. 2001;383:108–22.
11. Hotchkiss RN, An KN, Sowa DT, et al. An anatomic and mechanical study of the interosseous membrane of the forearm: pathomechanics of proximal migration of the radius. J Hand Surg Am. 1989;14(2 Pt 1):256–61.
12. Rabinowitz RS, Light TR, Harvey RM, et al. The role of the interosseous membrane and triangular fibrocartilage complex in forearm stability. J Hand Surg Am. 1994;19(3):385–93.
13. Manson TT, Pfaeffle HJ, Herdon JH, et al. Forearm rotation alters interosseous ligament strain distribution. J Hand Surg Am. 2000;25(6):1058–63.
14. Fester EW, Murray PM, Sanders TG, et al. The efficacy of magnetic resonance imaging and ultrasound in detecting disruptions of the forearm interosseous membrane: a cadaver study. J Hand Surg Am. 2002;27(3):418–24.
15. Chandler JW, Stabile KJ, Pfaeffle HJ, et al. Anatomic parameters for planning of interosseous ligament reconstruction using computer assisted techniques. J Hand Surg Am. 2003;28(1):111–6.
16. Marcotte AL, Osterman AL. Longitudinal radioulnar dissociation: identification and treatment of acute and chronic injuries. Hand Clin. 2007;23:195–208.
17. Martin BF. The oblique cord of the forearm. J Anat. 1958;92:609–15.
18. Tubbs RS, O'Neil Jr JT, Key CD, Zarzour JG, Fulghum SB, Kim EJ, et al. The oblique cord of the forearm in man. Clin Anat. 2007;20:411–5.
19. Patel BA. Form and function of the oblique cord (chorda obliqua) in anthropoid primates. Primates. 2005;46:47–57.
20. Forster A. Uber den morphologischen Wert der Chorda oblique antebrachii anterior und der Chorda oblique antebrachii posterior. Z Morphol Anthropol. 1905;8:62–79.

21. Watanabe H, Berger RA, Berglund LJ, Zobitz ME, An KN. Contribution of the interosseous membrane to distal radioulnar joint constraint. J Hand Surg Am. 2005;30A:1164–71.
22. Kihara H, Short WH, Werner FW, Fortino MD, Palmer AK. The stabilizing mechanism of the distal radioulnar joint during pronation and supination. J Hand Surg Am. 1995;20A:930–6.
23. Skahen 3rd JR, Palmer AK, Werner FW, et al. Reconstruction of the interosseous membrane of the forearm in cadavers. J Hand Surg Am. 1997;22(6):986–94.
24. Palmer AK, Werner FW. Biomechanics of the distal radioulnar joint. Clin Orthop Relat Res. 1984;187:26–35.
25. Birbeck DP, Failla JM, Hoshaw SJ, et al. The interosseous membrane affects load distribution in the forearm. J Hand Surg Am. 1997;22(6):975–80.
26. Halls AA, Travill A. Transmission of pressures across the elbow joint. Anat Rec. 1964;150:243–7.
27. Coleman DA, Blair WF, Shurr D. Resection of the radial head for fracture of the radial head. Long term follow up of seventeen cases. J Bone Joint Surg Am. 1987;69(3):385–92.
28. Goldberg I, Peylan J, Yosipovitch Z. Late results of excision of the radial head for an isolated closed fracture. J Bone Joint Surg Am. 1986;68(5):675–9.
29. Stephen IB. Excision of the radial head for closed fracture. Acta Orthop Scand. 1981;52(4):409–12.
30. Morrey BF, Chao EY, Hui FC. Biomechanical study of the elbow following excision of the radial head. J Bone Joint Surg Am. 1979;61(1):63–8.
31. Radin EL, Riseborough EJ. Fractures of the radial head. A review of eighty-eight cases and analysis of the indications for excision of the radial head and non-operative treatment. J Bone Joint Surg Am. 1966;48(6):1055–64.
32. McDougall A, White J. Subluxation of the inferior radio-ulnar joint complicating fracture of the radial head. J Bone Joint Surg Br. 1957;39(2):278–87.
33. Pfaeffle HJ, Fischer KJ, Manson TT, et al. Role of the forearm interosseous ligament: is it more than just longitudinal load transfer? J Hand Surg Am. 2000;25(4):683–8.
34. Swanson AB, Jaeger SH, La Rochelle D. Comminuted fractures of the radial head. The role of silicone-implant replacement arthroplasty. J Bone Joint Surg Am. 1981;63(7):1039–49.
35. Starch DW, Dabezies EJ. Magnetic resonance imaging of the interosseous membrane of the forearm. J Bone Joint Surg Am. 2001;83(2):235–8.
36. Failla JM, Jacobson J, van Holsbeeck M. Ultrasound diagnosis and surgical pathology of the torn interosseous membrane in forearm fractures/dislocations. J Hand Surg Am. 1999;24(2):257–66.
37. Smith AM, Urbanosky LR, Castle JA, et al. Radius pull test: predictor of longitudinal forearm instability. J Bone Joint Surg Am. 2002;84(11):1970–6.
38. Geel CW, Palmer AK. Radial head fractures and their effect on the distal radioulnar joint. A rationale for treatment. Clin Orthop Relat Res. 1992;275:79–84.
39. Harman TW, Graham TJ, Bamberger HB. Contemporary management of fractures of the radial head and neck with implant arthroplasty. Curr Opin Orthop. 2005;16:285–92.
40. Tejwani SG, Markolf KL, Benhaim P. Reconstruction of the interosseous membrane of the forearm with a graft substitute: a cadaveric study. J Hand Surg Am. 2005;30(2):326–34.
41. Sellman DC, Seitz Jr WH, Postak PD, et al. Reconstructive strategies for radioulnar dissociation: a biomechanical study. J Orthop Trauma. 1995;6:516–22.
42. Skahen 3rd JR, Palmer AK, Werner FW, et al. Reconstruction of the interosseous membrane of the forearm in cadavers. J Hand Surg Am. 1997;22A:986–94.
43. Ruch DS, Change DS, Koman LA. Reconstruction of longitudinal stability of the forearm after disruption of interosseous ligament and radial head excision (Essex-Lopresti lesion). J South Orthop Assoc. 1999;8:47–52.
44. Chloros GD, Wiesler ER, Ruch DS, Kuzma GR, et al. Reconstruction of Essex-Lopresti injury of the forearm: technical note. J Hand Surg Am. 2008;33A:124–30.
45. Skahen 3rd JR, Palmer AK, Werner FW, et al. Reconstruction of the interosseous membrane of the forearm in cadavers. J Hand Surg Am. 1997;22(6):986–94.
46. Pfaeffle HJ, Stabile KJ, Li ZM, et al. Reconstruction of the interosseous ligament restores normal forearm compressive load transfer in cadavers. J Hand Surg Am. 2005;30(2):319–25.
47. Tomaino MM, Pfaeffle J, Stabile K, et al. Reconstruction of the interosseous ligament of the forearm reduces load on the radial head in cadavers. J Hand Surg Br. 2003;28(3):267–70.
48. Sellman DC, Seitz Jr WH, Postak PD, et al. Reconstructive strategies for radioulnar dissociation: a biomechanical study. J Orthop Trauma. 1995;9(6):516–22.
49. Hey-Groves EW. Modern methods of treating fractures. 2nd ed. Bristol: John Wright and sons; 1921. p. 320.
50. Chen F, Culp RW, Schneider LH, Osterman AL. Revision of the ununited one bone forearm. J Hand Surg Am. 1998;23(6):1091–6.
51. Peterson CA, Maki S, Wood MB. Clinical results of the one-bone forearm. J Hand Surg Am. 1998;23(6):1091–6.
52. Allende C, Allende BT. Posttraumatic one bone forearm reconstruction. A report of seven cases. J Bone Joint Surg Am. 2004;86(2):364–9.
53. Murray PM. Free vascularized bone transfer in limb salvage surgery of the upper extremity. Hand Clin. 2004;20:203–11.
54. Dell PC, Sheppard JE. Vascularized bone grafts in the treatment of infected forearm nonunions. J Hand Surg Am. 1984;9(5):653–8.
55. Duffy GP, Wood MB, Rock MG, et al. Vascularized free fibula transfer combined with autografting for the management of fracture nonunions associated with radiation therapy. J Bone Joint Surg Am. 2000;82(4):544–54.
56. Taylor GI, Miller GD, Ham FJ. The free vascularized bone graft. A clinical extension of microvascular techniques. Plast Reconstr Surg. 1975;55(5):533–44.
57. Taylor GI. Microvascular free bone transfer. Orthop Clin North Am. 1977;8:425–47.
58. Taylor GI, Townsend P, Corlett R. Superiority of the deep circumflex iliac vessels as a supply for free groin flaps: clinical study. Plast Reconstr Surg. 1979;64:745.
59. Weiland AJ, Moore JR, Daniel RK. Vascularized bone autografts: experience with 41 cases. Clin Orthop. 1983;174:87.
60. Sempuku T, Tamai S, Mizumoto S, Yajima H. Vascularized tail bone grafts in rats. Plast Reconstr Surg. 1993;91(3):502–10.
61. Phemister DB. The fate of transplanted bone and regenerative powers of its various constituents. Surg Gynecol Obstet. 1914;19:303–33.
62. Cutting CB, McCarthy JG. Comparison of residual osseous mass between vascularized and nonvascularized onlay bone transfers. Plast Reconstr Surg. 1983;72(5):672–5.
63. Weiland AJ. Current concepts review vascularized free bone transplants. J Bone Joint Surg Am. 1981;63(1):166–9.
64. de Boer HH, Wood MB. Bone changes in the vascularized fibular graft. J Bone Joint Surg Br. 1989;71(3):374–8.
65. Han CS, Wood MB, Bishop AT, Cooney III WP. Vascularized bone transfer. J Bone Joint Surg Am. 1992;74(10):1441–9.
66. Enneking WF, Eady JL, Burchardt H. Autogenous cortical bone grafts in the reconstruction of segmental skeletal defects. J Bone Joint Surg Am. 1980;62(7):1039–58.
67. Mankin HJ, Gebhardt MC, Tomford WW. The use of frozen cadaveric allografts in the management of patients with bone tumors of the extremities. Orthop Clin North Am. 1987;18(2):275–89.
68. Hsu RW, Wood MB, Sim FH, Chao EY. Free vascularized fibular grafting for reconstruction after tumor resection. J Bone Joint Surg Br. 1997;70(1):36–42.

69. Shea KG, Coleman DA, Scott SM, et al. Microvascularized free fibula grafts for reconstruction of skeletal defects after tumor resection. J Pediatr Orthop. 1997;17(4):424–32.
70. Davis PK, Mazur JM, Coleman GN. A torsional strength comparison of vascularized and nonvascularized bone grafts. J Biomech. 1982;15(11):875–80.
71. Gao YH, Ketch LL, et al. Upper limb salvage with microvascular bone transfer for major long-bone segmental tumor resections. Ann Plast Surg. 2001;47:240–6.
72. Weiland AJ, Kleinert HE, Kutz J, Daniel RK. Free vascularized bone graft in surgery of the upper extremity. J Hand Surg Am. 1979;4A:129–44.
73. Gerwin M, Weiland AJ. Vascularized bone grafts to the upper extremity: indications and technique. Microsurgery. 1992; 8:509.
74. Yijima H, Tamai S, Ono H, Kizaki K. Vascularized bone grafts to the upper extremities. Plast Reconstr Surg. 1998;101:727.
75. Tang C. Reconstruction of the bones and joints of the upper extremity by vascularized free fibula graft: a report of 46 cases. J Reconstr Microsurg. 1992;8:285.
76. Taylor GI, Wilson KR, Rees MD, et al. The anterior tibial vessels and their role in epiphyseal and diaphyseal transfer of the fibula: experimental study and clinical applications. Br J Plast Surg. 1988;41:451.
77. Pho RWH. Free vascularized fibula transplantation for replacement of lower radius. J Bone Joint Surg Br. 1979;61B:362.
78. Tsai T, Ludwig L, Tonkin M. Vascularized fibula epiphyseal transfer: a clinical study. Clin Orthop. 1986;210:228.
79. Beppu M, Hanel DP, Johnston GHF, Carmo JM, Tsai TM. The osteocutaneous fibula flap: an anatomic study. J Reconstr Microsurg. 1992;8(3):215–23.
80. Ihara K, Doi K, Yamamoto M, et al. Free vascularized fibular grafts for large bone defects in the extremities after tumor excision. J Reconstr Microsurg. 1998;14(6):371–6.
81. Minanmi A, Kasashima T, Iwasaki N, et al. Vascularized fibula grafts. An experience of 102 patients. J Bone Joint Surg Br. 2000;82(7):1022–5.
82. Ceruso M, Falcone C, Innocenti M, et al. Skeletal reconstruction with a free vascularized fibula graft associated to bone allograft after resection of malignant bone tumor of limbs. Handchir Mikrochir Plast Chir. 2001;33(4):277–82.
83. Youdas JW, Wood MB, Cahalan TD, et al. A quantitative analysis of donor site morbidity after vascularized fibula transfer. J Orthop Res. 1988;6(5):621–9.
84. Shpitzer T, Neligan P, Boyd B, et al. Leg morbidity and function following fibular free flap harvest. Ann Plast Surg. 1997;38(5): 460–4.
85. Babovic S, Johnson CH, Finical SJ. Free fibula donor site morbidity: the Mayo experience with 100 consecutive harvests. J Reconstr Microsurg. 2000;16(2):107–10.
86. Vail TP, Urbaniak JR. Donor site morbidity with use of vascularized autogenous fibular grafts. J Bone Joint Surg Am. 1996;78(2):204–11.
87. Bodde EW, de Visser E, Duysens JE, et al. Donor site morbidity after free vascularized autogenous fibular transfer: subjective and quantitative analysis. Plast Reconstr Surg. 2003;111(7):2237–42.
88. Kellam JF, Jupiter JB. Diaphyseal fractures of the forearm. In: Browner BD, Jupiter JB, Levine AM, Trafton PG, editors. Skeletal trauma. 1st ed. Philadelphia: Saunders; 1992. p. 1095–122.
89. Parikh SN. Bone graft substitutes: past, present, future. J Postgrad Med. 2002;48:142.
90. Geesink RGT, Hoefnagels NHM, Bulstra SK. Osteogenic activity of OP-1 bone morphogenetic protein (BMP-7) in a human fibular defect. J Bone Joint Surg Br. 1999;81:710–8.
91. Boden SD, Zdeblick TA, Sandhu HS, Heim SE. The use of rhBMP-2 in interbody fusion cages. Spine. 2000;25:376–81.
92. Morrey BF, Schneeberger AG. Anconeus arthroplasty: a new technique for reconstruction of the radiocapitellar and/or proximal radioulnar joint. J Bone Joint Surg Am. 2002;84:1960–9.

Secondary Options in Failed Tissue Transfers About the Hand

25

Robert E. Schlenker and Jeffrey B. Friedrich

Abstract

Soft-tissue transfers after previous failed soft-tissue coverage can be quite challenging. This is especially true if the preferred donor graft or flap was utilized, but was unsuccessful. In general, the dorsum of the hand can be covered by split thickness skin grafts, and the volar aspect of the hand covered with full thickness skin grafts, given the different thickness of skin in these locations. However, if there are exposed tendons, nerves, or vessels, these will require more complex options in order to provide soft-tissue coverage. This chapter outlines some of the creative fallback options when primary treatment has failed. The patient should be counseled that these procedures may require multiple stages and may require further surgery (such as tenolysis and contracture release) later in order to increase function once the viability of the coverage is proven.

Keywords

Failed • Tissue • Transfer • Hand • Secondary • Options

Key Points

- The palmar skin and dorsal skin are distinctively different with respect to structure and function. Palmar skin is thick and durable facilitating gripping and pinching. Dorsal skin is thinner and more mobile allowing excursion of underlying extensor tendons and accommodating finger flexion.
- The replacement chosen for coverage of soft-tissue defects on the hand should follow the guidelines of the reconstructive ladder by utilizing the least invasive option available and compatible with the best functional recovery.
- The ultimate goal of secondary hand soft-tissue reconstruction is to provide stable, vascularized soft-tissue coverage which may require multiple staged procedures.
- The final strategy to reconstruction will also be influenced by other factors including the patient's age, occupational demands, desire for restoration of appearance, other injuries, and future plans.
- In most instances, the wound VAC serves as a bridge to final wound closure rather than a means of primary treatment, and may decrease the time from injury to definitive soft-tissue coverage.
- STSG's (meshed or nonmeshed) are usually reserved for coverage of the dorsum of the hand. FTSG's should be used when covering the palmar surface of the hand and, if possible, limited to

(continued)

R.E. Schlenker, MD • J.B. Friedrich, MD (✉)
Department of Surgery, Division of Plastic Surgery, University of Washington, 325 9th Avenue, Box 359796, Seattle, WA 98104-2499, USA
e-mail: jfriedri@u.washington.edu

S.F.M. Duncan (ed.), *Reoperative Hand Surgery*,
DOI 10.1007/978-1-4614-2373-7_25, © Springer Science+Business Media, LLC 2012

areas not requiring critical sensibility. Skin grafts should never be placed over areas of denuded bone, cartilage, tendon, nerves or blood vessels. In such instances, alternative means of coverage, such as a flap, are necessary.

- Dorsal metacarpal artery flaps are excellent options for coverage of soft-tissue defects of the fingers with exposed bone, joint or tendon (particularly on the dorsum of digits). The advantages of these flaps include the fact that they are sensate and can be done in a single stage.
- The radial forearm flap is an excellent match for the hand, as it is quite thin with very little subcutaneous fat, and its versatility allows it to reach nearly any part of the hand.
- The pedicled groin flap is an extremely reliable source of immediate coverage for any defect on any portion of the hand and wrist. It is ideal for providing soft-tissue coverage of large, full-thickness defects, as it provides a large area of skin and subcutaneous fat.
- When hand or forearm-based donor tissue is not sufficient for reconstruction of a hand defect and all other options on the reconstructive ladder have been eliminated, tissue from a distant source must be employed in the form of a free flap (radial forearm flap, lateral arm flap, anterolateral thigh flap).

Introduction

The soft-tissue envelope of the hand encloses a multitude of tendons, nerves, vessels, bones, and joints. There are many upper extremity insults which can compromise this soft-tissue envelope of the hand, resulting in significant soft-tissue defects including trauma, thermal injury, infection, and malignancy. The approach to these difficult injuries has changed over time from one of simply getting the wound covered to soft-tissue reconstruction targeted at restoring the aesthetic appearance and preserving hand function. Total viable skin coverage is of prime importance in the management of hand injuries and must be restored before secondary reconstruction of deeper structures.

When skin has been lost, the replacement chosen should follow the guidelines of the reconstructive ladder by utilizing the least invasive option available and compatible with the best functional recovery. Most hand surgeons initially employ local tissue flaps when primarily managing these soft-tissue defects, such as transposition flaps, rotational flaps, advancement flaps, cross-finger flaps, thenar flaps, or Moberg flaps. Occasionally, unpredictable problems may arise with these local flaps resulting in challenging salvage situations. The need for a second (more complex) operation prolongs morbidity, results in increased hospitalization, and compromises the extremity. This chapter describes the array of available coverage options following failure of local tissue flaps and provides a summary of current concepts in secondary hand soft-tissue reconstruction. We have attempted to provide, by figures, diagrams, and text the secondary coverage options which should increase the surgeon's repertoire and help achieve better end results.

The soft-tissue envelope of the hand is uniquely designed to provide us with tactile input from our environment, and as such, it must withstand an incredible amount of abuse and wear over a lifetime. The palmar skin and dorsal skin are distinctively different with respect to structure and function. The palmar skin is thick with fibrous septa attachments connecting the skin to the underlying fascia limiting motion during gripping and pinching. Dorsal skin is thinner, more elastic, and looser with areolar tissue between the skin and extensor tendons. Dorsal skin is more mobile than palmar as it must accommodate finger flexion. The unique structural, functional, and aesthetic requirements of the hand can also be its downfall when the soft-tissue envelope is compromised. Where other body parts have ample skin, fat, and muscle, allowing easy primary or secondary closure, the hand does not. Since the hand's moving parts are just beneath the skin's surface, the skin envelope must be elastic and nonadherent in order for the hand to function properly. Therefore, soft-tissue losses in the hand require originality of thought and ingenuity for correction by surgical reconstruction.

Wound VAC

Indications for wound VAC placement:
- Wounds in need of temporary coverage because immediate primary coverage is not advisable, not achievable, or contraindicated
- Bridge to final wound closure ("second-look" procedures, serial debridements, and between the time of final debridement and that of definitive coverage)
- Complex wounds with exposed bone, muscle, tendon, or hardware
- Immature wounds in need of further granulation tissue formation prior to definitive coverage (e.g., skin grafting, flap)
- Coverage of skin grafts and dermal replacements
- Closure through secondary intention

Contraindications for wound VAC placement:
- Contaminated wounds with necrotic tissue in need of debridement
- Infected wounds
- Wounds lacking adequate hemostasis
- Wounds with uncovered nerve coaptations or vessel anastomoses
- Unreliable patients in whom close outpatient monitoring of wound healing and regularly scheduled VAC changes may prove challenging

The emergence of negative pressure wound therapy with reticulated open cell foam (NPWT/ROCF) as delivered by V.A.C. Therapy (Kinetic Concepts Inc, San Antonio, TX) has revolutionized the treatment of complex wounds and established itself a rung on the reconstructive ladder. The wound VAC's biological effects are thought to be due to microstrain and macrostrain. Microstrain promotes revascularization and granulation tissue formation through the stimulatory effects on cell division, angiogenesis, and growth factor elaboration. From a macrostrain standpoint, the active removal of excessive interstitial fluid (edema) decompresses the extravascular space enhancing microcirculation within the injured tissue. The wound also benefits from the associated removal of microcontaminants, proinflammatory cytokines, and destructive proteases. Another important macrostrain effect is the facilitation of bacterial clearance from the wound, resulting in lower bacterial counts and decreased risk of infection [1–3].

Wound VAC's can primarily treat soft-tissue defects to closure by stimulating granulation tissue that ultimately epithelializes or facilitating healing through secondary intention. In most instances, the wound VAC serves as a bridge to final wound closure rather than a means of primary treatment, and may decrease the time from injury to definitive soft-tissue coverage. Wound VAC's are frequently used for temporary coverage of complex wounds when immediate primary coverage is not advisable, such as with wounds requiring serial debridements, those awaiting the demarcation of viable tissue, wounds with possible residual contamination, or where there is prolonged delay from injury until presentation. They are also useful when definitive coverage is not achievable, for instance, when a surgeon with sufficient technical expertise to accomplish free tissue transfer is not readily available or a wound is not ready for skin grafting due to poor vascularity. Immediate coverage may also be contraindicated in patients with multisystem trauma, patient instability preventing transport to the operating room, or those with significant medical comorbidities.

Wound VAC's, in some situations, may present a valid alternative to traditional free tissue coverage as they promote granulation tissue formation such that a skin graft can be supported. There is evidence in some centers of an overall decreased need for complex soft-tissue reconstructive procedures (e.g., free tissue transfer) to obtain wound coverage since the advent of the wound VAC. This has been associated with a higher rate of achieving coverage by skin graft, delayed primary closure, and secondary intention.

Operative Approach

Wound VAC's have become an important adjunct in the management of failed tissue transfer of the hand, even in the most complex wounds. It must be emphasized that basic wound management principles cannot be abandoned, and should precede wound VAC usage. Thorough operative debridement of all contaminated and devitalized tissue is mandatory prior to wound VAC placement. After the failed tissue transfer of the hand has been debrided, a "second-look" procedure may be indicated if the surgeon is concerned about the quality of debridement or further necrosis of tissue. In these instances, the wound VAC can be placed and serve as a bridge between debridements. The patient should return to the operating room within 48 h for reexploration of the wound, and serial debridements can occur at these regular intervals until the wound is ready for definitive treatment. The wound VAC can then serve once again as the bridge between the time of final debridement and that of definitive coverage.

If the surgeon feels that the resulting wound would be best managed through healing by secondary intention, the wound VAC should be continued until closure. Wounds treated in this manner require regularly scheduled wound VAC changes. In certain situations, particularly those where no tendons or bones are exposed within the wound, skin grafting may be the form of definitive treatment.

Wound VAC's can be continued postgrafting to ensure better skin graft take on the hand and should be left intact for 5 days to optimize graft adherence. When a more complex secondary coverage option is required, such as a flap, the wound VAC should be continued until the wound bed is ready and up to the time of definitive closure. A cautionary note should be given: in instances in which it is clear that skin grafting or secondary closure of a wound is not possible, the wound VAC should not be used to unnecessarily prolong the time to definitive coverage.

Wound VAC placement on the hand can be more difficult than other places on the body. Larger wounds isolated to the dorsum or palm are fairly easy, but obtaining an airtight seal around the irregular contour of the web spaces can be challenging. The commercially available VAC dressing kit (Kinetic Concepts Inc, San Antonio, TX) is usually all that is needed, although occasionally additional strips of Ioban™, Tegaderm™, and Mastisol® liquid adhesive are helpful in obtaining a seal. The sponge should be cut back to fit the wound without overlapping the surrounding intact skin in order to minimize skin maceration (Fig. 25.1).

Wound VAC's are often the dressing of choice over skin grafts because they create a moist environment, prevent shearing, protect the site from contamination, and evacuate transudate from the wound while the skin graft incorporates. Neovascularization of the graft is also assisted via the mechanical stress applied to the wound bed. After securing the skin graft to the wound bed, a nonadherent dressing is placed over the graft followed by the wound VAC sponge. The nonadherent dressing is necessary to prevent graft adherence to the sponge and disruption of the graft at the time of sponge removal [4].

Optimizing outcomes

- Wound must be suitable for application (operative debridement of all contaminated and devitalized tissue)
- Bleeding should be controlled before application of the wound VAC
- Wound VAC must be applied appropriately such that an airtight seal is created and maintained
- Wound VAC must be changed at regularly scheduled intervals (every 2–3 days) such that wound healing is closely monitored
- Wound VAC should be continued until the wound bed is ready for definitive closure (e.g., skin grafting, flap)
- Wound VAC should be applied with minimal sponge bulk to facilitate splint placement (if indicated) and the least possible adhesive draping to allow adequate mobilization

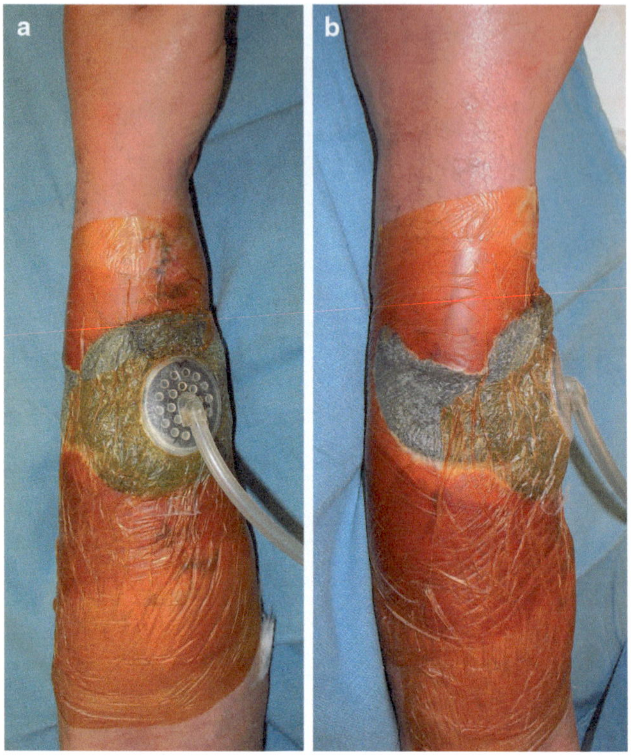

Fig. 25.1 Wound VAC placed over a forearm wound in preparation for skin grafting (**a**, **b**)

Complications and Side Effects

Complications related to wound VAC usage can result from its placement on wounds not suitable for their application. Necrotic tissue present underneath a wound VAC will hinder the wound healing process and slow progression to a healthy granulating bed capable of definitive closure. An even worse complication is the development of a local wound infection. Operative debridement of all devitalized tissue and thorough irrigation of the wound prior to wound VAC placement can help minimize these suboptimal outcomes. If nonviable tissue develops after wound VAC placement, it should be appropriately debrided at the time of VAC change, prior to the application of a new wound VAC. Similarly, an infected wound should never be covered by a wound VAC, but rather treated with nonocclusive dressings.

Wound VAC's inadvertently placed over an exposed vessel or wounds without adequate hemostasis can result in substantial blood loss. If hemorrhage within the wound is discovered, the wound VAC should be disconnected and the dressing immediately switched to a compressive dressing. Surgical reexploration may be required if hemostasis is not achieved.

Another common problem is the difficulty in obtaining an airtight seal, and the development of leaks within the system. Leaks should be dealt with in an expeditious manner and patched at the bedside with any remaining VAC adhesive drape or Tegaderm™. If the sponge has not been cut back to appropriately fit the wound, the surrounding intact skin can become macerated, thereby creating a potentially larger wound. Once skin breakdown has been identified, it is imperative that subsequent sponges be trimmed such that they fit adequately within the confines of the wound.

A common side effect of wound VAC usage is the patient discomfort associated with VAC changes. Immature wounds are more susceptible to painful VAC changes than those covered with a thick granulating bed. In such cases, patients may need to have their initial VAC changes performed in the operating room under sedation until bedside VAC changes become tolerable. A technique used at our institution involves turning the wound VAC off and injecting a 30 cc tube of 2% lidocaine jelly into the sponge. After the wound has been allowed to be in contact with the lidocaine-soaked sponge for 15 min, it can be removed with significantly less pain to the patient.

Postoperative Care

The postoperative care for wound VAC's involves troubleshooting any leaks that develop and maintaining an airtight seal throughout the course of its usage. Wound VAC's should be changed regularly at 2–3 day intervals such that wound healing can be closely monitored.

Clinical "pearls" and potential complications/pitfalls

- Wound VAC's expedite the healing process by decreasing edema, increasing local blood flow, promoting granulation tissue formation, and isolating the wound from the outside environment
- Wound VAC's should never be used in contaminated wounds with necrotic tissue, infected wounds, or wounds lacking adequate hemostasis
- Wound VAC's should be applied in such a way as to allow placement of an overlying splint (if indicated) and permit early hand mobilization
- Wound VAC's should be changed every 2–3 days

Skin Grafts: Autografts, Biologic and Synthetic Skin Substitutes

Autologous skin grafts are useful options for the reconstruction of certain defects that cannot be closed primarily. Several principles must be kept in mind when considering skin grafting the hand. Since all skin grafts undergo primary and secondary contraction, the implications of graft contracture on hand function must be taken into account. Full-thickness skin grafts (FTSG's) are preferred over split-thickness skin grafts (STSG's) in areas where graft contracture would limit mobility, such as joint creases. Skin grafts become firmly attached to their wound bed over time, so they are not suitable permanent coverage over areas requiring movement through a range greater than that of the overlying skin. Similarly, skin grafting should be avoided if there are any plans to operate on structures beneath the graft (e.g., tendon or bone grafting). Raw soft tissue with no exposed deep structures are amenable to coverage with a skin graft, however, when deep structures are exposed their ability to take a skin graft and the effects of skin graft coverage on function must be addressed. The periosteum of bone, cancellous bone, perichondrium, and paratenon are all capable of providing a well-vascularized bed, and skin grafts can be directly applied to them. Grafts should never be placed over areas of denuded bone, cartilage, tendon, nerves, or blood vessels. In such instances, alternative means of coverage, such as a flap, are necessary.

Indications for skin graft placement:

- Wounds with good underlying soft-tissue bed and adequate vascularity
- Simple wounds with no exposed deep structures

Contraindications for skin graft placement:

- Contaminated wounds with necrotic tissue in need of debridement
- Infected wounds
- Wounds lacking adequate hemostasis
- Future plans for secondary surgery on structure(s) beneath the graft (e.g., tendon grafting)
- Complex wounds with exposed bone, cartilage, tendon, nerves, blood vessels, or hardware

STSG's (meshed or nonmeshed) are usually reserved for coverage of the dorsum of the hand. Since dorsal skin is similar to skin found elsewhere on the body it can usually be adequately treated with a STSG. Palmar skin is not easily substituted, since it contains special dermal neural mechanoreceptors not present anywhere else on the body except the plantar foot. FTSG's should be used when covering the palmar surface of the hand and, if possible, limited to areas not requiring critical sensibility. STSG's should not be used on palmar surfaces of the hand unless there is no other choice or the coverage is considered to be temporary, with secondary resurfacing to be followed at a later date. FTSG's from the hypothenar eminence and lateral surface of the great toe are good for covering the palmar surface of fingers and fingertips, while the plantar arch of the foot can be utilized for coverage of larger areas on the palm. If a digit is irreparably damaged, it can serve as a valuable source of skin cover as well. These glabrous FTSG's provide a similar quality of

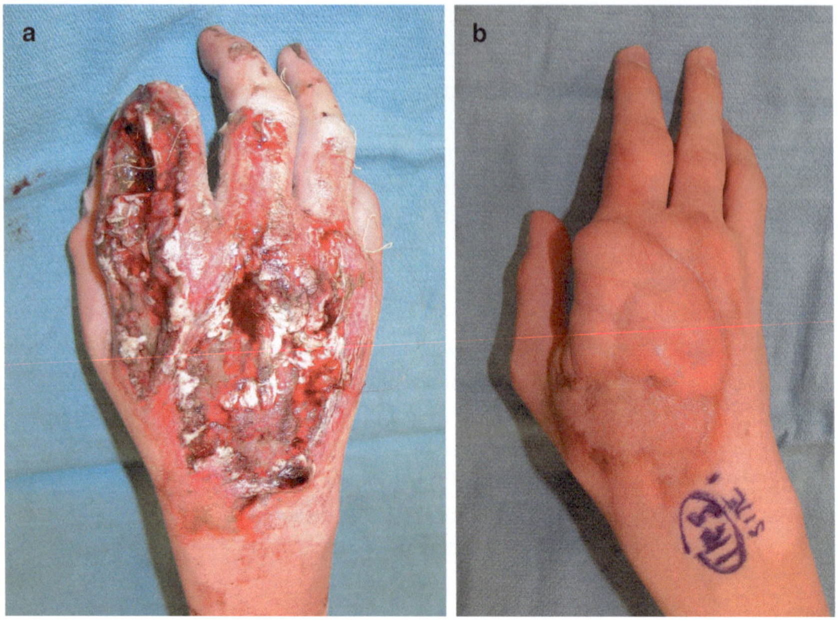

Fig. 25.2 Degloving injury of right hand (**a**). End result of wound covered with fillet of finger flap and skin graft (**b**)

coverage and potentially improved sensibility compared to nonglabrous skin.

Split-thickness skin grafts can be taken from anywhere on the body, although the color, texture, thickness of the dermis, and donor site morbidity of body locations vary considerably. The thicker the skin graft, the poorer the quality of the donor site after healing. As thicker grafts are desirable for the hand, it is best to harvest from areas of the body with thicker skin such as the posterolateral aspects of the trunk and thighs. Split-thickness skin grafts may be harvested as either "thin" grafts (0.008–0.010 in.) or "thick" grafts (0.016–0.020 in.). Deeper grafts increase the chance of reinnervation of Merkel's complexes and restoration of sensibility in the recipient site. Most wounds are best covered by intermediate thickness grafts approximately 0.015 in. in thickness. Thinner grafts of 0.010–0.012 in. may be best for wounds where graft survival is at risk.

In cases where there is significant skin loss (e.g., upper extremity degloving injury) or limited donor sites (e.g., large burns), temporary coverage can be achieved with skin substitutes to protect the recipient bed from desiccation and further trauma until definitive closure can occur. There have been many attempts in recent years to develop biologic and synthetic skin substitutes. Biologic skin substitutes include human allografts (cadaver skin) or xenografts (such as pig skin). Allografts become vascularized and initially "take" but are later rejected at approximately 4 days. Conversely, xenografts are rejected before becoming vascularized. The application of synthetic skin substitutes such as silicone polymers and composite membranes have also been described [5]. Additional research and progress will be needed before biologic and synthetic skin substitutes can be considered a reliable alternative.

Integra Dermal Regeneration Template (Integra® Lifesciences, Plainsboro, NJ) is a temporary bilayer skin substitute used for reconstruction of the dermis. The inner layer is composed a matrix framework (bovine collagen and shark chondroitin-6-sulfate) which forms a neodermis by promoting the migration of fibroblasts and endothelial cells into the scaffold. The outer layer is a silastic membrane which protects the new underlying cellular matrix by acting as a mechanical barrier to bacterial invasion and fluid loss. Once the neodermis has developed, the silicone layer is carefully peeled away and a thin skin graft is applied. Integra has been shown in small series to form a well-vascularized neodermis over avascular tissue (exposed bone, cartilage, tendons, and joints), which is then capable of taking a skin graft. It has been proposed that Integra provides protection of deep structures by restoring a gliding plane for tendons, allowing superior motion in the reconstructed area. The primary problem with these dermal substitutes is that they generally have to be applied 1–3 weeks before coverage with a STSG to allow for revascularization of the collagen matrix, thus necessitating two operations [6, 7].

Operative Approach

When covering the hand we prefer to harvest a sheet of good-quality skin at approximately 15/1,000 of an inch. After the sheet of split-thickness skin is harvested it is ready for application if it is to be used as a nonmeshed sheet graft. Whenever possible we prefer to cover wounds on the dorsum of the hand with sheet grafts (Figs. 25.2 and 25.3). However, if the

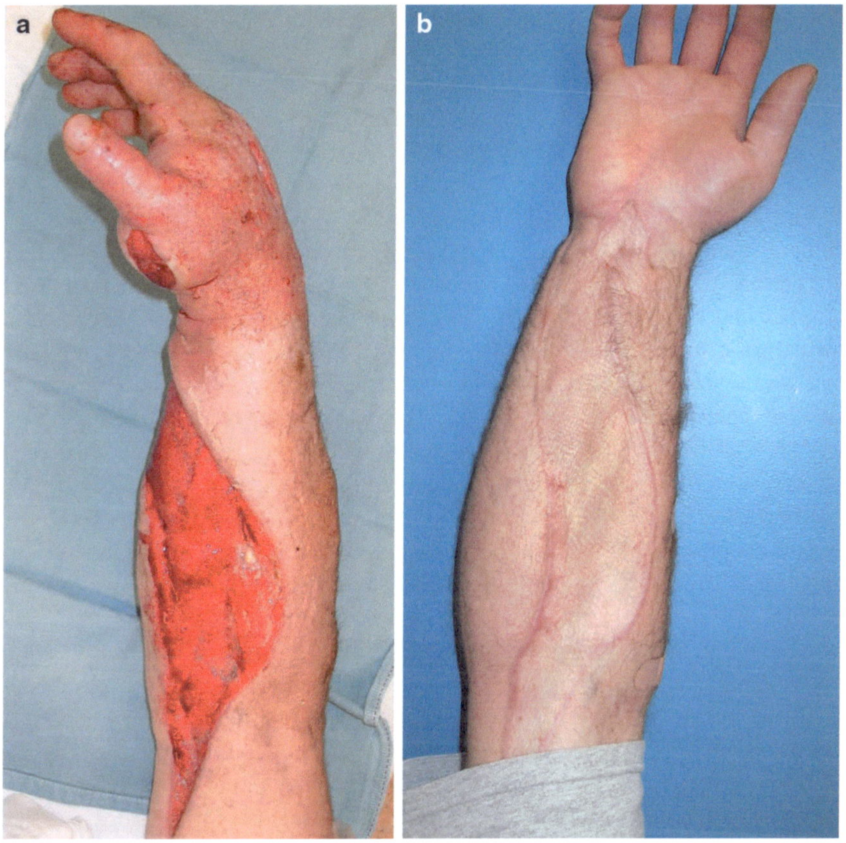

Fig. 25.3 Granulating wound extending over right forearm and onto thenar eminence initially treated with wound VAC therapy (**a**). End result of wound covered with STSG (**b**)

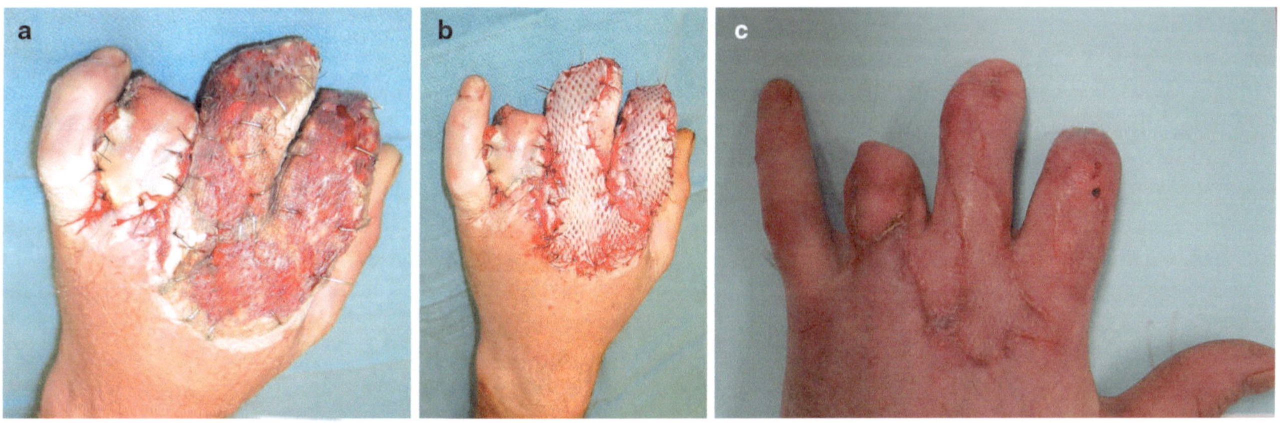

Fig. 25.4 Degloving injury of left hand (**a**, **b**). Expected result following split-thickness skin grafting of middle finger and index finger (**c**)

skin is to be placed as a meshed STSG, the surgeon must decide how much the graft is to be expanded. STSG's can be meshed in ratios from 1:1 to 9:1. We prefer to mesh STSG's at 1:1 or 2:1, because anything greater forms very large interstices which are not practical for coverage of the hand (Fig. 25.4).

A template, such as a piece of paper from a glove wrapper trimmed to the shape of the defect, can be helpful when determining exactly how much skin is needed for a FTSG. This is particularly helpful when multiple sites are to be covered with FTSG's, because the different smaller templates can be put together such that a single large template is made. It is ideal to place the axis of the ellipse in the direction of minimal tension and within a skin crease. All underlying fat and subcutaneous tissue must be removed from the undersurface of a FTSG because they will act as a barrier to vascularization and impede graft take. We try to achieve this at the time of graft excision by using a #10 scalpel to carefully lift off only the skin at the plane between the dermis and subcutaneous fatty tissue. The donor site is then primarily closed in standard fashion with buried subdermal sutures and a running subcuticular stitch. We prefer to "pie-crust" the FTSG to some degree by placing the graft on an upside down kidney basin and making several small incisions with a #15 scalpel. "Pie crusting" allows egress of fluid from under the graft.

The harvested graft is secured in place with suture or skin staples, and carefully tailored to the size of recipient site while being inset. We prefer insetting grafts with 4-0 chromic absorbable interrupted sutures. Once the graft has been applied it needs to be covered with some type of nonadherent dressing followed by a compressive bolster. Compressive dressings are important because incorporation is promoted by intimate apposition of the graft to the recipient bed. They should supply enough pressure to hold the graft in place, promote graft adherence, minimize excessive shearing motion at the graft–wound interface, and prevent hematoma or seroma accumulation underneath the graft. Although many types of compressive dressings exist, we prefer to use either a wound VAC or a stent ("tied-over bolster"). Wound VAC's are used over larger skin grafts and have the added benefit of evacuating transudate from the wound while the skin graft incorporates. They are ideal for use over difficult anatomic sites, such as those found on the hand, as they are able to conform to the uneven surfaces of the hand. Maintaining adherence of the skin graft to these sites is often difficult with the other compressive dressing techniques. Stents are constructed with cotton balls soaked in mineral oil, wrapped within a layer of nonadherent gauze, and secured in place with nylon sutures placed in the surrounding skin.

Compressive dressings are left in place for 5 days before removal as long as there is no erythema, foul-smelling drainage, fever, or other causes for concern. However, if it is anticipated that a hematoma or seroma may collect, such as with a sheet graft, the dressing should be removed at 24 h. Any fluid collections under the graft are evacuated by making stab incisions with a #11 scalpel and gently rolling a cotton-tipped applicator over the graft.

Complications and Side Effects

The main causes of graft failure include their placement on a recipient bed not ready for grafting, shearing forces, accumulation of fluid collections beneath the graft and infection. Necrotic tissue present within a recipient bed will hinder the wound healing process and impede graft take. Debridement of all devitalized tissue prior to skin graft placement can help minimize graft loss. Similarly, an infected wound should never be covered by a skin graft. If there is any question about the status of a wound, quantitative cultures should be obtained to determine the bacterial content prior to grafting. It has been established that 10,000 organisms/g of tissue is a critical level of contamination which will not support a skin graft.

It is imperative that grafts become vascularized for ultimate survival, and anything that acts as a barrier to this process will cause loss of the graft. The collection of blood or serum beneath the graft will compromise its survival by raising the graft from the bed and preventing revascularization. This complication can be avoided through meticulous hemostasis before applying the skin graft, and either meshing STSG's or "pie-crusting" FTSG's. Shearing forces result in movement of the graft on the bed and compromise its survival by interrupting revascularization. Postgrafting compressive dressings (bolster dressings, wound VAC's) optimize graft adherence to the recipient bed and minimize shearing forces.

Postoperative Care

The postoperative care for skin grafts involves maintaining adherence of the graft to the recipient bed with a compressive dressing for 5 days. In addition, immobilization of the hand in a splint is advised. Following removal of the compressive dressing STSG's should be covered with petroleum-impregnated gauze to prevent desiccation. The dressing should be changed once daily. After all graft interstices have filled in, the grafts should be kept lubricated with a moisturizing lotion or cream applied daily (or more frequently as needed to prevent drying of the skin). A compression garment may be recommended to help prevent scar contracture.

Optimizing outcomes

- Recipient site must be suitable for graft placement (operative debridement of all contaminated and devitalized tissue)
- Bleeding should be well controlled before application of graft
- Mesh or "pie-crust" graft to avoid accumulation of fluid underneath
- Immobilize hand as needed to optimize graft take
- Compressive dressing ×5 days to minimize shearing forces on graft

Clinical "pearls" and potential complications/pitfalls

- FTSG's contract less, are more durable, and have improved cosmetic results
- FTSG's are preferred over STSG's in areas where graft contracture would limit mobility
- FTSG's should be used when covering the palmar surface of the hand. STSG's (meshed or nonmeshed) are usually reserved for coverage of the dorsum of the hand
- Compressive dressings should be left in place for 5 days

Local Flaps: Dorsal Metacarpal Artery Flaps

Indications for dorsal metacarpal artery flaps:
- Wounds on the fingers where skin graft coverage is contraindicated due to exposed bone, joint cartilage, or tendon

Flaps perfused by the dorsal metacarpal artery system are finding expanded uses in hand reconstruction. Island skin flaps from the dorsal hand are excellent options for coverage of soft-tissue defects of the fingers with exposed bone, joint or tendon (particularly on the dorsum of digits). These flaps are nourished by the palmar-dorsal vascular connection in the hand at the level of the metacarpophalangeal (MP) joint, just distal to the extensor tendon juncturae. While the first and second dorsal metacarpal arteries are commonly used for these flaps, the other metacarpal arteries are also reliable with the exception of the fifth whose presence is not consistent [8]. The advantages of these flaps include the fact that they are sensate and can be done in a single stage. The dorsal metacarpal arteries are accompanied by venae comitantes which permit venous drainage of the flaps.

Operative Approach: First Dorsal Metacarpal Artery Flap (Kite flap)

The first dorsal metacarpal artery flap (FDMA flap) is an island pedicle flap proximally based off the first dorsal metacarpal artery (FDMA) and veins. When the pedicle is fully dissected it has a length up to 7 cm with a wide arc of rotation that allows it to resurface defects of the dorsal thumb and first web space. The FDMA arises from the radial artery just distal to the tendon of the extensor pollicis longus muscle and proximal to the point at which the radial artery pierces between the radial and ulnar heads of the first dorsal interosseous muscle. The artery runs over the fascial layer of the first dorsal interosseous muscle and divides into the radial branch to the thumb, the intermediate branch to the first web space, and the ulnar branch to the index finger. The ulnar branch courses distally between the ulnar head of the first dorsal interosseous muscle and the shaft of the second metacarpal, until it reaches the MP joint where it divides into a number of small vessels which supply the subdermal plexus over the dorsum of the proximal phalanx.

When designing a FDMA flap, the course of the FDMA and its ulnar branch are traced with a Doppler device and marked on the skin. The size of the defect is measured and its pattern transposed onto the radial side of the index finger between the MP joint and PIP joint. The skin incision is taken to the level of the fascia, and a wide swath of tissue is dissected along the course of the artery. In order to avoid damaging the artery or draining veins, the radial-sided periosteum of the second metacarpal and the fascia of the first dorsal interosseous muscle can be included in the flap dissection.

The flap is elevated from distal to proximal and from the ulnar to radial side. The paratenon must be left undisturbed in order to ensure skin graft take and free gliding of the extendor tendon. If a sensory flap is desired, a branch of the radial sensory nerve can be taken with the pedicle. The fascia is carefully lifted off the first dorsal interosseous muscle to near its base to allow rotation of the flap on its pedicle. The pedicle includes the fascia of the first dorsal interosseous muscle, the dorsal veins, and the radial sensory nerve. Once an adequate pedicle has been lifted, the flap is passed through a subcutaneous tunnel to reach the defect. The donor site is usually closed with a full-thickness skin graft (Fig. 25.5). Like other fasciocutaneous flaps, the skin portion of the FDMA flap can be eliminated so that it consists of fascia alone. In these cases, the donor site is closed primarily and the flap itself is covered with a skin graft [9–11].

Optimizing outcomes
- The flap should be centered over the ulnar branch of the FDMA
- Include the second metacarpal periosteum and first dorsal interosseous muscle fascia in the dissection to avoid injuring the artery or venae comitantes
- Avoid disrupting the extensor paratenon to facilitate skin graft take over the flap donor site
- Avoid vascular compression of the pedicle (twisting or kinking the pedicle when rotating the flap into position, passing pedicle through too tight of a subcutaneous tunnel)

Complications and Side Effects

Harvesting a FDMA flap can be more challenging than some of the other flaps described in this chapter due to the smaller caliber vessels supplying the flap. The best way to avoid injuring the vasculature is to include a generous portion of surrounding tissues when dissection along the course of the artery. The blood supply to the flap can become compromised if the pedicle become twisted or kinked when rotated into position. Similarly, vascular compression can result if the pedicle is passed through a subcutaneous tunnel which is too tight.

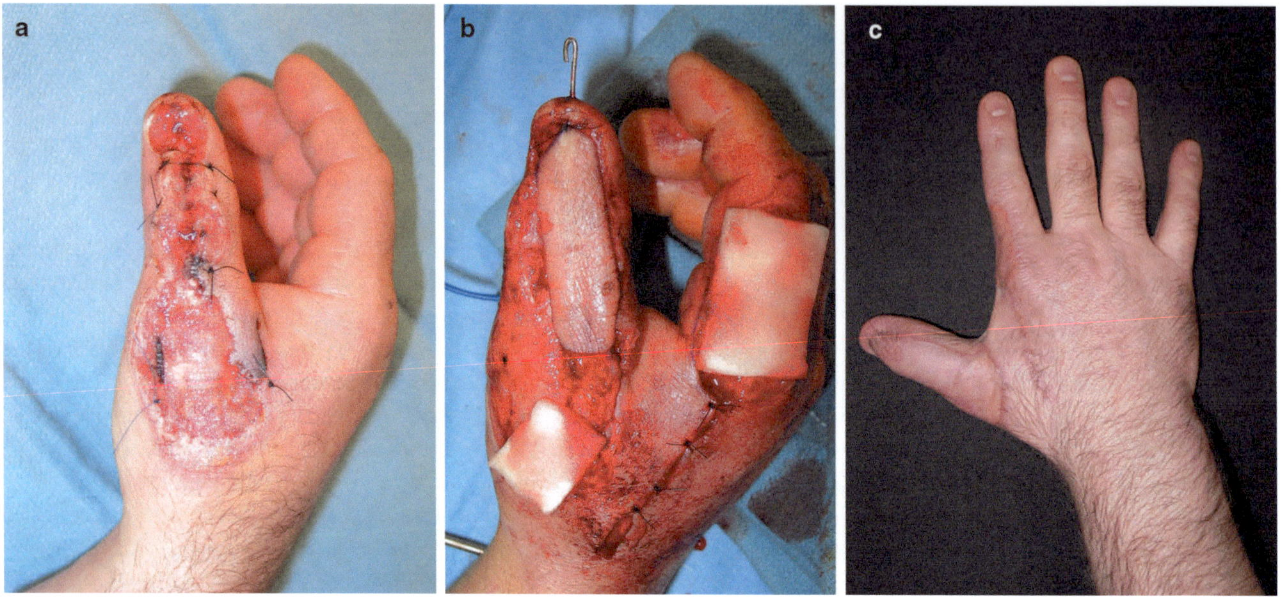

Fig. 25.5 Reconstruction of right thumb defect with a first dorsal metacarpal artery (FDMA) flap (**a–c**)

Postoperative Care

The postoperative care required for FDMA flaps is minimal. If a skin graft is placed over the donor site, this portion of the hand should be immobilized to facilitate graft take. If the donor site was primarily closed, then early active mobilization is appropriate.

Clinical "pearls" and potential complications/pitfalls

- Include surrounding tissue when dissecting along the course of the artery to avoid injuring the artery or venae comitantes
- Avoid compromising blood flow to the flap by twisting the pedicle during distal rotation or passing through too tight a subcutaneous tunnel

Regional Flaps: Radial Artery Forearm Flap

Regional flaps refer to coverage provided by tissues not immediately adjacent to the primary defect but from its vicinity. The pedicled reverse radial forearm flap continues to be regarded as one of the best reconstructive tools for the hand and its value to the field of hand surgery cannot be overestimated. The radial forearm flap is an excellent match for the hand, as it is quite thin with very little subcutaneous fat, and its versatility allows it to reach nearly any part of the hand. It provides excellent resurfacing for both palmar and dorsal hand and digit defects and can reach even the tips of the fingers. The advantages of this flap include the fact that it is a robust well-perfused flap capable of providing not only skin and subcutaneous tissue but also the durability of fascial coverage. The radial forearm flap can be harvested with skin and fascia (fasciocutaneous flap), skin alone (suprafascial flap), or with only fascia (fascia-alone flap). In addition, radial forearm flaps result in minimal functional problems and allow single stage reconstruction.

Indications for radial forearm flap:

– Wounds on any part of the hand not amenable to skin graft coverage due to exposed bone, joint cartilage, or tendon

Contraindications for radial forearm flap:

– Patients with an abnormal Allen's test
– Patients in whom there are forearm scars where the flap is to be designed

The primary disadvantages of this flap include sacrificing one of the two major arteries to the hand and poor donor site cosmesis. In nearly all cases of radial forearm flap harvest, the loss of the radial artery contribution to the circulation of the hand does not appear to have any detrimental effects. The flap donor defect frequently requires skin grafting which results in an aesthetically unpleasant scar. The desire to ameliorate these problems has led to important refinements of the radial forearm flap. This led to the development of suprafascial harvest of the radial forearm flap, thereby sparing the volar forearm fascia and allowing a smoother skin graft recipient site. Another option that allows better donor site appearance is the use of the radial forearm fascia-alone flap where the fascia is raised alone without the overlying skin. This version is harvested through a linear forearm incision which spares the overlying skin, and the flap itself is covered with a skin graft. Flaps that can be limited to skin paddles of only 4–6 cm in width can be closed primarily allowing a more acceptable donor site [12, 13].

Operative Approach

Prior to surgery, it is mandatory to perform an Allen test to ensure that flow is present and adequate through both the radial and ulnar arteries. A radial forearm flap must not be performed in patients with an abnormal Allen test which indicates deficient palmar arch circulation and digit perfusion that is dependent solely on the radial artery. Nearly all individuals without prior injuries or vascular disease have the ability to adequately perfuse the hand and digits with the ulnar artery alone.

When designing the radial forearm fasciocutaneous flap, the course of the radial artery is traced with an arterial Doppler device and marked out on the skin. The size of the defect in need of coverage is measured and its pattern transposed onto the forearm with a marking pen. The location of the flap on the forearm is determined by measuring the distance from the radial styloid to the closest edge of the defect on the hand. This distance represents the location for the distal edge of the flap and the flap designed should extend proximal to this point, such that the pedicle will have adequate length for rotation of the flap. The flap is usually designed as an ellipse centered over the course of the radial artery.

The margins of the flap are incised down to the level of the deep fascia. A skin incision is made extending distally from the flap margin over the course of the radial artery. The skin edges adjacent to the flap margin are elevated from the underlying deep fascia for approximately 1 cm circumferentially around the flap. The deep fascia is incised around the flap, and the flap is raised from the underlying muscles by dissecting within the loose areolar tissue beneath the fascia. It is important to dissect directly on top of the muscle (brachioradialis on the radial side and FCR on the ulnar side) to avoid separating the fascia from the skin. The placement of tacking sutures between the skin and fascia helps prevent separation, which could damage any perforating vessels. Any tendons encountered while elevating the flap in the proximal forearm must be carefully dissected to preserve their overlying paratenon. After the flap has been raised over the FCR, the radial artery and its venae comitantes will be seen within the intermuscular septum. Next, the lateral intermuscular septum is approached from the radial side by dissecting the flap off the brachioradialis muscle and tendon. The FCR and the brachioradialis muscles are retracted away from each other, and the intermuscular septum is incised parallel and deep to the radial artery. When retracting the brachioradialis muscle, it is important to identify and protect the sensory branch of the radial nerve located on the undersurface of the muscle. The radial artery is dissected distally through the previously made longitudinal skin incision. The pedicle should be dissected out as a unit without attempting to separate the veins from the radial artery. The radial artery and venae comitantes are ligated proximally and the flap transposed to the hand defect.

In order to ensure that the fingers as well as the flap remain perfused, we prefer to place an Acland clamp on the radial artery just proximal to the flap. If the flap and digits remain perfused, the radial artery can be safely divided. The pedicled flap can be tunneled underneath any intervening intact skin between the forearm incision and hand defect to be covered. Twisting or kinking the pedicle when rotating the flap into position is to be avoided. Additionally, if the flap is tunneled under an intact skin bridge, there must be enough laxity to prevent vascular compression of the pedicle. The margins of the flap are trimmed as needed to conform to the edge of the defect, and the flap is sutured into place. The longitudinal forearm incision is closed in layers (Fig. 25.6).

If the skin paddle is less than 6 cm the donor site can sometimes be closed primarily. Larger donor site must be covered with a split-thickness skin graft. We prefer to cover our STSG's for radial forearm flaps with a wound VAC, especially if the STSG has been placed over the paratenon of flexor tendons.

The poor appearance of the donor defect can be eliminated by utilizing the radial forearm fascia-alone flap. This flap provides durable thin coverage of the hand and avoids the need for skin grafting of the donor site. This version of the flap is also preferred in patients in whom a standard fasciocutaneous flap would be too bulky due to a thick skin and fat layer in the forearm. In this technique, the fascia is approached through a linear forearm incision and the skin is elevated off the underlying fascia. It is important to leave the network of small fascial vessels on the surface as well as a thin stippling of fat when dissecting the forearm skin and subcutaneous tissue off of the fascia. After the skin is elevated, the dissection deep to the fascia proceeds as described earlier for the fasciocutaneous flap. The forearm donor defect is closed as a straight line.

Complications and Side Effects

Although the radial forearm flap has a robust blood supply, flap failure or partial flap loss can occur from technical errors. Radial forearm flaps should not be attempted in patients in

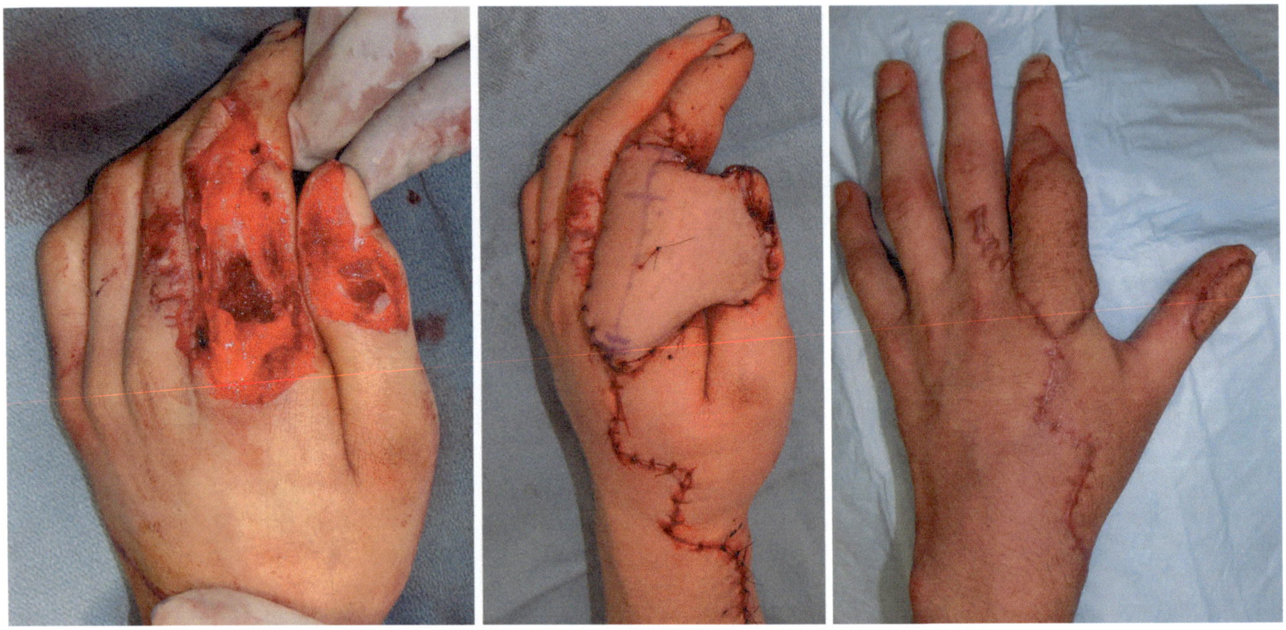

Fig. 25.6 Degloving injury involving left thumb and index finger (**a**). Reconstruction of multidigit degloving injury with pedicled radial forearm flap, including staged syndactyly release (**b**, **c**)

Optimizing outcomes

- Perform an Allen test on all patients being considered for a radial forearm flap
- The flap should be centered over the radial artery which can be located with an arterial Doppler device
- If planning on primarily closing the donor site (avoiding STSG) a skin paddle <6 cm wide should be designed
- Avoid separating the skin from the fascia while elevating the flap
- Avoid injuring the sensory branch of the radial nerve when retracting the brachioradialis muscle
- Avoid vascular compression of the pedicle (twisting or kinking the pedicle when rotating the flap into position, passing pedicle through a tight skin tunnel)

Clinical "pearls" and potential complications/pitfalls

- Perform an Allen test on all patients prior to surgery
- Avoid inadvertent separation of the fascia and overlying skin when elevating the flap which will injure the perforating vessels supplying the skin paddle
- Avoid compromising blood flow to the flap by twisting the pedicle during distal rotation or passing through a tight subcutaneous tunnel
- Consider a radial forearm fascia-alone flap for patients in whom a fasciocutaneous would be too bulky or when there are concerns about the donor site appearance

whom the local blood supply may have been disrupted by previous trauma or incisions within the planned flap skin paddle. When dissecting out the flap, care must be taken not to injure the radial artery or damage its perforating vessels to the skin and subcutaneous tissue. The blood supply to the flap can become compromised if the pedicle become twisted or kinked when rotated into position. Similarly, vascular compression can result if the pedicle is passed through a subcutaneous tunnel which is too tight. The most serious complication would be to divide the radial artery in a patient whose ulnar artery is unable to adequately perfuse a portion of the hand or digits. In these instances, acute ischemia of the hand will ensue, and it is critical to reconstruct the radial artery and abort the surgery. Noninvasive vascular studies to determine arterial dominance are usually unnecessary.

Postoperative Care

The postoperative care for radial forearm flaps requires immobilization of the wrist, MP joints and PIP joints to allow skin graft take. After approximately 1–2 weeks adequate skin graft take should be established and the patient can begin motion. Routine flap monitoring including flap color, capillary refill, Doppler signal, and temperature are required in the postoperative period.

Distant Flaps: Pedicled Groin Flap

Indications for pedicled groin flap:

- Wounds on any part of the hand not amenable to skin graft coverage due to exposed bone, joint cartilage, or tendon

Contraindications for pedicled groin flap:

- Patients in whom the superficial circumflex iliac artery (SCIA) may have been disrupted (groin scars overlying the area from which the flap is to be raised)
- Obese patients in whom the flap will be too bulky (especially in the midportion of the flap)
- Unreliable patients in whom it will be difficult to keep the extremity immobilized during the healing process

The pedicled groin flap is an extremely reliable distant flap and a source of immediate coverage for any defect on any portion of the hand and wrist. The groin flap is ideal for providing soft-tissue coverage of large, full-thickness defects, as it provides a large area of skin and subcutaneous fat. The advantages of this flap include the large length-to-width ratio, primary closure of the donor site, and the added benefit of permitting joint mobilization while in place. The groin flap is an axial flap based on the superficial circumflex iliac artery (SCIA), which has relatively constant anatomy. This vessel branches from the femoral artery within the femoral triangle, crosses over the sartorius muscle, and continues laterally approximately 2.5 cm inferior and parallel to the inguinal ligament. The SCIA crosses the sartorius muscle within its superficial fascia. The vessel ends lateral to the anterior superior iliac spine and supplies the skin below the iliac crest. The venous drainage of this region is through venae comitantes that drain to the femoral triangle [14, 15].

Operative Approach

The patient should be positioned supine on the operating room table with a bump under the hip from which the flap will be harvested. When designing the groin flap, the size of the defect in need of coverage should be measured and its pattern transposed onto the groin with a marking pen. The midline of the designed flap should be centered over the expected course of the SCIA which can be verified with an arterial Doppler device. The width of the flap that can be harvested and still allow primary closure of the groin is determined by flexing the hip and pinching together the skin edges in the inguinal crease. The margin of the flap is incised and undermined in the subcutaneous plane from a lateral to medial direction. At the lateral border of the sartorius, the muscle fascia should be incised and elevated along with the skin and subcutaneous tissue. Division of the deep fascia and the deep branch of the SCIA protects the SCIA and prevents tethering of the pedicle at the sartorius muscle. Dissection of the upper margin of the flap from the external oblique aponeurosis will often require sacrifice of the superficial inferior epigastric artery. The lateral femoral cutaneous nerve will be encountered over the medial border of the sartorius muscle, and must be preserved to prevent dysesthesia of the lateral thigh [16]. The nerve and its branches can be safely dissected from the undersurface of the flap and preserved, since they pass deep into the SCIA. Occasionally, the nerve or one of its branches may be superficial and need to be divided to properly elevate the flap. The deep dissection is usually terminated just medial to the sartorius muscle.

After all fascial incisions have been completed, the lateral portion of the flap is thinned of its excess bulk. Care must be taken when defatting the middle portion of the flap as not to injure the pedicle. Since the pedicle emerges through the deep fascia in the midline of the flap, the portion to be designed into a tube should not be thinned except at the margins.

Primary closure of the secondary defect can be easily accomplished as long as the flap is no larger than approximately 12 cm wide. Skin grafts may be necessary to close the secondary defect if a flap wider than 12 cm was utilized. Closure should begin at the lateral end and progress medially all the way to the pedicle (where the tubing of the flap originates). Flexing the operating room table at the hip will help facilitate closure of the wound. The flap is folded into a tube at the base and closed with interrupted sutures. The flap can be tubed in different directions to facilitate closure of either palmar or dorsal defects. It is important not to close the secondary defect too far medially or vascular compression of the pedicle within the base of the tube may occur. The hand is next brought to the groin and the distal margin of the flap is cut to conform to the edge of the defect. The flap is sutured in place beginning at the center point of the distal margin of the flap and then proceeding around both margins toward the base of the pedicle [17–19].

After the flap has been sutured in place, the extremity must be immobilized to prevent avulsion of the flap. We prefer to obtain immobilization by placing a rolled bandage between the limb and the abdomen, and then restraining the arm in position with an ace wrap wrapped around the torso. The arm can also be immobilized with an external fixator using pins in the radius and the iliac wing. Immobilization is most critical during the initial postoperative period when awakening and recovering from anesthesia, and can usually be removed by the first or second postoperative day.

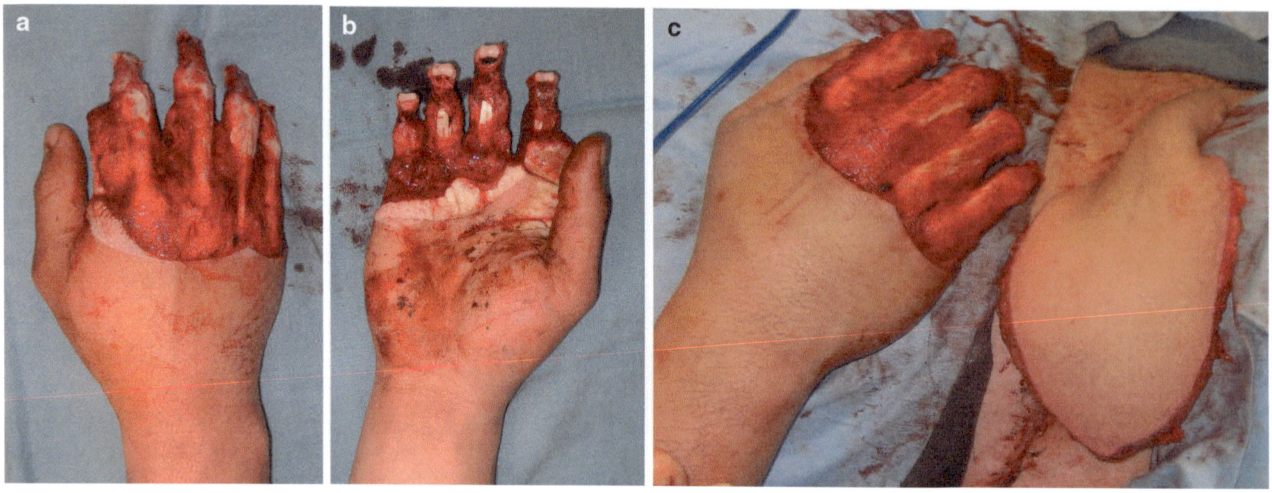

Fig. 25.7 Circumferential degloving injury of right second through fifth digits (**a**, **b**). Injured hand is brought to the groin in preparation for suturing the tubed groin flap in place. Donor site has been closed primarily (**c**)

Fig. 25.8 The groin flap, based on the superficial circumflex iliac artery (SCIA), provides immediate soft-tissue coverage for a full-thickness defect over the wrist (**a**, **b**)

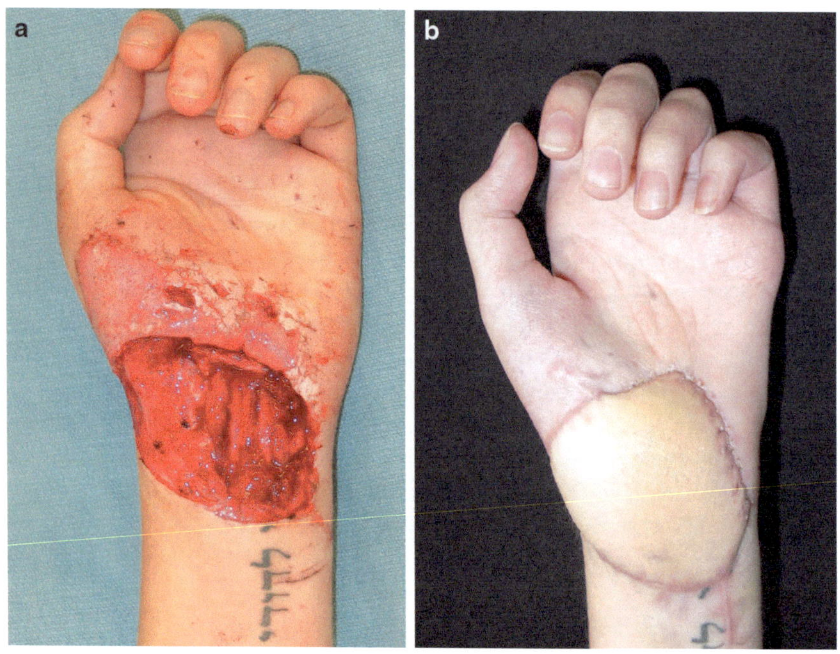

Unless any unanticipated circumstances occur, the flap can be safely divided and completely inset after 3 weeks. At this time, the flap should be adequately supplied by blood flow across the wound bed. Complete healing of all incisions is an indication that the flap is ready for division. Any question about the potential viability of the flap can be resolved by placing a rubber tourniquet around the tube pedicle and confirming that the flap remains perfused while the pedicle is occluded. After division of the flap, the proximal margin of the flap is cut to conform to the edge of the defect and sutured in place (Figs. 25.7 and 25.8).

Complications and Side Effects

Although the pedicled groin flap is extremely reliable, necrosis can occur from errors in flap construction. Alternative coverage options should be considered if the surgeon is unable to locate the vessel with the assistance of a Doppler device as the patient may not have a vessel of adequate size to support a flap. Similarly, groin flaps should be avoided in patients where the SCIA may have been disrupted, such as those who have scars in the region of their groin from previous hernia repairs or lymph node dissections. The most

Optimizing outcomes

- The flap should be centered over the SCIA which can be located with an arterial Doppler device
- The width of the flap that can be harvested while still allowing primary closure is determined by flexing the hip and pinching together the skin edges in the inguinal crease
- Deep fascia should be divided along the lateral margin of the sartorius muscle to prevent tethering and kinking of the pedicle as it pierces the fascia
- Avoid overly superficial dissection when elevating the flap, which places the pedicle at risk
- Preserve the lateral femoral cutaneous nerve to prevent post-op dysesthesias
- Defatting the lateral portion of the flap is safe
- Immobilize the extremity to prevent avulsion of the flap when the patient recovering from anesthesia
- Efforts should be made to have the patient safely mobilize their elbow and shoulder to prevent joint stiffness
- To confirm that a flap is ready for division a rubber tourniquet can be placed around the pedicle to ensure the flap remains perfused

serious complication is accidental division of the SCIA. Extreme care must be taken to not undermine the flap too superficially and damage this vessel. Care must also be taken when thinning the middle portion of the flap to avoid injury to the pedicle. If the deep branch of the SCIA is not divided as it goes deep into the sartorius, the flap can be tethered here. The pedicle can also become constricted within the base of the tube if the secondary defect is closed too far medially.

Problems during the postoperative period are related to dehiscence of the flap from the wound. In order to avoid this it is extremely important to immobilize the extremity when the patient is recovering from anesthesia. Arm straps or sutures should be utilized to prevent excessive traction that may disrupt the flap.

Problems may be encountered during the subsequent surgery at the time of flap division. Flaps that are divided prematurely can result in partial or total flap loss. Flaps are usually ready to be divided by 3 weeks: however, circumstances may arise where the flap has not incorporated appropriately and is not being adequately perfused by the recipient site.

Postoperative Care

The postoperative care for groin flaps involves initially immobilizing the extremity to prevent avulsion of the flap. Routine flap monitoring including checking the flap color,

Clinical "pearls" and potential complications/pitfalls

- Flaps should be limited to 12 cm in width to assure primary closure of the secondary donor defect. Thigh flexion facilitates closure
- Extreme care must be taken when elevating the flap and later when thinning the flap as not to injure the pedicle
- Preserve the lateral cutaneous nerve of the thigh to prevent postoperative thigh dysesthesia

capillary refill, and temperature are required. Following restraint removal the patient is shown which part of the flap to inspect for kinking and which positions are acceptable. The patient should be provided with instructions on how to safely exercise the elbow, shoulder, and possibly fingers during the time period required for flap incorporation in order to prevent the development of stiffness across these joints.

Free Flaps: Radial Forearm Flap, Lateral Arm Flap, Anterolateral Thigh Flap

Recent developments in microsurgical free tissue transfer have expanded the reconstructive possibilities available for hand surgeons and their patients. A wide variety of free flaps allows great versatility in the restoration of soft tissue and offers the potential to reconstruct nearly any defect of the upper extremity. When hand or forearm-based donor tissue is not sufficient for reconstruction of a hand defect and all other options on the reconstructive ladder have been eliminated, tissue from a distant source must be employed in the form of a free flap.

With the exception of small muscle flaps covered with a skin graft, such as the serratus anterior, most free muscle flaps are too bulky for the hand and impede function, even with muscle atrophy. For this reason, fascia-only flaps covered

Indications for free tissue transfer:

- Wounds on any part of the hand where skin graft coverage is contraindicated due to exposed bone, joint cartilage, or tendon

Contraindications for free tissue transfer:

- Free tissue transfer should not be used to salvage a limb with insufficient potential for eventual function
- Patients who have peripheral vascular disease
- Abnormal bleeding or clotting diatheses
- Cigarette smoking (relative contraindication)

with a skin graft and fasciocutaneous flaps are the best options for reconstruction of the hand, particularly when reconstructing the palm. They are thin and pliable, offer a superior cosmetic result, and facilitate later surgery through or under the flap. This is particularly true in the case of secondary tendon surgery, where the fascia contained in these flaps offers a good gliding surface for tendons.

When choosing a donor site for a fascia-only flap, skin color match is not a consideration, so the flap choice is dictated by donor site and surgeon preference. Common fascia flaps utilized for the hand include the radial forearm, lateral arm, temporoparietal, scapular, and anterolateral thigh fascial free flaps. If a larger piece of fascia is required than that can be harvested with the radial forearm or lateral arm flap, the anterolateral thigh (ALT) fascia free flap is an excellent choice. While a fascia flap covered with a skin graft generally works well, is thin, and allows good tendon gliding underneath, the appearance of the overlying skin graft can be undesirable.

The employment of a thin fasciocutaneous free flap can help solve the issue of bulk in the hand, and presents some improvement in appearance when compared to the fascia flap–skin graft combination. Since fasciocutaneous free flaps include a skin paddle, the choice of donor site becomes an important consideration. The free dorsalis pedis flap from the foot dorsum is ideally suited for the hand, especially the dorsal surface. Unfortunately, the donor site on the dorsal foot can be very troublesome and require further wound care or secondary surgery to obtain wound closure. Common fasciocutaneous free flaps utilized for the hand include the radial forearm and lateral arm free flaps. The ALT can be taken as a fasciocutaneous free flap, but these are usually too bulky for hand reconstruction. However, the fasciocutaneous version of the ALT flap can be useful when employed to simultaneously cover a large defect that extends onto the forearm.

Regardless of the type of free flap chosen, the primary issue in microvascular free tissue transfer is vascular access for vessel anastomoses. Although the upper extremity has a rich vascular supply, trauma may limit the available choices as a site outside the zone of injury should be chosen to perform the vascular anastomosis. The radial artery may occasionally be the only patent vessel to the hand when there has been a penetrating or crushing injury to the forearm or palmar surface of the hand. In most patients, the hand will maintain adequate perfusion if only one of the major arteries (radial or ulnar) is patent. If the hand is viable and either one of these pulses is strong, arteriography is usually unnecessary. On the other hand, an arteriogram should be performed if there is any question regarding the status of hand perfusion.

When covering defects isolated to the hand, anastomosis is usually performed to either the radial or ulnar artery. The radial artery in the snuffbox can be used when covering the radial side of the hand or dorsal surface. It is safer to perform an end-to-side anastomosis; however, an end-to-end anastomosis to the radial artery at this level should not compromise circulation to the hand if both the radial and ulnar arteries are patent. For coverage of defects involving both the hand and forearm, the radial, ulnar, or brachial arteries (within the antecubital fossa) can be used. A proximal end-to-side anastomosis to the brachial artery is preferable if there is significant trauma to the forearm. Venous anastomosis can be accomplished with either venae comitantes or subcutaneous veins.

Free Flaps: Radial Artery Forearm Flap

The radial forearm free flap possesses ideal characteristics for hand reconstruction. Although the radial forearm flap is an excellent free flap, it can usually be used as pedicled flap based on reversed flow through the distal radial artery and venae comitantes. Occasionally, the size and the shape of the defect may necessitate using a free radial forearm flap either from the contralateral forearm.

Operative Approach

The initial part of the free flap dissection follows the same steps outlined earlier in this chapter for the pedicled radial forearm flap. The radial artery provides a large caliber vessel for anastomosis. The venae comitantes offer reliable drainage, but superficial cutaneous veins can be incorporated into larger flaps [20, 21].

Free Flaps: Lateral Arm Flap

The lateral arm free flap has consistently demonstrated utility in providing coverage of hand wounds. It is very useful in covering small defects of the hand and works very well in the first web space. In thin patients, it can be used to cover degloving injuries of the thumb. The lateral arm flap is raised from the posterolateral aspect of the distal upper arm. The harvest is straightforward, with distinct tissue planes and a constant anatomy, and can be taken from the ipsilateral arm using the same tourniquet. Advantages of this flap over the radial forearm flap are that it avoids the sacrifice of a major vessel as its pedicle is an end artery which is not essential to the blood supply of the upper limb. In addition, the donor site can often be closed primarily. Fascia up to 9×12 cm may be used. The primary disadvantages of the lateral arm flap are its limited size and the short (5–7 cm) and small diameter (1.5–2 mm) pedicle. Other disadvantages include the donor site scar on the lateral arm and anesthesia of the lateral forearm due to transection of the posterior cutaneous nerve of the forearm.

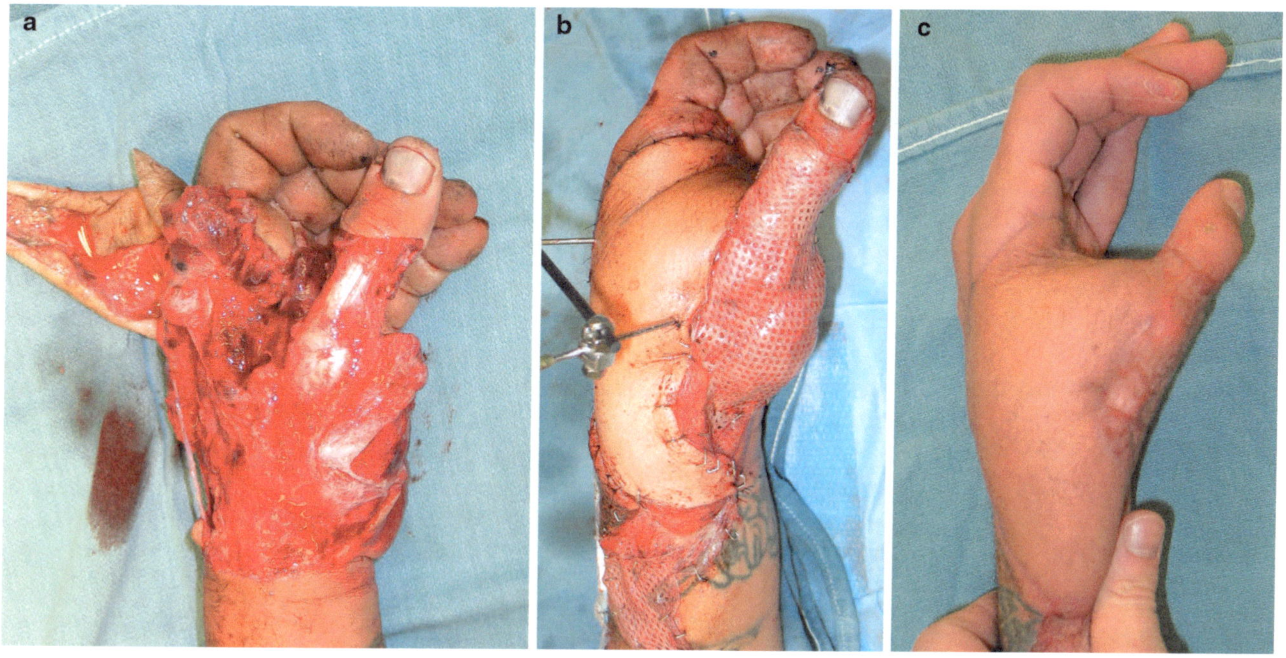

Fig. 25.9 Complex injury to the hand and wrist reconstructed with a free lateral arm fasciocutaneous flap and STSG (**a**–**c**)

The flap is based on the posterior radial collateral artery, one of the two terminal branches of the profunda brachii artery. The posterior cutaneous nerve of the arm contained within the flap can be used to reinnervate the flap if necessary. Donor sites up to 7 cm in width can be closed primarily. Larger donor sites require skin grafting which can be unsightly. The flap is relatively thin, but can still require debulking. The fascia-only flap obviates the need for later debulking procedures and results in better donor site scars [22–26].

Operative Approach

The lateral arm flap may be harvested in the supine, lateral, or prone position. A sterile tourniquet is applied high on the upper arm after preparation to the axilla. The lateral intermuscular septum is identified by a line marking its course from the deltoid tubercle to the lateral epicondyle. A point 10 cm cephalad to the lateral epicondyle is marked as this is the location of the dominant posterior fascial branch. If a fasciocutaneous flap is to be harvested, an ellipse of skin centered directly over the distal half of the marked intermuscular septum is designed.

The posterior margin skin of the flap is incised down to the level of the fascia. The posterior skin edge of the flap is elevated from the underlying fascia until the midline of the triceps tendon is reached. The posterior fascia is incised along the midline of the tendon and elevated from the triceps in a posterior to anterior direction. The fascia and skin can be sutured to each other to prevent disrupting the perforating vessels from the fascia to the skin. Perforators are visible within the fascia and can be followed to their origin from the posterior radial collateral artery at the base of the lateral intermuscular septum. Once the posterior radial collateral artery is identified, care must be taken when separating it from the surrounding tissues to prevent injury to the radial nerve which lies anterior to the vessel. The radial nerve runs between the origin of the brachialis and brachioradialis muscles, and must be retracted and preserved during dissection. The anterior margin incision of the ellipse is then made and the anterior fascia is elevated in a similar manner from the brachialis and brachioradialis muscles.

After dissecting posteriorly and anteriorly, the flap can be elevated away from the lateral humerus. The lateral intermuscular septum is elevated by sharp dissection off the periosteum of the humerus from distally to proximal. The posterior cutaneous nerve of the arm and the posterior cutaneous nerve of the forearm pass superficially within the intermuscular septum and are encountered during the part of the dissection. The deeper posterior cutaneous nerve of the forearm can be dissected from the septum and protected to avoid a sensory deficit in the forearm. The more superficial posterior cutaneous nerve of the arm, which enters the skin flap proximally and superficial to the triceps fascia, can be divided proximally and later used to reinnervate the flap. Division of this nerve results in an area of decreased sensation along the posterior lateral aspect of the distal arm. Once adequate pedicle length is attained, the posterior radial collateral artery and venae comitantes are divided proximally. If the secondary defect is less than 7 cm wide, it can be closed primarily over a drain; otherwise, a skin graft must be placed over the donor site. If a fascia-only flap is harvested a split-thickness skin graft is placed over the transferred fascia once adequate hemostasis is obtained (Fig. 25.9).

Optimizing outcomes

- The flap should be centered over the distal half of the lateral intermuscular septum which contains the posterior radial collateral artery and venae comitantes
- If planning on primarily closing the donor site a skin paddle <7 cm wide should be designed
- Avoid separating the skin from the fascia while elevating the flap which will damage the perforating vessels
- Carefully separate the posterior radial collateral artery from the surrounding tissues to prevent injury of the radial nerve
- If possible, preserve the posterior cutaneous nerve of the forearm to prevent sensory deficit in the forearm

Clinical "pearls" and potential complications/pitfalls

- Flap should be centered over the lateral intermuscular septum and include the point 10 cm cephalad to the lateral epicondyle which is the approximate location of the dominant posterior fascial branch supplying the skin
- Flap skin paddles should be limited to 7 cm in width if planning on primarily closing the donor site
- Avoid inadvertent separation of the fascia and overlying skin when elevating the flap which will injure the perforating vessels supplying the skin paddle
- Preserve the posterior cutaneous nerve of the forearm to prevent sensory deficit in the forearm

Free Flaps: Anterolateral Thigh Flap

The ALT flap is an extremely versatile flap that has broad applicability in upper extremity and hand reconstruction. The ALT flap is based on the descending branch of the lateral circumflex femoral artery and can be harvested as a skin and subcutaneous, fasciocutaneous, musculocutaneous, or fascial flap. The thickness of the flap can be varied to better match the contour of the hand being reconstructed. Advantages of this flap are that it has a long vascular pedicle (8–12 cm in length) with large caliber vessels and the surface area of flap that can be harvested is very large (15 × 20 cm). Furthermore, it can be harvested as a sensate flap to allow for protective sensation by taking the lateral cutaneous nerve of the thigh. Donor sites that can be closed primarily will leave a linear scar on the anterior thigh. If a large area is harvested the donor sites must be covered with a split-thickness skin graft which will worsen the cosmetic outcome and may be unacceptable to certain patients [27–32].

Operative Approach

The patient is placed in the supine position which will allow access to the flap harvest site and exposure of the surgical site on the hand. A line is drawn from the anterior superior iliac spine to the lateral border of the patella, and starting at the midpoint of this line the descending branch of the lateral circumflex femoral artery is mapped out using a Doppler device. Alternative coverage options should be considered if the surgeon is unable to locate the vessel with the assistance of a Doppler as the descending branch of the lateral circumflex femoral artery must be patent for this flap to work. Perforators generally cluster within 3–4 cm inferolateral to the midpoint. After the vessel and perforators are marked, an appropriately sized flap is designed with its center around the perforating vessels.

After the skin paddle is marked, the skin is incised down to the deep fascia overlying the rectus femoris and vastus lateralis muscles. The fascia is incised and taken off with the skin and subcutaneous tissue when harvesting a fasciocutaneous flap. The flap is elevated initially from its medial border and dissection is continued medial to lateral until the skin perforators are identified. The skin perforators can be used as a landmark and followed down to the main pedicle within the intermuscular septum between the rectus femoris and vastus lateralis muscles. The flap is next elevated from its lateral border until the main pedicle is encountered. The intermuscular septum is then entered, and the pedicle is carefully dissected back to its origin from the descending branch of the lateral circumflex femoral artery. The lateral cutaneous nerve of the thigh sits in the subcutaneous tissue just above the deep fascia at the superior border of the flap along the line connecting the anterior superior iliac spine to the lateral patella. This nerve can be divided proximally and later used to reinnervate the flap. Once adequate pedicle length is attained, the descending branch of the lateral circumflex femoral artery and venae comitantes are divided proximally. After transection of the pedicle, the flap is transferred to the defect, anastomosed to the recipient vessels, and inset after successful reperfusion. If the skin paddle is less than approximately 9 cm wide, the donor site can be closed primarily over a drain, while wider donor sites must be covered with a split-thickness skin graft. If a fascia-only flap is harvested, a skin graft is placed over the transferred fascia once adequate hemostasis is obtained.

Complications and Side Effects

Free tissue transfer has the same possible donor and recipient site complications as previously described regional and

Optimizing outcomes

- Inability to locate a patent vessel with the arterial Doppler device is considered a contraindication to proceeding with the flap elevation
- The flap should be centered over a line drawn between the anterior superior iliac spine and lateral border of the patella
- Avoid separating the skin from the fascia while elevating the flap which will damage the perforating vessels
- If planning on primarily closing the donor site (avoiding STSG) a skin paddle <9 cm wide should be designed
- Elevation should begin at the medial border of the flap and dissected medially to lateral until the pedicle within the intermuscular septum is identified

Clinical "pearls" and potential complications/pitfalls

- The descending branch of the lateral circumflex femoral artery and its perforators should be mapped out using a Doppler device prior to designing the flap
- Skin paddle should be centered over a line drawn between the anterior superior iliac spine and lateral border of the patella, and include the cluster of perforators located within 3–4 cm inferolateral to the midpoint of this line
- Flap skin paddles should be limited to 9 cm in width if planning on primarily closing the donor site

distant flaps (e.g., hematoma, seroma, donor site morbidity), in addition to the potential risks and complications associated with microsurgery. Microsurgery is complex and technically demanding, but with recent advances in microsurgical technique free flap failure rates in experienced hands are now less than 5%. When considering a patient for free flap reconstruction the patient must be medically prepared and in reasonable health for the proposed surgery which are often lengthy procedures. The surgeon should rule out the presence of significant cardiovascular, respiratory, hepatic, or renal dysfunction, and abnormal bleeding or clotting diatheses.

The most common causes of flap loss are associated with arterial or venous thrombosis. It is important to minimize handling of the vessels which should only be manipulated by holding the adventitial tissue on the outermost aspect of the vessel wall. It is equally important to avoid significant traction on the vessels during their dissection. Manipulation of the lumen should be kept to a minimum to avoid intimal damage.

The pedicle should be of sufficient length such that the anastomosis is not under excessive tension, and is free of acute bends or twists. Care should be taken to prevent back-wall suturing of the vessel or entrapment of prothrombotic adventitial elements. When using the ALT flap, the vascular pedicle often is intramuscular (vastus lateralis), rather than in the intermuscular septum. This can significantly prolong the dissection.

Postoperative Care

Free flaps require careful monitoring postoperatively by assessing color, capillary refill time, and temperature. At our institution, we place an implantable venous Doppler probe adjacent to the venous anastomoses to assist with flap monitoring. However, an external arterial Doppler probe can also be used to assess vascular flow within the pedicle and on the skin paddle over a cutaneous perforator. The patient should be kept warm and well hydrated during the postoperative period, and vasoconstrictive agents should be avoided. The use of an anticoagulant agent such as dextran, heparin, or aspirin can be administered depending on the microsurgeon's preference. Signs of arterial insufficiency include pale flap color, reduction in flap temperature, slow capillary refill, and loss of flap turgor. Signs of venous insufficiency include congestion (purple or blue color), swelling, and brisk capillary refill. A change in the character of the Doppler signals may also indicate vascular occlusion. Immediate release of the flap from the inset may be required if venous congestion is noted postoperatively. A low threshold of returning free flaps with perfusion problems for reexploration is advantageous as salvage rates are considerably greater with early identification and treatment.

Conclusion

The treatment of wounds on the hand resulting from failure of local tissue flaps is a challenging aspect of hand surgery, and achieving good outcomes requires intimate knowledge of the available coverage options. When a patient suffers from failure of a tissue transfer on the hand, the surgeon must carefully assess the wound and make a number of important decisions when formulating a comprehensive reconstructive plan that will provide optimal form and function. The assessment of the injury should take into account the status of the wound (clean or dirty), whether deep structures (bone, joints, hardware, tendon, nerves, or blood vessels) are exposed, and the presence or absence of fractures. The ultimate goal of secondary hand soft-tissue reconstruction is to provide stable, vascularized soft-tissue coverage which may require multiple staged procedures. The reconstructive surgeon must ensure that the tissue chosen is of sufficient size to cover the defect and that the benefits of the procedure chosen outweigh any disadvantages. The final strategy to reconstruction will also be influenced by other factors including the patient's age, occupational demands, desire for restoration of appearance, other injuries, and future plans.

References

1. Morykwas MJ, Argenta LC, Shelton-Brown EI, McGuirt W. Vacuum-assisted closure: a new method for wound control and treatment: animal studies and basic foundation. Ann Plast Surg. 2000;45(3):332–4.
2. Webb LX, Pape H-C. Current thought regarding the mechanism of action of negative pressure wound therapy with reticulated open cell foam. J Orthop Trauma. 2008;22(10):S135–7.
3. Tarkin IS. The versatility of negative pressure wound therapy with reticulated open cell foam for soft tissue management after severe musculoskeletal trauma. J Orthop Trauma. 2008;22(10): S146–51.
4. Schneider AM, Morykwas MJ, Argenta LC. A new and reliable method of securing skin grafts to the difficult recipient bed. Plast Reconstr Surg. 1998;102(4):1195–8.
5. Jones I, Currie L, Martin R. A guide to biological skin substitutes. Br J Plast Surg. 2002;55(3):185–93.
6. Dantzer E, Braye FM. Reconstructive surgery using an artificial dermis (Integra): results with 39 grafts. Br J Plast Surg. 2001;54(8):659–64.
7. Verolino P, Casoli V, Masia D, Delia G, Isacu C, Castede JC. A skin substitute (Integra) in a successful delayed reconstruction of a severe injured hand. Burns. 2008;34(2):284–7.
8. Gregory H, Heitmann C, Germann G. The evolution and refinements of the distally based dorsal metacarpal artery (DMCA) flaps. J Plast Reconstr Aesthet Surg. 2007;60(7):731–9.
9. Foucher G, Braun JB. A new island flap transfer from the dorsum of the index to the thumb. Plast Reconstr Surg. 1979;63(3):344–9.
10. Earley MJ, Milner RH. Dorsal metacarpal flaps. Br J Plast Surg. 1987;40(4):333–41.
11. Chang SC, Chen SL, Chen TM, Chuang CJ, Cheng TY, Wang HJ. Sensate first dorsal metacarpal artery flap for resurfacing extensive pulp defects of the thumb. Ann Plast Surg. 2004;53(5):449–54.
12. Mühlbauer W, Herndl E, Stock W. The forearm flap. Plast Reconstr Surg. 1982;70(3):336–44.
13. Kaufman MR, Jones NF. The reverse radial forearm flap for soft tissue reconstruction of the wrist and hand. Tech Hand Up Extrem Surg. 2005;9(1):47–51.
14. Smith PJ, Foley B, McGregor IA, Jackson IT. The anatomical basis of the groin flap. Plast Reconstr Surg. 1972;49(1):41–7.
15. Hester Jr TR, Nahai F, Beegle PE, Bostwick III J. Blood supply of the abdomen revisited, with emphasis on the superficial inferior epigastric artery. Plast Reconstr Surg. 1984;74(5):657–70.
16. Moscona AR, Hirshowitz B. Meralgia paresthetica as a complication of the groin flap. Ann Plast Surg. 1980;4(2):161–3.
17. Schlenker JD. Important considerations in the design and construction of groin flaps. Ann Plast Surg. 1980;5(5):353–7.
18. Wray RC, Wise DM, Young VL, Weeks PM. The groin flap in severe hand injuries. Ann Plast Surg. 1982;9(6):459–62.
19. Chuang DC, Colony LH, Chen HC, Wei FC. Groin flap design and versatility. Plast Reconstr Surg. 1989;84(1):100–7.
20. Médard de Chardon V, Balaguer T, Chignon-Sicard B, Riah Y, Ihrai T, Dannan E, Lebreton E. The radial forearm free flap: a review of microsurgical options. J Plast Reconstr Aesthet Surg. 2009;62(1):5–10.
21. Jones NF, Jarrahy R, Kaufman MR. Pedicled and free radial forearm flaps for reconstruction of the elbow, wrist, and hand. Plast Reconstr Surg. 2008;121(3):887–98.
22. Song R, Song Y, Yu Y, Song Y. The upper arm free flap. Clin Plast Surg. 1982;9(1):27–35.
23. Katsaros J, Schusterman M, Beppu M, Banis Jr JC, Acland RD. The lateral upper arm flap: anatomy and clinical applications. Ann Plast Surg. 1984;12(6):489–500.
24. Katsaros J, Tan E, Zoltie N, Barton M, Dr. Venugopalsrinivasan, Venkataramakrishnan. Further experience with the lateral arm free flap. Plast Reconstr Surg. 1991;87(5):902–10.
25. Yousif NJ, Warren R, Matloub HS, Sanger JR. The lateral arm fascial free flap: its anatomy and use in reconstruction. Plast Reconstr Surg. 1990;86(6):1138–45.
26. Lanzetta M, Bernier M, Chollet A, St-Laurent JY. The lateral forearm flap: an anatomic study. Plast Reconstr Surg. 1997;99(2):460–4.
27. Song YG, Chen GZ, Song YL. The free thigh flap: a new free flap concept based on the septocutaneous artery. Br J Plast Surg. 1984;37(2):149–59.
28. Javaid M, Cormack GC. Anterolateral thigh free flap for complex soft tissue hand reconstructions. J Hand Surg Br. 2003;28(1):21–7.
29. Koshima I, Nanba Y, Tsutsui T, Takahashi Y. New anterolateral thigh perforator flap with a short pedicle for reconstruction of defects in the upper extremities. Ann Plast Surg. 2003;51(1):30–6.
30. Wang HT, Erdmann D, Fletcher JW, Levin LS. Anterolateral thigh flap technique in hand and upper extremity reconstruction. Tech Hand Up Extrem Surg. 2004;8(4):257–61.
31. Adani R, Tarallo L, Marcoccio I, Cipriani R, Gelati C, Innocenti M. Hand reconstruction using the thin anterolateral thigh flap. Plast Reconstr Surg. 2005;116(2):467–73.
32. Wang HT, Fletcher JW, Erdmann D, Levin LS. Use of the anterolateral thigh free flap for upper-extremity reconstruction. J Hand Surg Am. 2005;30(4):859–64.

Index

S.F.M. Duncan (ed.), *Reoperative Hand Surgery*,
DOI 10.1007/978-1-4614-2373-7, © Springer Science+Business Media, LLC 2012

D

G

H

I

J

K

L

M

U

MIX
Papier aus verantwortungsvollen Quellen
Paper from responsible sources
FSC® C105338

FSC
www.fsc.org

If you have any concerns about our products,
you can contact us on
ProductSafety@springernature.com

In case Publisher is established outside the EU,
the EU authorized representative is:
Springer Nature Customer Service Center GmbH
Europaplatz 3, 69115 Heidelberg, Germany

Printed by Libri Plureos GmbH
in Hamburg, Germany